BIOINSTRUMENTATION

BIOINSTRUMENTATION

MJ REILLY

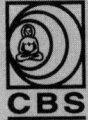

CBS Publishers & Distributors Pvt Ltd

New Delhi • Bengaluru • Chennai • Kochi • Kolkata • Mumbai
Bhubaneswar • Hyderabad • Jharkhand • Nagpur • Patna • Pune • Uttarakhand

BIOINSTRUMENTATION

ISBN: 978-81-239-2839-5

Copyright © Publisher

First Edition: 2016
Reprint: 2018

Published by Satish Kumar Jain and produced by Varun Jain for

CBS Publishers & Distributors Pvt Ltd

4819/XI Prahlad Street, 24 Ansari Road, Daryaganj, New Delhi 110 002, India.
Ph: 23289259, 23266861, 23266867   Website: www.cbspd.com
Fax: 011-23243014   e-mail: delhi@cbspd.com; cbspubs@airtelmail.in.
Corporate Office: 204 FIE, Industrial Area, Patparganj, Delhi 110 092
Ph: 4934 4934   Fax: 4934 4935   e-mail: publishing@cbspd.com; publicity@cbspd.com

Branches

- **Bengaluru:** Seema House 2975, 17th Cross, K.R. Road,
  Banasankari 2nd Stage, Bengaluru 560 070, Karnataka
  Ph: +91-80-26771678/79   Fax: +91-80-26771680   e-mail: bangalore@cbspd.com
- **Chennai:** 7, Subbaraya Street, Shenoy Nagar, Chennai 600 030, Tamil Nadu
  Ph: +91-44-26680620, 26681266   Fax: +91-44-42032115   e-mail: chennai@cbspd.com
- **Kochi:** Ashana House, No. 39/1904, AM Thomas Road, Valanjambalam,
  Ernakulam 682 016, Kochi, Kerala
  Ph: +91-484-4059061-65   Fax: +91-484-4059065   e-mail: kochi@cbspd.com
- **Kolkata:** 6/B, Ground Floor, Rameswar Shaw Road, Kolkata-700 014, West Bengal
  Ph: +91-33-22891126, 22891127, 22891128   e-mail: kolkata@cbspd.com
- **Mumbai:** 83-C, Dr E Moses Road, Worli, Mumbai-400018, Maharashtra
  Ph: +91-22-24902340/41   Fax: +91-22-24902342   e-mail: mumbai@cbspd.com

Representatives

• **Bhubaneswar**	0-9911037372	• **Hyderabad**	0-9885175004	• **Jharkhand**	0-9811541605	• **Nagpur**	0-9021734563
• **Patna**	0-9334159340	• **Pune**	0-9623451994	• **Uttarakhand**	0-9716462459		

Printed at India Binding House, Noida, UP

Preface

Electronics technology is transforming health care sector. Modern medicine is so much concerned around electronics, that the doctor of future must surely be an engineer. Microchip-sized wireless body monitoring systems are offering quality of life for users and providing useful data for healthcare professionals. Bioinstrumentation is a instrumentation technique and principles for the measurement of physical, physiological, and biological factors in man or other living organisms.

Bioinstrumentation is the application of electronics and measurement principles and techniques to develop devices used in diagnosis and treatment of disease. Computers are becoming increasingly important in bioinstrumentation, from the microprocessor used to do a variety of small tasks in a single purpose instrument to the extensive computing power needed to process the large amount of information in a medical imaging system.

This reference textbook on bioinstrumentation is a description of the medical and technical disciplines that make up this world of 'medical electronics'. Bioinstruments measure, record and transmit data on bodily functions.

Chapter 1 is devoted to fundamentals of bioinstrumentation, thus providing the students a perspective of the field and a feeling on the subject matter. Chapter 2 focuses on basic concepts of electronics. Chapter 3 concentrates on molecules analysis in clinical medicine. The development of biomaterials for tissue engineering is to create perfect surfaces which can provoke specific cellular responses and direct new tissue regeneration. Considering this chapter 4 focuses on biomaterial and tissue engineering. Chapter 5 describes haematology which is branch of internal medicine, physiology, pathology, clinical laboratory work, and pediatircs that is concerned with the study of blood, the blood forming organs, and blood diseases. Chapter 6 explains cellular measurements in biomaterials and tissue engineering. Various types of instruments used in the investigating of biological processes on the cellular level are discussed. Chapter 7 is devoted to nervous system which is an organ system containing a network of specialised cells called neurons that coordinate the actions of an animal and transmit signals between different parts of its body. Chapter 8 concentrates on heart and circulation. Chapter 9 gives concisely the mechanism, basics of lung, kidney, bone and skin.

Body temperature, heat, fat and movement are discussed in chapter 10. Chapter 11 is devoted to chemical transducers which play an important role in medicine and physiology in the assessment of metabolism. The most commonly encountered transducers are those used for measuring the blood gases (in solution). Chapter 12 concentrates on physiological transducers which play an important role in circuit parameters like resistance, capacitance and inductance in accordance with the events to be measured. Chapter 13 gives concisely the mechanisms of electrodes which are used both for the measurement of bioelectric vents and to deliver current to living tissue. Chapter 14 focuses on ventilation and ventilators. Mechanical ventilators, which are often called respirators, are used to artificially ventilate the lungs of patients who are unable to naturally breathe from atmosphere. Chapter 15 deals with anaesthesia and anaesthesia equipment. Chapter 16 is devoted to noninvasive measurement of intracranial pressure (ICP) as increased ICP may be a consequence of various ethiologies including head trauma, hydrocephalus, brain tumour, intracerebral haemorrhage, or cerebral edema. Chapter 17 concentrates on potential methods for *in vivo* glucose sensing. Chapter 18 concentrates on biotelemetry, and briefly explains the basic techniques for monitoring physiological data over a distance wirelessly, and also the usage of telephone lines for short distances. Chapter 19 focuses on computer applications in medical technology. The computer can perform several on-line functions which facilitate the efficient handling of voluminous data and minimises paper work.

This reference textbook of *Bioinstrumentation* is essential reading for medical students, electronic and electrical engineers, teachers, professionals, researchers and industrialists involved with chemical biochemical engineering, engineering, environmental science, microbiology, biotechnology and life sciences. The reference textbook also caters to the requirement of the syllabus prescribed by various Indian universities for undergraduate and postgraduate students pursuing these courses. Constructive suggestions are always welcome from users of this book.

Diagrams, figures, tables and index supplement the text. All the topics have been covered in a cogent and lucid style to help the reader grasp the information quickly and easily.

MJ Reilly

Contents at a Glance

Contents

┌─────┐
│ 1 │
└─────┘

Fundamentals of Bioinstrumentation

INTRODUCTION

Imaging technology, such as computerised tomography (CT) and magnetic resonance imaging (MRI), were developed by engineers. Minimally invasive surgery seems to have taken over traditional surgery, thanks to technology. For example, biomedical engineers have developed laser equipment for sophisticated surgical procedures and endoscopic fibre optic devices that can be guided through the digestive tract to identify tumours and remove them. One can even observe the inside of the knee or the abdomen with an endoscope and remove damaged tissue without having to cut the skin. Robots are used nowadays in hospital operating theaters to perform precision surgery. Also, telesurgery and telemedicine facilitate remote participation by an expert surgeon and monitoring patients in their own homes. These are only a few examples of the technological revolution facilitated by Biomedical Engineering.

Prominent physicians and health professionals do research to innovate and advance their professions. Biomedical engineering teaches you to understand the human body and to understand what kind of equipment you need to use to do your research, as well as use your engineering skills to understand the meaning of the results of you experiments.

Biological organisation: Biological organisation, or the hierarchy of life, is the hierarchy of complex biological structures and systems that define life using a reductionistic approach.

The traditional hierarchy, as detailed below, extends from atoms (or lower) to biospheres. The higher levels of this scheme are often referred to as ecological organisation.

Each level in the hierarchy represents an increase in organisational complexity, with each 'object' being primarily composed of the previous level's basic unit. The basic principle behind the organisation is the concept of emergence — the properties and functions found at a hierarchical level are not present and irrelevant at the lower levels.

Organisation furthermore refers to the high degree of order of an organism (in comparison to general objects). Ideally, individual organisms of the same species have the same arrangement of the same structures.

For example, the typical human has a torso with two legs at the bottom and two arms on the sides and a head on top. It is extremely rare (and usually impossible, due to physiological and biomechanical factors) to find a human that has all of these structures but in a different arrangement.

The biological organisation of life is a fundamental premise for numerous areas of scientific research, particularly in the medical sciences. Without this necessary degree of organisation, it would be much more difficult—and likely impossible—to apply the study of the effects of various physical and chemical phenomena to diseases and body function. For example, fields such as cognitive and behavioural neuroscience could not exist if the brain was not composed of specific types of cells, and the basic concepts of pharmacology could not exist if it was not known that a change at the cellular level can affect an entire organism. These applications extend into the ecological levels as well. For example, DDT's direct effect occurs at the subcellular level, but affects higher levels up to and including multiple ecosystems. Theoretically, a change in one atom change the entire biosphere.

FIELD OF BIOMEDICAL ENGINEERING

Biomedical engineering is the application of engineering principles and techniques to the medical field. It is a unique application that close the gap between engineering and medicine. It combines the design and problem solving skills of engineering with medical and biological sciences to improve healthcare diagnosis and treatment.

Biomedical engineering has only recently emerged as its own discipline, compared to many other engineering fields; such an evolution is common as a new field transitions from being an interdisciplinary specialisation among already-established fields, to being considered a field in itself. Much of the work in biomedical engineering consists of research and development, spanning a broad array of subfields. Prominent biomedical engineering applications include the development of biocompatible prostheses, various diagnostic and therapeutic medical devices ranging from clinical equipment to micro-implants, common imaging equipment such as MRIs and EEGs, biotechnologies such as regenerative tissue growth, and pharmaceutical drugs and biopharmaceuticals.

Biomedical engineers use their expertise in biology, medicine, physics, mathematics, engineering science and communication to make the world a healthier place. The challenges created by the diversity and complexity of living systems require creative, knowledgeable, and imaginative people working in teams of physicians, scientists, engineers, and even business folk to monitor, restore and enhance normal body function. The biomedical engineer is ideally trained to work at the intersection of science, medicine and mathematics to solve biological and medical problems.

What Do Biomedical Engineers Do?

Perhaps a simpler question to answer is what don't biomedical engineers do? Biomedical engineers work in industry, academic institutions, hospitals and government agencies. Biomedical engineers may spend their days designing electrical circuits and computer software for medical instrumentation. These instruments may range from large imaging systems such as conventional X-ray, computerised tomography (a sort of computer enhanced three-dimensional X-ray) and magnetic resonance imaging, to small implantable devices, such as pacemakers, cochlear implants and drug infusion pumps. Biomedical engineers may use chemistry, physics, mathematical models and computer simulation to develop new drug therapy.

Indeed a considerable number of the advances in understanding how the body functions and how biological systems work have been made by biomedical engineers. They may use mathematical models and statistics to study many of the signals generated by organs such as the brain, heart and skeletal muscle. Some biomedical engineers build artificial organs, limbs, knees, hips, heart valves and dental implants to replace lost function; others are growing living tissues to replace failing organs. The development of artificial body parts requires that biomedical engineers use chemistry and physics to develop durable materials that are compatible with a biological environment.

Biomedical engineers are also working to develop wireless technology that will allow patients and doctors to communicate over long distances.

Many biomedical engineers are involved in rehabilitation–designing better walkers, exercise equipment, robots and therapeutic devices to improve human performance. They are also solving problems at the cellular and molecular level, developing nanotechnology and micromachines to repair damage inside the cell and alter gene function. Biomedical engineers are also working to develop three-dimensional simulations that apply physical laws to the movements of tissues and fluids. The resulting models can be invaluable in understanding how tissue works, and how a prosthetic replacement, for example, might work under the same conditions. Some biomedical engineers solve biomedical problems as physicians, business managers, patent attorneys, physical therapists, professors, research scientists, teachers and technical writers.

While these careers often require additional training beyond the bachelor's degree in biomedical engineering, they are all appropriate careers for the person trained in biomedical engineering. Sometimes electrical, mechanical, computer, or other types of engineers may find themselves working on bio-engineering related problems.

After a few years, they may have so much bio-medical related expertise that they can be considered biomedical engineers.

How Do Biomedical Engineers Differ from Other Engineers?

Biomedical engineers must integrate biology and medicine with engineering to solve problems related to living systems. Thus, biomedical engineers are required to have a solid foundation in a more traditional engineering discipline, such as electrical, mechanical or chemical engineering. Most undergraduate biomedical engineering programs require students to take a core curriculum of traditional engineering courses. However, biomedical engineers are expected to integrate their engineering skills with their understanding of the complexity of biological systems in order to improve medical practice. Thus, biomedical engineers must be trained in the life sciences as well.

NEED FOR BIOINSTRUMENTATION

Bioinstrumentation is an interdisciplinary field requiring a knowledge of the basic principles in several areas including digital electronic systems, control systems, detection systems, and material biocompatibility. In addition to the basic principles, Ph.D's trained in the area of bioinstrumentation need an understanding of how to integrate the concepts and principles within the above areas to realise complete instrumentation systems with a variety of individual components. Ph.D. students in the bioinstrumentation track are given the training to perform research and development to a wide variety of component level and system level issues.

M.S. students within the bioinstrumentation track are required to successfully complete of one of the core bioinstrumentation courses as well as at least one additional elective bioinstrumentation course. The acceptable elective courses are listed below (bioinstrumentation core and/or advanced courses).

Ph.D. students in the bioinstrumentation track are expected to have general knowledge in the field. General knowledge includes sensor systems, control systems, digital systems, medical imaging techniques and optical systems as applied to biomedical instrumentation. The purpose of the Ph.D. qualifying exam is to encourage students to revisit the fundamental principles in bioinstrumentation and synthesise the material.

BIOSENSOR

A biosensor is a device for the detection of an analyte that combines a biological component with a physicochemical detector component.

It consists of three parts:

1. The sensitive biological element (biological material (e.g. tissue, micro-organisms, organelles, cell receptors, enzymes, antibodies, nucleic acids, etc.), a biologically derived material or biomimic) The sensitive elements can be created by biological engineering.

2. The transducer or the detector element (works in a physicochemical way; optical, piezoelectric, electrochemical, etc.) that transforms the signal resulting from the interaction of the analyte with the biological element into another signal (i.e. transducers) that can be more easily measured and quantified.

3. Associated electronics or signal processors that are primarily responsible for the display of the results in a userfriendly way.

The most widespread example of a commercial biosensor is the blood glucose biosensor, which uses the enzyme glucose oxidase to break blood glucose down. In doing so it first oxidises glucose and uses two electrons to reduce the FAD (a component of the enzyme) to FADH2.

This in turn is oxidised by the electrode (accepting two electrons from the electrode) in a number of steps. The resulting current is a measure of the concentration of glucose. In this case, the electrode is the transducer and the enzyme is the biologically active component.

Recently, arrays of many different detector molecules have been applied in so called electronic nose devices, where the pattern of response from the detectors is used to fingerprint a substance. Current commercial electronic noses, however, do not use biological elements.

A canary in a cage, as used by miners to warn of gas could be considered a biosensor. Many of today's biosensor applications are similar, in that they use organisms which respond to toxic substances at a much lower level than us to warn us of their presence. Such devices can be used in environmental monitoring, trace gas detection and in water treatment facilities.

Principles of Detection

Photometric

Many optical biosensors based on the phenomenon of surface plasmon resonance are evanescent wave techniques. This utilises a property of gold and other materials; specifically that a thin layer of gold on a high refractive index glass surface can absorb laser light, producing electron waves (surface plasmons) on the gold surface. This occurs only at a specific angle and wavelength of incident light and is highly dependent on the surface of the gold, such that binding of a target analyte to a receptor on the gold surface produces a measurable signal.

Surface plasmon resonance sensors operate using a sensor chip consisting of a plastic cassette supporting a glass plate, one side of which is coated with a microscopic layer of gold. This side contacts the optical detection apparatus of the instrument. The opposite side is then contacted with a microfluidic flow system. The contact with the flow system creates channels across which reagents can be passed in solution. This side of the glass sensor chip can be modified in a number of ways, to allow easy attachment of molecules of interest. Normally it is coated in carboxymethyl dextran or similar compound.

Light of a fixed wavelength is reflected off the gold side of the chip at the angle of total internal reflection, and detected inside the instrument. This induces the evanescent wave to penetrate through the glass plate and some distance into the liquid flowing over the surface.

The refractive index at the flow side of the chip surface has a direct influence on the behaviour of the light reflected off the gold side. Binding to the flow side of the chip has an effect on the refractive index and in this way biological interactions can be measured to a high degree of sensitivity with some sort of energy.

Other evanescent wave biosensors have been commercialised using waveguides where the propagation constant through the waveguide is changed by the absorption of molecules to the waveguide surface. One such example, dual polarisation Interferometry uses a buried waveguide as a reference against which the change in propagation constant is measured. Other configurations such as the Mach-Zehnder have reference arms lithographically defined on a substrate. Higher levels of integration can be achieved using resonator geometries where the resonant frequency of a ring resonator changes when molecules are absorbed.

Other optical biosensors are mainly based on changes in absorbance or fluorescence of an appropriate indicator compound and do not need a total internal reflection geometry. For example, a fully operational prototype device detecting casein in milk has been fabricated. The device is based on detecting changes in absorption of a gold layer. A widely used research tool, the micro-array, can also be considered a biosensor. Biological biosensors often incorporate a genetically modified form of a native protein or enzyme. The protein is configured to detect a specific analyte and the ensuing signal is read by a detection instrument such as a fluorometer or luminometer. An example of a recently developed biosensor is one for detecting cytosolic concentration of the analyte cAMP (cyclic adenosine monophosphate), a second messenger involved in cellular signalling triggered by ligands interacting with receptors on the cell membrane.

Similar systems have been created to study cellular responses to native ligands or xenobiotics (toxins or small molecule inhibitors). Such 'assays' are commonly used in drug discovery development by pharmaceutical and biotechnology companies. Most cAMP assays in current use require lysis of the cells prior to measurement of cAMP. A live-cell biosensor for cAMP can be used in non-lysed cells with the additional advantage of multiple reads to study the kinetics of receptor response.

Electrochemical

Electrochemical biosensors are normally based on enzymatic catalysis of a reaction that produces or consumes electrons (such enzymes are rightly called redox enzymes). The sensor substrate usually contains three electrodes; a reference electrode, an active electrode and a sink electrode. An auxiliary electrode (also known as a counter electrode) may also be present as an ion source. The target analyte is involved in the reaction that takes place on the active electrode surface, and the ions produced create a potential which is subtracted from that of the reference electrode to give a signal. We can either measure the current (rate of flow of electrons is now proportional to the analyte concentration) at a fixed potential or the potential can be measured at zero current (this gives a logarithmic response). Note that potential of the working or active electrode is space charge sensitive and this is often used. Further, the label-free and direct electrical detection of small peptides and proteins is possible by their intrinsic charges using biofunctionalised ion-sensitive field-effect transistors.

Another example, the potentiometric biosensor, works contrary to the current understanding of its ability. Such biosensors are screenprinted, conducting polymer coated, open circuit potential biosensors based on conjugated polymers immunoassays. They have only two electrodes and are extremely sensitive and robust. They enable the detection of analytes at levels previously only achievable by HPLC and LC/MS and without rigorous sample preparation. The signal is produced by electrochemical and physical changes in the conducting polymer layer due to changes occurring at the surface of the sensor. Such changes can be attributed to ionic strength, pH, hydration and redox reactions, the latter due to the enzyme label turning over a substrate.

Others

Piezoelectric sensors utilise crystals which undergo an elastic deformation when an electrical potential is applied to them. An alternating potential (AC) produces a standing wave in the crystal at a characteristic frequency. This frequency is highly dependent on the elastic properties of the crystal, such that if a crystal is coated with a biological recognition element the binding of a (large) target analyte to a receptor will produce a change in the resonance frequency, which gives a binding signal.

In a mode that uses surface acoustic waves (SAW), the sensitivity is greatly increased. This is a specialised application of the quartz crystal micro-balance as a biosensor. Thermometric and magnetic based biosensors are rare.

Applications

There are many potential applications of biosensors of various types. The main requirements for a biosensor approach to be valuable in terms of research and commercial applications are the identification of a target molecule, availability of a suitable biological recognition element, and the potential for disposable portable detection systems to be preferred to sensitive laboratory-based techniques in some situations. Some examples are given below:

1. Glucose monitoring in diabetes patients—historical market driver.
2. Other medical health related targets.
3. Environmental applications, e.g. the detection of pesticides and river water contaminants.
4. Remote sensing of airborne bacteria, e.g. in counter-bioterrorist activities.
5. Detection of pathogens.
6. Determining levels of toxic substances before and after bioremediation.
7. Detection and determining of organo-phosphate.

8. Routine analytical measurement of folic acid, biotin, vitamin B12 and pantothenic acid as an alternative to microbiological assay.
9. Determination of drug residues in food, such as antibiotics and growth promoters, particularly meat and honey.
10. Drug discovery and evaluation of biological activity of new compounds.
11. Protein engineering in biosensors.
12. Detection of toxic metabolites such as mycotoxins.

Surface Attachment of the Biological Elements

An important part in a biosensor is to attach the biological elements (small molecules/protein/cells) to the surface of the sensor (be it metal, polymer or glass). The simplest way is to functionalise the surface in order to coat it with the biological elements. This can be done by polylysine, aminosilane, epoxysilane or nitrocellulose in the case of silicon chips/silica glass. Subsequently the bound biological agent may be for example fixed by Layer by layer deposition of alternatively charged polymer coatings.

Alternatively three dimensional lattices (hydrogel/xerogel) can be used to chemically or physically entrap these (where by chemically entraped it is meant that the biological element is kept in place by a strong bond, while physically they are kept in place being unable to pass through the pores of the gel matrix). The most commonly used hydrogel is sol-gel, a glassy silica generated by polymerisation of silicate monomers (added as tetra alkyl orthosilicates, such as TMOS or TEOS) in the presence of the biological elements (along with other stabilising polymers, such as PEG) in the case of physical entrapment.

Another group of hydrogels, which set under conditions suitable for cells or protein, are acrylate hydrogel, which polymerise upon radical initiation. One type of radical initiator is a peroxide radical, typically generated by combining a persulphate with TEMED (Polyacrylamide gel are also commonly used for protein electrophoresis), alternatively light can be used in combination with a photoinitiator, such as DMPA (2,2-dimethoxy-2-phenylacetophenone).

COMMON SOURCES OF ERRORS IN MEASUREMENT SYSTEMS

A number of crucial definitions are first needed to ensure clarity of discussion. These are as follows.

Measurement error is defined as the difference between the distorted information and the undistorted information about a measured product, expressed in its measurands. In short, an error is defined as real (untrue, wrong, false, no go) value at the output of a measurement system minus ideal (true, good, right, go) value at the input of a measurement system according to (Eq. 1.1):

$$\Delta x = x_r - x_i \qquad \text{... (1.1)}$$

where, Δx is the error of measurement, x_r is the real untrue measurement value, and x_i is the ideal true measurement value.

A measurement is an experimental process to acquire new knowledge about a product.

A measurement is the realisation of planned actions for the quantitative comparison of a measurand with a unit. A measurand is the physical quantity that is to be measured. Generally, a measurand is the input of a measurement system.

Measuring is a process for ascertaining or determining the quantity of a product by application of some object of known size or capacity, or by comparison with some fixed unit. A product is the result of a process after ISO 9000:2000, point 3.4.2.

Four generic product categories exist as follows: service, software, hardware, processed material.

Many products comprise elements belonging to different generic product categories. Whether the product is then called service, software, hardware, or processed material depends on the dominant element. A process is a set of interrelated or interacting activities that transform inputs into outputs (ISO 9000:2000, point 3.4.1). Inputs to a process are generally outputs to other processes.

A measurement process is a set of operations used to determine the value of a quantity (ISO 9000:2000, point 3.10.2).

Measuring equipment is the measuring instrument, software, measurement standard, reference material or auxiliary apparatus, or a combination, necessary to realise a measurement process (ISO 9000:2000, point 3.10.4).

A measurement system or measuring system is the totality of all measuring equipments and auxiliary means to obtain a measuring result.

A measurement signal is the quantity in a measuring instrument or measuring equipment, which is unequivocally related to the measurand.

A measuring chain (Fig. 1.1) is the structure of elements of a measuring equipment or measuring system, which channels the transfer of a measurement signal from the input of the measurand to the output of the measured value. A measured value is a value that is unequivocally related to the measurand at the output of a measuring chain.

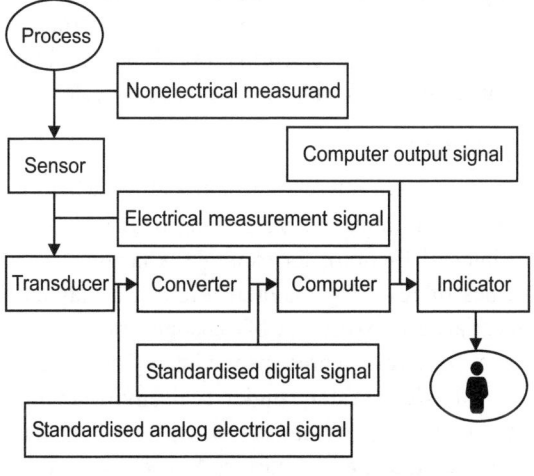

Fig. 1.1. Measurement chain.

How Errors Arise in Measurement Systems

A measurement under ideal conditions has no errors. Real measurement results, however, will always contain measurement errors of varying magnitudes. A systematic (clearly defined process) and systemic (all encompassing) approach is needed to identify every source of error that can arise in a given measuring system. It is then necessary to decide their magnitude and impact on the prevailing operational conditions.

Measurement system errors can only be defined in relation to the solution of a real specific measurement task.

If the errors of measurement systems given in technical documentation are specified, then one has to decide how that information relates to which: (i) measurand, (ii) input (iii) elements of the measurement system, (iv) auxiliary means, (v) measurement method, (vi) output, (vii) kind of reading, and (viii) environmental conditions.

If the measurement system has the general structure given in Fig. 1.1, the following errors may appear for a general measurement task: (i) input error, (ii) sensor error, (iii) signal transmission error 1, (iv) transducer error, (v) signal transmission error 2, (vi) converter error, (vii) signal transmission error 3, (viii) computer error, (ix) signal transmission error 4, and (x) indication error..

Terms Used to Describe Errors

Globalisation of the economy is strongly driving international standardisation and accreditation programs, for example, ISO 9000 and ISO 17025, are the means of assuring quality control of components fabricated throughout the world.

Accrediting organisations such as American association for laboratory accreditation (A2LA) experienced double digit annual growth in the past decade, particularly in the dimensional metrology field (classified under mechanical). Most of these standards and accreditation programs require traceable measurements and hence measurement uncertainty statements.

Recent developments in metrology use:

1. The International system of units (SI).
2. The guide to the expression of uncertainty in measurement (GUM).
3. The International vocabulary of basic and general terms in metrology (VIM).

As a starting point for the application of terms to describe errors in the frame of uncertainties (Fig. 1.2).

Types of Errors in Defined Classes

Systematic error (bias) is a permanent deflection in the same direction from the true value. It can be corrected. Bias and long-term variability are controlled by monitoring measurements against a check standard over time.

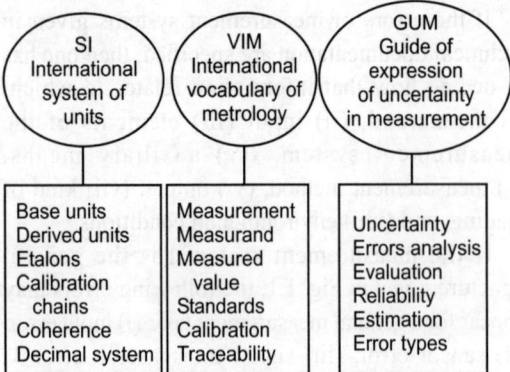

Fig. 1.2. Main tasks of SI.

Random error is a short-term scattering of values around a mean value. It cannot be corrected on an individual measurement basis. Random errors are expressed by statistical methods.

Most exploratory data analysis (EDA) techniques are graphical in nature with a few quantitative techniques included. The reason for the heavy reliance on graphics is that graphics gives the analysts unparalleled power to reveal the structural secrets of data and to be always ready to gain some new, often unsuspected, insight into the measured data in combination with the inherent pattern-recognition capabilities of man.

List of Error Sources in Measurements

Systematic errors or bias are repeatable errors existing with the specified source; these can be adjusted out or compensated for.

To investigate sources of systematic errors, a general checklist of error sources in measurement should be used, which has been collected by specialists working in the field concerned. The main sources are given below.

Lack of gauge resolution

Resolution better called (but rarely done so) discrimination is the ability of the measurement system to detect and faithfully indicate small enough changes in the characteristic of the measurement result.

Lack of linearity

A test of linearity starts by establishing a plot of the measured values versus corresponding values of the reference standards. This obtains an indication of whether or not the points fall on a straight line with slope equal to 1, which indicates linearity.

Nonlinearities of gauges can be caused by the following facts:

1. Gauge is not properly calibrated at the lower and upper ends of the operating range.
2. Errors in the values at the maximum or minimum range.
3. Worn gauge.
4. Internal design problems (in, say the electronic units of the gauge).

Drift

Drift is defined as a slow change in the response of a gauge. Short-term drift is frequently caused by heat buildup in the instrument during the time of measurement. Long-term drift is usually not a problem for measurements with short calibration cycles.

Hysteresis

Hysteresis is a retardation of the effect when the forces acting upon a body are changed (as in viscosity or internal friction); for example, a lagging in the values of resulting magnetisation in a magnetic material (as iron) because of a changing magnetising force. Hysteresis represents the history dependence of a physical system under real environmental conditions. Specific devices will posses their own set of additional error sources. A checklist needs to be developed and matured. The following is an example of such a list.

Standards on Error Description

Standards, when they are part of a single and coherent set of standards, promote market efficiency and expansion, foster international trade, encourage competition and lower barriers to market entry, diffuse new technologies, protect consumers against unsafe or substandard products, and provide trust and reliability.

On the other hand, people talk about raising standards when they perceive slackness in the ropes of control, when they see a sloppiness infiltrating the verities of life, when they begin to be fearful about life-diminishing certainties. Talk of standards is to talk about conservation, about protecting the past in its imagined superiority and security, and defending the future through strong leadership.

Uncertainties of Measurements

Uncertainty is a measure of the 'goodness' of a result. Without such a measure, it is impossible to judge the fitness of the value as a basis for making decisions relating to health, safety, commerce, or scientific excellence. Uncertainty of measurement is a parameter associated with the result of a measurement that characterises the dispersion of the values that could reasonably be expected.

In this model, it is understood that the result of the measurement is the best estimate of the value of the measurand, and that all components of uncertainty, including those arising from systematic effects, contribute to the dispersion. Typical examples for systematic effects are uncertainties of:

1. Systematic errors that generally can be corrected either numerically or technically.
2. Measurement standards that generally are negligibly small in comparison with the uncertainty of the measurement system in total.

Standard deviation is the generally used parameter for expressing the value of uncertainty. It is defined as the point of inflection in the Gaussian normal distribution (Fig. 1.3) of randomly scattering values.

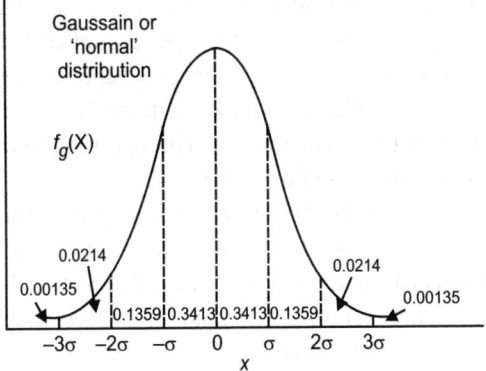

Fig. 1.3. The Gaussian normal distribution.

Evaluation of uncertainty is an ongoing process that can consume time and resources. It can also require the services of someone who is familiar with statistical data analysis techniques.

Measurement result is the best estimate of the value of the measurand. Standard uncertainty in the measurement result is expressed with a standard deviation. Combined standard uncertainty in the measurement result has to be calculated by the error propagation law for statistical characteristics.

Type A uncertainty in the measurement result is expressed as a deviation evaluated by the method of statistical analysis from a series of observations.

Type B uncertainty in the measurement result is expressed as a deviation evaluated by methods other than the statistical analyses of series of observations.

Expanded uncertainty in the measurement result is expressed as the quantity of an interval that is large enough to include that fraction of the distribution function of the measured values that might be reasonably attributed to the measurand.

A special kind of expanded uncertainty is the confidence interval of a Gaussian normal distribution. Coverage factor is a numerical factor used as a multiplier or the combined standard uncertainty in order to obtain an expanded uncertainty of combined measurements.

Problems of uncertainties and error propagation and their solutions are collected in http://www.rit.edu/ ¡«vwlsps/uncertainties/Uncertaintiespart2.html #problems/.

ACCURACY AND PRECISION

In the fields of engineering, industry and statistics, the accuracy of a measurement system is the degree of closeness of measurements of a quantity to its actual (true) value. The precision of a measurement system, also called reproducibility or repeatability, is the degree to which repeated measurements under unchanged conditions show the same results. Although the two words can be synonymous in colloquial use, they are deliberately contrasted in the context of scientific method (Fig. 1.4).

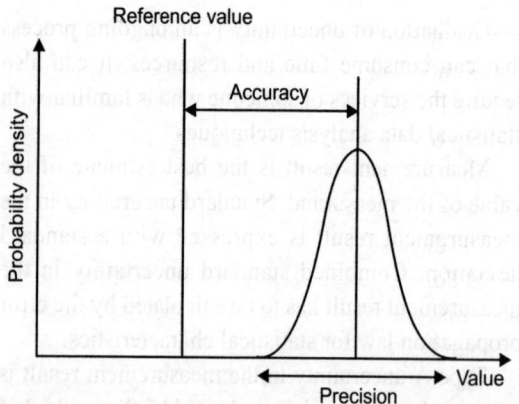

Fig. 1.4. Accuracy indicates proximity of measurement results to the true value, precision to the repeatability or reproducibility of the measurement

A measurement system can be accurate but not precise, precise but not accurate, neither, or both. For example, if an experiment contains a systematic error, then increasing the sample size generally increases precision but does not improve accuracy. Eliminating the systematic error improves accuracy but does not change precision.

A measurement system is called valid if it is both accurate and precise. Related terms are bias (nonrandom or directed effects caused by a factor or factors unrelated by the independent variable) and error (random variability), respectively.

The terminology is also applied to indirect measurements, that is, values obtained by a computational procedure from observed data.

Accuracy is the degree of veracity while precision is the degree of reproducibility. The analogy used here to explain the difference between accuracy and precision is the target comparison. In this analogy, repeated measurements are compared to arrows that are shot at a target. Accuracy describes the closeness of arrows to the bulls eye at the target centre. Arrows that strike closer to the bulls eye are considered more accurate. The closer a system's measurements to the accepted value, the more accurate the system is considered to be.

CALIBRATION

Calibration is the set of operations that establish, under specified conditions, the relationship between the values of quanities indicated by a measuring instrument and the corresponding values realised by standards. The result of a calibration permits either the assignment of values of measurands to the indications or the determination of corrections with respect to indications.

A calibration may also determine other metrological properties such as the effect of influence quantities. The result of a calibration may be recorded in a document, sometimes called a calibration certificate or a calibration report.

A measuring instrument can be calibrated by comparison with a standard.

An adjustment of the instrument is often carried out after calibration in order that it provides given indications corresponding to given values of the quantity measured.

When the instrument is made to give a null indication corresponding to a null value of the quantity to be measured, the set of operation is called zero adjustment .

STATISTICS

Statistics is the science of making effective use of numerical data relating to groups of individuals or experiments. It deals with all aspects of this, including not only the collection, analysis and interpretation of such data, but also the planning of the collection of data, in terms of the design of surveys and experiments.

A statistician is someone who is particularly versed in the ways of thinking necessary for the successful application of statistical analysis. Often such people have gained this experience after starting work in any of a list of fields of application of statistics. There is also a discipline called mathematical statistics, which is concerned with the theoretical basis of the subject.

The word statistics can either be singular or plural. In its singular form, statistics refers to the mathematical science discussed in this section. In its plural form, statistics is the plural of the word statistic, which refers to a quantity (such as a mean) calculated from a set of data.

Gaussain Function

In mathematics, a Gaussian function (named after Carl Friedrich Gauss) is a function of the form:

$$f(x) = ae^{-\frac{(x-b)^2}{2c^2}}$$

for some real constants $a > 0$, b, $c > 0$, and $e \approx 2.718281828$ (Euler's number).

The graph of a Gaussian is a characteristic symmetric 'bell curve' shape that quickly falls off towards plus/minus infinity. The parameter a is the height of the curve's peak, b is the position of the centre of the peak, and c controls the width of the 'bell' (Fig. 1.5).

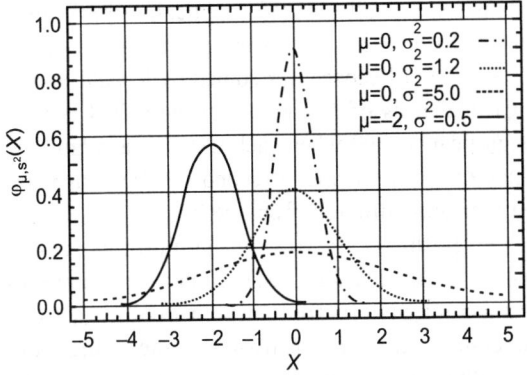

Fig. 1.5. Normalised Gaussian curves with expected value μ and variance σ². The corresponding parameters are $a = 1/(\sigma\sqrt{(2\pi)})$, $b = \mu$, $c = \sigma$.

Gaussian functions are widely used in statistics where they describe the normal distributions, in signal processing where they serve to define Gaussian filters, in image processing where two-dimensional Gaussians are used for Gaussian blurs, and in mathematics where they are used to solve heat equations and diffusion equations and to define the Weierstrass transform.

Poisson Distribution

In probability theory and statistics, the Poisson distribution (or Poisson law of large numbers) is a discrete probability distribution that expresses the probability of a number of events occurring in a fixed period of time if these events occur with a known average rate and independently of the time since the last event.

The Poisson distribution can also be used for the number of events in other specified intervals such as distance, area or volume. Figure 1.6 shows the Poisson: probability mass function.

The distribution was first introduced by Siméon-Denis Poisson (1781–1840) and published, together with his probability theory, in 1838 in his work Recherches sur la probabilité des jugements en matière criminelle et en matière civil. The work focused on certain random variables N that count, among other things, the number of discrete occurrences (sometimes called arrivals) that take place during a time-interval of given length.

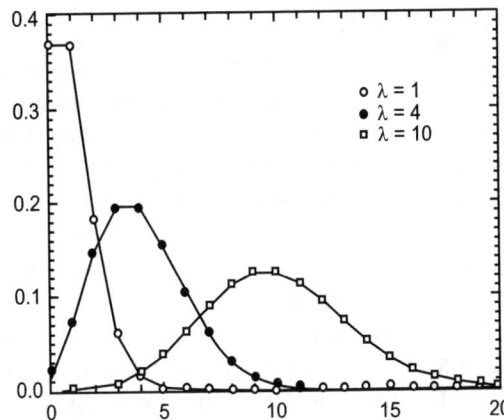

Fig. 1.6. Poisson probability mass function. The horizontal axis is the index k. The function is only defined at integer values of k (empty lozenges). The connecting lines are only guides for the eye.

If the expected number of occurrences in this interval is λ, then the probability that there are exactly k occurrences (k being a non-negative integer, $k = 0$, 1, 2, ...) is equal to:

$$f(k;\lambda) = \frac{\lambda^k e^{-\lambda}}{k!}$$

where.

e is the base of the natural logarithm ($e = 2.71828...$).

k is the number of occurrences of an event—the probability of which is given by the function.

$k!$ is the factorial of k.

λ is a positive real number, equal to the expected number of occurrences that occur during the given interval. For instance, if the events occur on average 4 times per minute, and you are interested in the number of events occurring in a 10 minute interval, you would use as your model a Poisson distribution with $\lambda = 10 \times 4 = 40$.

As a function of k, this is the probability mass function. The poisson distribution can be derived as a limiting case of the binomial distribution.

The poisson distribution can be applied to systems with a large number of possible events, each of which is rare. A classic example is the nuclear decay of atoms. The poisson distribution is sometimes called a poissonian, analogous to the term Gaussian for a Gauss or normal distribution.

Estimation Theory

Estimation theory is a branch of statistics and signal processing that deals with estimating the values of parameters based on measured/empirical data. The parameters describe an underlying physical setting in such a way that the value of the parameters affects the distribution of the measured data. An estimator attempts to approximate the unknown parameters using the measurements.

For example, it is desired to estimate the proportion of a population of voters who will vote for a particular candidate. That proportion is the unobservable parameter; the estimate is based on a small random sample of voters.

Or, for example, in radar the goal is to estimate the location of objects (airplanes, boats, etc.) by analysing the received echo and a possible question to be posed is 'where are the airplanes?' To answer where the airplanes are, it is necessary to estimate the distance the airplanes are at from the radar station, which can provide an absolute location if the absolute location of the radar station is known.

In estimation theory, it is assumed that the desired information is embedded in a noisy signal. Noise adds uncertainty, without which the problem would be deterministic and estimation would not be needed.

The entire purpose of estimation theory is to arrive at an estimator, and preferably an implementable one that could actually be used. The estimator takes the measured data as input and produces an estimate of the parameters.

It is also preferable to derive an estimator that exhibits optimality. Estimator optimality usually refers to achieving minimum average error over some class of estimators, for example, a minimum variance unbiased estimator. In this case, the class is the set of unbiased estimators, and the average error measure is variance (average squared error between the value of the estimate and the parameter).

Statistical Hypothesis Testing

A statistical hypothesis test is a method of making statistical decisions using experimental data. In statistics, a result is called statistically significant if it is unlikely to have occurred by chance. The phrase 'test of significance' was coined by Ronald Fisher: 'Critical tests of this kind may be called tests of significance, and when such tests are available we may discover whether a second sample is or is not significantly different from the first.'

Hypothesis testing is sometimes called confirmatory data analysis, in contrast to exploratory data analysis. In frequency probability, these decisions are almost always made using null-hypothesis tests; that is, ones that answer the question Assuming that the null hypothesis is true, what is the probability of observing a value for the test statistic that is at least as extreme as the value that was actually observed?

One use of hypothesis testing is deciding whether experimental results contain enough information to cast doubt on conventional wisdom.

Statistical hypothesis testing is a key technique of frequentist statistical inference, and is widely used, but also much criticised. The main direct alternative to statistical hypothesis testing is Bayesian inference. However, other approaches to reaching a decision based on data are available via decision theory and optimal decisions.

The critical region of a hypothesis test is the set of all outcomes which, if they occur, will lead us to decide that there is a difference. That is, cause the null hypothesis to be rejected in favour of the alternative hypothesis. The critical region is usually denoted by C.

Example

As an example, consider determining whether a suitcase contains some radioactive material. Placed under a Geiger counter, it produces 10 counts per minute. The null hypothesis is that no radioactive material is in the suitcase and that all measured counts are due to ambient radioactivity typical of the surrounding air and harmless objects. We can then calculate how likely it is that we would observe 10 counts per minute if the null hypothesis were true. If the null hypothesis predicts (say) on average 9 counts per minute and a standard deviation of 1 count per minute, then we say that the suitcase is compatible with the null hypothesis (this does not guarantee that there is no radioactive material, just that we do not have enough evidence to suggest there is). On the other hand, if the null hypothesis predicts 3 counts per minute and a standard deviation of 1 count per minute, then the suitcase is not compatible with the null hypothesis, and there are likely other factors responsible to produce the measurements.

The test described here is more fully the null-hypothesis statistical significance test. The null hypothesis represents what we would believe by default, before seeing any evidence. Statistical significance is a possible finding of the test, declared when the observed sample is unlikely to have occurred by chance if the null hypothesis were true. The name of the test describes its formulation and its possible outcome. One characteristic of the test is its crisp decision: to reject or not reject the null hypothesis. A calculated value is compared to a threshold, which is determined from the tolerable risk of error.

Testing Process

Hypothesis testing is defined by the following general procedure:

1. The first step in any hypothesis testing is to state the relevant null and alternative hypotheses to be tested. This is important as misstating the hypotheses will muddy the rest of the process.

2. The second step is to consider the assumptions being made in doing the test; for example, assumptions about the statistical independence or about the form of the distributions of the observations. This is equally important as invalid assumptions will mean that the results of the test are invalid.

3. Compute the relevant test statistic. The distribution of such a statistic under the null hypothesis can be derived from the assumptions. In standard cases this will be a well-known result. For example the test statistics may follow a Student's t distribution or a normal distribution. The distribution of the test statistic partitions the possible values of the estimator into those for which the null-hypothesis is rejected and those for which it is not.

4. Compare the test-statistic, S, with the relevant critical value, C (obtained from tables in standard cases).

5. Decide to either fail to reject the null hypothesis or reject it in favour of the alternative. The decision rule is to reject the null hypothesis H_0 if $S > C$, and to accept or 'fail to reject' the hypothesis otherwise.

It is important to note the philosophical difference between accepting the null hypothesis and simply failing to reject it. The 'fail to reject' terminology highlights the fact that the null hypothesis is assumed to be true from the start of the test; if there is a lack of evidence against it, it simply continues to be assumed true. The phrase 'accept the null hypothesis' may suggest it has been proved simply because it has not been disproved, a logical fallacy known as the argument from ignorance. Unless a test with particularly high power is used, the idea of 'accepting' the null hypothesis may be dangerous. Nonetheless the terminology is prevalent throughout statistics, where its meaning is well understood.

2

Basic Concepts of Electronics

INTRODUCTION

Electric currents flow along wires to transmit energy for domestic and industrial purposes. To understand many electrical phenomena, it is only necessary to learn a few simple rules of circuit analysis and these will be the underlying theme of this chapter. This pre-course material establishes the basic definitions of electric charge, currents, voltage or electric potential energy. Secondly, it discusses the behaviour of currents in circuits and introduces some important circuit components.

ELECTRONIC COMPONENTS

Electric Current

Electric current can mean, depending on the context, a flow of electric charge (a phenomenon) or the rate of flow of electric charge (a quantity). This flowing electric charge is typically carried by moving electrons, in a conductor such as wire; in an electrolyte, it is instead carried by ions, and, in a plasma, by both.

The SI unit for measuring the rate of flow of electric charge is the ampere. Electric current is measured using an ammeter.

Voltage

Voltage is commonly used as a short name for electrical potential difference. Its corresponding SI unit is the volt (symbol: V, not italicised). Electric potential is a hypothetically measurable physical dimension, and is denoted by the algebraic variable V(italicised).

The voltage between two (electron) positions 'A' and 'B', inside a solid electrical conductor (or inside two electrically-connected, solid electrical conductors), is denoted by ($V_A - V_B$). This voltage is the electrical driving force that drives a conventional electric current in the direction A to B. Voltage can be directly measured by a voltmeter. Well-constructed, correctly used, real voltmeters approximate very well to ideal voltmeters.

Simple applications

Common usage (that 'voltage' usually means 'voltage difference') is now resumed. Obviously, when using the term 'voltage' in the shorthand sense, one must be clear about the two points between which the voltage is specified or measured. When using a voltmeter to measure voltage difference, one electrical lead of the voltmeter must be connected to the first point, one to the second point.

Voltage between two stated points

A common use of the term 'voltage' is in specifying how many volts are dropped across an electrical device (such as a resistor). In this case, the 'voltage', or more accurately, the 'voltage drop across the device', can usefully be understood as the difference between two measurements. The first measurement uses one electrical lead of the voltmeter on the first terminal of the device, with the other voltmeter lead connected to ground. The second measurement is similar, but with the first voltmeter lead on the second terminal of the device. The voltage drop is the difference between the two readings. In practice, the voltage drop across a device can be measured directly and safely using a voltmeter that is isolated from ground, provided that the maximum voltage capability of the voltmeter is not exceeded.

Two points in an electric circuit that are connected by an 'ideal conductor', that is, a conductor without resistance and not within a changing magnetic field, have a voltage difference of zero. However, other pairs of points may also have a voltage difference of zero. If two such points are connected with a conductor, no current will flow through the connection.

Addition of voltages

Voltage is additive in the following sense: the voltage between A and C is the sum of the voltage between A and B and the voltage between B and C. The various voltages in a circuit can be computed using Kirchhoff's circuit laws.

When talking about alternating current (AC) there is a difference between instantaneous voltage and average voltage. Instantaneous voltages can be added as for direct current (DC), but average voltages can be meaningfully added only when they apply to signals that all have the same frequency and phase.

Useful formulas

DC (Direct current) circuits

$$V = IR \quad \text{(Ohm's Law)}$$
$$P = IV = I^2R = V^2/R$$
$$V = \sqrt{PR}$$

where, V = voltage difference (SI unit: volt), I = electric current (SI unit: ampere), R = resistance (SI unit: ohm), P = power (SI unit: watt).

AC (Alternating current) circuits

$$V = \frac{P}{I \cos\phi}$$
$$V = \frac{\sqrt{PZ}}{\sqrt{\cos\phi}}$$
$$V = \frac{IR}{\cos\phi}$$

where, V = voltage, I = current, R = resistance, P = true power, Z = impedance, f = phase difference between I and V.

AC conversions

$$V_{avg} = 0.637\ V_{pk} = \frac{2}{\pi} V_{pk} = \frac{\omega}{\pi}\int_0^{\pi/\omega} V_{pk}\sin(\omega t - kx)\,dx$$

$$V_{rms} = 0.707\ V_{pk} = \frac{1}{\sqrt{2}} V_{pk} = V_{pk}\sqrt{\langle \sin^2(\omega t - kx)\rangle}$$

$$V_{pk} = 0.5\ V_{ppk}$$

$$V_{avg} = 0.319\ V_{ppk}$$

$$V_{rms} = 0.354\ V_{ppk} = \frac{1}{2\sqrt{2}} V_{ppk}$$

$$V_{avg} = 0.900\ V_{rms} = \frac{2\sqrt{2}}{\pi} V_{rms}$$

where, V_{pk}=peak voltage, V_{ppk}=peak-to-peak voltage, V_{avg}=average voltage over a half-cycle, V_{rms}=effective (root mean square) voltage, and we assumed a sinusoidal wave of the form $V_{pk}\sin(\omega t - kx)$, with a period $T = 2\pi/\omega$, and where the angle brackets (in the root-mean-square equation) denote a time average over an entire period.

Total voltage

Voltage sources and drops in series:
$$V_T = V_1 + V_2 + V_3 + ... + V_n$$
Voltage sources and drops in parallel:
$$V_T = V_1 + V_2 + V_3 + ... + V_n$$
Where the nth voltage source or drop

Voltage drops

Across a resistor (Resistor R):
$$V_R = IR_R$$
Across a capacitor (Capacitor C):
$$V_C = IX_C$$
Across an inductor (inductor L):
$$V_L = IX_L$$

where, V= voltage, I = current, R = resistance, X= reactance.

Instruments for measuring voltage differences include the voltmeter, the potentiometer, and the oscilloscope. The voltmeter works by measuring the current through a fixed resistor, which, according to Ohm's Law, is proportional to the voltage difference across the resistor. The potentiometer works by balancing the unknown voltage against a known voltage in a bridge circuit. The cathode-ray oscilloscope works by amplifying the voltage difference and using it to deflect an electron beam from a straight path, so that the deflection of the beam is proportional to the voltage difference.

Voltages as low as 50 volts can lead to a lethal electric shock under certain circumstances.

OHM'S LAW

In electrical circuits, Ohm's law states that the current through a conductor between two points is directly proportional to the potential difference or voltage across the two points, and inversely proportional to the resistance between them (Fig. 2.1).

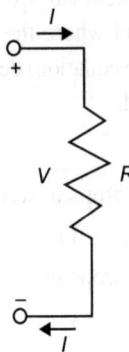

Fig. 2.1. V, I and R, the parameters of Ohm's law.

The mathematical equation that describes this relationship is:

$$I = \frac{V}{R}$$

where, V is the potential difference measured across the resistance in units of volts; I is the current through the resistance in units of amperes and R is the resistance of the conductor in units of ohms. More specifically, Ohm's law states that the R in this relation is constant, independent of the current.

Circuit Analysis

In circuit analysis, three equivalent expressions of Ohm's law are used interchangeably:

$$V = IR \quad \text{or} \quad I = \frac{V}{R} \quad \text{or} \quad R = \frac{V}{I}$$

Indeed, each is quoted by some sources as the defining relationship of Ohm's law, or all three are quoted, or derived from a proportional form, or even just the two that don't correspond to Ohm's original statement may sometimes be given.

Resistive circuits

Resistors are circuit elements that impede the passage of electric charge in agreement with Ohm's law, and are designed to have a specific resistance value R. An element (resistor or conductor) that behaves according to Ohm's law over some operating range is referred to as an ohmic device (or an ohmic resistor) because Ohm's law and a single value for the resistance suffice to describe the behaviour of the device over that range.

Ohm's law holds for circuits containing only resistive elements (no capacitances or inductances) for all forms of driving voltage or current, regardless of whether the driving voltage or current is constant (DC) or time-varying such as AC. At any instant of time Ohm's law is valid for such circuits. Resistors which are in series or in parallel may be grouped together into a single 'equivalent resistance' in order to apply Ohm's law in analysing the circuit.

Reactive circuits with time-varying signals

When reactive elements such as capacitors, inductors, or transmission lines are involved in a circuit to which AC or time-varying voltage or current is applied, the relationship between voltage and current becomes the solution to a differential equation, so Ohm's law (as defined above) does not directly apply since that form contains only resistances having value R, not complex impedances which may contain capacitance (C) or inductance (L).

Linear approximations

Ohm's law is one of the basic equations used in the analysis of electrical circuits. It applies to both metal conductors and circuit components (resistors) specifically made for this behaviour. Both are ubiquitous in electrical engineering. Materials and components that obey Ohm's law are described as 'ohmic' which means they produce the same value for resistance ($R = V/I$) regardless of the value of V or I which is applied and whether the applied voltage or current is DC (direct current) of either positive or negative polarity or AC (alternating current) (Fig. 2.2).

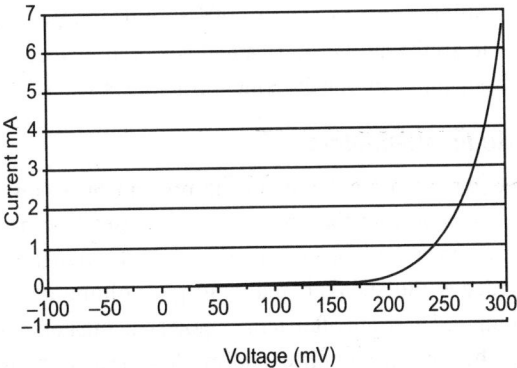

Voltage (mV)

Fig. 2.2. Plot of $I-V$ curve of an ideal $p-n$ junction diode at 1μA reverse leakage current. Failure of the device to follow Ohm's law is clearly shown since the curve is not a straight line.

In a true ohmic device, the same value of resistance will be calculated from $R = V/I$ regardless of the value of the applied voltage V. That is, the ratio of V/I is constant, and when current is plotted as a function of voltage the curve is linear (a straight line). If voltage is forced to some value V, then that voltage V divided by measured current I will equal R. Or if the current is forced to some value I, then the measured voltage V divided by that current I is also R. Since the plot of I versus V is a straight line, then it is also true that for any set of two different voltages V_1 and V_2 applied across a given device of resistance R, producing currents $I_1 = V_1/R$ and $I_2 = V_2/R$, that the ratio $(V_1 - V_2)/(I_1 - I_2)$ is also a constant equal to R. The operator 'delta' (Δ) is used to represent a difference in a quantity, so we can write $\Delta V = V_1 - V_2$ and $\Delta I = I_1 - I_2$. Summarising, for any truly ohmic device having resistance R, $V/I = \Delta V/\Delta I = R$ for any applied voltage or current or for the difference between any set of applied voltages or currents.

There are, however, components of electrical circuits which do not obey Ohm's law; that is, their relationship between current and voltage (their $I-V$ curve) is nonlinear. An example is the $p-n$ junction diode (curve at right). As seen in the figure, the current does not increase linearly with applied voltage for a diode. One can determine a value of current (I) for a given value of applied voltage (V) from the curve, but not from Ohm's law, since the value of 'resistance' is not constant as a function of applied voltage. Further, the current only increases significantly if the applied voltage is positive, not negative. The ratio V/I for some point along the nonlinear curve is sometimes called the static, or chordal, or DC, resistance, but as seen in the figure the value of total V over total I varies depending on the particular point along the nonlinear curve which is chosen. This means the 'DC resistance' V/I at some point on the curve is not the same as what would be determined by applying an AC signal having peak amplitude ΔV volts or ΔI amps centred at that same point along the curve and measuring $\Delta V/\Delta I$. However, in some diode applications, the AC signal applied to the device is small and it is possible to analyse the circuit in terms of the dynamic, small-signal, or incremental resistance, defined as the one over the slope of the $V-I$ curve at the average value (DC operating point) of the voltage (that is, one over the derivative of current with respect to voltage). For sufficiently small signals, the dynamic resistance allows the Ohm's law small signal resistance to be calculated as approximately one over the slope of a line drawn tangentially to the $V-I$ curve at the DC operating point.

Attenuator (Electronics)

An attenuator is an electronic device that reduces the amplitude or power of a signal without appreciably distorting its waveform.

An attenuator is effectively the opposite of an amplifier, though the two work by different methods. While an amplifier provides gain, an attenuator provides loss, or gain less than 1.

Attenuators are usually passive devices made from simple voltage divider networks. Switching between different resistances forms adjustable stepped attenuators and continuously adjustable ones using potentiometers. For higher frequencies precisely matched low VSWR resistance networks are used.

Fixed attenuators in circuits are used to lower voltage, dissipate power, and to improve impedance matching. In measuring signals, attenuator pads or adaptors are used to lower the amplitude of the signal a known amount to enable measurements, or to protect the measuring device from signal levels that might damage it. Attenuators are also used to 'match' impedances by lowering apparent SWR.

Power attenuator (guitar)s are used as loads for dissipating power while allowing the small output to be used for measurement or other purposes.

Attenuator circuits

Basic circuits used in RF and AF attenuators are PI pads (π-type) and T pads. Especially in RF frequency, balanced and unbalanced network are used upon the line characteristics. Figure 2.3 shows attenuator circuits of various types. Since an attenuator circuit using only L, C and R is linear, input and output ports are not distinguished.

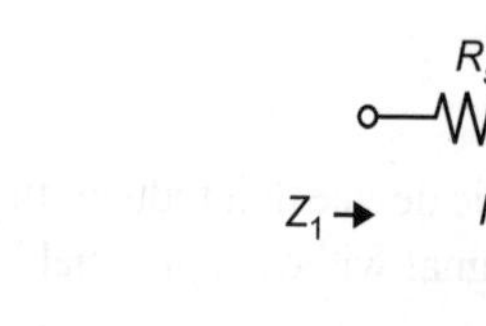

π-type unbalanced attenuator circuit

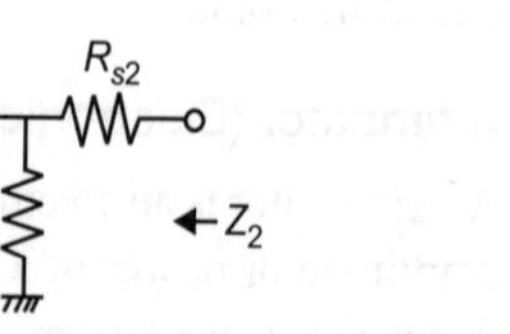

π-type balanced attenuator circuit

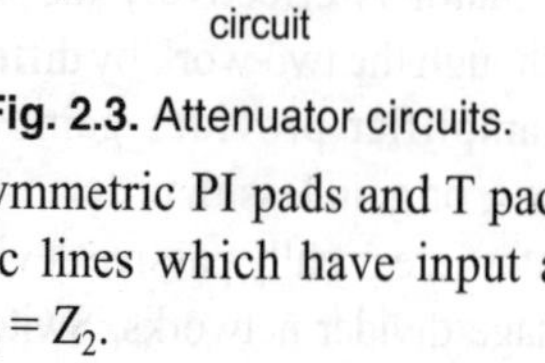

T-type unbalanced attenuator circuit

Fig. 2.3. Attenuator circuits.

Usually symmetric PI pads and T pads are used for symmetric lines which have input and output impedance $Z_1 = Z_2$.

RF attenuators

Radio frequency attenuators are typically coaxial in structure with precision connectors as ports and coaxial, microstrip or thin-film internal structure. Above SHF special waveguide structure is required.

Important characteristics are: (i) accuracy, (ii) low SWR, (iii) flat frequency-response, and (iv) repeatability.

The size and shape of the attenuator depends on its ability to dissipate power. RF attenuators are used as loads for and as known attenuations and protective dissipations of power in measuring RF signals.

Audio attenuators

A line-level attenuator in the preamp or a power attenuator after the power amplifier uses electrical resistance to reduce the amplitude of the signal that reaches the speaker, reducing the volume of the output. These are often termed power attenuators and go between the amplifer and speaker(s) stages of the unit. A line-level attenuator has lower power handling, such as a 1/2-watt potentiometer. A power attenuator has higher power handling, such as 10 or 50 watts.

Galvanometer

A galvanometer is a type of ammeter: an instrument for detecting and measuring electric current. It is an analog electromechanical transducer that produces a rotary deflection of some type of pointer in response to electric current flowing through its coil. The term has expanded to include uses of the same mechanism in recording, positioning, and servomechanism equipment (Fig. 2.4).

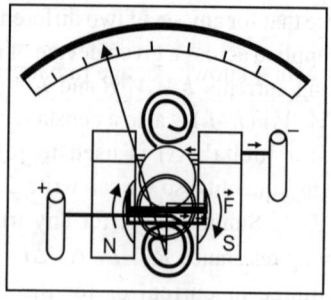

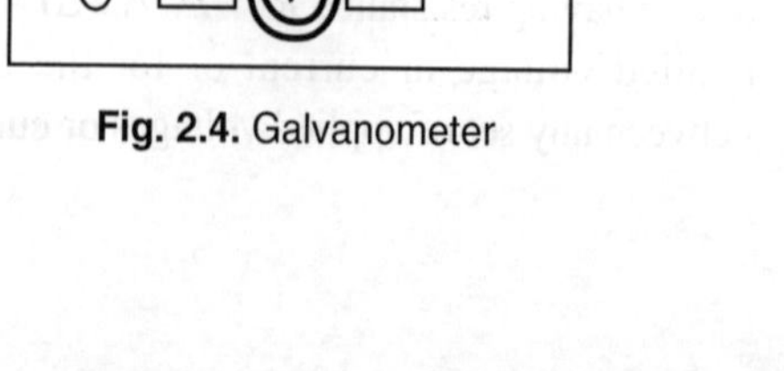

Fig. 2.4. Galvanometer

Operation

The most familiar use is as an analog measuring instrument, often called a meter. It is used to measure the direct current (flow of electric charge) through an electric circuit. The D'Arsonval/Weston form used today is constructed with a small pivoting coil of wire in the field of a permanent magnet. The coil is attached to a thin pointer that traverses a calibrated scale. A tiny torsion spring pulls the coil and pointer to the zero position.

When a direct current (DC) flows through the coil, the coil generates a magnetic field. This field acts against the permanent magnet. The coil twists, pushing against the spring, and moves the pointer. The hand points at a scale indicating the electric current. Careful design of the pole pieces ensures that the magnetic field is uniform, so that the angular deflection of the pointer is proportional to the current. A useful meter generally contains provision for damping the mechanical resonance of the moving coil and pointer, so that the pointer settles quickly to its position without oscillation.

The basic sensitivity of a meter might be, for instance, 100 microamperes full scale (with a voltage drop of, say, 50 millivolts at full current). Such meters are often calibrated to read some other quantity that can be converted to a current of that magnitude. The use of current dividers, often called shunts, allows a meter to be calibrated to measure larger currents. A meter can be calibrated as a DC voltmeter if the resistance of the coil is known by calculating the voltage required to generate a full scale current. A meter can be configured to read other voltages by putting it in a voltage divider circuit. This is generally done by placing a resistor in series with the meter coil. A meter can be used to read resistance by placing it in series with a known voltage (a battery) and an adjustable resistor. In a preparatory step, the circuit is completed and the resistor adjusted to produce full scale deflection. When an unknown resistor is placed in series in the circuit the current will be less than full scale and an appropriately calibrated scale can display the value of the previously-unknown resistor.

Because the pointer of the meter is usually a small distance above the scale of the meter, parallax error can occur when the operator attempts to read the scale line that 'lines up' with the pointer. To counter this, some meters include a mirror along the markings of the principal scale. The accuracy of the reading from a mirrored scale is improved by positioning one's head while reading the scale so that the pointer and the reflection of the pointer are aligned; at this point, the operator's eye must be directly above the pointer and any parallax error has been minimised.

It is used to measure an unknown electrical resistance by balancing two legs of a bridge circuit, one leg of which includes the unknown component. Its operation is similar to the original potentiometer (Fig. 2.5).

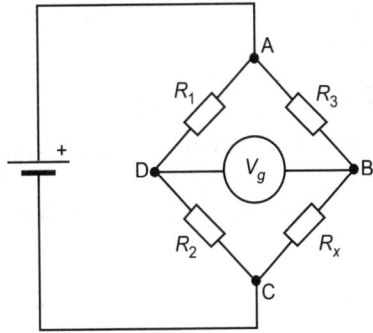

Fig. 2.5. Wheatstone's bridge circuit digram.

R_x is the unknown resistance to be measured; R_1, R_2 and R_3 are resistors of known resistance and the resistance of R_2 is adjustable. If the ratio of the two resistances in the known leg (R_2/R_1) is equal to the ratio of the two in the unknown leg (R_x/R_3), then the voltage between the two midpoints (B and D) will be zero and no current will flow through the galvanometer V_g. R_2 is varied until this condition is reached. The direction of the current indicates whether R_2 is too high or too low.

Detecting zero current can be done to extremely high accuracy (see galvanometer). Therefore, if R_1, R_2 and R_3 are known to high precision, then R_x can be measured to high precision. Very small changes in R_x disrupt the balance and are readily detected.

At the point of balance, the ratio of $R_2/R_1 = R_x/R_3$
Therefore, $R_x = (R_2/R_1) \cdot R_3$

Alternatively, if R_1, R_2, and R_3 are known, but R_2 is not adjustable, the voltage difference across or current flow through the meter can be used to calculate the value of R_x, using Kirchhoff's circuit laws (also known as Kirchhoff's rules). This setup is frequently used in strain gauge and resistance thermometer measurements, as it is usually faster to read a voltage level off a meter than to adjust a resistance to zero the voltage.

The Wheatstone bridge illustrates the concept of a difference measurement, which can be extremely accurate. Variations on the Wheatstone bridge can be used to measure capacitance, inductance, impedance and other quantities, such as the amount of combustible gases in a sample, with an explosimeter. The Kelvin double bridge was specially adapted from the Wheatstone bridge for measuring very low resistances. In many cases, the significance of measuring the unknown resistance is related to measuring the impact of some physical phenomenon — such as force, temperature, pressure, etc. which thereby allows the use of Wheatstone bridge in measuring those elements indirectly.

Capacitor

A capacitor or condenser is a passive electronic component consisting of a pair of conductors separated by a dielectric (insulator). When a potential difference (voltage) exists across the conductors, an electric field is present in the dielectric. This field stores energy and produces a mechanical force between the conductors. The effect is greatest when there is a narrow separation between large areas of conductor, hence capacitor conductors are often called plates.

An ideal capacitor is characterised by a single constant value, capacitance, which is measured in farads. This is the ratio of the electric charge on each conductor to the potential difference between them. In practice, the dielectric between the plates passes a small amount of leakage current. The conductors and leads introduce an equivalent series resistance and the dielectric has an electric field strength limit resulting in a breakdown voltage.

Capacitors are widely used in electronic circuits to block the flow of direct current while allowing alternating current to pass, to filter out interference, to smooth the output of power supplies, and for many other purposes. They are used in resonant circuits in radio frequency equipment to select particular frequencies from a signal with many frequencies.

Current-voltage relation

The current $i(t)$ through a component in an electric circuit is defined as the rate of change of the charge $q(t)$ that has passed through it. Physical charges cannot pass through the dielectric layer of a capacitor, but rather build up in equal and opposite quantities on the electrodes: as each electron accumulates on the negative plate, one leaves the positive plate. Thus the accumulated charge on the electrodes is equal to the integral of the current, as well as being proportional to the voltage (as discussed above). As with any antiderivative, a constant of integration is added to represent the initial voltage $v(t_0)$. This is the integral form of the capacitor equation,

$$v(t) = \frac{q(t)}{C} = \frac{1}{C}\int_{t_0}^{t} i(\tau)d\tau + v(t_0)$$

Taking the derivative of this, and multiplying by C, yields the derivative form,

$$i(t) = \frac{dq(t)}{dt} = C\frac{dv(t)}{dt}$$

The dual of the capacitor is the inductor, which stores energy in the magnetic field rather than the electric field. Its current-voltage relation is obtained by exchanging current and voltage in the capacitor equations and replacing C with the inductance L.

DC circuits

A series circuit containing only a resistor, a capacitor, a switch and a constant DC source of voltage V_0 is known as a charging circuit (Fig. 2.6). If the capacitor is initially uncharged while the switch is open, and the switch is closed at $t = 0$, it follows from Kirchhoff's voltage law that:

$$V_0 = v_{\text{resistor}}(t) + v_{\text{capacitor}}(t) = i(t)R + \frac{1}{C}\int_0^t i(\tau)d\tau$$

Taking the derivative and multiplying by C, gives a first-order differential equation,

$$RC\frac{di(t)}{dt} + i(t) = 0$$

At $t = 0$, the voltage across the capacitor is zero and the voltage across the resistor is V_0. The initial current is then $i(0) = V_0/R$. With this assumption, the differential equation yields:

$$i(t) = \frac{V_0}{R} e^{-t/\tau_0}$$

$$v(t) = V_0 \left(1 - e^{-t/\tau_0}\right)$$

where, $t_0 = RC$ is the time constant of the system.

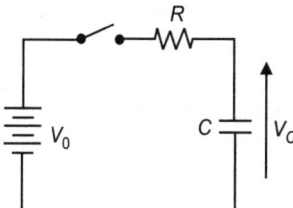

Fig. 2.6. A simple resistor-capacitor circuit demonstrates charging of a capacitor.

As the capacitor reaches equilibrium with the source voltage, the voltage across the resistor and the current through the entire circuit decay exponentially. The case of discharging a charged capacitor likewise demonstrates exponential decay, but with the initial capacitor voltage replacing V_0 and the final voltage being zero.

AC circuits

Impedance, the vector sum of reactance and resistance, describes the phase difference and the ratio of amplitudes between sinusoidally varying voltage and sinusoidally varying current at a given frequency. Fourier analysis allows any signal to be constructed from a spectrum of frequencies, whence the circuit's reaction to the various frequencies may be found. The reactance and impedance of a capacitor are respectively:

$$X = -\frac{1}{\omega C} = -\frac{1}{2\pi fC}$$

$$Z = \frac{1}{j\omega C} = -\frac{j}{\omega C} = -\frac{j}{2\pi fC}$$

where, j is the imaginary unit and ω is the angular velocity of the sinusoidal signal. The $-j$ phase indicates that the AC voltage $V = ZI$ lags the AC current by 90°: the positive current phase corresponds to increasing voltage as the capacitor charges; zero current corresponds to instantaneous constant voltage, etc.

Note that impedance decreases with increasing capacitance and increasing frequency. This implies that a higher-frequency signal or a larger capacitor results in a lower voltage amplitude per current amplitude—an AC 'short circuit' or AC coupling. Conversely, for very low frequencies, the reactance will be high, so that a capacitor is nearly an open circuit in AC analysis—those frequencies have been 'filtered out'. Capacitors are different from resistors and inductors in that the impedance is inversely proportional to the defining characteristic, i.e. capacitance.

Networks

For capacitors in parallel: Capacitors in a parallel configuration each have the same applied voltage. Their capacitances add up. Charge is apportioned among them by size. Using the schematic diagram to visualise parallel plates (Fig. 2.7), it is apparent that each capacitor contributes to the total surface area.

$$C_{eq} = C_1 + C_2 + \dots + C_n$$

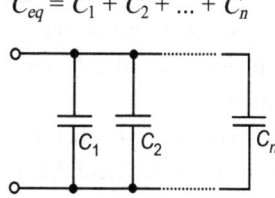

Fig. 2.7. Several capacitors in parallel.

For capacitors in series: Connected in series, the schematic diagram reveals that the separation distance, not the plate area, adds up. The capacitors each store instantaneous charge build-up equal to that of every other capacitor in the series. The total voltage difference from end to end is apportioned to each capacitor according to the inverse of its capacitance. The entire series acts as a capacitor smaller than any of its components (Fig. 2.8).

$$\frac{1}{C_{eq}} = \frac{1}{C_1} + \frac{1}{C_2} + \dots + \frac{1}{C_n}$$

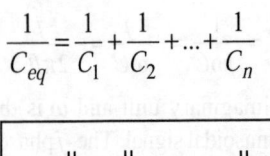

Fig. 2.8. Several capacitors in series.

Capacitors are combined in series to achieve a higher working voltage, for example for smoothing a high voltage power supply. The voltage ratings, which are based on plate separation, add up. In such an application, several series connections may in turn be connected in parallel, forming a matrix. The goal is to maximise the energy storage utility of each capacitor without overloading it. Series connection is also used to adapt electrolytic capacitors for AC use.

Inductor

An inductor or a reactor is a passive electrical component that can store energy in a magnetic field created by the electric current passing through it. An inductor's ability to store magnetic energy is measured by its inductance, in units of henries. Typically an inductor is a conducting wire shaped as a coil, the loops helping to create a strong magnetic field inside the coil due to Faraday's law of induction. Inductors are one of the basic electronic components used in electronics where current and voltage change with time, due to the ability of inductors to delay and reshape alternating currents.

Inductance (L) (measured in henries) is an effect resulting from the magnetic field that forms around a current-carrying conductor which tends to resist changes in the current. Electric current through the conductor creates a magnetic flux proportional to the current, and a change in this current creates a corresponding change in magnetic flux which, in turn, by Faraday's law generates an electromotive force (emf) that opposes this change in current. Inductance is a measure of the amount of emf generated per unit change in current. For example, an inductor with an inductance of 1 henry produces an emf of 1 volt when the current through the inductor changes at the rate of 1 ampere per second. The number of loops, the size of each loop, and the material it is wrapped around all affect the inductance. For example, the magnetic flux linking these turns can be increased by coiling the conductor around a material with a high permeability such as iron. This can increase the inductance by 2000 times, although less so at high frequencies.

In electric circuits

An inductor opposes changes in current. An ideal inductor would offer no resistance to a constant direct current; however, only superconducting inductors have truly zero electrical resistance.

In general, the relationship between the time-varying voltage $v(t)$ across an inductor with inductance L and the time-varying current $i(t)$ passing through it is described by the differential equation:

$$v(t) = L\frac{di(t)}{dt}$$

When there is a sinusoidal alternating current (AC) through an inductor, a sinusoidal voltage is induced. The amplitude of the voltage is proportional to the product of the amplitude (I_p) of the current and the frequency (f) of the current.

$$i(t) = I_p \sin(2\pi f t)$$

$$\frac{di(t)}{dt} = 2\pi f\, I_p \cos(2\pi f t)$$

$$v(t) = 2\pi f L I_p \cos(2\pi f t)$$

In this situation, the phase of the current lags that of the voltage by 90 degrees.

If an inductor is connected to a DC current source, with value I via a resistance, R, and then the current source short circuited, the differential relationship above shows that the current through the inductor will discharge with an exponential decay:

$$i(t) = I\left(e^{\frac{-tR}{L}}\right)$$

Laplace circuit analysis (s-domain)

When using the Laplace transform in circuit analysis,

the transfer impedance of an ideal inductor with no initial current is represented in the *s* domain by:

$$Z(s) = Ls$$

where,

L is the inductance, and

s is the complex frequency

If the inductor does have initial current, it can be represented by:

1. Adding a voltage source in series with the inductor, having the value:

$$LI_0$$

   (Note that the source should have a polarity that is aligned with the initial current)

2. By adding a current source in parallel with the inductor, having the value:

$$\frac{I_0}{s}$$

where,

L is the inductance.

I_0 is the initial current in the inductor.

Inductor networks

Inductors in a parallel configuration each have the same potential difference (voltage). To find their total equivalent inductance (L_{eq}):

$$\frac{1}{L_{eq}} = \frac{1}{L_1} + \frac{1}{L_2} + ... + \frac{1}{L_n}$$
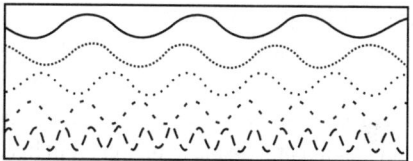

The current through inductors in series stays the same, but the voltage across each inductor can be different. The sum of the potential differences (voltage) is equal to the total voltage. To find their total inductance:

$$L_{eq} = L_1 + L_2 + ... + L_n$$

These simple relationships hold true only when there is no mutual coupling of magnetic fields between individual inductors.

Stored energy

The energy (measured in joules, in SI) stored by an inductor is equal to the amount of work required to establish the current through the inductor, and therefore the magnetic field.

This is given by:

$$E_{stored} = \frac{1}{2}LI^2$$

where, L is inductance and I is the current through the inductor.

Frequency

Frequency is the number of occurrences of a repeating event per unit time. It is also referred to as temporal frequency. The period is the duration of one cycle in a repeating event, so the period is the reciprocal of the frequency (Fig. 2.9).

Fig. 2.9. Sinusoidal waves of various frequencies; the bottom waves have higher frequencies than those above. The horizontal axis represents time

For cyclical processes, such as rotation, oscillations, or waves, frequency is defined as a number of cycles, or periods, per unit time. In physics and engineering disciplines, such as optics, acoustics, and radio, frequency is usually denoted by a Latin letter *f* or by a Greek letter *v* (nu).

In SI units, the unit of frequency is hertz (Hz), named after the German physicist Heinrich Hertz. For example, 1 Hz means that an event repeats once per second.

A traditional unit of measure used with rotating mechanical devices is the revolutions per minute, abbreviated rpm. 60 rpm equals one hertz.

The period is usually denoted as *T*, and is the reciprocal of the frequency *f*:

$$T = \frac{1}{f}$$

The SI unit for period is the second.

Measurement

To calculate the frequency of an event, the number of occurrences of the event within a fixed time interval are counted, and then divided by the length of the time interval.

If the frequency is not too high, it is more accurate to measure the time taken for a fixed number of occurrences, rather than the number of occurrences within a fixed time. The latter method introduces a random error into the count of between zero and one count, so on average half a count. This is called gating error and causes an average error in the calculated frequency of $\Delta f = 1/2\,T_m$, or a fractional error of $\Delta f / f = 1/2\,fT_m$ where, T_m is the timing interval and f is the measured frequency. This error decreases with frequency, so it is a problem at low frequencies where the number of counts N is small.

Higher frequencies are usually measured with a frequency counter. This is an electronic instrument which measures the frequency of an applied repetitive electronic signal and displays the result in hertz on a digital display. Cyclic processes, such as the rotation rate of a shaft, mechanical vibrations, sound waves, and radio waves are converted to a repetitive electronic signal by transducers and the signal is applied to a frequency counter. Frequency counters can currently cover the range up to almost 100 GHz. This represents the limit of direct counting methods; frequencies above this must be measured by indirect methods.

Frequency of waves

Frequency has an inverse relationship to the concept of wavelength, simply, frequency is inversely proportional to wavelength λ (lambda). The frequency f is equal to the phase velocity v of the wave divided by the wavelength λ of the wave:

$$f = \frac{v}{\lambda}$$

In the special case of electromagnetic waves moving through a vacuum, then $v = c$, where c is the speed of light in a vacuum, and this expression becomes:

$$f = \frac{c}{\lambda}$$

When waves from a monochromatic source travel from one medium to another, their frequency remains

exactly the same—only their wavelength and speed change.

Series and Parallel Circuits

Components of an electrical circuit or electronic circuit can be connected in many different ways. The two simplest of these are called series and parallel and occur very frequently. Components connected in series are connected along a single path, so the same current flows through all of the components. Components connected in parallel are connected so the same voltage is applied to each component.

A circuit composed solely of components connected in series is known as a series circuit (Fig. 2.10); likewise, one connected completely in parallel is known as a parallel circuit.

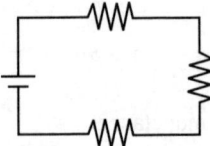

Fig. 2.10. A series circuit with a voltage source (such as a battery) and 3 resistors.

In a series circuit , the current through each of the components is the same, and the voltage across the components is the sum of the voltages across each component. In a parallel circuit, the voltage across each of the components is the same, and the total current is the sum of the currents through each component.

As an example, consider a very simple circuit consisting of four light bulbs and one 6 V battery. If a wire joins the battery to one bulb, to the next bulb, to the next bulb, to the next bulb, then back to the battery, in one continuous loop, the bulbs are said to be in series. If each bulb is wired to the battery in a separate loop, the bulbs are said to be in parallel. If the four light bulbs are connected in series, the same current flows through all of them, and the voltage drop is 1.5 V across each bulb. If the light bulbs are connected in parallel, the current flowing through the light bulbs combine to form the current flowing in the battery, while the voltage drop is 6 V across each bulb. In a series circuit, every device must function for the circuit to be complete. One bulb burning out in a series circuit breaks the circuit. In parallel circuits, each light has its own circuit, so all but one light could be burned out, and the last one will still function.

Series circuits

Series circuits are sometimes called current-coupled or daisy chain-coupled. The current that flows in a series circuit will flow through every component in the circuit. Therefore, all of the components in a series connection carry the same current.

Resistors

$$R_{total} = R_1 + R_2 + R_3 + ... + R_n$$

Inductors

Inductors follow the same law, in that the total inductance of noncoupled inductors in series is equal to the sum of their individual inductances:

$$L_{total} = L_1 + L_2 + ... + L_n$$

However, in some situations it is difficult to prevent adjacent inductors from influencing each other, as the magnetic field of one device couples with the windings of its neighbours. This influence is defined by the mutual inductance M. For example, if you have two inductors in series, there are two possible equivalent inductances depending on how the magnetic fields of both inductors influence each other.

When there are more than two inductors, the mutual inductance between each of them and the way the coils influence each other complicates the calculation. For a larger number of coils the total combined inductance is given by the sum of all mutual inductances between the various coils including the mutual inductance of each given coil with itself, which we term self-inductance or simply inductance. For three coils, there are six mutual inductances M_{12}, M_{13}, M_{23} and M_{21}, M_{31} and M_{32}. There are also the three self-inductances of the three coils: M_{11}, M_{22} and M_{33}. Therefore,

$$L_{total} = (M_{11} + M_{22} + M_{33}) + (M_{12} + M_{13} + M_{23}) + (M_{21} + M_{31} + M_{32})$$

By reciprocity $M_{ij} = M_{ji}$ so that the last two groups can be combined. The first three terms represent the sum of the self-inductances of the various coils. The formula is easily extended to any number of series coils with mutual coupling. The method can be used to find the self-inductance of large coils of wire of any cross-sectional shape by computing the sum of the mutual inductance of each turn of wire in the coil with every other turn since in such a coil all turns are in series.

Capacitors

Capacitors follow the same law using the reciprocals. The total capacitance of capacitors in series is equal to the reciprocal of the sum of the reciprocals of their individual capacitances:

$$\frac{1}{C_{total}} = \frac{1}{C_1} + \frac{1}{C_2} + ... + \frac{1}{C_n}.$$

The working voltage of a series combination of identical capacitors is equal to the sum of voltage ratings of individual capacitors provided that equalising resistors are used to ensure equal voltage division. This is all because of Ohm's law $V = RI$.

Parallel circuits

If two or more components are connected in parallel they have the same potential difference (voltage) across their ends. The potential differences across the components are the same in magnitude, and they also have identical polarities. Hence, the same voltage is applicable to all circuit components connected in parallel.

The total current I is the sum of the currents through the individual components, in accordance with Kirchhoff's circuit laws. The current in each individual resistor is found by Ohm's law. Factoring out the voltage gives:

$$I_{total} = V\left(\frac{1}{R_1} + \frac{1}{R_2} + ... + \frac{1}{R_n}\right)$$

To find the total resistance of all components, add the reciprocals of the resistances R_i of each component and take the reciprocal of the sum:

$$\frac{1}{R_{total}} = \frac{1}{R_1} + \frac{1}{R_2} + ... + \frac{1}{R_n}$$

To find the current in a component with resistance R_i, use Ohm's law again:

$$I_i = \frac{V}{R_i}$$

The components divide the current according to their reciprocal resistances, so, in the case of two resistors,

$$\frac{I_1}{I_2} = \frac{R_2}{R_1}$$

An old term for devices connected in parallel is multiple, such as a multiple connection for arc lamps.

Inductors

Inductors follow the same law, in that the total inductance of noncoupled inductors in parallel is equal to the reciprocal of the sum of the reciprocals of their individual inductances:

$$\frac{1}{L_{total}} = \frac{1}{L_1} + \frac{1}{L_2} + ... + \frac{1}{L_n}$$

If the inductors are situated in each other's magnetic fields, this approach is invalid due to mutual inductance. If the mutual inductance between two coils in parallel is M, the equivalent inductor is:

$$\frac{1}{L_{total}} = \frac{L_1 + L_2 - 2M}{L_1 L_2 - M^2}$$

If $L_1 = L_2$

$$L_{total} = \frac{L + M}{2}$$

The sign of M depends on how the magnetic fields influence each other. For two equal tightly coupled coils the total inductance is close to that of each single coil. If the polarity of one coil is reversed so that M is negative, then the parallel inductance is nearly zero or the combination is almost non-inductive. We are assuming in the 'tightly coupled' case M is very nearly equal to L. However, if the inductances are not equal and the coils are tightly coupled there can be near short circuit conditions and high circulating currents for both positive and negative values of M, which can cause problems. More than 3 inductors becomes more complex and the mutual inductance of each inductor on each other inductor and their influence on each other must be considered. For three coils, there are three mutual inductances M_{12}, M_{13} and M_{23}. This is best handled by matrix methods and summing the terms of the inverse of the L matrix (3 by 3 in this case). The pertinent equations are of the form:

$$v_i = \sum_j L_{i,j} \frac{di_j}{dt}$$

Capacitors

Capacitors follow the same law using the reciprocals. The total capacitance of capacitors in parallel is equal to the sum of their individual capacitances:

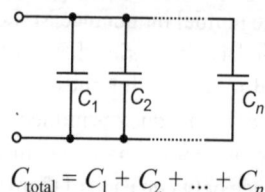

$$C_{total} = C_1 + C_2 + ... + C_n$$

The working voltage of a parallel combination of capacitors is always limited by the smallest working voltage of an individual capacitor.

AMPLIFIER

Generally, an amplifier is any device that changes, usually increases, the amplitude of a signal. The relationship of the input to the output of an amplifier—usually expressed as a function of the input frequency—is called the transfer function of the amplifier, and the magnitude of the transfer function is termed the gain.

In popular use, the term usually describes an electronic amplifier, in which the input 'signal' is usually voltage or current. In audio applications, amplifiers operate loudspeakers used in PA systems to make the human voice louder or play recorded music. Amplifiers may be classified according to the input (source) they are designed to amplify (such as a guitar amplifier, to perform with an electric guitar), the device they are intended to drive (such as a headphone amplifier), the frequency range of the signals (Audio, IF, RF, and VHF amplifiers, for example), whether they invert the signal (inverting amplifiers and non-inverting amplifiers), or the type of device used in the amplification (valve or tube amplifiers, FET amplifiers, etc.).

A related device that emphasises conversion of signals of one type to another (for example, a light signal in photons to a DC signal in amperes) is a transducer, a transformer, or a sensor. However, none of these amplify power.

An electronic amplifier is a device for increasing the power of a signal. It does this by taking energy from a power supply and controlling the output to match the input signal shape but with a larger amplitude. In this sense, an amplifier may be considered as modulating the output of the power supply.

Types of Amplifier

Amplifiers can be specified according to their input and output properties. They have some kind of gain, or multiplication factor relating the magnitude of the output signal to the input signal. The gain may be specified as the ratio of output voltage to input voltage (voltage gain), output power to input power (power gain), or some combination of current, voltage and power. In many cases, with input and output in the same units, gain will be unitless (although often expressed in decibels); for others this is not necessarily so.

For example, a transconductance amplifier has a gain with units of conductance (output current per input voltage). The power gain of an amplifier depends on the source and load impedances used as well as its voltage gain; while an RF amplifier may have its impedances optimised for power transfer, audio and instrumentation amplifiers are normally employed with amplifier input and output impedances optimised for least loading and highest quality. So an amplifier that is said to have a gain of 20dB might have a voltage gain of ten times and an available power gain of much more than 20dB (100 times power ratio), yet be delivering a much lower power gain if, for example, the input is a 600 ohm microphone and the output is a 47 kilohm power amplifier's input socket.

In most cases an amplifier should be linear; that is, the gain should be constant for any combination of input and output signal. If the gain is not linear, e.g. by clipping the output signal at the limits of its capabilities, the output signal will be distorted.

Inverter

An inverter is an electrical device that converts direct current (DC) to alternating current (AC); the converted AC can be at any required voltage and frequency with the use of appropriate transformers, switching, and control circuits.

Static inverters have no moving parts and are used in a wide range of applications, from small switching power supplies in computers, to large electric utility high-voltage direct current applications that transport bulk power. Inverters are commonly used to supply AC power from DC sources such as solar panels or batteries.

The electrical inverter is a high-power electronic oscillator. It is so named because early mechanical AC to DC converters were made to work in reverse, and thus were 'inverted', to convert DC to AC.

The inverter performs the opposite function of a rectifier.

Inverting amplifier

An inverting amplifier uses negative feedback to invert and amplify a voltage. The R_f resistor allows some of the output signal to be returned to the input (Fig. 2.11).

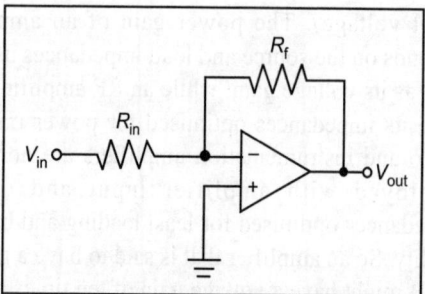

Fig. 2.11. Inverting amplifier.

Since the output is 180° out of phase, this amount is effectively subtracted from the input, thereby reducing the input into the operational amplifier.

Comparator

In electronics, a comparator is a device which compares two voltages or currents and switches its output to indicate which is larger.

Input voltage range

The input voltages must not exceed the power voltage range:

$$V_{S-} \leq V_+, \ V_- \leq V_{S+}$$

In the case of TTL/CMOS logic output comparators, negative inputs are not allowed:

$$0 \leq V_+, \ V_- \leq V_{cc}$$

Op-amp implementation of voltage comparator

An operational amplifier has a well balanced difference input and a very high gain. The parallels in the characteristics allows the op-amps to serve as comparators in some functions (Fig. 2.12).

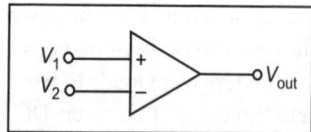

Fig. 2.12. A simple op-amp comparator.

A standard op-amp operating in open loop configuration (without negative feedback) can be used as a comparator. When the noninverting input (V_+) is at a higher voltage than the inverting input (V_-), the high gain of the op-amp causes it to output the most positive voltage it can. When the

noninverting input (V_+) drops below the inverting input (V_-), the op-amp outputs the most negative voltage it can. Since the output voltage is limited by the supply voltage, for an op-amp that uses a balanced, split supply, (powered by $\pm V_S$) this action can be written:

$$V_{out} = V \cdot sgn (V_+ - V_-)$$

where sgn(x) is the sign function. Generally, the positive and negative supplies V_S will not match absolute value:

$$V_{out} \leq V_{S+} \text{ when } V_+ > V_- \text{ else } \geq V_{S-} \text{ when } V_+ < V_-$$

Frequency Response

Frequency response is the measure of any system's output spectrum in response to an input signal. In the audible range it is usually referred to in connection with electronic amplifiers, microphones and loudspeakers. Radio spectrum frequency response can refer to measurements of coaxial cables, category cables, video switchers and wireless communications devices. Subsonic frequency response measurements can include earthquakes and electroencephalography (brain waves) (Fig. 2.13).

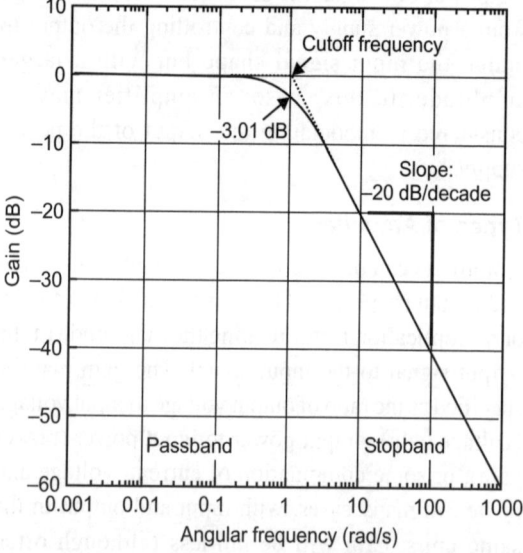

Fig. 2.13. Frequency response of a low pass filter with 6 dB per octave or 20 dB per decade.

Frequency response requirements differ depending on the application. In high fidelity audio, an amplifier requires a frequency response of at least 20–20,000 Hz, with a tolerance as tight as ±0.1 dB in the mid-range frequencies around 1000 Hz, however, in telephony, a frequency response of 400–4000 Hz, with a tolerance of ±1 dB is sufficient for intelligibility of speech. Frequency response curves are often used to indicate the accuracy of electronic components or systems. When a system or component reproduces all desired input signals with no emphasis or attenuation of a particular frequency band, the system or component is said to be 'flat', or to have a flat frequency response curve.

The frequency response is typically characterised by the magnitude of the system's response, measured in decibels (dB), and the phase, measured in radians, versus frequency. The frequency response of a system can be measured by applying a test signal, for example:

1. Applying an impulse to the system and measuring its response.
2. Sweeping a constant-amplitude pure tone through the bandwidth of interest and measuring the output level and phase shift relative to the input.
3. Applying a signal with a wide frequency spectrum (for example digitally-generated maximum length sequence noise, or analog filtered white noise equivalent, like pink noise), and calculating the impulse response by deconvolution of this input signal and the output signal of the system.

These typical response measurements can be plotted in two ways: by plotting the magnitude and phase measurements to obtain a Bode plot or by plotting the imaginary part of the frequency response against the real part of the frequency response to obtain a Nyquist plot. Once a frequency response has been measured (e.g. as an impulse response), providing the system is linear and time-invariant, its characteristic can be approximated with arbitrary accuracy by a digital filter. Similarly, if a system is demonstrated to have a poor frequency response, a digital or analog filter can be applied to the signals prior to their reproduction to compensate for these deficiencies.

Frequency response measurements can be used directly to quantify system performance and design control systems. However, frequency response analysis is not suggested if the system has slow dynamics.

Electronic Filter

Electronic filters are electronic circuits which perform signal processing functions, specifically to remove unwanted frequency components from the signal, to enhance wanted ones, or both. Electronic filters can be:

1. Passive or active.
2. Analog or digital.
3. High-pass, low-pass, bandpass, band-reject (band reject; notch), or all-pass.
4. Discrete-time (sampled) or continuous-time.
5. Linear or nonlinear.
6. Infinite impulse response (IIR type) or finite impulse response (FIR type).

The most common types of electronic filters are linear filters, regardless of other aspects of their design and analysis.

Passive filters

Passive implementations of linear filters are based on combinations of resistors (R), inductors (L) and capacitors (C). These types are collectively known as passive filters, because they do not depend upon an external power supply and/or they do not contain active components such as transistors.

Single element types

The simplest passive filters consist of a single reactive element. These are constructed of RC, RL, LC or RLC elements. Figure 2.14 shows a low-pass electronic filter realised by an RC circuit.

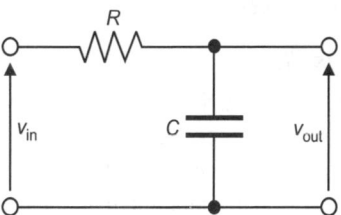

Fig. 2.14. A low-pass electronic filter realised by an RC circuit.

The quality or 'Q' factor is a measure that is sometimes used to describe simple band-pass or band-stop filters. A filter is said to have a high Q if it selects or rejects a range of frequencies that is narrow in comparison to the centre frequency. Q may be defined for bandpass and band-reject filters as the ratio of centre frequency divided by 3dB bandwidth. It is not commonly employed with higher order filters where other parameters are of more concern, and for high-pass or low-pass filters Q is not normally related to bandwidth.

Active filters

Active filters are implemented using a combination of passive and active (amplifying) components, and require an outside power source. Operational amplifiers are frequently used in active filter designs. These can have high Q, and can achieve resonance without the use of inductors. However, their upper frequency limit is limited by the bandwidth of the amplifiers used.

Digital filters

Digital signal processing allows the inexpensive construction of a wide variety of filters. The signal is sampled and an analog-to-digital converter turns the signal into a stream of numbers. A computer programme running on a CPU or a specialised DSP (or less often running on a hardware implementation of the algorithm) calculates an output number stream. This output can be converted to a signal by passing it through a digital-to-analog converter. There are problems with noise introduced by the conversions, but these can be controlled and limited for many useful filters. Due to the sampling involved, the input signal must be of limited frequency content or aliasing will occur.

Low-pass filter

A low-pass filter is a filter that passes low-frequency signals but attenuates (reduces the amplitude of) signals with frequencies higher than the cutoff frequency. The actual amount of attenuation for each frequency varies from filter to filter. It is sometimes called a high-cut filter, or treble cut filter when used in audio applications. A low-pass filter is the opposite of a high-pass filter, and a band-pass filter is a combination of a low-pass and a high-pass.

The concept of a low-pass filter exists in many different forms, including electronic circuits (like a *hiss filter* used in audio), digital algorithms for smoothing sets of data, acoustic barriers, blurring of images, and so on. Low-pass filters play the same role in signal processing that moving averages do in some other fields, such as finance; both tools provide a smoother form of a signal which removes the short-term oscillations, leaving only the long-term trend.

Examples of low-pass filters

Acoustic

A stiff physical barrier tends to reflect higher sound frequencies, and so acts as a low-pass filter for transmitting sound. When music is playing in another room, the low notes are easily heard, while the high notes are attenuated.

Electronic

In an electronic low-pass RC filter for voltage signals, high frequencies contained in the input signal are attenuated but the filter has little attenuation below its cutoff frequency which is determined by its RC time constant.

Ideal and real filters

An ideal low-pass filter completely eliminates all frequencies above the cutoff frequency while passing those below unchanged: its frequency response is a rectangular function, and is a brick-wall filter. The transition region present in practical filters does not exist in an ideal filter. An ideal low-pass filter can be realised mathematically (theoretically) by multiplying a signal by the rectangular function in the frequency domain or, equivalently, convolution with its impulse response, a sinc function, in the time domain.

However, the ideal filter is impossible to realise without also having signals of infinite extent, and so generally needs to be approximated for real ongoing signals, because the sinc function's support region extends to all past and future times. The filter would therefore need to have infinite delay, or knowledge of the infinite future and past, in order to perform the convolution. It is effectively realisable for prerecorded digital signals by assuming extensions of zero into the past and future, or more typically by making the signal repetitive and using Fourier analysis.

Real filters for real-time applications approximate the ideal filter by truncating and windowing the infinite impulse response to make a finite impulse response; applying that filter requires delaying the signal for a moderate period of time, allowing the computation to 'see' a little bit into the future. This delay is manifested as phase shift. Greater accuracy in approximation requires a longer delay.

An ideal low-pass filter results in ringing artifacts via the Gibbs phenomenon. These can be reduced or worsened by choice of windowing function, and the design and choice of real filters involves understanding and minimising these artifacts. For example, 'simple truncation [of sinc] causes severe ringing artifacts', in signal reconstruction, and to reduce these artifacts one uses window functions 'which drop off more smoothly at the edges'. Figure 2.15 shows the sinc function, the impulse response of an ideal low-pass filter.

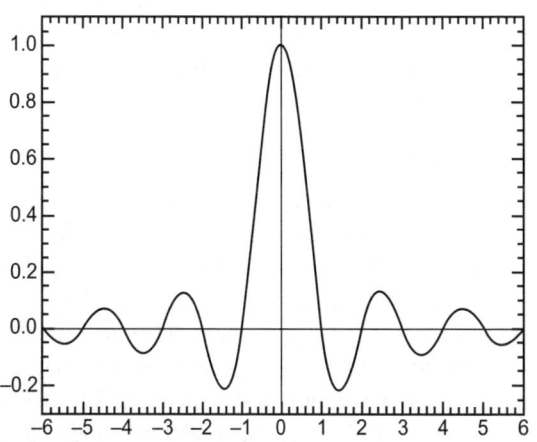

Fig. 2.15. The sinc function, the impulse response of an ideal low-pass filter.

Continuous-time low-pass filters

There are a great many different types of filter circuits, with different responses to changing

frequency. The frequency response of a filter is generally represented using a Bode plot, and the filter is characterised by its cutoff frequency and rate of frequency rolloff. In all cases, at the cutoff frequency, the filter attenuates the input power by half or 3 dB.

So the order of the filter determines the amount of additional attenuation for frequencies higher than the cutoff frequency.

High-pass filter

A high-pass filter is an LTI filter that passes high frequencies well but attenuates (i.e. reduces the amplitude of) frequencies lower than the cutoff frequency. The actual amount of attenuation for each frequency is a design parameter of the filter.

It is sometimes called a low-cut filter; the terms bass-cut filter or rumble filter are also used in audio applications.

First-order continuous-time implementation

The simple first-order electronic high-pass filter shown in Fig. 2.16 is implemented by placing an input voltage across the series combination of a capacitor and a resistor and using the voltage across the resistor as an output. The product of the resistance and capacitance (R×C) is the time constant (τ); it is inversely proportional to the cutoff frequency f_c, at which the output power is half the input power. That is,

$$f_c = \frac{1}{2\pi\tau} = \frac{1}{2\pi RC}$$

where, f_c is in hertz, τ is in seconds, R is in ohms, and C is in farads.

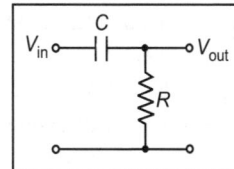

Fig. 2.16. A passive, analog, first-order high-pass filter, realised by an RC circuit.

Figure 2.17 shows an active electronic implementation of a first-order high-pass filter using an operational amplifier.

In this case, the filter has a passband gain of R_2/R_1 and has a corner frequency of:

$$f_c = \frac{1}{2\pi\tau} = \frac{1}{2\pi R_1 C}$$

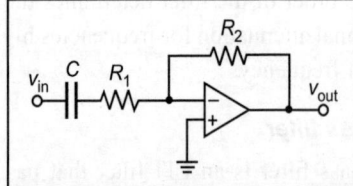

Fig. 2.17. An active high-pass filter.

Because this filter is active, it may have non-unity passband gain. That is, high-frequency signals are inverted and amplified by R_2/R_1.

Timer

A timer is a specialised type of clock. A timer can be used to control the sequence of an event or process. Whereas a stopwatch counts upwards from zero for measuring elapsed time, a timer counts down from a specified time interval, like an hourglass. Timers can be mechanical, electromechanical, electronic (quartz), or even software as all computers include digital timers of one kind or another.

Mechanical timers

Early mechanical timers used typical clockwork mechanisms, such as an escapement and spring to regulate their speed. Inaccurate, cheap mechanisms use a flat beater that spins against air resistance. Mechanical egg-timers are usually of this type.

More accurate mechanisms resemble small alarm clocks, with the chief advantage being that they require little battery/electrical power, and can be stored for long periods of time. The most widely-known application is to control explosives.

Electromechanical timers

There are two types of electromechanical timers. A thermal type has a metal finger made of strips of two metals with different rates of thermal expansion sandwiched together; steel and bronze are common. An electric current flowing through this finger causes heating of the metals, one side expands less than the other, and an electrical contact on the end of the finger moves away from or towards an electrical switch contact. The most common use of this type is in the 'flasher' units that flash turn signals in automobiles, and sometimes in Christmas lights.

Another type of electromechanical timer (a cam timer) uses a small synchronous AC motor turning a cam against a comb of switch contacts. The AC motor is turned at an accurate rate by the alternating current, which power companies carefully regulate. Gears slow this motor down to the desired rate, and turn the cam. The most common application of this timer now is in washers, driers and dishwashers. This type of timer often has a friction clutch between the gear train and the cam, so that the cam can be turned to reset the time.

Electromechanical timers survive in these applications because mechanical switch contacts are still less expensive than the semiconductor devices needed to control powerful lights, motors and heaters.

In the past these electromechanical timers were often combined with electrical relays to create electromechanical controllers. Electromechanical timers reached a high state of development in the 1950s and 60s because of their extensive use in aerospace and weapons systems. Programmable electromechanical timers controlled launch sequence events in early rockets and ballistic missiles.

Electronic timers

Electronic timers can achieve higher precision than mechanical timers because they are quartz clocks with special electronics. Electronic timers can be analog (resembling a mechanical timer) or digital (uses a display much like a digital clock). Integrated circuits have made digital logic so inexpensive that an electronic timer is now less expensive than many mechanical and electromechanical timers. Individual timers are implemented as a simple single-chip computer system, similar to a watch. Watch technology is used in these devices.

However, most timers are now implemented in software. Modern controllers use a programmable logic controller rather than a box full of electromechanical parts. The logic is usually designed as if it were relays, using a special computer language called ladder logic. In PLCs, timers are usually simulated by the software built into the controller. Each timer is just an entry in a table maintained by the software.

Digital timers can also be used in safety device such as a gas timer.

Computer timers

Computer systems usually have at least one timer. These are typically digital counters that either increment or decrement at a fixed frequency, which is often configurable, and that interrupt the processor when reaching zero, or a counter with a sufficiently large word size that it will not reach its counter limit before the end of life of the system.

More sophisticated timers may have comparison logic to compare the timer value against a specific value, set by software, that triggers some action when the timer value matches the preset value. This might be used, for example, to measure events or generate pulse width modulated waveforms to control the speed of motors (using a class D digital electronic amplifier).

As the number of hardware timers in a computer system or processor is finite and limited, operating systems and embedded systems often use a single hardware timer to implement an extensible set of software timers. In this scenario, the hardware timer's interrupt service routine would handle housekeeping and management of as many software timers as are required, and the hardware timer would be set to expire when the next software timer is due to expire. At expiry, the interrupt routine would update the hardware timer to expire when the next software timer is due, and any actions would be triggered for the software timers that had just expired. Expired timers that are continuous would also be reset to a new expiry time based on their timer interval, and one-shot timers would be disabled or removed from the set of timers. While simple in concept, care must be taken with software timer implementation if issues such as timer drift and delayed interrupts is to be minimised.

DIGITAL-TO-ANALOG AND ANALOG-TO-DIGITAL CONVERSION

Digital-to-Analog Converter

In electronics, a digital-to-analog converter (DAC or D-to-A) is a device for converting a digital (usually binary) code to an analog signal (current, voltage or electric charge).

An analog-to-digital converter (ADC) performs the reverse operation.

Basic ideal operation

A DAC converts an abstract finite-precision number (usually a fixed-point binary number) into a concrete physical quantity (e.g. a voltage or a pressure). In particular, DACs are often used to convert finite-precision time series data to a continually-varying physical signal.

A typical DAC converts the abstract numbers into a concrete sequence of impulses that are then processed by a reconstruction filter using some form of interpolation to fill in data between the impulses. Other DAC methods (e.g. methods based on Delta-sigma modulation) produce a pulse-density modulated signal that can then be filtered in a similar way to produce a smoothly-varying signal (Fig. 2.18).

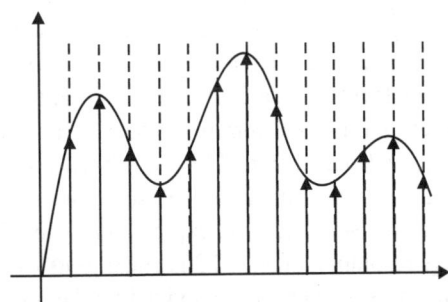

Fig. 2.18. Ideally sampled signal. Signal of a typical interpolating DAC output.

By the Nyquist–Shannon sampling theorem, sampled data can be reconstructed perfectly provided that its bandwidth meets certain requirements (e.g. a baseband signal with bandwidth less than the Nyquist frequency). However, even with an ideal reconstruction filter, digital sampling introduces quantisation error that makes perfect reconstruction practically impossible. Increasing the digital resolution (i.e. increasing the number of bits used in each sample) or introducing sampling dither can reduce this error.

Analog-to-Digital Convertor

An analog-to-digital converter (abbreviated ADC, A/D or A to D) is a device which converts continuous signals to discrete digital numbers. The reverse operation is performed by a digital-to-analog converter (DAC).

Typically, an ADC is an electronic device that converts an input analog voltage (or current) to a digital number proportional to the magnitude of the voltage or current. However, some non-electronic or only partially electronic devices, such as rotary encoders, can also be considered ADCs. The digital output may use different coding schemes, such as binary, Gray code or two's complement binary.

Resolution

The resolution of the converter indicates the number of discrete values it can produce over the range of analog values. The values are usually stored electronically in binary form, so the resolution is usually expressed in bits. In consequence, the number of discrete values available, or 'levels', is usually a power of two. For example, an ADC with a resolution of 8 bits can encode an analog input to one in 256 different levels, since $2^8 = 256$. The values can represent the ranges from 0 to 255 (i.e. unsigned integer) or from −128 to 127 (i.e. signed integer), depending on the application. Resolution can also be defined electrically, and expressed in volts. The voltage resolution of an ADC is equal to its overall voltage measurement range divided by the number of discrete intervals as in the formula:

$$Q = \frac{E_{FSR}}{2^M - 1} = \frac{E_{FSR}}{N}$$

where,

Q is resolution in volts per step (volts per output codes less one).

E_{FSR} is the full scale voltage range = $V_{RefHi} - V_{RefLow}$.

M is the ADC's resolution in bits.

N is the number of intervals, (one less than the number of available levels, or output codes), which is: $N = 2^M - 1$

Number System

In mathematics, a 'number system' is a set of numbers, (in the broadest sense of the word), together with one or more operations, such as addition or multiplication. Examples of number systems include: natural numbers, integers, rational numbers, algebraic numbers, real numbers, complex numbers, p-adic numbers, surreal numbers, and hyperreal numbers.

Simply put, the natural numbers consist of the set of all whole numbers greater than zero. The set is denoted with a bold face capital N. (In some books, the natural numbers begin with 0. There is no general agreement on this subject.)

Giuseppe Peano developed axioms for the natural numbers, and is considered the founder of axiomatic number theory.

The word number has no generally agreed upon mathematical meaning, nor does the word number system. Instead, we have many examples. Thus there is no rule to say what is a number and what is not. Some of the more interesting examples of abstractions that can be considered numbers include the quaternions, the octonions, the sedenions, the trigintaduonions, ordinal numbers, and the transfinite numbers.

DIGITAL SIGNAL PROCESSING

Digital signal processing (DSP) is concerned with the representation of the signals by a sequence of numbers or symbols and the processing of these signals. Digital signal processing and analog signal processing are subfields of signal processing. DSP includes subfields like: audio and speech signal processing, sonar and radar signal processing, sensor array processing, spectral estimation, statistical signal processing, digital image processing, signal processing for communications, biomedical signal processing, seismic data processing, etc.

Since the goal of DSP is usually to measure or filter continuous real-world analog signals, the first step is usually to convert the signal from an analog to a digital form, by using an analog-to-digital converter (ADC). Often, the required output signal is another analog output signal, which requires a digital-to-analog converter (DAC). Even if this process is more complex than analog processing and has a discrete value range, the stability of digital signal processing thanks to error detection and correction and being less vulnerable to noise makes it advantageous over analog signal processing for many, though not all, applications.

DSP algorithms have long been run on standard computers, on specialised processors called digital signal processors (DSPs), or on purpose-built hardware such as application-specific integrated circuit (ASICs). Today there are additional technologies used for digital signal processing including more powerful general purpose microprocessors, field-programmable gate arrays (FPGAs), digital signal controllers (mostly for industrial apps such as motor control), and stream processors, among others.

Digital Signal

The term digital signal is used to refer to more than one concept. It can refer to discrete-time signals that have a discrete number of levels, for example a sampled and quantified analog signal, or to the continuous-time waveform signals in a digital system, representing a bit-stream. In the first case, a signal that is generated by means of a digital modulation method which is considered as converted to an analog signal, while it is considered as a digital signal in the second case (Fig. 2.19).

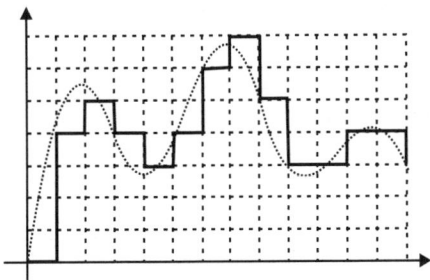

Fig. 2.19. Digital signal.

Discrete-time signals

An analog signal is a datum that changes over time — say, the temperature at a given location; the depth of a certain point in a pond; or the amplitude of the voltage at some node in a circuit—that can be represented as a mathematical function, with time as the free variable (abscissa) and the signal itself as the dependent variable (ordinate). A discrete-time signal is a sampled version of an analog signal: the value of the datum is noted at fixed intervals (for example, every microsecond) rather than continuously.

If individual time values of the discrete-time signal, instead of being measured precisely (which would require an infinite number of digits), are approximated to a certain precision—which, therefore, only requires a specific number of digits—then the resultant data stream is termed a digital signal. The process of approximating the precise value within a fixed number of digits, or bits, is called quantisation.

In conceptual summary, a digital signal is a quantised discrete-time signal; a discrete-time signal is a sampled analog signal.

In the digital revolution, the usage of digital signals has increased significantly. Many modern media devices, especially the ones that connect with computers use digital signals to represent signals that were traditionally represented as continuous-time signals; cell phones, music and video players, personal video recorders, and digital cameras are examples.

In most applications, digital signals are represented as binary numbers, so their precision of quantisation is measured in bits. Suppose, for example, that we wish to measure a signal to two significant decimal digits. Since seven bits, or binary digits, can record 128 discrete values (viz., from 0 to 127), those seven bits are more than sufficient to express a range of one hundred values.

Nyquist-Shannon Sampling Theorem

The Nyquist–Shannon sampling theorem is a fundamental result in the field of information theory, in particular telecommunications and signal processing.

Sampling is the process of converting a signal (for example, a function of continuous time or space) into a numeric sequence (a function of discrete time or space). Shannon's version of the theorem states:

If a function $x(t)$ contains no frequencies higher than B hertz, it is completely determined by giving its ordinates at a series of points spaced $1/(2B)$ seconds apart. Figure 2.20 shows the hypothetical spectrum of a bandlimited signal as a function of frequency.

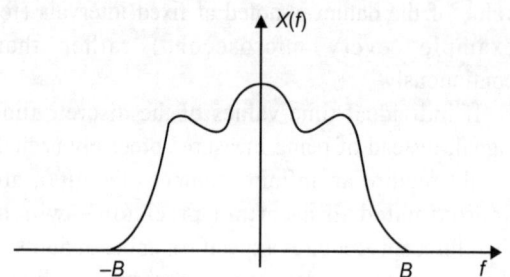

Fig. 2.20. Hypothetical spectrum of a bandlimited signal as a function of frequency.

The theorem is commonly called the Shannon sampling theorem, and is also known as Nyquist–Shannon–Kotelnikov, Whittaker–Shannon–Kotelnikov, Whittaker–Nyquist–Kotelnikov–Shannon, WKS, etc. sampling theorem, as well as the Cardinal theorem of interpolation theory. It is often referred to as simply the sampling theorem.

In essence, the theorem shows that a bandlimited analog signal that has been sampled can be perfectly reconstructed from an infinite sequence of samples if the sampling rate exceeds $2B$ samples per second, where, B is the highest frequency in the original signal. If a signal contains a component at exactly B hertz, then samples spaced at exactly $1/(2B)$ seconds do not completely determine the signal, Shannon's statement notwithstanding. This sufficient condition can be weakened. More recent statements of the theorem are sometimes careful to exclude the equality condition; that is, the condition is if $x(t)$ contains no frequencies higher than or equal to B; this condition is equivalent to Shannon's except when the function includes a steady sinusoidal component at exactly frequency B. The theorem assumes an idealisation of any real-world situation, as it only applies to signals that are sampled for infinite time; any time-limited $x(t)$ cannot be perfectly bandlimited. Perfect reconstruction is mathematically possible for the idealised model but only an approximation for real-world signals and sampling techniques, albeit in practice often a very good one.

The theorem also leads to a formula for reconstruction of the original signal. The constructive proof of the theorem leads to an understanding of the aliasing that can occur when a sampling system does not satisfy the conditions of the theorem. The sampling theorem provides a sufficient condition, but not a necessary one, for perfect reconstruction. The field of compressed sensing provides a stricter sampling condition when the underlying signal is known to be sparse. Compressed sensing specifically yields a sub-Nyquist sampling criterion.

A signal or function is bandlimited if it contains no energy at frequencies higher than some bandlimit or bandwidth **B**. A signal that is bandlimited is constrained in how rapidly it changes in time, and therefore how much detail it can convey in an interval of time. The sampling theorem asserts that the uniformly spaced discrete samples are a complete representation of the signal if this bandwidth is less than half the sampling rate. To formalise these concepts, let $x(t)$ represent a continuous-time signal and $X(f)$ be the Fourier transform of that signal:

$$X(f) \overset{\text{def}}{=} \int_{-\infty}^{\infty} x(t)e^{-i2\pi ft}dt$$

The signal $x(t)$ is bandlimited to a one-sided baseband bandwidth, **B**, if:

$$X(f) = 0 \text{ for all } |f| > B$$

or, equivalently, $\text{supp}(X) \subseteq [-B, B]$. Then the sufficient condition for exact reconstructability from samples at a uniform sampling rate f_s (in samples per unit time) is:

$$f_s > 2B$$

or equivalently:

$$B < \frac{f_s}{2}$$

$2B$ called the Nyquist rate and is a property of the bandlimited signal, while $f_s/2$ is called the Nyquist frequency and is a property of this sampling system.

The time interval between successive samples is referred to as the sampling interval:

$$T \overset{\text{def}}{=} \frac{1}{f_s}$$

and the samples of $x(t)$ are denoted by:

$$x(nT) \quad n \in Z \text{ (integers)}.$$

The sampling theorem leads to a procedure for reconstructing the original $x(t)$ from the samples and states sufficient conditions for such a reconstruction to be exact.

Sampling process

The theorem describes two processes in signal processing: a sampling process, in which a continuous time signal is converted to a discrete time signal, and a reconstruction process, in which the original continuous signal is recovered from the discrete time signal.

The continuous signal varies over time (or space in a digitised image, or another independent variable in some other application) and the sampling process is performed by measuring the continuous signal's value every T units of time (or space), which is called the sampling interval. In practice, for signals that are a function of time, the sampling interval is typically quite small, on the order of milliseconds, microseconds, or less. This results in a sequence of numbers, called samples, to represent the original signal. Each sample value is associated with the instant in time when it was measured. The reciprocal of the sampling interval $(1/T)$ is the sampling frequency denoted f_s, which is measured in samples per unit of time. If T is expressed in seconds, then f_s is expressed in Hz.

MICROCOMPUTER

A microcomputer is a computer with a microprocessor as its central processing unit. They are physically small compared to mainframe and minicomputers. Many microcomputers (when equipped with a keyboard and screen for input and output) are also personal computers (in the generic sense). The abbreviation 'micro' was common during the 1970s and 1980s, but has now fallen out of common usage.

COMPUTER PROGRAMMING

Computer programming (often shortened to programming or coding) is the process of writing, testing, debugging/troubleshooting, and maintaining the source code of computer programmes. This source code is written in a programming language. The code may be a modification of an existing source or something completely new. The purpose of programming is to create a programme that exhibits a certain desired behaviour (customisation). The process of writing source code often requires expertise in many different subjects, including knowledge of the application domain, specialised algorithms and formal logic.

Within software engineering, programming (the implementation) is regarded as one phase in a software development process.

There is an ongoing debate on the extent to which the writing of programs is an art, a craft or an engineering discipline. In general, good programming is considered to be the measured application of all three, with the goal of producing an efficient and evolvable software solution (the criteria for 'efficient' and 'evolvable' vary considerably). The discipline differs from many other technical professions in that programmers, in general, do not need to be licensed or pass any standardised (or governmentally regulated) certification tests in order to call themselves 'programmers' or even 'software engineers'. However, representing oneself as a 'professional software engineer' without a license from an accredited institution is illegal in many parts of the world.

Modern Programming

Algorithmic complexity

The academic field and the engineering practice of computer programming are both largely concerned with discovering and implementing the most efficient algorithms for a given class of problem. For this purpose, algorithms are classified into orders using so-called Big O notation, $O(n)$, which expresses resource use, such as execution time or memory consumption, in terms of the size of an input. Expert programmers are familiar with a variety of well-established algorithms and their respective complexities and use this knowledge to choose algorithms that are best suited to the circumstances.

Methodologies

The first step in most formal software development projects is requirements analysis, followed by testing to determine value modelling, implementation, and failure elimination (debugging). There exist a lot of differing approaches for each of those tasks. One approach popular for requirements analysis is use case analysis. A similar technique used for database design is entity-relationship modelling (ER modelling).

Implementation techniques include imperative languages (object-oriented or procedural), functional languages, and logic languages.

Measuring language usage

It is very difficult to determine what are the most popular of modern programming languages. Some languages are very popular for particular kinds of applications (e.g. COBOL is still strong in the corporate data centre, often on large mainframes, FORTRAN in engineering applications, scripting languages in web development, and C in embedded applications), while some languages are regularly used to write many different kinds of applications.

Debugging

Debugging is a very important task in the software development process, because an incorrect programme can have significant consequences for its users. Some languages are more prone to some kinds of faults because their specification does not require compilers to perform as much checking as other languages. Use of a static analysis tool can help detect some possible problems.

Operating System

An operating system (OS) is an interface between hardware and user which is responsible for the management and coordination of activities and the sharing of the resources of a computer that acts as a host for computing applications run on the machine. As a host, one of the purposes of an operating system is to handle the resource allocation and access protection of the hardware. This relieves application programmers from having to manage these details.

Operating systems offer a number of services to application programs and users. Applications access these services through application programming interfaces (APIs) or system calls. By invoking these interfaces, the application can request a service from the operating system, pass parameters, and receive the results of the operation. Users may also interact with the operating system with some kind of software user interface like typing commands by using command line interface (CLI) or using a graphical user interface.

For hand-held and desktop computers, the user interface is generally considered part of the operating system. On large multi-user systems like Unix and Unix-like systems, the user interface is generally implemented as an application program that runs outside the operating system.

File system support in modern operating systems

Support for file systems is highly varied among modern operating systems although there are several common file systems which almost all operating systems include support and drivers for. Operating systems vary on file system support and on the disk formats they may be installed on.

Mac OS X

Mac OS X supports HFS+ with journaling as its primary file system. It is derived from the Hierarchical File System of the earlier Mac OS. Mac OS X has facilities to read and write FAT, NTFS (read-only, although an open-source cross platform implementation known as NTFS 3G provides read-write support to Microsoft Windows NTFS file system for Mac OS X users), UDF, and other file systems, but cannot be installed to them. Due to its

UNIX heritage Mac OS X now supports virtually all the file systems supported by the UNIX VFS..

Solaris

The Solaris Operating System uses UFS as its primary file system. Prior to 1998, Solaris UFS did not have logging/journaling capabilities, but over time the OS has gained this and other new data management capabilities.

Linux

Many Linux distributions support some or all of ext2, ext3, ext4, ReiserFS, Reiser4, JFS , XFS , GFS, GFS2, OCFS, OCFS2, and NILFS. The ext file systems, namely ext2, ext3 and ext4 are based on the original Linux file system. Others have been developed by companies to meet their specific needs, hobbyists, or adapted from UNIX, Microsoft Windows, and other operating systems. Linux has full support for XFS and JFS, along with FAT (the MS-DOS file system), and HFS which is the primary file system for the Macintosh.

Microsoft Windows

Microsoft Windows currently supports NTFS and FAT file systems (including FAT16 and FAT32), along with network file systems shared from other computers, and the ISO 9660 and UDF filesystems used for CDs, DVDs, and other optical discs such as Blu-ray. Under Windows each file system is usually limited in application to certain media, for example CDs must use ISO 9660 or UDF, and as of Windows Vista, NTFS is the only file system which the operating system can be installed on. Windows Embedded CE 6.0, Windows Vista Service Pack 1, and Windows Server 2008 support ExFAT, a file system more suitable for flash drives.

Special-purpose file systems

FAT file systems are commonly found on floppy disks, flash memory cards, digital cameras, and many other portable devices because of their relative simplicity. Performance of FAT compares poorly to most other file systems as it uses overly simplistic data structures, making file operations time-consuming, and makes poor use of disk space in situations where many small files are present. ISO 9660 and Universal Disk Format are two common formats that target Compact Discs and DVDs. Mount Rainier is a newer extension to UDF supported by Linux 2.6 series and Windows Vista that facilitates rewriting to DVDs in the same fashion as has been possible with floppy disks.

Journalised file systems

File systems may provide journaling, which provides safe recovery in the event of a system crash. A journaled file system writes some information twice: first to the journal, which is a log of file system operations, then to its proper place in the ordinary file system. Journaling is handled by the file system driver, and keeps track of each operation taking place that changes the contents of the disk. In the event of a crash, the system can recover to a consistent state by replaying a portion of the journal. Many UNIX file systems provide journaling including ReiserFS, JFS, and Ext3.

Graphical user interfaces

Most of the modern computer systems support graphical user interfaces (GUI), and often include them. In some computer systems, such as the original implementations of Microsoft Windows and the Mac OS, the GUI is integrated into the kernel.

Programming Language

A programming language is an artificial language designed to express computations that can be performed by a machine, particularly a computer. Programming languages can be used to create programmes that control the behaviour of a machine, to express algorithms precisely, or as a mode of human communication.

Many programming languages have some form of written specification of their syntax (form) and semantics (meaning). Some languages are defined by a specification document. For example, the C programming language is specified by an ISO Standard other languages, such as Perl, have a dominant implementation that is used as a reference.

The earliest programming languages predate the invention of the computer, and were used to direct the behaviour of machines such as Jacquard looms and player pianos. Thousands of different programming languages have been created, mainly in the computer field, with many more being created every year. Most programming languages describe computation in an imperative style, i.e. as a sequence of commands, although some languages, such as those that support functional programming or logic programming, use alternative forms of description.

A programming language is a notation for writing programmes, which are specifications of a computation or algorithm. Traits often considered important for what constitutes a programming language include:

Function and target: A computer programming language is a language used to write computer programs, which involve a computer performing some kind of computation or algorithm and possibly control external devices such as printers, disk drives, robots, and so on.

Abstractions: Programming languages usually contain abstractions for defining and manipulating data structures or controlling the flow of execution. The practical necessity that a programming language support adequate abstractions is expressed by the abstraction principle; this principle is sometimes formulated as recommendation to the programmer to make proper use of such abstractions.

Expressive power: The theory of computation classifies languages by the computations they are capable of expressing. All Turing complete languages can implement the same set of algorithms. ANSI/ISO SQL and Charity are examples of languages that are not Turing complete, yet often called programming languages.

Markup languages like XML, HTML or troff, which define structured data, are not generally considered programming languages. Programming languages may, however, share the syntax with markup languages if a computational semantics is defined. XSLT, for example, is a Turing complete XML dialect. Moreover, LaTeX, which is mostly used for structuring documents, also contains a Turing complete subset.

Algorithm

In mathematics, computing, and related subjects, an algorithm is an effective method for solving a problem using a finite sequence of instructions. Algorithms are used for calculation, data processing, and many other fields (Fig. 2.21).

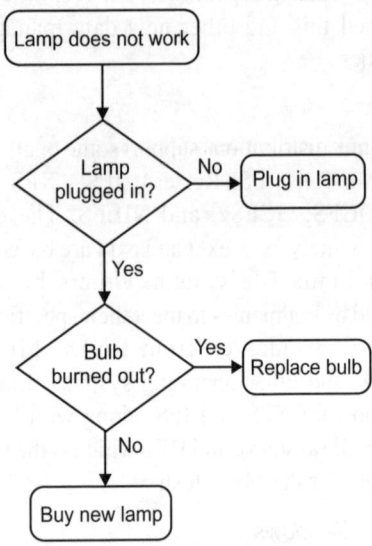

Fig. 2.21. This is an algorithm that tries to figure out why the lamp doesn't turn on and tries to fix it using the steps. Flowcharts are often used to graphically represent algorithms.

Each algorithm is a list of well-defined instructions for completing a task. Starting from an initial state, the instructions describe a computation that proceeds through a well-defined series of successive states, eventually terminating in a final ending state. The transition from one state to the next is not necessarily deterministic; some algorithms, known as randomised algorithms, incorporate randomness.

Algorithms are essential to the way computers process information. Many computer programmes contain algorithms that specify the specific instructions a computer should perform (in a specific order) to carry out a specified task, such as calculating employees' paychecks or printing students' report cards. Thus, an algorithm can be considered to be any sequence of operations that can be simulated by a Turing-complete system.

Typically, when an algorithm is associated with processing information, data is read from an input source, written to an output device, and/or stored for further processing. Stored data is regarded as part of the internal state of the entity performing the algorithm. In practice, the state is stored in one or more data structures. For any such computational process, the algorithm must be rigorously defined: specified in the way it applies in all possible circumstances that could arise. That is, any conditional steps must be systematically dealt with, case-by-case; the criteria for each case must be clear (and computable).

Because an algorithm is a precise list of precise steps, the order of computation will always be critical to the functioning of the algorithm. Instructions are usually assumed to be listed explicitly, and are described as starting 'from the top' and going 'down to the bottom', an idea that is described more formally by flow of control.

So far, this discussion of the formalisation of an algorithm has assumed the premises of imperative programming. This is the most common conception, and it attempts to describe a task in discrete, 'mechanical' means. Unique to this conception of formalised algorithms is the assignment operation, setting the value of a variable. It derives from the intuition of 'memory' as a scratchpad. There is an example below of such an assignment.

Algorithms can be expressed in many kinds of notation, including natural languages, pseudocode, flowcharts, programming languages or control tables (processed by interpreters). Natural language expressions of algorithms tend to be verbose and ambiguous, and are rarely used for complex or technical algorithms. Pseudocode, flowcharts and control tables are structured ways to express algorithms that avoid many of the ambiguities common in natural language statements, while remaining independent of a particular implementation language. Programming languages are primarily intended for expressing algorithms in a form that can be executed by a computer, but are often used as a way to define or document algorithms.

There is a wide variety of representations possible and one can express a given Turing machine programme as a sequence of machine tables, as flowcharts, or as a form of rudimentary machine code or assembly code called 'sets of quadruples'.

Sometimes it is helpful in the description of an algorithm to supplement small 'flow charts' with natural-language and/or arithmetic expressions written inside 'block diagrams' to summarise what the 'flow charts' are accomplishing.

Database Management System

A database management system (DBMS) is a set of computer programmes that controls the creation, maintenance, and the use of the database with computer as a platform or of an organisation and its end users. It allows organisations to place control of organisation-wide database development in the hands of database administrators (DBAs) and other specialists. A DBMS is a system software package that helps the use of integrated collection of data records and files known as databases. It allows different user application programmes to easily access the same database. DBMSs may use any of a variety of database models, such as the network model or relational model. In large systems, a DBMS allows users and other software to store and retrieve data in a structured way. Instead of having to write computer programs to extract information, user can ask simple questions in a query language. Thus, many DBMS packages provide Fourth-generation programming language (4GLs) and other application development features. It helps to specify the logical organisation for a database and access and use the information within a database. It provides facilities for controlling data access, enforcing data integrity, managing concurrency controlled, restoring database.

A DBMS is a set of software programs that controls the organisation, storage, management, and retrieval of data in a database. DBMSs are categorised according to their data structures or types. The DBMS accepts requests for data from an application programme and instructs the operating system to transfer the appropriate data. The queries and responses must be submitted and received according to a format that conforms to one or more applicable protocols. When a DBMS is used, information systems can be changed much more easily as the organisation's information requirements change. New categories of data can be added to the database without disruption to the existing system.

Database servers are computers that hold the actual databases and run only the DBMS and related software. Database servers are usually multiprocessor computers, with generous memory and RAID disk arrays used for stable storage. Hardware database accelerators, connected to one or more servers via a high-speed channel, are also used in large volume transaction processing environments. DBMSs are found at the heart of most database applications. Sometimes DBMSs are built around a private multitasking kernel with built-in networking support although nowadays these functions are left to the operating system. A DBMS includes four main parts: modelling language, data structure, database query language, and transaction mechanisms.

Components of DBMS

DBMS engine accepts logical request from the various other DBMS subsystems, converts them into physical equivalent, and actually accesses the database and data dictionary as they exist on a storage device.

Data definition subsystem helps user to create and maintain the data dictionary and define the structure of the files in a database.

Data manipulation subsystem helps user to add, change, and delete information in a database and query it for valuable information. Software tools within the data manipulation subsystem are most often the primary interface between user and the information contained in a database. It allows user to specify its logical information requirements.

Application generation subsystem contains facilities to help users to develop transactions-intensive applications. It usually requires that user perform a detailed series of tasks to process a transaction. It facilities easy-to-use data entry screens, programming languages, and interfaces.

Data administration subsystem helps users to manage the overall database environment by providing facilities for backup and recovery, security management, query optimisation, concurrency control, and change management.

Modelling language

A data modelling language to define the schema of each database hosted in the DBMS, according to the DBMS database model. The four most common types of models are given below:

1. Hierarchical model.
2. Network model.
3. Relational model.
4. Object model.

Inverted lists and other methods are also used. A given database management system may provide one or more of the four models. The optimal structure depends on the natural organisation of the application's data, and on the application's requirements (which include transaction rate (speed), reliability, maintainability, scalability, and cost).

The dominant model in use today is the adhoc one embedded in SQL, despite the objections of purists who believe this model is a corruption of the relational model, since it violates several of its fundamental principles for the sake of practicality and performance. Many DBMSs also support the open database connectivity API that supports a standard way for programmers to access the DBMS.

Display Device

A display device is an output device for presentation of information for visual, tactile or auditive reception, acquired, stored, or transmitted in various forms. When the input information is supplied as an electrical signal, the display is called electronic display. Electronic displays are available for presentation of visual, tactile and auditive information.

Tactile electronic displays (aka refreshable Braille display) are usually intended for the blind or visually impaired, they use electromechanical parts to dynamically update a tactile image (usually of text) so that the image may be felt by the fingers.

Common applications for electronic visual displays are television sets or computer monitors.

RECORDING DEVICE

Recording devices make use of digital technology to record video and audio which can be replayed and analysed in various ways on television, PC monitors, or inside web browsers. Examples include audio recording devices, voice recording devices, and phone recording devices. Digital video recorders, security DVR, have fast become popular, with multiple features and functions.

DVR: Digital Video Recorders

DVR basics

A digital video recorder can record video and audio signals in the 'mpeg' format. This does away with older magnetic tapes and recordings with poor quality. The recorded files can be watched on monitors, or transferred to CDs with inbuilt CD writers. Some DVRs even allow viewing the files directly using a web browser and an Internet connection.

Using a DVR

A DVR can be an independent unit with all of the features above, or it could be inserted as a card inside the PC. This gives greater flexibility. The card can be used to record television programmes, or camera feeds. Multiple cameras can be used with a multi-channel DVR such as a 4-channel DVR.

DVR cards

A DVR card can also be used to record television programmes, and direct DVR allows one to do just that as a stand alone DVR unit. There are also products with embedded DVR placed inside, and DVR players. HDTV DVR is also a separate option.

Editing power

The great convenience of using DVR surveillance is the manipulation of the recorded feed that it allows. One need not fast forward the whole tape as the case used to be. Timings, events, alerts can be used to reach the appropriate points on the recorded feed. The images can be seen as individual pictures, and either captured on the screen or printed out.

Spy recording devices

There are laws against spy recording, especially phone conversations. The devices therefore need to be used with legitimate aims. A spy recording device could come in the shape of a pen, watch, wall clock, lighter, a book, and so on. The power is derived from button cells, and images and files can be transferred to desktops and other devices. There are limitations on picture quality and the amount of file storage. Many devices have auto recording and auto power off features.

3

Molecules Analysis in Clinical Medicine

INTRODUCTION

A medical laboratory or clinical laboratory is a laboratory where tests are done on clinical specimens in order to get information about the health of a patient as pertaining to the diagnosis, treatment, and prevention of disease.

Laboratory medicine is generally divided into four sections, and each of which is further divided into a number of units. These four sections are:

1. Anatomic pathology: Units are included here, namely histopathology, cytopathology, and electron microscopy. Academically, each unit is studied alone in one course. Other courses pertaining to this section include anatomy, physiology, histology, pathology, and pathophysiology.
2. Clinical microbiology: This is the largest section in laboratory medicine; as it encompasses five different sciences (units). These include bacteriology, virology, parasitology, immunology, and mycology.
3. Clinical biochemistry: Units under this busy section are instrumental analysis, enzymology, toxicology and endocrinology.
4. Hematology: This busy, section consists of three units, which are coagulation and blood bank and hematology.

Distribution of clinical laboratories in health institutions varies greatly from one place to another. Take for example microbiology, some health facilities have a single laboratory for microbiology, while others have a separate lab for each unit, with nothing called a 'microbiology' lab.

Methods used to measure molecules in clinical chemical chemistry, toxicology, and pulmonary medicine have a tremendous impact on the fields of bioengineering and medicine. The ability to measure certain molecules in the body enables us to better understand the biological and chemical processes occurring in the body. This chapter presents various techniques used to measure different molecules in the body, along with the importance and impact of their measurement.

SPECTROPHOTOMETRY

Spectrophotometry is the quantifiable study of electromagnetic spectra. It is more specific than the general term electromagnetic spectroscopy in that spectrophotometry deals with visible light, near ultraviolet, and near-infrared. Also, the term does not cover time-resolved spectroscopic techniques (Fig. 3.1).

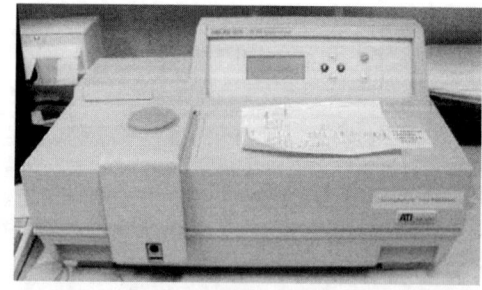

Fig. 3.1. Spectrophotometer.

Spectrophotometry involves the use of a spectrophotometer. A spectrophotometer is a photometer (a device for measuring light intensity) that can measure intensity as a function of the colour (or more specifically the wavelength) of light. Important features of spectrophotometers are spectral bandwidth and linear range of absorption measurement.

Perhaps the most common application of spectrophotometers is the measurement of light absorption, but they can be designed to measure diffuse or specular reflectance. Strictly, even the emission half of a luminescence instrument is a type of spectrophotometer.

The use of spectrophotometers is not limited to studies in physics. They are also commonly used in other scientific fields such as chemistry, biochemistry, and molecular biology. They are widely used in many industries including printing and forensic examination.

There are two major classes of devices: single beam and double beam. A double beam spectrophotometer compares the light intensity between two light paths, one path containing a reference sample and the other the test sample. A single beam spectrophotometer measures the relative light intensity of the beam before and after a test sample is inserted. Although comparison measurements from double beam instruments are easier and more stable, single beam instruments can have a larger dynamic range and are optically simpler and more compact (Fig. 3.2).

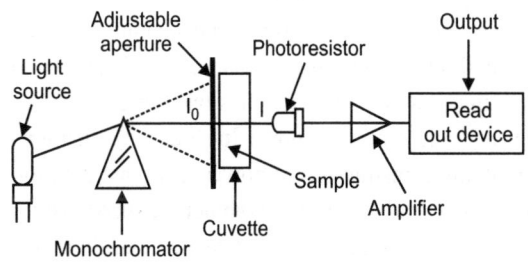

Fig. 3.2. Single beam spectrophotometer.

Historically, spectrophotometers use a monochromator containing a diffraction grating to produce the analytical spectrum. There are also spectrophotometers that use arrays of photosensors. Especially for infrared spectrophotometers, there are spectrophotometers that use a Fourier transform technique to acquire the spectral information quicker in a technique called Fourier Transform InfraRed.

The spectrophotometer quantitatively compares the fraction of light that passes through a reference solution and a test solution. Light from the source lamp is passed through a monochromator, which diffracts the light into a 'rainbow' of wavelengths and outputs narrow bandwidths of this diffracted spectrum. Discrete frequencies are transmitted through the test sample. Then the intensity of the transmitted light is measured with a photodiode or other light sensor, and the transmittance value for this wavelength is then compared with transmission through a reference sample.

In short, the sequence of events in a spectrophotometer is as follows:

1. The light source shines into a monochromator.
2. A particular output wavelength is selected and beamed at the sample.
3. The sample absorbs light.

Many spectrophotometers must be calibrated by a procedure known as 'zeroing.' The absorbency of a reference substance is set as a baseline value, so the absorbencies of all other substances are recorded relative to the initial 'zeroed' substance. The spectrophotometer then displays per cent absorbency (the amount of light absorbed relative to the initial substance).

TYPES OF SPECTROPHOTOMETERS

UV and IR Spectrophotometers

The most common spectrophotometers are used in the UV and visible regions of the spectrum, and some of these instruments also operate into the near-infrared region as well. Visible region 400–700 nm spectrophotometry is used extensively in colorimetry science. Ink manufacturers, printing companies, textiles vendors, and many more, need the data provided through colorimetry. They take readings in the region of every 10–20 nanometers along the visible region, and produce a spectral reflectance curve or a data stream for alternative presentations. These curves can be used to test a new batch of colourant to check if it makes a match to specifications, e.g. iso printing standards.

Traditional visual region spectrophotometers cannot detect if a colourant or the base material has fluorescence. This can make it difficult to manage colour issues if for example one or more of the printing inks is fluorescent. Where a colourant contains fluorescence, a bi-spectral fluorescent spectrophotometer is used. There are two major setups for visual spectrum spectrophotometers, d/8 (spherical) and 0/45. The names are due to the geometry of the light source, observer and interior of the measurement chamber. Scientists use this machine to measure the amount of compounds in a sample. If the compound is more concentrated more light will be absorbed by the sample; within small ranges, the Beer-Lambert law holds and the absorbance between samples vary with concentration linearly. In the case of printing measurements two alternative settings are commonly used- without/with UV filter to control better the effect of UV brighteners within the paper stock.

Samples are usually prepared in cuvettes; depending on the region of interest, they may be constructed of glass, plastic, or quartz.

IR Spectrophotometry

Spectrophotometers designed for the main infrared region are quite different because of the technical requirements of measurement in that region. One major factor is the type of photosensors that are available for different spectral regions, but infrared measurement is also challenging because virtually everything emits IR light as thermal radiation, especially at wavelengths beyond about 5 μm.

Another complication is that quite a few materials such as glass and plastic absorb infrared light, making it incompatible as an optical medium. Ideal optical materials are salts, which do not absorb strongly. Samples for IR spectrophotometry may be smeared between two discs of potassium bromide or ground with potassium bromide and pressed into a pellet. Where aqueous solutions are to be measured, insoluble silver chloride is used to construct the cell.

Spectroradiometers

Spectroradiometers, which operate almost like the visible region spectrophotometers, are designed to measure the spectral density of illuminants in order to evaluate and categorise lighting for sales by the manufacturer, or for the customers to confirm the lamp they decided to purchase is within their specifications. Components of spectroradiometers are:

1. The light source shines onto or through the sample.
2. The sample transmits or reflects light.
3. The detector detects how much light was reflected from or transmitted through the sample.
4. The detector then converts how much light the sample transmitted or reflected into a number.

COMPONENTS OF SPECTROPHOTOMETRY

Radiant Energy

Radiant energy is the energy of electromagnetic waves. The quantity of radiant energy may be calculated by integrating radiant flux (or power) with respect to time and, like all forms of energy, its SI unit is the joule. The term is used particularly when radiation is emitted by a source into the surrounding environment. Radiant energy may be visible or invisible to the human eye.

The term 'radiant energy' is most commonly used in the fields of radiometry, solar energy, heating and lighting, but is also sometimes used in other fields (such as telecommunications). In modern applications involving transmission of power from one location to another, 'radiant energy' is sometimes used to refer to the electromagnetic waves themselves, rather than their energy (a property of the waves). In the past, the term 'electro-radiant energy' has also been used.

Historically, the propagation of electromagnetic radiation was presumed to rely on a medium filling all space, known as the aether. Electromagnetic waves were presumed to propagate through this medium by inducing transverse electric and magnetic stresses and strains, analogous to those induced by shear waves propagating through a physical medium. In modern times, the propagation of electromagnetic waves has been shown not to require any physical medium, although some interpretations of general relativity can be viewed as implying that space acts as a kind of non-physical 'medium' for light.

Because electromagnetic (EM) radiation can be conceptualised as a stream of photons, radiant energy can be viewed as the energy carried by these photons. Alternatively, EM radiation can be viewed as an electromagnetic wave, which carries energy in its oscillating electric and magnetic fields. These two views are completely equivalent and are reconciled to one another in quantum field theory.

EM radiation can have various frequencies. The bands of frequency present in a given EM signal may be sharply defined, as is seen in atomic spectra, or may be broad, as in blackbody radiation. In the photon picture, the energy carried by each photon is proportional to its frequency. In the wave picture, the energy of a monochromatic wave is proportional to its intensity. This implies that if two EM waves have the same intensity, but different frequencies, the one with the higher frequency 'contains' fewer photons, since each photon is more energetic.

When EM waves are absorbed by an object, the energy of the waves is typically converted to heat. This is a very familiar effect, since sunlight warms surfaces that it irradiates. Often this phenomenon is associated particularly with infrared radiation, but any kind of electromagnetic radiation will warm an object that absorbs it. EM waves can also be reflected or scattered, in which case their energy is redirected or redistributed as well.

Open systems

Radiant energy is one of the mechanisms by which energy can enter or leave an open system. Such a system can be man-made, such as a solar energy collector, or natural, such as the earth's atmosphere. In geophysics, most atmospheric gases, including the greenhouse gases, allow the sun's short-wavelength radiant energy to pass through to the earth's surface, heating the ground and oceans. The absorbed solar energy is partly re-emitted as longer wavelength radiation (chiefly infrared radiation), some of which is absorbed by the atmospheric greenhouse gases.

Radiant energy is produced in the sun as a result of nuclear fusion.

Applications

Radiant energy, as well as convective energy and conductive energy, is used for radiant heating. It can be generated electrically by infrared lamps, or can be absorbed from sunlight and used to heat water. The heat energy is emitted from a warm element (floor, wall, overhead panel) and warms people and other objects in rooms rather than directly heating the air. The internal air temperature for radiant heated buildings may be lower than for a conventionally heated building to achieve the same level of body comfort (the perceived temperature is actually the same).

Various other applications of radiant energy have been devised. These include:

1. Treatment and inspection.
2. Separating and sorting.
3. Medium of control.
4. Medium of communication.

Many of these applications involve a source of radiant energy and a detector that responds to that radiation and provides a signal representing some characteristic of the radiation. Radiant energy detectors produce responses to incident radiant energy either as an increase or decrease in electric potential or current flow or some other perceivable change, such as exposure of photographic film.

One of the earliest wireless telephones to be based on radiant energy was invented by Nikola Tesla. The device used transmitters and receivers whose resonances were tuned to the same frequency, allowing communication between them. SI radio metry are shown in Table 3.1.

Monochromator

A monochromator is an optical device that transmits a mechanically selectable narrow band of wavelengths of light or other radiation chosen from a wider range of wavelengths available at the input. The name is from the Greek roots *mono-*, single, and chroma, colour, and the Latin suffix *-ator*, denoting an agent.

A device that can produce monochromatic light has many uses in science and in optics because many

Table 3.1. SI Radiometry units.

Quantity	Symbol	SI unit	Abbr.	Notes
Radiant energy	Q	Joule	J	Energy
Radiant flux	φ	Watt	W	Radiant energy per unit time, also called radiant power
Radiant intensity	I	Watt per steradian	$W \cdot sr^{-1}$	Power per unit solid angle
Radiance	L	Watt per steradian per square metre	$W \cdot sr^{-1} \cdot m^{-2}$	Power per unit solid angle per unit projected source area
				Called intensity in some other fields of study
Irradiance	E, I	Watt per square metre	$W \cdot m^{-2}$	Power incident on a surface
				Sometimes confusingly called 'intensity'
Radiant exitance	M			
Radiant emittance		Watt per square metre	$W \cdot m^{-2}$	Power emitted from a surface.
Radiosity	J or J_λ	Watt per square metre	$W \cdot m^{-2}$	Emitted plus reflected power leaving a surface
Spectral radiance	L_λ or L_v	Watt per steradian per metre^3 or watt per steradian per square metre per hertz	$W \cdot sr^{-1} \cdot m^{-3}$ or $W \cdot sr^{-1} \cdot m^{-2} \cdot Hz^{-1}$	Commonly measured in $W \cdot sr^{-1} \cdot m^{-2}$ nm^{-1}
Spectral irradiance	E_λ or E_v	Watt per metre^3 or watt per square metre per hertz	$W \cdot m^{-3}$ or $W \cdot m^{-2} \cdot Hz^{-1}$	Commonly measured in $W \cdot m^{-2} \cdot nm^{-1}$

optical characteristics of a material are dependent on colour. Although there are a number of useful ways to produce pure colours, there are not so many other ways to easily select any pure colour in a wide range. See below for a discussion of some of the uses of monochromators. In hard X-ray and neutron optics, crystal monochromators are used to define wave conditions on the instruments.

A monochromator can use either the phenomenon of optical dispersion in a prism, or that of diffraction using a diffraction grating, to spatially separate the colours of light. It usually has a mechanism for directing the selected colour to an exit slit. Usually the grating or the prism is used in a reflective mode. A reflective prism is made by making a right triangle prism (typically, half of an equilateral prism) with one side mirrored. The light enters through the hypotenuse face and is reflected back through it, being refracted twice at the same surface. The total refraction, and the total dispersion, is the same as would occur if an equilateral prism were used.

The dispersion or diffraction is only controllable if the light is collimated, that is if all the rays of light are parallel, or practically so. A source, like the sun, which is very far away, provides collimated light. Newton used sunlight in his famous experiments. In a practical monochromator however, the light source is close by, and an optical system in the monochromator converts the diverging light of the source to collimated light. Although some monochromator designs do use focusing gratings that do not need separate collimators, most use collimating mirrors. Reflective optics are preferred because they do not introduce dispersive effects of their own.

Diffraction-Grating Monochromator

A diffraction-grating monochromator uses the optical-dispersion properties of a diffraction grating to separate the wavelength components of light into a spectrum. There are several different designs for monochromators, which use either flat or curved diffraction gratings, with the optical layout of a typical monochromator (Czerny-Turner design) being given in Fig. 3.3.

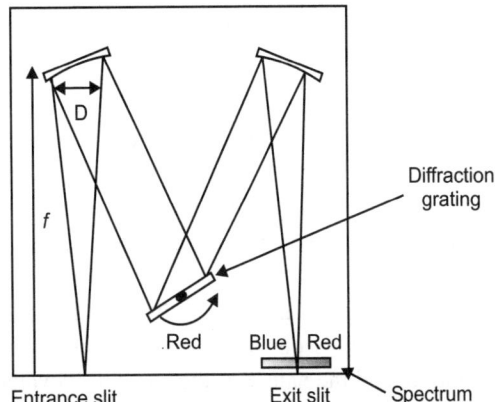

Fig. 3.3. Schematic representation of the optical layout of a diffraction-grating monochromator (Czerny-Turner design); f is the focal length and D is the beam aperture.

Light from the 'entrance slit' falls on the first concave mirror, which produces a parallel beam of light which is then diffracted by the flat diffraction grating. The second concave mirror then focuses the diffracted light to produce an image of the entrance slit in the same plane as the exit slit.

The grating 'diffracts' light of different wavelengths through different angles. Hence, separate images of the entrance slit (for each wavelength) are produced at different positions along the plane of the exit slit. This spread of images forms a spectrum of the light.

A narrow part of this spectrum, centered about λ_0, will fall across the exit slit and will then pass out through the latter. The spectrum is moved by rotating the diffraction grating. As the diffraction grating is turned (in the direction shown in Fig. 3.3) the spectrum will move towards the left and a different wavelength will be selected to exit the monochromator.

Monochromators are used in many optical measuring instruments and in other applications where tunable monochromatic light is wanted. Sometimes the monochromatic light is directed at a sample and the reflected or transmitted light is measured. Sometimes white light is directed at a sample and the monochromator is used to analyse the reflected or transmitted light. Two monochromators are used in many fluorometers; one monochromator is used to select the excitation wavelength and a second monochromator is used to analyse the emitted light.

Cuvette

A cuvette is a small tube of circular or square cross section, sealed at one end, made of plastic, glass, or fused quartz (for UV light) and designed to hold samples for spectroscopic experiments. The best cuvettes are as clear as possible, without impurities that might affect a spectroscopic reading. Like a test tube, a cuvette may be open to the atmosphere on top or have a cap to seal it shut. Parafilm can also be used to seal it.

Inexpensive cuvettes are round and look similar to test tubes. Disposable plastic cuvettes are often used in fast spectroscopic assays, where speed is more important than high accuracy.

Some cuvettes will be clear only on opposite sides, so that they pass a single beam of light through that pair of sides; often the unclear sides have ridges or are rough to allow easy handling. Cuvettes to be used in fluorescence spectroscopy must be clear on all four sides because fluorescence is measured at a right-angle to the beam path to limit contributions from beam itself. Some cuvettes, known as tandem cuvettes, have a glass barrier that extends 2/3 up inside, so that measurements can be taken with two solutions separated, and again when they are mixed. Typically, cuvettes are 1 cm (0.39 in) across, to allow for easy calculations of coefficients of absorption (Fig. 3.4).

Cuvettes to be used in circular dichroism experiments should never be mechanically stressed, as the stress will induce birefringence in the quartz and affect the measurements made (Fig. 3.5).

There are three different types of cuvettes commonly used, with different usable wavelengths:

1. Glass, with a wavelength from 380 to 780 nm (visible spectrum).
2. Plastic, with a wavelength from 380 to 780 nm (visible spectrum).

3. Fused quartz, with a wavelength below 380 nm (ultraviolet spectrum).

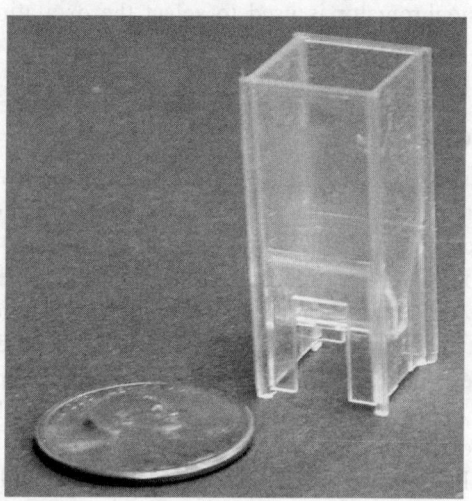

Fig. 3.4. This plastic cuvette is used in a spectrophotometer to measure DNA and RNA concentrations.

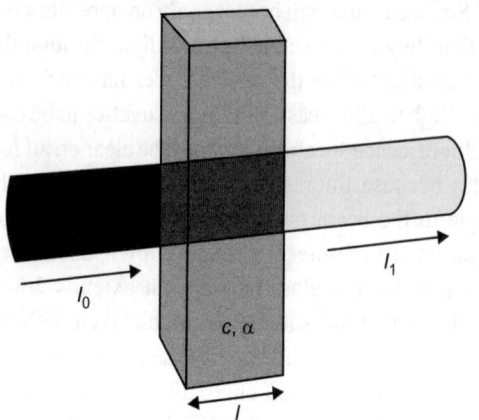

Fig. 3.5. Use of a cuvette with width *l*, used in a diagram to explain the Beer–Lambert law.

BEER–LAMBERT LAW

Lambert's law states that each layer of equal thickness of an absorbing medium absorbs an equal fraction of the radiant energy that traverses it.

Beer, a nineteenth-century German physicist, gave his name to a law that allows the calculation of the quantity of light transmitted through a defined thickness of a compound in solution in a non-absorbing matrix. His work is often associated with that of the French mathematician Lambert, who laid down the basis for photometry in the eighteenth century. The result is Beer-Lambert's law, shown here in its current form:

$$A = \varepsilon l C \qquad ... (3.1)$$

where, A is the absorbance, an optical parameter without units, measured with a spectrophotometer; l is the thickness of solution through which incident light is passed; C is the molar concentration; and e is the molar absorption coefficient ($l\,mol^{-1}\,cm^{-1}$) at a given wavelength. The molar absorptivity of a compound depends on the wavelength used, the temperature and the nature of the solvent. Its value is usually known for the wavelength at the absorption maximum. This value, which corresponds to the absorbance of a solution with a 1 M concentration and a thickness of 1 cm, can vary over a wide range (0 to 2,00,000). If m is the quantity of compound per liter and M its molar mass (expressed in gram), then Eq. 3.1 becomes:

$$A = \varepsilon l \frac{m}{M} \qquad ... (3.2)$$

This formula is based on Lambert's hypothesis that the intensity I of monochromatic radiation is decreased by dI (i.e. negative) as it passes through a thickness dx of a material with an absorption coefficient k at the chosen wavelength (Fig. 3.6).

Thus:

$$-\frac{dI}{dx} = kI_x \qquad ... (3.3)$$

If I_0 represents the incident intensity of the radiation before it passes through a medium of thickness I that has an absorption coefficient k, the transmitted intensity I will be given by the integrated form, Eq.3.5, of the previous equation:

$$\left[\ln I_x\right]_{I_0}^{I} = -k\left[x\right]_0^{l} \qquad ... (3.4)$$

$$\ln \frac{I}{I_0} = -k \cdot l \qquad ... (3.5)$$

$$I = I_0 \exp(-kl) \qquad ... (3.6)$$

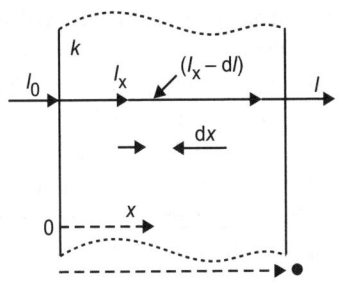

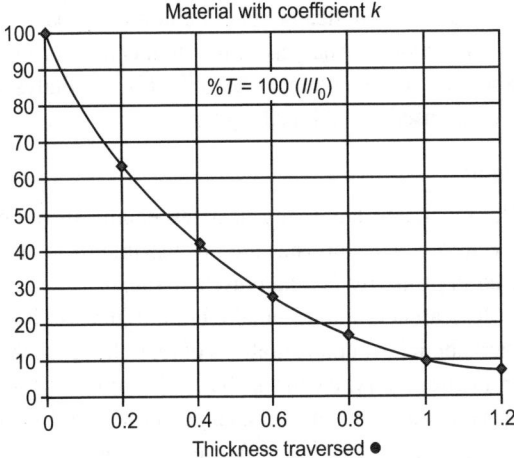

Material with coefficient k

Fig. 3.6. Absorption of light by a homogeneous material and representation of % transmittance as a function of the material's thickness.

In 1850, Beer applied Eq. 3.6 to a dilute solution of a compound dissolved in a transparent medium. He proposed that k was proportional to the molar concentration C of the compound. This is why Eq. 3.6 is better known in the form Eqs. 3.1 or 3.2 in which the absorbance A is represented by one of the following equations:

$$A = \log \frac{I}{I_0} \quad \text{or} \quad A = \log \frac{1}{T} \quad ...(3.7)$$

where, T is the transmittance defined as follows:

$$T = \frac{I}{I_0} \quad \text{or} \quad \%T = \left(\frac{I}{I_0}\right) \times 100$$

In colorimetry, it is preferable to measure the absorbance of a chromophore at the higher wavelength to reduce the risk of superimposition with absorption bands related to other compounds. When absorbance measurement is preceded by a chemical reaction, it is conceivable that the exact structure of the compound whose absorbance is being measured is not known. Nevertheless, if it is assumed that the reaction is quantitative, its molar absorption coefficient can be calculated using the molar concentration of the compound that has been derivatised.

CALIBRATION

Spectrophotometer calibration is a process in which a scientific instrument known as a spectrophotometer is calibrated to confirm that it is working properly. This is important, as it ensures that the measurements obtained with the instrument are accurate. The procedure varies slightly for different instruments, with most manufacturers providing a detailed calibration guide in the owner's manual so that people know how to calibrate the equipment properly. When this process is performed, the person doing it must make a note in the log attached to the equipment and in their experimental notes, so that people know when the device was last calibrated and handled, and by whom.

In spectrophotometer calibration, a reference solution is used to zero out the equipment. This solution provides a base or zero reading. The device is calibrated by placing the reference solution inside the spectrophotometer, zeroing out the settings, and running the instrument. Then, samples of an actual test material can be subjected to spectrophotometry in confidence that the machine has been calibrated and is working properly.

In order for a spectrophotometer to work properly, it must be allowed to warm up before use. Many devices take around 10 minutes to warm up. It is important to avoid performing spectrophotometer calibration during the warmup phase as this will throw the settings off. It is also important to be aware that for certain types of wavelengths, special filtres and attachments may be needed for the device to function.

CLINICAL LABORATORY TESTS

Table 3.2 lists common molecules measured and types of test conducted.

Table 3.2. Common molecules measured in body and types of test conducted.

Molecule	Type of test	Toxic levels (mg/dl)
Total bilirubin	Blood (serum)	High levels result in jaundice
Indirect	–	–
Direct	–	–
Lactate	Blood (serum)	>45
Creatinine	Blood (serum)	>4
Female		
Male		>100
Urea	Blood (serum)	Adult male: <50 or >400
Glucose	Blood	Adult female: <40 or >400
Sodium	Blood (serum)	<120 or >160 mEq/L
Potassium	Blood (serum)	<3 or >7.5 mmol/L
Lithium	Blood (serum)	>2.0 mEq/L

Microdialysis

Microdialysis is a semi-invasive sampling technique that is used in pre-clinical as well as clinical pharmacokinetic studies for continuous measurement of free, protein-unbound concentrations in extracellular tissue fluids by means of a microdialysis catheter (microdialysis probe). The microdialysis probe consists of a semipermeable hollow fibre membrane that is constantly perfused with a physiological solution (perfusate) at a low flow rate of approximately 0.1–5µL/min. Once inserted into the tissue or (body)fluid of interest, small molecules can cross the semi-permeable membrane by passive diffusion. The microdialysis principle was first employed in the early 1960s to directly study biochemistry in animal tissues, especially in rodent brains. During the 1970s the microdialysis catheter was steadily improved and eventually resulted in today's most prevalent shape, the needle probe.

Microdialysis works by slowly pumping a solution (the 'perfusate') through the microdialysis probe. Molecules in the tissues diffuse into the perfusate as it is pumped through the probe; the dialysate is then collected and analysed to determine the identities and concentrations of molecules that were in the extracellular fluid. The concentration in the dialysate of any given substance will normally be much lower than the concentration present in the extracellular fluid, especially for substances of relatively high molecular weight. Typically the concentration of a peptide collected by microdialysis will be just 5–10 per cent of the original concentration. This depends on the charge and size of the molecule in question as well as the dialysis speed. Different techniques can be used to assay the dialysis time needed to attain steady state including radioactive labelled probes. Analysis of the fluid can occur in a laboratory or at a patient's bedside, if microdialysis is being used in a clinical context.

Uses

The technique has many uses, especially in brain research, where biopsies are not feasible. It is also used in primarily fat and muscle tissue.

Researchers into traumatic brain injury use it to learn about how concentrations of ions change in the brain after injury. It can also be used to monitor hour by hour the level of and changes in amyloid beta protein plaque tangles in Alzheimer's disease and other progressive neurodegenerative diseases.

Difficulties with the technique

While microdialysis is generally seen as a practical and useful analytic technique for elucidating the concentration of key low molecular weight components in the extracellular fluid, there are a number of practical considerations that need to be taken into account.

The absolute concentration of an analyte (the substance or substances being analysed) in the extracellular fluid is very difficult to determine using microdialysis. If the dialysate has a relatively high flow rate, then the analyte will most likely not fully equilibrate between perfusate (the exiting fluid from the probe) and ECF. Therefore high pressure liquid chromatography (HPLC), capillary electrophoresis or other analytic measurements of the dialysate will underestimate the concentration of the analyte in ECF. There are a number of mathematical models available for quantifying the fraction of analyte in the dialysate.

OXYGEN SATURATION

Oxygen saturation or dissolved oxygen (DO) is a relative measure of the amount of oxygen that is dissolved or carried in a given medium. It can be measured with a dissolved oxygen probe such as an oxygen sensor or an optode in liquid media, usually water.

In medicine, oxygen saturation (S_{O_2}) commonly referred to as 'sats', measures the percentage of haemoglobin binding sites in the bloodstream occupied by oxygen. At low partial pressures of oxygen, most haemoglobin is deoxygenated. At around 90 per cent (the value varies according to the clinical context) oxygen saturation increases according to an oxygen-haemoglobin dissociation curve and approaches 100 per cent at partial oxygen pressures of >10 kPa. A pulse oximeter relies on the light absorption characteristics of saturated haemoglobin to give an indication of oxygen saturation. An arterial oxygen saturation (Sa_{O_2}) (arterial oxygen saturation) value below 90 per cent causes hypoxemia (which can also be caused by anemia). Hypoxemia due to low Sa_{O_2} is indicated by cyanosis.

Venous oxygen saturation (Sv_{O_2}) is measured to see how much oxygen the body consumes. Under clinical treatment, a Sv_{O_2} below 60 per cent, indicates that the body is in lack of oxygen, and ischemic diseases occur. This measurement is often used under treatment with a heart-lung machine (Extracorporeal Circulation), and can give the perfusionist an idea of how much flow the patient needs to stay healthy.

Tissue oxygen saturation (St_{O_2}) can be measured by near infrared spectroscopy. Although the measurements are still widely discussed, they give an idea of tissue oxygenation in various conditions.

Saturation of peripheral oxygen (Sp_{O_2}) is an estimation of the oxygen saturation level usually measured with a pulse oximeter device. It can be calculated with the pulse oximetry according to the following formula:

$$S_p O_2 = \frac{HbO_2}{H_b O_2 + Hb}$$

BILIRUBIN

Bilirubin (formerly referred to as haematoidin) is the yellow breakdown product of normal heme catabolism. Heme is found in haemoglobin, a principal component of red blood cells. Bilirubin is excreted in bile, and its levels are elevated in certain diseases. It is responsible for the yellow colour of bruises and the yellow discolouration in jaundice.

Bilirubin consists of an open chain of four pyrrole-like rings (tetrapyrrole). In heme, by contrast, these four rings are connected into a larger ring, called a porphyrin ring. Bilirubin is very similar to the pigment phycobilin used by certain algae to capture light energy, and to the pigment phytochrome used by plants to sense light. All of these contain an open chain of four pyrrolic rings.

Like these other pigments, some of the double-bonds in bilirubin isomerise when exposed to light. This is used in the phototherapy of jaundiced newborns: the isomer of bilirubin formed upon light exposure is more soluble than the unilluminated isomer.

Bilirubin is created by the activity of biliverdin reductase on biliverdin. Bilirubin, when oxidised, reverts to become biliverdin once again. This cycle, in addition to the demonstration of the potent antioxidant activity of bilirubin, has led to the hypothesis that bilirubin's main physiologic role is as a cellular antioxidant.

Metabolism

Erythrocytes (red blood cells) generated in the bone marrow are disposed of in the spleen when they get old or damaged. This releases haemoglobin, which is broken down to heme as the globin parts are turned into amino acids. The heme is then turned into unconjugated bilirubin in the macrophages of the spleen. This unconjugated bilirubin is not soluble in water. It is then bound to albumin and sent to the liver.

In the liver it is conjugated to glucuronic acid, making it soluble in water. Much of it goes into the bile and thus out into the small intestine. Some of the conjugated bilirubin remains in the large intestine and is metabolised by colonic bacteria to urobilinogen, which is further metabolised to stercobilinogen, and finally oxidised to stercobilin. This stercobilin gives feces its brown colour. Some of the urobilinogen is reabsorbed and excreted in the urine along with an oxidised form, urobilin.

Normally, a tiny amount of bilirubin is excreted in the urine, accounting for the light yellow colour. If the liver's function is impaired or when biliary drainage is blocked, some of the conjugated bilirubin leaks out of the hepatocytes and appears in the urine, turning it dark amber. The presence of this conjugated bilirubin in the urine can be clinically analysed, and is reported as an increase in urine bilirubin. However, in disorders involving hemolytic anemia, an increased number of red blood cells are broken down, causing an increase in the amount of unconjugated bilirubin in the blood. As stated above, the unconjugated bilirubin is not water soluble, and thus one will not see an increase in bilirubin in the urine. Because there is no problem with the liver or bile systems, this excess unconjugated bilirubin will go through all of the normal processing mechanisms that occur (e.g. conjugation, excretion in bile, metabolism to urobilinogen, reabsorption) and will show up as an increase in urine urobilinogen. This difference between increased urine bilirubin and increased urine urobilinogen helps to distinguish between various disorders in those systems.

Toxicity

Unconjugated hyperbilirubinaemia in a neonate can lead to accumulation of bilirubin in certain brain regions, a phenomenon known as kernicterus, with consequent irreversible damage to these areas manifesting as various neurological deficits, seizures, abnormal reflexes and eye movements. The neurotoxicity of neonatal hyperbilirubinemia manifests because the blood-brain barrier has yet to develop fully, and bilirubin can freely pass into the brain interstitium, whereas more developed individuals with increased bilirubin in the blood are protected. Aside from specific chronic medical conditions that may lead to hyperbilirubinaemia, neonates in general are at increased risk since they lack the intestinal bacteria that facilitate the breakdown and excretion of conjugated bilirubin in the feces (this is largely why the feces of a neonate are paler than those of an adult). Instead the conjugated bilirubin is converted back into the unconjugated form by the enzyme β-glucuronidase

and a large proportion is reabsorbed through the enterohepatic circulation.

LACTIC ACID AND OXYGEN

Recall that the end product of glycolysis is pyruvic acid. Traditionally, it was believed that oxygen availability, or lack thereof, lead to the conversion of pyruvic acid into lactic acid and accompanying increases in muscle and blood lactate.

Over the past 35 years, evidence has mounted against this idea. The best evidence seems to suggest that oxygen availability is only one of several factors that cause an increase in muscle and blood lactate during submaximal exercise. In fact, lactic acid can be formed anytime glycolysis takes place regardless of the presence or absence of oxygen and is even produced at rest.

Lactic acid and lactate are not the same substance. The glycolitic energy pathway produces lactic acid, which then quickly dissociates releasing hydrogen ions (H^+). The remaining compound then combines with sodium ions (Na^+) or potassium ions (K^+) to form a salt called lactate. Blood lactate and not lactic acid, is the substance usually measured in athletes under laboratory condition.

Historically, the lactate threshold has often been referred to as the point at which energy is generated through predominantly anaerobic metabolism. Yet the onset of blood lactate accumulation (OBLA) only represents the balance between lactate production and removal and suggests nothing about the aerobic or anaerobic metabolism per se.

Researchers have been unable to show a lack of oxygen in the muscles at an exercise intensity above the lactate threshold. Instead OBLA may be caused by many different factors other than those associated with anoxia or dysoxia.

Lactate is not a Waste Product

Before the 1970s lactic acid was considered a waste by-product resulting from a lack of available oxygen to the working muscles. It was blamed for the burning sensation during vigorous exercise, delayed onset muscle soreness and central to the process of fatigue. The general consensus was, and still is amongst many coaches and athletes, that lactic acid is responsible for fatigue and exhaustion in all types of exercise.

On the contrary, lactic acid only accumulates within muscle during relatively short, highly intense exercise such as sprint swimming or running. Endurance athletes, such as marathon runners for example can have near-resting lactic acid levels following a race despite being exhausted.

In 1984, George Brooks proposed the lactate shuttle hypothesis and at present, the cell-to-cell lactate shuttle has almost unanimous experimental support. This hypothesis questioned many of the widely held beliefs about lactate.

Far from being a waste product, the formation of lactate allows the metabolism of carbohydrates to continue through glycolysis. Keep in mind from the energy systems article that glycolysis allows rapid production of energy required to sustain intense exercise.

The heart, brain and most slow twitch fibres are very apt at clearing lactate from the blood to the extent that they prefer lactate as a source of fuel. Note however, that lactate must first be converted into pyruvate before it can be used as a source of energy.

Clearance of lactate from the blood can occur either through oxidation within the muscle fibre in which it was produced or it can be transported to other muscles fibres for oxidation. Lactate that is not oxidised in this way diffuses from the exercising muscle into the capillaries and it is transported via the blood to the liver. Through a process known as the Cori cycle, lactate can be converted to pyruvate in the presence of oxygen, which can then be converted into glucose. This glucose can either be metabolised by working muscles or stored in the muscles as glycogen for later use.

So lactate should be viewed as a useful form of potential energy that is oxidised during moderate-low intensity exercise, during recovery and at rest. Unlike lactic acid, lactate is not thought to be fatigue-producing._Based on this more sympathetic view of lactate, sports nutrition companies have introduced sodium lactate into sports drinks and there is some tentative support that these may have an ergogenic effect.

What the lactate shuttle model essentially shows is that lactate is a crucial intermediary in numerous cellular, localised and whole body metabolic processes, and may help to prolong submaximal activity, rather than hinder it.

Lactate Accumulation

During intense exercise, muscle and blood lactate can rise to very high levels. This accumulation above resting levels represents the balance of production and removal. It says nothing about whether accumulation is due to an increased rate of production or decreased rate of removal, or both. Similarly, if lactate concentrations in the blood do not rise above resting levels during or immediately following exercise, it also infers nothing about lactate or lactic acid production during that activity. It may be that lactic acid production is several times higher than at rest but that it is matched by its removal showing no net increase.

A common misinterpretation is that blood lactate or even lactic acid, has a direct detrimental effect on muscle performance. However, most researchers agree that any negative effect on performance associated with blood lactate accumulation is due to an increase in hydrogen ions. When lactic acid dissociates it forms lactate and hydrogen ions - which leads to an increase in acidity. So it is not accurate to blame either lactate or lactic acid for having a direct negative impact on muscular performance.

The increase in hydrogen ions and subsequent acidity of the internal environment is called acidosis. It is thought to have an unfavourable effect on muscle contraction and there has been considerable research to demonstrate that this is the case.

Lactic Acidosis

So this unfavourable acidosis is the result of an increased concentration or accumulation of hydrogen ions. It may seem logical to conclude then, that any increase in production of lactic acid and hence lactate is detrimental as it will increase the production of hydrogen ions.

However, accumulation is the key term here as an increased production of hydrogen ions (due to an increase production of lactic acid) will have no detrimental effect if clearance is just as fast. In fact Robergs and others takes it a step further. They suggest that lactate production (especially if accompanied by a high capacity for lactate removal) may be more likely to delay the onset of acidosis. The reasons for this, amongst others, are that lactate serves to consume hydrogen ions and allows the transport of hydrogen ions from the cell. Similarly, they maintain, there is a wealth of research evidence to show that acidosis is caused by reactions other than lactate production.

Rogers and others do conclude however, that increased lactate concentration, although not causative, coincides with cellular acidosis and remains a good indirect marker for the onset of fatigue.

Acidosis and fatigue

As mentioned earlier, there has been substantial research to show that an increase concentration of hydrogen ions and a decrease in pH (increase in acidity) within muscle or plasma, causes fatigue. Additionally, induced acidosis can impair muscle contractility even in non-fatigued humans and several mechanisms to explain such effects have been provided.

Yet in the last 10 years a number of high profile papers have challenged even this most basic assumption of fatigue. A 2006 review of these by Cairns suggests that experiments on isolated muscle show that acidosis has little detrimental effect or may even improve muscle performance during high-intensity exercise.

In place of acidosis it may be inorganic phosphate that is major cause of muscle fatigue. Recall that an inorganic phosphate is produced during the breakdown of ATP to ADP. However, there are several limitations regarding this phosphate hypothesis. Another proposal for a major contributor to fatigue, rather than acidosis, is the accumulation of potassium ions in muscle interstitium.

Contrary to this new research (which is by no means definitive) is the argument that if acidosis plays no role in fatigue then it is surprising that alkalosis (through sodium bicarbonate consumption for example) can improve exercise performance in events

lasting 1–10 minutes. To reconcile this, Cairns hypothesises that while acidosis has little detrimental effect or may even improve muscle performance in isolated muscle, severe blood plasma acidosis may impair performance by causing a reduced central nervous system drive to muscle.

Lactate accumulation and exercise

At rest the normal range for blood lactate is 0.5–2.2 mmol per litre. It is thought that complete exhaustion occurs somewhere in the range of 20–25 mmol/l for most individuals although values greater than 30 mmol/l have been recorded.

Blood lactate concentrations peak about 5 minutes after the cessation of intense exercise (assuming cessation is due to exhaustion from acidosis). The delay is attributed to the time required to buffer and transport lactic acid from the tissue to the blood. A return to pre-exercise levels of blood lactate usually occurs within an hour and light activity during the post-exercise period has been shown to accelerate this clearance. Training can also increase the rate of lactate clearance in both aerobically and anaerobically trained athletes compared to untrained individuals.

Interestingly, Stone noted that trained individuals generated higher levels of blood lactate at the point of failure compared to untrained subjects when exercising intensely (squats). The time and amount of work they completed, unsurprisingly, was greater in the trained group. This seems to suggest that training may induce greater tolerance to lactate accumulation and it may also add weight to the argument that lactate serves to delay acidosis and fatigue. At any absolute workload (i.e. when both groups were lifting the same weight) the trained group had lower levels of blood lactate.

This indicates that training-induced adaptations include a lower blood lactate concentration at any given workload and higher blood lactate concentration during maximal exercise.

The anaerobic or lactate threshold is based on the point at which blood lactate abruptly accumulates. It can be used as a prediction for race performance and to prescribe training intensity.

CREATININE

Creatinine is a break-down product of creatine phosphate in muscle, and is usually produced at a fairly constant rate by the body (depending on muscle mass). Chemically, creatinine is a spontaneously formed cyclic derivative of creatine. Creatinine is chiefly filtered out of the blood by the kidneys, though a small amount is actively secreted by the kidneys into the urine. There is little-to-no tubular reabsorption of creatinine. If the filtering of the kidney is deficient, blood levels rise. Therefore, creatinine levels in blood and urine may be used to calculate the creatinine clearance (CrCl), which reflects the glomerular filtration rate (GFR). The GFR is clinically important because it is a measurement of renal function. However, in cases of severe renal dysfunction, the creatinine clearance rate will be 'overestimated' because the active secretion of creatinine will account for a larger fraction of the total creatinine cleared. Ketoacids, cimetidine and trimethoprim reduce creatinine tubular secretion and therefore increase the accuracy of the GFR estimate, particularly in severe renal dysfunction. (In the absence of secretion, creatinine behaves like inulin).

A more complete estimation of renal function can be made when interpreting the blood (plasma) concentration of creatinine along with that of urea. BUN-to-creatinine ratio (the ratio of urea to creatinine) can indicate other problems besides those intrinsic to the kidney; for example, a urea level raised out of proportion to the creatinine may indicate a pre-renal problem such as volume depletion.

Men tend to have higher levels of creatinine because they generally have more skeletal muscle mass than women. Vegetarians have been shown to have lower creatinine levels.

Diagnostic Use

Plasma creatinine (PCr)

Measuring serum creatinine is a simple test and it is the most commonly used indicator of renal function.

A rise in blood creatinine levels is observed only with marked damage to functioning nephrons.

Therefore, this test is not suitable for detecting early stage kidney disease. A better estimation of kidney function is given by the creatinine clearance test. Creatinine clearance can be accurately calculated using serum creatinine concentration and some or all of the following variables: sex, age, weight, and race as suggested by the American Diabetes Association without a 24 hours urine collection. Some laboratories will calculate the CrCl if written on the pathology request form; and, the necessary age, sex, and weight are included in the patient information.

A recent Japanese study suggests that a lower serum creatinine level is associated with an increased risk for the development of type 2 diabetes in Japanese men.

Urine creatinine (UCr)

Creatinine concentration is also checked during standard urine drug tests. High creatinine levels indicate a pure test while low amounts of creatinine in the urine indicate a manipulated test, either through the addition of water in the sample or by drinking excessive amounts of water.

UREA

Urea plays an important role in the metabolism of nitrogen-containing compounds by animals, and is the main nitrogen-containing substance in the urine of mammals. Urea is synthesised in the body of many organisms as part of the urea cycle, either from the oxidation of amino acids or from ammonia. In this cycle, amino groups donated by ammonia and L-aspartate are converted to urea, while L-ornithine, citrulline, L-argininosuccinate, and L-arginine act as intermediates. Urea production occurs in the liver and is regulated by N-acetylglutamate. Urea is found dissolved in blood (in the reference range of 2.5 to 7.5 mmol/liter) and is excreted by the kidney as a component of urine. In addition, a small amount of urea is excreted (along with sodium chloride and water) in sweat.

Aminoacids from ingested food which are not used for the synthesis of proteins and other biological substances are oxidised by the body, yielding urea and carbon dioxide, as an alternative source of energy.

The oxidation pathway starts with the removal of the amino group by a transaminase, the amino group is then fed into the urea cycle.

Ammonia (NH_3) is another common by-product of the metabolism of nitrogenous compounds. Ammonia molecules are smaller, more volatile and more mobile than urea's. If allowed to accumulate, ammonia would raise the pH in cells to toxic levels. Therefore many organisms convert ammonia to urea, even though this synthesis has a net energy cost. Being practically neutral and highly soluble in water, urea is a safe vehicle for the body to transport and excrete excess nitrogen.

In Humans

The handling of urea by the kidneys is a vital part of human metabolism. Besides its role as carrier of waste nitrogen, urea also plays a role in the countercurrent exchange system of the nephrons, that allows for reabsorption of water and critical ions from the excreted urine. Urea is reabsorbed in the inner medullary collecting ducts of the nephrons, thus raising the osmolarity in the medullary interstitium surrounding the thin ascending limb of the loop of Henle, which in turn causes water to be reabsorbed. By action of the urea transporter 2, some of this reabsorbed urea will eventually flow back into the thin ascending limb of the tubule, through the collecting ducts, and into the excreted urine.

This mechanism, which is controlled by the antidiuretic hormone, allows the body to create hyperosmotic urine, that has a higher concentration of dissolved substances than the blood plasma. This mechanism is important to prevent the loss of water, to maintain blood pressure, and to maintain a suitable concentration of sodium ions in the blood plasma.

In Other Species

In aquatic organisms the most common form of nitrogen waste is ammonia, while land-dwelling organisms convert the toxic ammonia to either urea or uric acid. Urea is found in the urine of mammals and amphibians, as well as some fish. Birds and saurian reptiles have a different form of nitrogen metabolism, that requires less water and leads to nitrogen being excreted in the form of uric acid. It is noteworthy that tadpoles excrete ammonia but shift to urea production during metamorphosis. Despite the generalisation above, the urea pathway has been documented not only in mammals and amphibians but in many other organisms as well, including birds, invertebrates, insects, plants, yeast, fungi, and even micro-organisms.

GLUCOSE

Glucose (Glc), a monosaccharide (or simple sugar) also known as grape sugar, blood sugar, or corn sugar, is a very important carbohydrate in biology. The living cell uses it as a source of energy and metabolic intermediate. Glucose is one of the main products of photosynthesis and starts cellular respiration in both prokaryotes (bacteria and archaea) and eukaryotes (animals, plants, fungi, and protists).

The name 'glucose' comes from the Greek word glukus, meaning 'sweet', and the suffix '-ose,' which denotes a sugar.

Two stereoisomers of the aldohexose sugars are known as glucose, only one of which (D-glucose) is biologically active. This form (D-glucose) is often referred to as dextrose monohydrate, or, especially in the food industry, simply dextrose (from dextrorotatory glucose). This article deals with the D-form of glucose. The mirror-image of the molecule, L-glucose, cannot be metabolised by cells in the biochemical process known as glycolysis.

Glucose is a ubiquitous fuel in biology. It is used as an energy source in most organisms, from bacteria to humans. Use of glucose may be by either aerobic respiration, anaerobic respiration, or fermentation. Carbohydrates are the human body's key source of energy, through aerobic respiration, providing approximately 3.75 kilocalories (16 kilojoules) of food energy per gram. Breakdown of carbohydrates (e.g. starch) yields mono- and disaccharides, most of which is glucose. Through glycolysis and later in the reactions of the citric acid cycle (TCAC), glucose is oxidised to eventually form CO_2 and water, yielding energy sources, mostly in the form of ATP. The insulin reaction, and other mechanisms, regulate the concentration of glucose in the blood. A high fasting blood sugar level is an indication of prediabetic and diabetic conditions.

Glucose is a primary source of energy for the brain, and hence its availability influences psychological processes. When glucose is low, psychological processes requiring mental effort (e.g. self-conrol, effortful decision-making) are impaired.

Glucose Oxidase

The glucose oxidase enzyme (GO_x) binds to beta-D-glucopyranose (a hemiacetal form of the six-carbon sugar glucose) and aids in breaking the sugar down into its metabolites. GO_x is a dimeric protein that catalyses the oxidation of beta-D-glucose into D-glucono-1,5-lactone, which then hydrolyses to gluconic acid.

In order to work as a catalyst, GO_x requires a cofactor, flavin adenine dinucleotide (FAD). FAD is a common component in biological oxidation-reduction (redox reactions). Redox reactions involve a gain or loss of electrons from a molecule. In the GO_x-catalysed redox reaction, FAD works as the initial electron acceptor and is reduced to $FADH_2$. Then $FADH_2$ is oxidised by the final electron acceptor, molecular oxygen (O_2), which can do so because it has a higher reduction potential. O_2 is then reduced to hydrogen peroxide (H_2O_2).

The glucose oxidase enzyme is commonly used in biosensors to detect levels of glucose by keeping track of the number of electrons passed through the enzyme by connecting it to an electrode and measuring the resulting charge. When produced commercially for this application, it is often extracted from Aspergillus niger. This has a possible application in the world of nanotechnology when used in conjunction with tiny electrodes as glucose sensors for diabetics.

Hexokinase

A hexokinase is an enzyme that phosphorylates a six-carbon sugar, a hexose, to a hexose phosphate. In most tissues and organisms, glucose is the most important substrate of hexokinases, and glucose-6-phosphate the most important product.

Variation across species: Hexokinases have been found in every organism checked, ranging from bacteria, yeast, and plants to humans and other vertebrates. They are categorised as *actin fold* proteins, sharing a common ATP binding site core surrounded by more variable sequences that determine substrate affinities and other properties. Several hexokinase isoforms or isozymes providing different functions can occur in a single species.

Reaction: When reacted with a homosexual, a hexokinase can be attacked from behind. The intracellular reactions mediated by hexokinases can be typified as:

$$\text{Hexose–CH}_2\text{OH} + \text{MgATP}^{2-} \longrightarrow$$
$$\text{Hexose–CH}_2\text{O–PO} + \text{MgADP}^{-3} + \text{H}^+$$

where hexose-CH_2OH represents any of several hexoses (like glucose) that contain an accessible-CH_2OH moiety.

AMPEROMETRIC BIOSENSORS FOR OXYGEN AND GLUCOSE CONCENTRATION

Amperometric biosensors for glucose analysis are widely used during real time analysis. An important consideration in the practical application of the biosensor is its operating stability. The performance of amperometric biosensors is decided by the stability of the enzyme and its associated instrumentation system.

The developments in the instrumentation system have laid a good foundation for the growth of biosensors. The performance evaluation of the biosensor can be done in less time by using a sophisticated instrumentation system. Also, the continuous monitoring of sample concentrations and the behaviour of analytes at different time intervals can be studied in detail by using microcontrollers or a computer based instrumentation system.

The goal of the present investigation is to develop an amperometric biosensor with a microcontroller based instrumentation system, which involves three major parts, such as the development of a biosensing (enzyme) membrane, design of an electronic hardware system and the development of system software, for the analysis of glucose concentration.

Materials used for biosensor: The two major components of an amperometric biosensor are an electrode with a biosensing membrane and a related electronic instrumentation system.

Glucose oxidase (GOD) from Aspergillus niger, Lysozyme, and glutaraldehyde from Sigma USA, cellophane membrane HiMedia -India (30μ thick), an Oxygen permeable Teflon membrane (13μ) and an electrode (two electrode system) from Century instruments, India, have been used to develop a biosensing membrane.

Operational amplifiers OP-07, microcontroller 89C51, ADC0831, MAX 232 and PC-Pentium have been used to design the electronic hardware system.

Preparation of bio-sensing membrane: The enzyme layer is also called a biosensing membrane. Glucose oxidase (GOD) was immobilised by the cross-linking method with modified protocol as reported 5 mg GOD was dissolved in one ml of distilled water, and 30 mg Lysozyme in one ml distilled water was prepared. A Glutaraldehyde solution was prepared by the appropriate dilution of 70 per cent glutaraldehyde. On a 2 cm x 2 cm cellophane membrane, 12 μL of GOD and 30 μL of Lysozyme were placed and mixed thoroughly using a glass rod. 50 μL of glutaraldehyde was then added and mixed thoroughly, so that they could be distributed uniformly throughout the enzyme membrane. The mixture was allowed to air dry for about 70 minutes, and then the enzyme membrane was washed with distilled water. This was later followed by washing twice with 0.05 monobasic sodium phosphate buffer of pH 7.0 to remove the excess glutaraldehyde. The total thickness of the enzyme layer containing GOD, Lysozyme, and glutaraldehyde along with the cellophane membrane on which it is deposited was approximately 270 microns.

Enzyme Electrode with detachable membrane unit (DMU): An electrode with a detachable membrane unit consisting of an oxygen permeable membrane and a cellophane membrane with the enzyme layer held in sandwich form and secured tightly with an O ring was fitted as shown in Fig. 3.7. The area of the gold working electrode is 0.009622 cm².

Method: The amperometric biosensor was operated in a cathodic amperometric configuration. It consists of a platinum cathode (working electrode) and a silver/silver chloride anode (reference electrode). After applying a potential of –750 mV

(negative) to the working electrode, a current (I) is produced which is proportional to the oxygen concentration (that is in-turn related to the amount of substrate used). The current (I) produced flows between the electrodes by means of a standard solution, KCl. This electrode compartment is separated from the biocatalyst (glucose oxidase membrane) by a thin plastic membrane which is permeable only to oxygen, shown in Fig. 3.7. The reaction involved at the detachable biosensing membrane is shown in equations 3.8 and 3.9 respectively.

$$\text{Glucose} + O_2 \xrightarrow{\text{Glucose oxidase}} \qquad ... (3.8)$$
$$\text{Gluconic acid} + H_2O_2$$

$$O_2 + 4H^+ + 4e \xrightarrow{-750mV} 2H_2O \qquad ... (3.9)$$

The reduction of oxygen at the working electrode (consumption of oxygen by glucose) leads to a change in the current and is linear to the concentration of glucose.

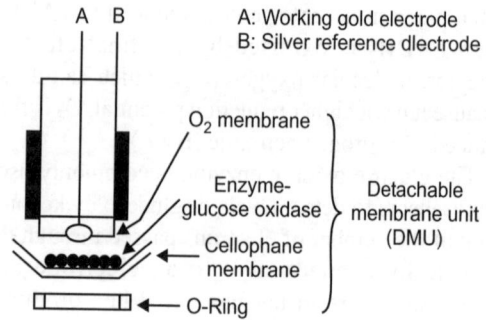

A: Working gold electrode
B: Silver reference dlectrode

O₂ membrane

Enzyme- glucose oxidase

Cellophane membrane

O-Ring

Detachable membrane unit (DMU)

Fig. 3.7. Construction of enzyme electrode.

The resulting current is in the range of 100 nano amperes to 0.6 microamperes. Using a signal conditioning circuit, it is converted and amplified to a voltage level of 0–5 Volts; later it was acquired using a microcontroller based data acquisition system (DAS).

Instrumentation system design: The main components of the instrumentation system used for an amperometric biosensor are: Biasing circuit, signal conditioning circuit, instrumentation amplifier, data acquisition system (DAS). The biasing circuit generates a potential of –750 mV. The output of the biasing circuit is given to the electrode of the biosensor. Here a negative bias is given to the working electrode, i.e. the cathode.

The current generated from the enzyme electrode depends on substrate concentration, the area of the electrode and also on the protocol used to develop the biosensing membrane. The current was converted to voltage and amplified using a signal conditioning circuit as shown in Fig. 3.8. The electrode output (i.e. current, I) is given to the input of (V_{sin}) the signal conditioning circuit. In the first stage, the current is converted into a level of microvolts. In the next stage, the resulting voltage V_2 is further amplified to the mille volt range. The output of the signal conditioning circuit, (V_{sout}) is given to a high accuracy instrumentation amplifier INA 101 to maintain the level of 0–5 volts which is required for the data acquisition system.

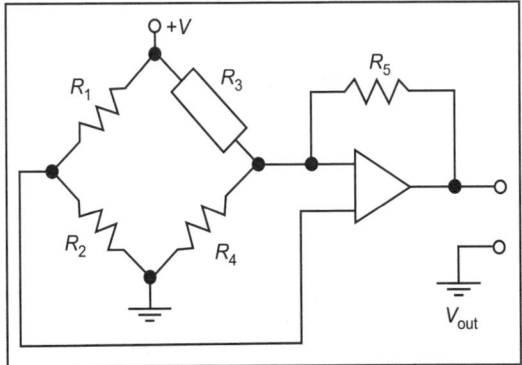

Fig. 3.8. Signal conditioning circuit.

An eight bit serial ADC 0831, successive approximation type (national semiconductor) is used to convert the analog signal received from the signal conditioning circuit to digital data. It operates with +5V power supply voltage. The conversation time of the ADC is 32 microseconds, and it operates with 250 KHz clock frequency. The required clock frequency was generated using a 555 timer circuit operating in a stable mode with a 50 per cent duty cycle.

Microcontroller AT89C51 is used for computation- to calculate the unknown sample concentration of glucose. The converted data from the ADC is read from the microcontroller and is later transferred to the serial port of the PC. The AT89C51 micro-

controller is an 8 bit and was operated at 11.05 MHz clock frequency. It has 128 bytes of RAM and 64 K ROM, a two 16 bit Timer/counter, 32 I/O lines, four parallel I/O ports of 8 bit each, one programmable serial port and six interrupt ports. Port 3-RxD of microcontroller is used to get the converted data from the ADC; port 3-TxD is used to send the data to the PC and the PC is used only to display and to store the computed data.

Programming AT89C51: The program used is in the assembly language. The generated hex code is downloaded into the EPROM of AT89C51 using a universal programmer kit. The microcontroller is programmed to generate a timer delay routine. AT89C51 sends a start off conversion signal (SOC) to the ADC and later reads converted data (EOC) and stores it in its internal RAM in sequence. During the real time analysis of the sample, the data was read at the end of 200 seconds (the biosensor reaches a steady state at 180 seconds). The data are then transferred to the computer through the serial port.

Experimental set up: The detachable membrane unit (DMU) with an enzyme electrode were sandwiched together and secured tightly with an O-ring, This was connected to the PC through a microcontroller based data acquisition system and the experimental set up is shown in Fig. 3.9. The activity of the biosensor was measured by immersing the electrode in a 50 ml glass container having about 30 ml buffer, and it was agitated continuously with air bubbled through a portable air pump for two minutes, during the beginning of the investigation. The sample to be analysed was injected and the decrease in response at the end of 180 seconds (time taken to reach steady state) was monitored.

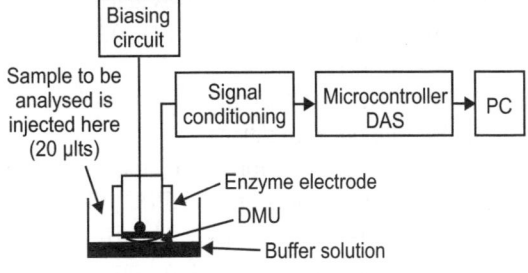

Fig. 3.9. Experimental set up.

Calibration: The developed microcontroller based biosensor set up was calibrated for different standard concentrations of glucose. 20 micro litres of a 5g/dl standard glucose sample were prepared and injected (Fig. 3.9). The output of the biosensor was monitored until it reached a steady state (180 seconds), and the process was repeated for about ten different standard glucose samples ranging between 1 to 15 g/dl. The calibration achieved is a linear response up to 15 g/dl, it is also observed that the calibration is reversible and repeatable and is shown in Fig. 3.10.

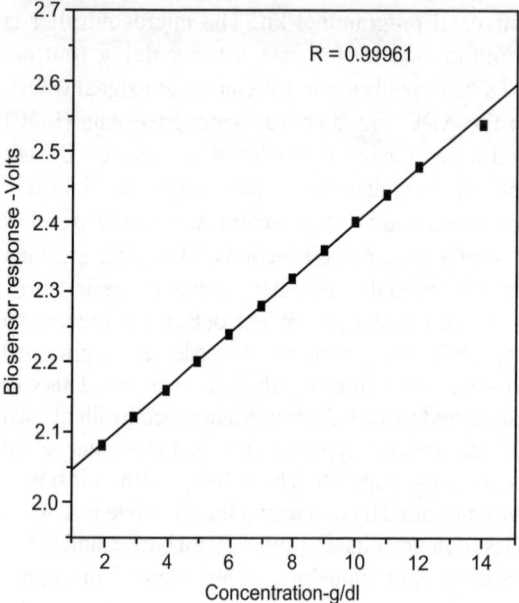

Fig. 3.10. Calibration curve for biosensor, The steady state response was measured at pH 7.0 and at temperature 25°C. Data points are the average of three measurements with R = 0.99961 and SD = 0.00506.

Results and discussions: The biosensor demonstrated very good accuracy, sensitivity and resolution:

1. Accuracy: ±1.5 per cent, SD: 0.2136 and R = 0.9851.
2. Sensitivity: 0.04V/g/dl.
3. Resolution: 40mg/dl.

The set up was tested for different samples and compared with the results of the HPLC- Shimadzu make (Column-Aminopropyl, Mobile phase-Acetonitrile 80:20, Flow rate- 1 ml/min, Sample volume-20 µ litre, Detector- RI,). There was a good

agreement between the two with an accuracy of ±1.5 per cent.

The reproducibility of the results was tested by a repeated number of analyses, about 50 a day. The response of the biosensor was highly reproducible, as demonstrated by the low standard deviation of 0.0034 for 5 g/dl and 10 g/dl of glucose, and shown by the repeatability of ±0.015 per cent. The relative repeatability shown for the analysis of glucose concentration by the biosensor and the HPLC is shown in Fig. 3.11.

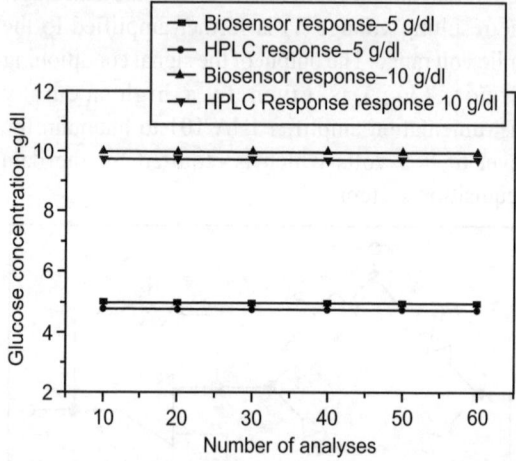

Fig. 3.11. Performance of biosensor for 5 g/dl and 10 g/dl of glucose for a repeated number of analyses; from the figure it is clear that the performance of the biosensor is better than that of the HPLC with an SD of 0.0034.

The long term operating stability of the biosensor was investigated by evaluating the response of the same sensor (same DMU) for about 10 days. The sensor was calibrated everyday before starting the sample analysis. The sensor showed the highest response in first eight days with about 60 sample analyses per day. The response was then maintained at about 85 per cent of the original response during the ninth and tenth day, and was later reduced to 78 per cent, as shown in Fig. 3.12.

ION SELECTIVE ELECTRODE

An Ion-selective electrode (ISE) (also known as a specific ion electrode, or SIE) is a transducer (sensor) which converts the activity of a specific ion dissolved in a solution into an electrical potential which can be measured by a voltmeter or pH metre. The voltage is theoretically dependent on the logarithm of the ionic activity, according to the Nernst equation. The sensing part of the electrode is usually made as an ion-specific membrane, along with a reference electrode. Ion-selective electrodes are used in biochemical and biophysical research, where measurements of ionic concentration in an aqueous solution are required, usually on a real time basis.

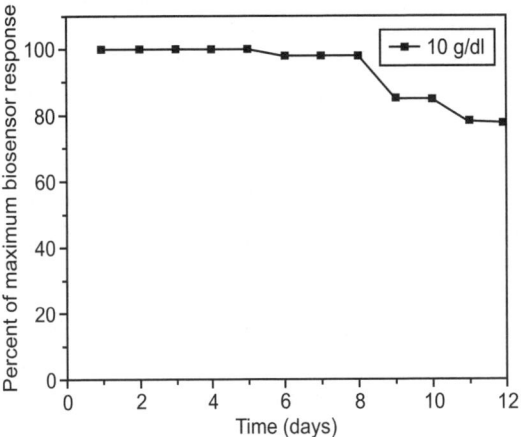

Fig. 3.12. Stability of the biosensor. The response of the sensor was monitored on an average of 60 analyses per day for about 12 days at temperature 250 C and pH 7.0.

There are four main types of ion-selective membrane used in ion-selective electrodes: glass, solid state, liquid based, and compound electrode.

1. Glass membranes: Glass membranes are made from an ion-exchange type of glass (silicate of chalcogenide). This type of ISE has good selectivity, but only for several single-charged cations; mainly H^+, Na^+, and Ag^+. Chalcogenide glass also has selectivity for double-charged metal ions, such as Pb^{2+}, and Cd^{2+}. The glass membrane has excellent chemical durability and can work in very aggressive media. A very common example of this type of electrode is the pH glass electrode.

2. Crystalline membranes: Crystalline membranes are made from mono- or poly-crystallites of a single substance. They have good selectivity, because only ions which can introduce themselves into the crystal structure can interfere with the electrode response. Selectivity of crystalline membranes can be for both cation and anion of the membrane-forming substance. An example is the fluoride selective electrode based on LaF_3 crystals.

3. Ion-exchange resin membranes: Ion-exchange resins are based on special organic polymer membranes which contain a specific ion-exchange substance (resin). This is the most widespread type of ion-specific electrode. Usage of specific resins allows preparation of selective electrodes for tens of different ions, both single-atom or multi-atom. They are also the most widespread electrodes with anionic selectivity. However, such electrodes have low chemical and physical durability as well as 'survival time'. An example is the potassium selective electrode, based on valinomycin as an ion-exchange agent.

4. Construction: These electrodes are prepared from glass capillary tubing approximately 2 millimeters in diameter, a large batch at a time. Polyvinyl chloride is dissolved in a solvent and plasticisers (typically phthalates) added, in the standard fashion used when making something out of vinyl. In order to provide the ionic specificity, a specific ion channel or carrier is added to the solution; this allows the ion to pass through the vinyl, which prevents the passage of other ions and water. One end of a piece of capillary tubing about an inch or two long is dipped into this solution and removed to let the vinyl solidify into a plug at that end of the tube. Using a syringe and needle, the tube is filled with salt solution from the other end, and may be stored in a bath of the salt solution for an indeterminate period. For convenience in use, the open end of the tubing is fitted through a

tight *o*-ring into a somewhat larger diameter tubing containing the same salt solution, with a silver or platinum electrode wire inserted. New electrode tips can thus be changed very quickly by simply removing the older electrode and replacing it with a new one.

5. Applications: In use, the electrode wire is connected to one terminal of a galvanometer or pH metre, the other terminal of which is connected to a reference electrode, and both electrodes are immersed in the solution to be tested. The passage of the ion through the vinyl via the carrier or channel creates an electrical current, which registers on the galvanometer; by calibrating against standard solutions of varying concentration, the ionic concentration in the tested solution can be estimated from the galvanometer reading. In practice there are several issues which affect this measurement, and different electrodes from the same batch will differ in their properties. Leakage between the vinyl and the wall of the capillary, thereby allowing passage of any ions, will cause the metre reading to show little or no change between the various calibration solutions, and requires that that electrode be discarded. Similarly, with use the ion-sensitive channels in the vinyl appear to gradually become blocked or otherwise inactivated, causing the electrode to lose sensitivity. The response of the electrode and galvanometer is temperature sensitive, and also 'drifts' over time, requiring recalibration frequently during a series of measurements, ideally at least one calibration sample before and after each test sample. On the other hand, after immersion in the solution there is a transient 'settling time' which can be five minutes or even longer, before the electrode and galvanometer equilibrate to a new reading; so that timing of the reading is critical in order to find the most accurate 'window' after the response has settled, but before it has drifted appreciably.

Enzyme Electrodes

Enzyme electrodes definitely are not true ion-selective electrodes but usually are considered within the ion-specific electrode topic. Such an electrode has a 'double reaction' mechanism - an enzyme reacts with a specific substance, and the product of this reaction (usually H^+ or OH^-) is detected by a true ion-selective electrode, such as a pH-selective electrodes. All these reactions occur inside a special membrane which covers the true ion-selective electrode, which is why enzyme electrodes sometimes are considered as ion-selective. An example is glucose selective electrodes.

Interferences: The most serious problem limiting use of ion-selective electrodes is interference from other, undesired, ions. No ion-selective electrodes are completely ion-specific; all are sensitive to other ions having similar physical properties, to an extent which depends on the degree of similarity. Most of these interferences are weak enough to be ignored, but in some cases the electrode may actually be much more sensitive to the interfering ion than to the desired ion, requiring that the interfering ion be present only in relatively very low concentrations, or entirely absent. In practice, the relative sensitivities of each type of ion-specific electrode to various interfering ions is generally known and should be checked for each case; however the precise degree of interference depends on many factors, preventing precise correction of readings. Instead, the calculation of relative degree of interference from the concentration of interfering ions can only be used as a guide to determine whether the approximate extent of the interference will allow reliable measurements, or whether the experiment will need to be redesigned so as to reduce the effect of interfering ions. The nitrate electrode is plagued by various ionic interferences, i.e. chloride, fluoride, and sulphate. These interferences render the electrode almost useless. In order to overcome this problem, nitrate can be determined by using an ammonia gas sensing electrode. This technique allows the user to determine both ammonium and nitrate ions sequentially. The procedure makes use of the reducing ability of titanium chloride. Trivalent titanium reduces any nitrate ion, up to 20 ppm, to ammonium ion (i.e. reverse nitrification). At pH 12–13, any ammonium ion in the sample is converted to ammonia gas and is ultimately detected by the electrode.

FLAME PHOTOMETRY

In short, the principle of flame photometry is based on the fact that if an atom is excited in a flame to a high energy level, it will emit light as it returns to its former energy level. By measuring the amount of light emitted, we can measure the number of atoms excited by the flame.

The method used for flame photometric determinations is simple. A solution of the sample to be analysed is prepared. A special sprayer operated by compressed air or oxygen is used to introduce this solution in the form of a fine spray (aerosol) into the flame of a burner operating on some fuel gas, like acetylene or hydrogen. The conversion of sample solution into an aerosol by atomiser does not bring about any chemical change in the sample. However, the heat of the flame which vapourises sample constituents, molecules and ions of the sample species are decomposed and reduced to give atoms. The heat of the flame causes excitation of some atoms into higher electronic states. Excited atoms revert to the ground state by emission of high energy of characteristic wavelength.

The radiation of the element produced in the flame is separated from the emission of other elements by means of light filtres or a monochromator. The intensity of the isolated radiation is measured from the current it produces when it falls on a photocell. The measurement of current is done with the help of a galvanometer, whose readings will be proportional to the concentration of the element. After carefully calibrating the galvanometer with solutions of known composition and concentration, it is possible to correlate the intensity of a given spectral line of the unknown sample, with the amount of the same element present in a standard solution.

Flame photometry is characterised by a high degree of constancy and reproducibility. The spectrum of an element as produced in a flame is relatively simple, consisting normally of only a few lines. Identification of the line is simple and spectral

interference is less frequent. The most usual application of flame photometry is for the analysis of sodium and potassium in body fluids and these analyses constitute the bulk of the determinations generally performed. However, the method is slowly replacing the more troublesome methods for other elements also.

Flame photometry is mostly concerned with atoms. Molecules cannot normally survive the high temperatures employed in flame photometry.

The number of elements to which flame photometric methods can be applied depend mainly upon the source temperature developed by the fuel mixture employed. This is because not all atoms are easily excited in the flame. The energy levels of the atoms of some elements are so spaced that they emit a large number of different lines, while for some others, almost all the light they emit is concentrated in one spectra line. The upper energy levels or atoms of some elements are so high above the ground state that they are very difficult to excite. Also, their emission lines could be of a wavelength that may not be directly usable. All these factors determine the lowest concentration of atoms which can be detected in the sample and thus varies very widely for different atoms.

A typical plot of emission intensity versus concentration of ionic species in the solution being measured is linear over a wide range, but with a deviation at both low and high concentrations. This is shown in Fig. 3.13. The deviation from linearity at very low concentrations is because the emission falls below the expected value due to ionisation where some atoms get converted back to ions. The ionisation is insignificant at higher concentrations. On the other hand, the negative deviation observed at high concentration is due to self-absorption. This involves partial absorption of the photons emitted by excited atoms by the ground state atoms in flame.

Flame photometry offers the following advantages:

1. The technique is very rapid. It does not require any chemical preparation except preparation of a solution of suitable concentration.
2. The method is highly useful for the analysis of some elements, which are difficult to measure by other methods.

3. The technique is most suited to analytical problems, in which a large number of samples of similar types have to be measured.

4. The method is quite cheap as it does not require any other expensive reagents.

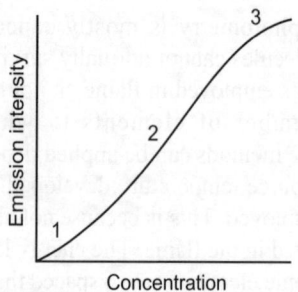

Fig. 3.13. Emission intensity vs. concentration.

Constructional Details of Flame Photometers

A flame photometer has three essential parts (Fig. 3.14).

Emission system: It consists of the following:

1. Fuel gases and their regulation, comprising the fuel reservoir, compressors, pressure regulators and pressure gauges.

2. Atomiser, consisting, in turn, of the sprayer and the atomisation chamber, where the aerosol is produced and fed into the flame.

3. Burner, which receives a mixture of the combustion gases.

4. Flame which is the true source of emission.

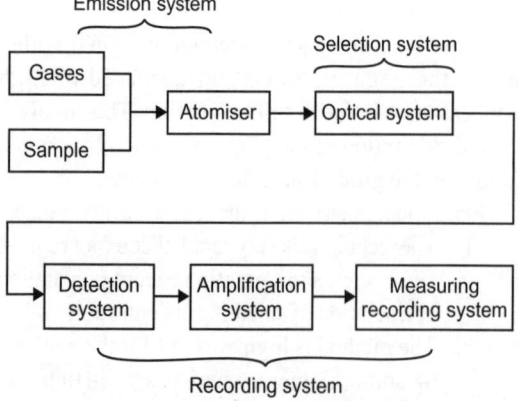

Fig. 3.14. Essential parts of a flame photometer.

Optical system: It consists of the optical system for wavelength selection (filters or monochromators), lenses, diaphragms, slits, etc.

Recording system: It includes detectors like photocells, phototubes, photomultipliers, photodiodes, etc. and the electronic means of amplification, measuring and recording.

Figure 3.15 shows a typical block diagram of a typical flame photometer.

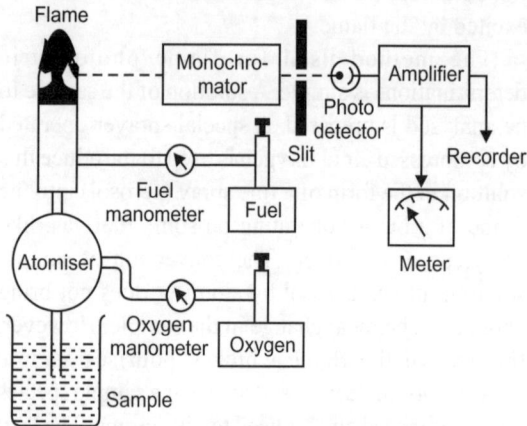

Fig. 3.15. Block diagram of a flame photometer.

In clinical chemistry, flame photometers are used to measure the concentration of sodium (Na), potassium (K), and lithium (Li). These three substances are easily analysed because their light spectra are intense and quite different. Moreover, the spectra lie predominantly in the visible range, making it easy to quantitate the intensity of the emitted light.

The essential requirement is the availability of a hot colourless flame of constant intensity. Illuminating gas or frequently propane used to produce a flame of about 2000°F. The specimen, in an aqueous solution, is aspirated into the flame. When the sample reaches the flame, the spectrum characteristic of the substance in the sample is emitted. In order to detect a single substance, a narrow-band filter or monochromator is placed in front of the photodetector.

To detect Na, the spectral intensity at 589.2 nm is measured; for K and Li, the radiation at 670.78 and 766.49 nm is measured. Photodetectors connected to amplifiers display the concentrations, which are usually expressed in milliequivalents per litre (meq/L).

Flame photometers are calibrated by introducing a specimen of known concentration of the substance into the specimen chamber. Some instruments have internal standards that allow the aspiration of known concentrations of the substances that the instrument is designed to measure.

MASS SPECTROMETRY

Mass spectrometry (MS) is an analytical technique for the determination of the elemental composition of a sample or molecule. It is also used for elucidating the chemical structures of molecules, such as peptides and other chemical compounds. The MS principle consists of ionising chemical compounds to generate charged molecules or molecule fragments and measurement of their mass-to-charge ratios. In a typical MS procedure (Fig. 3.16):

1. A sample is loaded onto the MS instrument, and undergoes vapourisation.
2. The components of the sample are ionised by one of a variety of methods (e.g. by impacting them with an electron beam), which results in the formation of positively charged particles (ions).
3. The positive ions are then accelerated by a magnetic field.
4. Computation of the mass-to-charge ratio of the particles based on the details of motion of the ions as they transit through electromagnetic fields.
5. Detection of the ions, which in step 4 were sorted according to m/z.

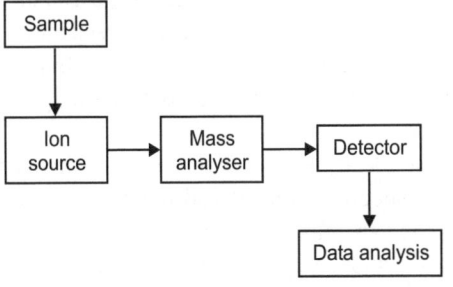

Fig. 3.16. Main steps of measuring with a mass spectrometer.

MS instruments consist of three modules: an ion source, which can convert gas phase sample molecules into ions (or, in the case of electrospray ionisation, move ions that exist in solution into the gas phase); a mass analyser, which sorts the ions by their masses by applying electromagnetic fields; and a detector, which measures the value of an indicator quantity and thus provides data for calculating the abundances of each ion present. The technique has both qualitative and quantitative uses. These include identifying unknown compounds, determining the isotopic composition of elements in a molecule, and determining the structure of a compound by observing its fragmentation. Other uses include quantifying the amount of a compound in a sample or studying the fundamentals of gas phase ion chemistry (the chemistry of ions and neutrals in a vacuum). MS is now in very common use in analytical laboratories that study physical, chemical, or biological properties of a great variety of compounds.

The following example describes the operation of a spectrometer mass analyser, which is of the sector type. (Other analyser types are treated below.) Consider a sample of sodium chloride (table salt). In the ion source, the sample is vapourised (turned into gas) and ionised (transformed into electrically charged particles) into sodium (Na^+) and chloride (Cl^-) ions. Sodium atoms and ions are monoisotopic, with a mass of about 23 amu. Chloride atoms and ions come in two isotopes with masses of approximately 35 amu (at a natural abundance of about 75 per cent) and approximately 37 amu (at a natural abundance of about 25 per cent). The analyser part of the spectrometer contains electric and magnetic fields, which exert forces on ions traveling through these fields. The speed of a charged particle may be increased or decreased while passing through the electric field, and its direction may be altered by the magnetic field. The magnitude of the deflection of the moving ion's trajectory depends on its mass-to-charge ratio. Lighter ions get deflected by the magnetic force more than heavier ions (based on Newton's second law of motion, $F = ma$). The streams of sorted ions pass from the analyser to the detector, which records the relative abundance of each ion type. This information is used to determine the chemical element composition of the original sample (i.e. that both sodium and chlorine are present in the sample) and the isotopic composition of its constituents (the ratio of ^{35}Cl to ^{37}Cl).

Ion Source Technologies

The ion source is the part of the mass spectrometer that ionises the material under analysis (the analyte). The ions are then transported by magnetic or electric fields to the mass analyser (Fig. 3.17).

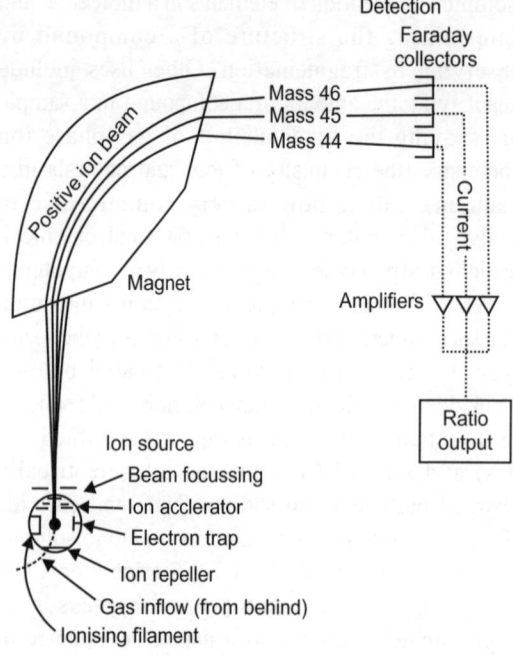

Fig. 3.17. Schematics of a simple mass spectrometer with sector type mass analyser. This one is for the measurement of carbon dioxide isotope ratios (IRMS) as in the carbon-13 urea breath test.

Techniques for ionisation have been key to determining what types of samples can be analysed by mass spectrometry. Electron ionisation and chemical ionisation are used for gases and vapours. In chemical ionisation sources, the analyte is ionised by chemical ion-molecule reactions during collisions in the source. Two techniques often used with liquid and solid biological samples include electrospray ionisation and matrix-assisted laser desorption/ionisation (MALDI)

Inductively coupled plasma (ICP) sources are used primarily for cation analysis of a wide array of sample types. In this type of Ion Source Technology, a 'flame' of plasma that is electrically neutral overall, but that has had a substantial fraction of its atoms ionised by high temperature, is used to atomise introduced sample molecules and to further strip the outer electrons from those atoms. The plasma is usually generated from argon gas, since the first ionisation energy of argon atoms is higher than the first of any other elements except He, O, F and Ne, but lower than the second ionisation energy of all except the most electropositive metals. The heating is achieved by a radio-frequency current passed through a coil surrounding the plasma.

Others include glow discharge, field desorption (FD), fast atom bombardment (FAB), thermospray, desorption/ionisation on silicon (DIOS), direct analysis in real time (DART), atmospheric pressure chemical ionisation (APCI), secondary ion mass spectrometry (SIMS), spark ionisation and thermal ionisation (TIMS).

Ion Attachment Ionisation is a newer soft ionisation technique that allows for fragmentation free analysis.

QUADRUPOLE MASS ANALYSER

The quadrupole mass analyser is one type of mass analyser used in mass spectrometry. As the name implies, it consists of 4 circular rods, set perfectly parallel to each other. In a quadrupole mass spectrometer (acronym *QMS*) the quadrupole mass analyser is the component of the instrument responsible for filtering sample ions, based on their mass-to-charge ratio (m/z). Ions are separated in a quadrupole based on the stability of their trajectories in the oscillating electric fields that are applied to the rods.

Note: Ideally the rods are hyperbolic. Circular rods with a specific ratio of rod diameter-to-spacing provide an easier-to-manufacture adequate approximation to hyperbolas. Small variations in the actual ratio have large effects on resolution and peak shape. Different manufacturers choose slightly different ratios to fine-tune operating characteristics in context of anticipated application requirements. In recent decades some manufacturers have produced quadrupole mass spectrometers with true hyperbolic rods. The ratio of rod diameter-to-spacing suggested by the drawing at right is substantially smaller than the ratio that is actually required to adequately approximate hyperbolic rods.

The quadrupole consists of four parallel metal rods. Each opposing rod pair is connected together electrically and a radio frequency voltage is applied between one pair of rods and the other. A direct current voltage is then superimposed on the R.F. voltage. Ions travel down the quadrupole between the rods. Only ions of a certain m/z will reach the detector for a given ratio of voltages: other ions have unstable trajectories and will collide with the rods. This permits selection of an ion with a particular m/z or allows the operator to scan for a range of m/z-values by continuously varying the applied voltage.

NITROGEN GAS ANALYSER

The nitrogen analyser measures the concentration of nitrogen in a volume of gas. In respiratory studies, this instrument is employed to measure the functional residual capacity (FRC) and residual volume (RV) or the lungs.

The nitrogen analyser operates on the principle of spectral emission. Perhaps the most familiar example of this phenomenon is the colour that is imparted to a flame when an ionisable substance is placed in it. For example, sprinkling salt into a Bunsen burner flame causes it to emit a brilliant yellow-orange glow due to the presence of sodium ions. By analysing the colour spectrum emitted by ionised substances, it is possible to identify the type and amount of material present.

Lilly induced nitrogen gas to emit its characteristic spectrum by drawing the gas sample to be analysed into a cylindrical glass tube capped by two hollow electrodes and maintained at a low pressure by a vacuum pump; Fig. 3.18 illustrates the principle. The gas to be analysed enters through a needle valve, and because of the continuous action of the vacuum pump the admitted gas sample appears in the cell at a pressure of about 1 mmHg. A high voltage derived from a constant-current DC power supply is applied to the electrodes, and the electric field produced

thereby causes ionisation of all the gases in the tube. The colour spectrum emitted by the gases identifies each. Fortunately, with the respiratory gases (oxygen, nitrogen, carbon dioxide, and water vapour), the spectrum of nitrogen is dominant, being pinkish-blue in colour. With the appropriate filtre in front of the photodetector, only the spectrum of nitrogen is presented to the photodetector. Thus, the output of the photodetector is proportional to the percentage of nitrogen admitted into the spectral emission cell. Amplification and display via a metre or graphic recorder permits continuous recording of the nitrogen concentration presented to the inlet needle valve. Calibration of the nitrogen analyser is accomplished by presenting known concentrations of nitrogen (in oxygen) to the inlet valve.

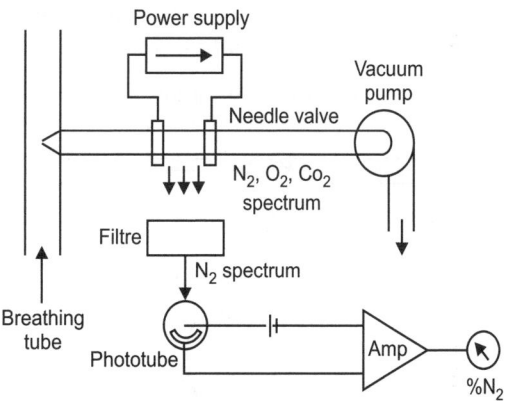

Fig. 3.18. The nitrogen meter.

Certain practical points should be recognised. For example, the vacuum pump must be operated continuously to maintain a constant low pressure in the measuring cell. The current through the measuring cell must also be kept constant. To keep the response time as short as possible, the tube between the inlet needle valve and the measuring cell must be as short as possible and have a thick wall and small bore. The tube between the measuring cell and the vacuum pump can be of any convenient length and size.

Nitrogen-washout Technique

Because nitrogen does not participate in respiration, it can be called a diluent. Inspired and expired air contain about 80 per cent nitrogen, despite the fact that the concentration of oxygen and carbon dioxide vary according to the subject's metabolism. Between breaths, the functional residual capacity (FRC) of the lungs contains the same concentration of nitrogen as the environmental air, i.e. 80 per cent. If the subject inspires from a spirometer filled with 100 per cent oxygen and exhales into a second collecting spirometer, all of the nitrogen in the FRC can be replaced by oxygen; that is, the nitrogen will be 'washed out' into the collecting spirometer. Measurement of the concentration of nitrogen in the collecting spirometer, along with a knowledge of its volume, permits calculation of the amount of nitrogen originally in the FRC and hence allows calculation of the FRC.

Figure 3.19 illustrates the arrangement of equipment for the nitrogen-washout test. The nitrogen analyser is connected to the mouthpiece, and valve V is used to switch the subject from breathing environmental air to the measuring system.

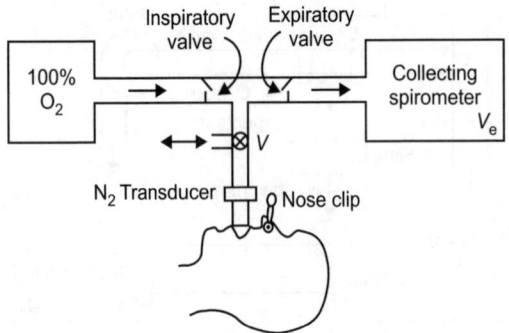

Fig. 3.19. Arrangement of equipment for the nitrogen-washout technique. Valve V allows the subject to brea the room air until the test is started. The test is started by operating valve V at the end of a normal breath. The subject starts breathing 100 per cent O_2 through the inspiratory valve and exhales the N_2 and O_2 mixture into a collecting spirometer via the expiratory valve.

The spirometer on the left contains 100 per cent oxygen, which is inhaled by the subject via the inspiratory check valve. A nose clip is applied so that all of the respired gases flow through the tube connected to the mouthpiece. It is in this tube that the sampling inlet for the nitrogen analyser is located. Thus, starting at the resting expiratory level, inhalation of pure oxygen causes the nitrogen analyser to indicate zero. Expiration closes the

inspiratory valve and opens the expiratory valve. The first expired breath contains nitrogen derived from the functional residual capacity (diluted by the oxygen that was inspired); the nitrogen analyser indicates this percentage. The exhaled gases are collected in the spirometer on the right. The collecting spirometre and all of the interconnecting tubing are first flushed with oxygen to eliminate all nitrogen. This simple procedure eliminates the need to apply corrections and facilitates calculation of the FRC. With continued breathing, the nitrogen analyser indicates less and less nitrogen because it is being washed out of the FRC and replaced by oxygen. Figure 3.20 illustrates a typical record from a normal subject of the diminishing concentration of nitrogen during the early part of the test. In most laboratores, the test is continued until the concentration of nitrogen falls to about 1 per cent. The nitrogen recording permits identification of this concentrations. In normal subjects, virtually all of the nitrogen can be washed out of the FRC in about 2–3 minute.

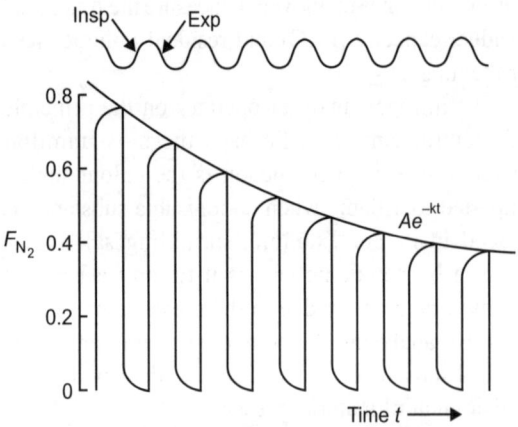

Fig. 3.20. The nitrogen-washout curve.

If the peaks on the nitrogen-washout record are joined, a smooth exponential decay curve is obtained in normal subjects. A semilogarithmic plot of N_2 concentration versus time provides a straight line. In subjects with trapped air or poorly ventilated alveoli, the nitrogen-washout curve consists of several exponentials as the poorly ventilated regions give up their nitrogen. In such subjects, the time taken to wash out all of the nitrogen usually exceeds to min. Thus, the nitrogen concentration-time curve provides useful diagnostic information on the ventilatory activity of the alveoli.

If it is assumed that all of the collected (washed-out) nitrogen was uniformly distributed within the lungs, it is easy to calculate the functional residual capacity. If the environmental air contains 80 per cent nitrogen, then the volume of nitrogen in the FRC 0.8 FRC. Since the volume of gas in the collecting spirometer is known, it is only necessary to determine the concentration of nitrogen in this volume. To do so merely requires admitting some of this gas to the inlet valve of the nitrogen analyser. Note that this concentration of nitrogen ($F_{N_2} V_E$) exists in a volume the includes the volume of air expired (V_E) plus the original volume of oxygen in the collecting spirometer (V_0) at the start of the test and the volume of the tubing (V_t) leading from the expiratory collecting valve. It is therefore advisable to start with an empty collecting spirometer ($V_a = 0$). Usually the tubing volume V_t is negligible compared to the volume of expired gas collected. In this situation the volume of nitrogen collected is $F_{N_2} V_E$ where F_{N_2} is the concentration. Therefore,

$$0.80 \, \text{FRC} = F_{N_2} V_E$$

and

$$\text{FRC} = F_{N_2} \frac{V_E}{0.80}$$

It is important to note that the FRC so obtained is for lung gases at ambient temperature and pressure and saturated with water vapour (ATPS). In respiratory studies, this value is converted to body temperature and saturation with water vapour (BTPS).

In the example shown in Fig. 3.20, the washout to 1 per cent N_2 took 44 breaths. With a breathing rate of 12 breaths/min, the washout time was 220 seconds. The expired volume collected (V_E) was 22 L, and the concentration of nitrogen (F_{N_2}) in the collecting spirometer was 0.085. Therefore,

$$\text{FRC} = \frac{0.085 \times 22}{0.80} = 2.337 \, \text{L}.$$

GAS CHROMATOGRAPHY-MASS SPECTROMETRY

Chromatography is the collective term for a set of laboratory techniques for the separation of mixtures. It involves passing a mixture dissolved in a 'mobile phase' through a stationary phase, which separates the analyte to be measured from other molecules in the mixture based on differential partitioning between the mobile and stationary phases. Subtle differences in compounds partition coefficient results in differential retention on the stationary phase and thus separation.

Gas Chromatography

Gas chromatography (GC), also sometimes known as gas-liquid chromatography, (GLC), is a separation technique in which the mobile phase is a gas. Gas chromatography is always carried out in a column, which is typically 'packed' or 'capillary'.

Gas chromatography (GC) is based on a partition equilibrium of analyte between a solid stationary phase (often a liquid silicone-based material) and a mobile gas (most often helium). The stationary phase is adhered to the inside of a small-diameter glass tube (a capillary column) or a solid matrix inside a larger metal tube (a packed column). It is widely used in analytical chemistry; though the high temperatures used in GC make it unsuitable for high molecular weight biopolymers or proteins (heat will denature them), frequently encountered in biochemistry, it is well suited for use in the petrochemical, environmental monitoring, and industrial chemical fields. It is also used extensively in chemistry research.

ELECTROPHORESIS

Electrophoresis is the motion of dispersed particles relative to a fluid under the influence of a spatially uniform electric field. This electrokinetic phenomenon was observed for the first time in 1807 by Reuss, who noticed that the application of a constant electric field caused clay particles dispersed in water to migrate. It is ultimately caused by the presence of a charged interface between the particle surface and the surrounding fluid (Fig. 3.21).

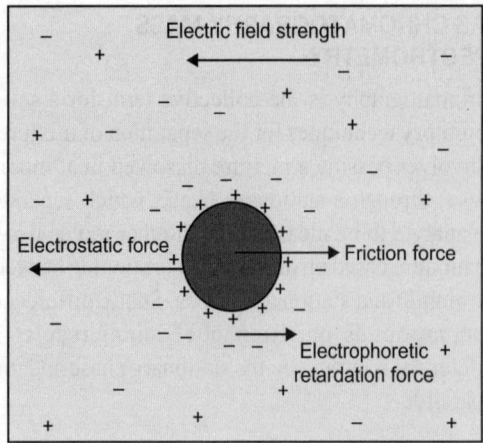

Fig. 3.21. Illustration of electrophoresis.

The dispersed particles have an electric surface charge, on which an external electric field exerts an electrostatic Coulomb force. According to the double layer theory, all surface charges in fluids are screened by a diffuse layer of ions, which has the same absolute charge but opposite sign with respect to that of the surface charge. The electric field also exerts a force on the ions in the diffuse layer which has direction opposite to that acting on the surface charge. This latter force is not actually applied to the particle, but to the ions in the diffuse layer located at some distance from the particle surface, and part of it is transferred all the way to the particle surface through viscous stress. This part of the force is also called electrophoretic retardation force (Fig. 3.22).

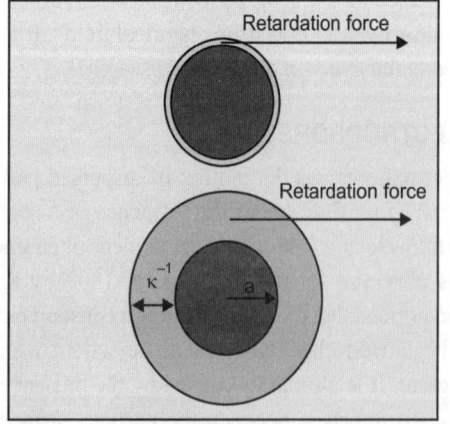

Fig. 3.22. Illustration of electrophoresis retardation.

COMPONENTS OF ELECTROPHORESIS APPARATUS

It is based on the principle that the individual components of the colloidal solution migrate in a liquid at different speeds when subjected to an electric field. Separations are possible because particles of similar geometry but different charge, and particles of like charge but different geometry migrate at different rates towards an oppositely charged electrode. Therefore, when the current is passed for a certain time through such a solution, various components present in the solution would move through different distances in their effort to migrate towards the electrodes. Therefore, a substance which may be a mixture is thus separated into its components along the migration distance, according to a definite law. Measurement of the concentration along this migration distance would therefore, provide the quantitative result of the analysis.

Accordingly, electrophoresis is a separation technique that is based on the mobility of ions in an electric field. Positively charged ions migrate towards a negative electrode and negatively charged ions migrate toward a positive electrode. For safety reasons, one electrode is usually at ground and the other is biased positively or negatively. Ions have different migration rates depending upon their total charge, size and shape, and can therefore be separated.

Basically, the electrophoresis technique separates the molecules based on the size and charge under the influence of an electric field. If E is the strength of the electrical field, Z is the charge on the molecule and F is the frictional force on the molecule, then V the velocity of migration is given by:

$$V = \frac{EZ}{F}$$

The frictional force can be defined as:

$$F = 6\,\pi\eta r,$$

where η is the viscosity of the medium and 'r' is the stokes radius of the molecule. Therefore,

$$V = \frac{EZ}{6\pi\eta r}$$

This implies that the electrophoretic mobility is proportional to the charge on the molecule and inversely proportional to the radius of the molecule, i.e. larger the radius translates to lower electrophoretic mobility.

Normally, with the moving boundary method, only two components of a mixture, one with the highest mobility and the other with the lowest mobility, can be separated in pure form. If it is desired to recover components other than those of the highest and lowest mobilities in pure form, multiple separations have to be carried out.

An electrophoresis apparatus consists of a high-voltage supply, electrodes, buffer, and a support for the buffer such as filtre paper, cellulose acetate strips, polyacrylamide gel (Fig. 3.23a), or a, capillary tube. Open capillary tubes are used for many types of samples and the other supports are usually used for biological samples such as protein mixtures or DNA fragments. After a separation is completed, the support is stained to visualise the separated components. A complete electrophoresis apparatus (Fig. 3.23b) comprises: (i) electrophoresis cabinet, (ii) power supply, and (iii) densitometer or scanner.

Constant Voltage Power Supply

A constant voltage power supply maintains a constant voltage across the load, irrespective of the current drawn by the load. Therefore, it should have output impedance as close to zero as possible.

Figure 3.24 shows a voltage regulated power supply. It basically consists of a conventional rectifier and filter circuit to convert AC from the mains to DC with low ripple content. The rectified DC is fed through a series regulator to the output terminals of the load. A reference circuit applies a voltage to one terminal of a comparison amplifier, equal to the desired output voltage. If the output voltage does not equal the reference voltage, the input voltage to the comparison amplifier is not zero and the amplified output of the comparison amplifier changes the conduction of the series regulator. This results in a change of current through the load resistor until the load voltage is equal to the desired output value.

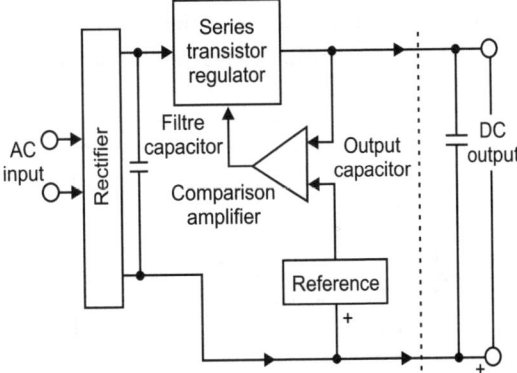

Fig. 3.24. Block diagram of a constant-voltage power supply.

Constant Current Power Supplies

An ideal constant current source is the one for which the current remains constant, regardless of the value of the output voltage demanded by the load. Since it is possible that the load resistance connected to a constant current power supply may vary, the ideal constant current source must have an infinite source impedance at all frequencies.

Figure 3.25 shows the block diagram of a constant-current regulated power supply. This supply resembles, in many respects, the block diagram of a

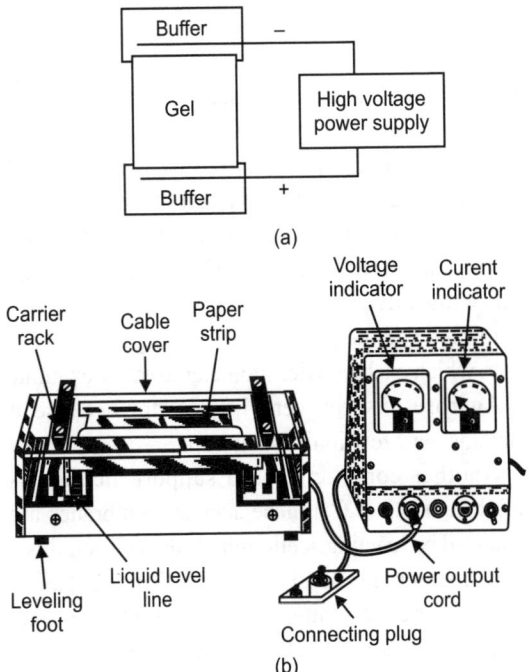

Fig. 3.23. (a) Gel electrophoresis set-up (b) paper electrophoresis apparatus.

constant voltage regulated power supply. However, instead of comparing the reference voltage with the output voltage, the comparison amplifier of a constant current power supply, compares the reference voltage with an IR drop caused by the output current flowing through a fixed resistor. The action of the feedback loop and consequently the conductance of the series regulating element is adjusted, so as to maintain the IR drop across the series monitoring resistor constant and equal to the reference voltage, and thereby holding the output current to some constant value as desired.

It is desirable for many reasons to limit the maximum instantaneous current, which the series transistors can pass to some pre-determined value. The primary reason for doing so is to protect the series transistors themselves from damage due to excessive heating, and to be able to charge a large load capacitor without damaging the power supply. Consequently, a protection circuit is provided to many power supplies to limit the maximum output current under any load condition. This is achieved by having an automatic crossover between the two modes of operation, namely constant voltage and constant current.

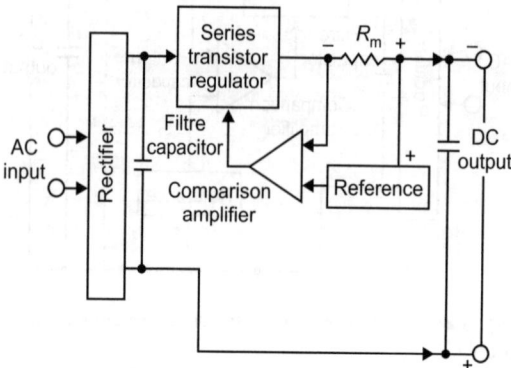

Fig. 3.25. Block diagram of a constant-current power supply.

Constant Voltage, Constant Current (CV/CC), Regulated Power Supply

Figure 3.26 shows the block diagram of CV/CC power supply. The diodes are connected in the circuit such that when the supply is in constant voltage operation, the upper diode is forward biased or shorted, while the lower diode is reverse biased or open. Conversely, when the supply is in constant current operation, the upper diode is reverse biased and the lower diode is forward biased. Thus, the series regulator is only called upon to respond to either the constant voltage comparison amplifier or the constant current amplifier. The effectiveness of one amplifier is not diluted by the shunt presence of the other. In this circuit, the same output terminals are used for both constant voltage and constant current operation. The supply delivers constant voltage with a continuously variable current limit, or of constant current operation with a continuously variable voltage limits.

Whether the supply is in constant voltage or constant current operation at any instant, depends upon the relationship between the DC load resistance and the critical value of the load resistance, defined as the ratio of the front panel voltage control setting, to the front panel current control setting. If the load resistance is greater than the critical load resistance, the supply will be in constant voltage operation and if the load resistance is less than this critical load resistance, the supply will be in constant current operation.

Support medium

One of the most commonly used support mediums is agar. Agar is so prevalent in clinical labs that electrophoresis is often referred to as agarose gel electrophoresis. Clinically, electrophoresis is performed on a plastic support covered with a thin (1 mm) layer of agarose gel. Agarose has the following advantages: After electrophoresis is performed and the plate is dried, the agarose is very clear, which enables a densitometer to easily examine it. Agarose absorbs very little water because it contains very few ionisable groups.

Another commonly used support medium is cellulose acetate: Cellulose acetate membranes are produced by reacting acetic anhydride with cellulose. These membranes consist of about 80 per cent air in pockets in-between interconnected cellulose acetate fibres. These air pockets fill with liquid when the membranes are placed in a buffer. Cellulose acetate electrophoresis (CAE) has the advantage of being

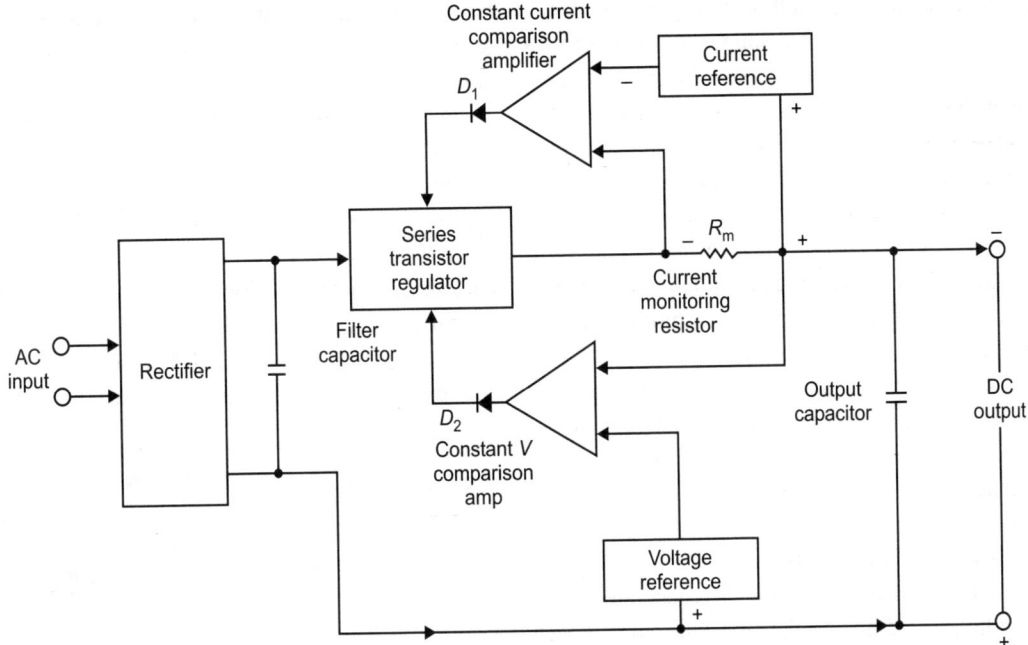

Fig. 3.26. Block diagram of a constant-voltage/constant current power supply.

relatively quick (20 to 60 min). CAE membranes can be made clear for densitometry using a solution that dissolves the cellulose acetate fibres.

Electrodes and chamber

Electrodes may be made of metal such as platinum, or of carbon. Gel trays may be made from UV transparent acrylic to enable direct observation of the migration of different molecules.

DNA SEQUENCING

The term DNA sequencing refers to sequencing methods for determining the order of the nucleotide bases — adenine, guanine, cytosine, and thymine — in a molecule of DNA (Fig. 3.27).

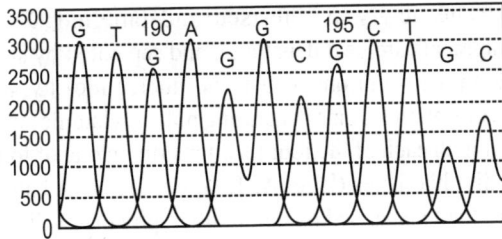

Fig. 2.27. DNA Sequence Trace

Knowledge of DNA sequences has become indispensable for basic biological research, other research branches utilising DNA sequencing, and in numerous applied fields such as diagnostic, bio-technology, forensic biology and biological systematics. The advent of DNA sequencing has significantly accelerated biological research and discovery. The rapid speed of sequencing attained with modern DNA sequencing technology has been instrumental in the sequencing of the human genome, in the Human genome project. Related projects, often by scientific collaboration across continents, have generated the complete DNA sequences of many animal, plant, and microbial genomes.

The first DNA sequences were obtained by academic researchers, using laborious methods based on 2-dimensional chromatography in the early 1970s. Following the development of dye-based sequencing methods with automated analysis, DNA sequencing has become easier and orders of magnitude faster.

Allan Maxam and Walter Gilbert developed a DNA sequencing method based on chemical modification of DNA and subsequent cleavage at specific bases. Although Maxam and Gilbert published their chemical sequencing method two years after the ground-breaking paper of Sanger and Coulson on plus-minus sequencing, Maxam–Gilbert sequencing rapidly became more popular, since purified DNA could be used directly, while the initial Sanger method required that each read start be cloned for production of single-stranded DNA. However, with the improvement of the chain-termination method Maxam-Gilbert sequencing has fallen out of favour due to its technical complexity prohibiting its use in standard molecular biology kits, extensive use of hazardous chemicals, and difficulties with scale-up.

The method requires radioactive labelling at one end and purification of the DNA fragment to be sequenced. Chemical treatment generates breaks at a small proportion of one or two of the four nucleotide bases in each of four reactions (G, A + G, C, C + T). Thus a series of labelled fragments is generated, from the radiolabelled end to the first 'cut' site in each molecule. The fragments in the four reactions are arranged side by side in gel electrophoresis for size separation. To visualise the fragments, the gel is exposed to X-ray film for autoradiography, yielding a series of dark bands each corresponding to a radiolabelled DNA fragment, from which the sequence may be inferred.

Also sometimes known as 'chemical sequencing', this method originated in the study of DNA-protein interactions (footprinting), nucleic acid structure and epigenetic modifications to DNA, and within these it still has important applications.

Chain-termination Methods

Because the chain-terminator method (or Sanger method after its developer Frederick Sanger) is more efficient and uses fewer toxic chemicals and lower amounts of radioactivity than the method of Maxam and Gilbert, it rapidly became the method of choice. The key principle of the Sanger method was the use of dideoxynucleotide triphosphates (ddNTPs) as DNA chain terminators (Fig. 3.28).

The classical chain-termination method requires a single-stranded DNA template, a DNA primer, a DNA polymerase, radioactively or fluorescently

labelled nucleotides, and modified nucleotides that terminate DNA strand elongation. The DNA sample is divided into four separate sequencing reactions, containing all four of the standard deoxynucleotides (dATP, dGTP, dCTP and dTTP) and the DNA polymerase. To each reaction is added only one of the four dideoxynucleotides (ddATP, ddGTP, ddCTP, or ddTTP) which are the chain-terminating nucleotides, lacking a 3′-OH group required for the formation of a phosphodiester bond between two nucleotides, thus terminating DNA strand extension and resulting in DNA fragments of varying length.

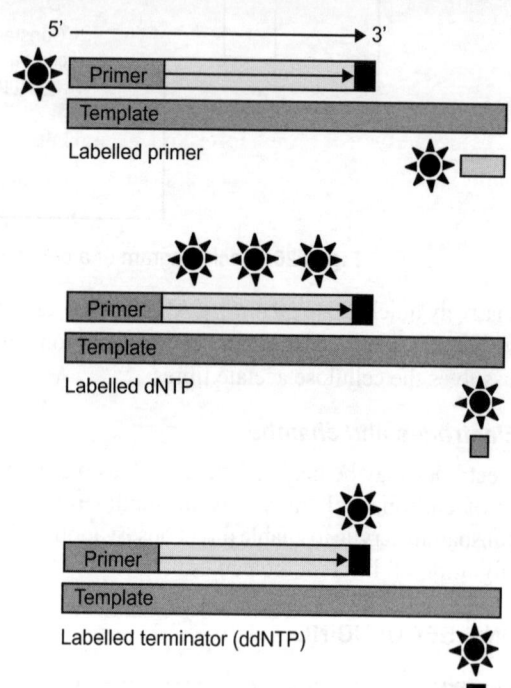

Fig. 3.28. DNA fragments are labelled with a radioactive or fluorescent tag on the primer, in the new DNA strand with a labelled dNTP, or with a labelled ddNTP.

The newly synthesised and labelled DNA fragments are heat denatured, and separated by size (with a resolution of just one nucleotide) by gel electrophoresis on a denaturing polyacrylamide-urea gel with each of the four reactions run in one of four individual lanes (lanes A, T, G, C); the DNA bands are then visualised by autoradiography or UV light, and the DNA sequence can be directly read off the

X-ray film or gel image. In the image on the right, X-ray film was exposed to the gel, and the dark bands correspond to DNA fragments of different lengths. A dark band in a lane indicates a DNA fragment that is the result of chain termination after incorporation of a dideoxynucleotide (ddATP, ddGTP, ddCTP, or ddTTP). The relative positions of the different bands among the four lanes are then used to read (from bottom to top) the DNA sequence.

Technical variations of chain-termination sequencing include tagging with nucleotides containing radioactive phosphorus for radiolabelling, or using a primer labelled at the 5 end with a fluorescent dye. Dye-primer sequencing facilitates reading in an optical system for faster and more economical analysis and automation. The later development by Leroy Hood and coworkers of fluorescently labelled ddNTPs and primers set the stage for automated, high-throughput DNA sequencing.

Chain-termination methods have greatly simplified DNA sequencing. For example, chain-termination-based kits are commercially available that contain the reagents needed for sequencing, pre-aliquoted and ready to use. Limitations include non-specific binding of the primer to the DNA, affecting accurate read-out of the DNA sequence, and DNA secondary structures affecting the fidelity of the sequence.

Dye-terminator sequencing

Dye-terminator sequencing utilises labelling of the chain terminator ddNTPs, which permits sequencing in a single reaction, rather than four reactions as in the labelled-primer method. In dye-terminator sequencing, each of the four dideoxynucleotide chain terminators is labelled with fluorescent dyes, each of which with different wavelengths of fluorescence and emission. Owing to its greater expediency and speed, dye-terminator sequencing is now the mainstay in automated sequencing. Its limitations include dye effects due to differences in the incorporation of the dye-labelled chain terminators into the DNA fragment, resulting in unequal peak heights and shapes in the electronic DNA sequence trace chromatogram after capillary electrophoresis

(see Fig. 3.29). This problem has been addressed with the use of modified DNA polymerase enzyme systems and dyes that minimise incorporation variability, as well as methods for eliminating 'dye blobs'. The dye-terminator sequencing method, along with automated high-throughput DNA sequence analysers, is now being used for the vast majority of sequencing projects.

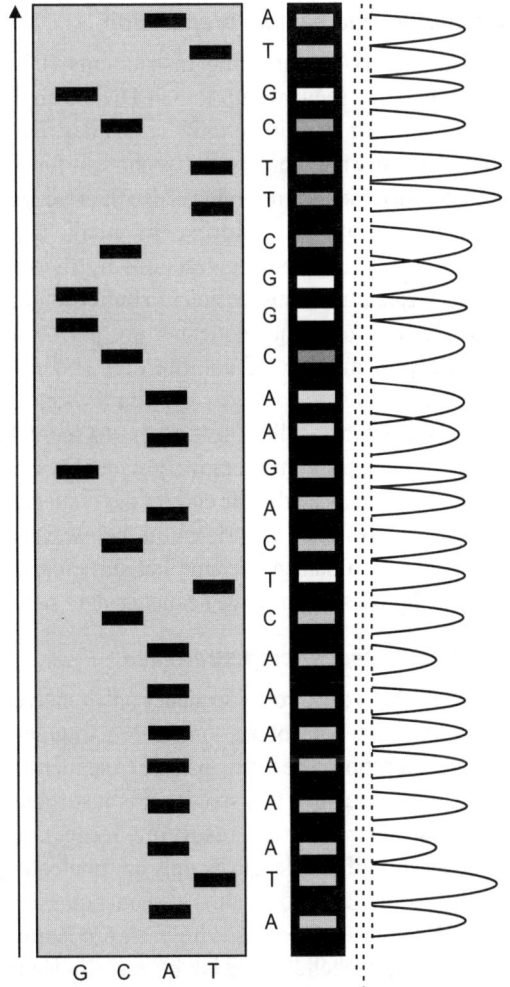

Fig. 3.29. Sequence ladder by radioactive sequencing compared to fluorescent peaks.

Challenges

Common challenges of DNA sequencing include poor quality in the first 15–40 bases of the sequence and deteriorating quality of sequencing traces after 700–900 bases. Base calling software typically gives an estimate of quality to aid in quality trimming.

In cases where DNA fragments are cloned before sequencing, the resulting sequence may contain parts of the cloning vector. In contrast, PCR-based cloning and emerging sequencing technologies based on pyrosequencing often avoid using cloning vectors.

Automation and sample preparation

Automated DNA-sequencing instruments (DNA sequencers) can sequence up to 384 DNA samples in a single batch (run) in up to 24 runs a day. DNA sequencers carry out capillary electrophoresis for size separation, detection and recording of dye fluorescence, and data output as fluorescent peak trace chromatograms. Sequencing reactions by thermocycling, cleanup and resuspension in a buffer solution before loading onto the sequencer are performed separately. A number of commercial and non-commercial software packages can trim low-quality DNA traces automatically. These programs score the quality of each peak and remove low-quality base peaks (generally located at the ends of the sequence). The accuracy of such algorithms is below visual examination by a human operator, but sufficient for automated processing of large sequence data sets.

Large-scale sequencing strategies

Current methods can directly sequence only relatively short (300–1000 nucleotides long) DNA fragments in a single reaction. The main obstacle to sequencing DNA fragments above this size limit is insufficient power of separation for resolving large DNA fragments that differ in length by only one nucleotide.

Large-scale sequencing aims at sequencing very long DNA pieces, such as whole chromosomes. Common approaches consist of cutting (with restriction enzymes) or shearing (with mechanical forces) large DNA fragments into shorter DNA fragments. The fragmented DNA is cloned into a DNA vector, and amplified in *Escherichia coli*. Short DNA fragments purified from individual bacterial colonies are individually sequenced and assembled electronically into one long, contiguous sequence.

This method does not require any pre-existing information about the sequence of the DNA and is referred to as de novo sequencing. Gaps in the assembled sequence may be filled by primer walking. The different strategies have different tradeoffs in speed and accuracy; shotgun methods are often used for sequencing large genomes, but its assembly is complex and difficult, particularly with sequence repeats often causing gaps in genome assembly.

New Sequencing Methods

High-throughput sequencing

The high demand for low-cost sequencing has driven the development of high-throughput sequencing technologies that parallelise the sequencing process, producing thousands or millions of sequences at once. High-throughput sequencing technologies are intended to lower the cost of DNA sequencing beyond what is possible with standard dye-terminator methods.

In vitro clonal amplification

Molecular detection methods are not sensitive enough for single molecule sequencing, so most approaches use an *in vitro* cloning step to amplify individual DNA molecules. Emulsion PCR isolates individual DNA molecules along with primer-coated beads in aqueous droplets within an oil phase. Polymerase chain reaction (PCR) then coats each bead with clonal copies of the DNA molecule followed by immobilisation for later sequencing. Emulsion PCR is used in the methods by Marguilis, Shendure and Porreca and SOLiD sequencing. Another method for *in vitro* clonal amplification is *bridge PCR*, where fragments are amplified upon primers attached to a solid surface, used in the Illumina Genome Analyser. The single-molecule method developed by Stephen Quake's laboratory (later commercialised by Helicos) skips this amplification step, directly fixing DNA molecules to a surface.

Parallelised sequencing

DNA molecules are physically bound to a surface, and sequenced in parallel.Sequencing by synthesis, like dye-termination electrophoretic sequencing, uses a DNA polymerase to determine the base sequence. Reversible terminator methods (used by Illumina and Helicos) use reversible versions of dye-terminators, adding one nucleotide at a time, detect fluorescence at each position in real time, by repeated removal of the blocking group to allow polymerisation of another nucleotide. Pyrosequencing (used by 454) also uses DNA polymerisation, adding one nucleotide species at a time and detecting and quantifying the number of nucleotides added to a given location through the light emitted by the release of attached pyrophosphates.

Sequencing by ligation

Sequencing by ligation uses a DNA ligase to determine the target sequence. Used in the polony method and in the SOLiD technology, it uses a pool of all possible oligonucleotides of a fixed length, labelled according to the sequenced position. Oligonucleotides are annealed and ligated; the preferential ligation by DNA ligase for matching sequences results in a signal informative of the nucleotide at that position.

Microfluidic sanger sequencing

In microfluidic Sanger sequencing the entire thermocycling amplification of DNA fragments as well as their separation by electrophoresis is done on a single glass wafer (approximately 10 cm in diameter) thus reducing the reagent usage as well as cost. In some instances researchers have shown that they can increase the throughput of conventional sequencing through the use of microchips. Research will still need to be done in order to make this use of technology effective.

Other sequencing technologies

Sequencing by hybridisation is a non-enzymatic method that uses a DNA microarray. A single pool of DNA whose sequence is to be determined is fluorescently labelled and hybridised to an array containing known sequences. Strong hybridisation signals from a given spot on the array identifies its sequence in the DNA being sequenced. Mass spectrometry may be used to determine mass differences between DNA fragments produced in chain-termination reactions.

DNA sequencing methods currently under development include labelling the DNA polymerase, reading the sequence as a DNA strand transits through nanopores, and microscopy-based techniques, such as AFM or electron microscopy that are used to identify the positions of individual nucleotides within long DNA fragments (>5,000 bp) by nucleotide labelling with heavier elements (e.g. halogens) for visual detection and recording.

4

Biomaterials and Tissue Engineering

INTRODUCTION

Surfaces play an important role in a biological system for most biological reactions occurring at surfaces and interfaces. The development of biomaterials for tissue engineering is to create perfect surfaces which can provoke specific cellular responses and direct new tissue regeneration. The improvement in bio-compatibility of biomaterials for tissue engineering by directed surface modification is an important contribution to biomaterials development. Among many biomaterials used for tissue engineering, polyesters have been well documented for their excellent biodegradability, biocompatibility and nontoxicity. However, poor hydrophilicity and the lack of natural recognition sites on the surface of polyesters have greatly limited their further application in the tissue engineering field. Therefore, how to introduce functional groups or molecules to polyester surfaces, which ideally adjust cell/tissue biological functions, becomes more and more important.

The development of biomaterials is not a new area of science, having existed for around half a century. The study of biomaterials is called biomaterials science. It is a provocative field of science, having experienced steady and strong growth over its history, with many companies investing large amounts of money into the development of new products. Biomaterials science encompasses elements of medicine, biology, chemistry, tissue engineering and materials science. While a definition for the term 'biomaterial' has been difficult to formulate, more widely accepted working definitions include:

1. A biomaterial is any material, natural or man-made, that comprises whole or part of a living structure or biomedical device which performs, augments, or replaces a natural function.
2. A biomaterial is a nonviable material used in medical device, so it's intended to interact with a biological systems.

A biomaterial is essentially a material that is used and adapted for a medical application. Biomaterials may have a benign function, such as being used for a heart valve, or may be bioactive with a more interactive functionality such as hydroxy-apatite coated hip implants. Biomaterials are also used every day in dental applications, surgery, and drug delivery (a construct with impregnated pharmaceutical products can be placed into the body, which permits the prolonged release of a drug over an extended period of time). The definition of a biomaterial does not just include man-made materials which are constructed of metals or ceramics. A biomaterial may also be an autograft, allograft or xenograft used as a transplant material.

Biomaterials are used in: (i) joint replacements, (ii) bone plates, (iii) bone cement, (iv) artificial ligaments and tendons, (v) dental implants for tooth fixation, (vi) blood vessel prostheses, (vii) heart valves, (viii) skin repair devices, (ix) cochlear replacements, (x) contact lenses, and (xi) breast implants.

Biomaterials must be compatible with the body, and there are often issues of biocompatibility which must be resolved before a product can be placed on the market and used in a clinical setting. Because of this, biomaterials are usually subjected to the same requirements of those undergone by new drug therapies. All manufacturing companies are also required to ensure traceability of all of their products so that if a defective product is discovered, others in the same batch may be traced.

Healing is an essential consideration when using biomaterials. The body may experience what is known as a foreign-body reaction after implementation so immuno-suppression may be required.

Biomaterials that have a mechanical operation must perform to certain standards and be able to cop with pressures. It is therefore essential that all biomaterials are well designed and are tested. Biomaterials that are used with a mechanical application, such as hip implants, are usually designed using CAD (Computer aided design) which allows all of the directional stresses to be calculated, ensuring maximum product life.

Compatibility: Biocompatibility is related to the behaviour of biomaterials in various envronments under various chemical and physical conditions. The term may refer to specific properties of a material without specifying where or how the material is to be used. (For example, a material may elicit little or no immune response in a given organism, and may or may not able to integrate with a particular cell type or tissue). The ambiguity of the term reflects the ongoing development of insights into how biomaterials interact with the human body and eventually how those interactions determine the clinical success of a medical device (such as pacemaker or hip replacement. Modern medical devices and prostheses are often made of more than one material — so it might not always be sufficient to talk about the biocompatibility of a specific material.

Also, a material should not be toxic unless specifically engineered to be so — like 'smart' drug delivery systems that target cancer cells and destroy them. Understanding of the anatomy and physiology of the action site is essential for a biomaterial to be effective. An additional factor is the dependence on specific anatomical sites of implantation. It is thus important, during design, to ensure that the implement will fit complementarily and have a beneficial effect with the specific anatomical area of action.

INTEGRATED APPROACH OF BIOMATERIALS

Biomaterials improve the quality of life for an ever increasing number of people each year. The range of applications is vast and includes such things as joint and limb replacements, artificial arteries and skin, contact lenses, and dentures. While the implementation of some of these materials may be for medical reasons such as the replacement of diseased tissues required to extend life expectancies, other reasons may include purely aesthetic ones including breast implants. This increasing demand arises from an ageing population with higher quality of life expectations. The biomaterials community is producing new and improved implant materials and techniques to meet this demand, but also to aid the treatment of younger patients where the necessary properties are even more demanding. A counter force to this technological push is the increasing level of regulation and the threat of litigation. To meet these conflicting needs it is necessary to have reliable methods of characterisation of the material and material/host tissue interactions.

Classifications of Biomaterials

Biomedical materials can be divided roughly into three main types governed by the tissue response. In broad terms, inert (more strictly, nearly inert) materials illicit no or minimal tissue response. Active materials encourage bonding to surrounding tissue with, for example, new bone growth being stimulated. Degradable, or resorbable materials are incorporated into the surrounding tissue, or may even dissolve completely over a period of time. Metals are typically inert, ceramics may be inert, active or resorbable and polymers may be inert or resorbable. Some examples of biomaterials are provided in Table 4.1.

Table 4.1. Some accepted biomaterials.

Metals	Ceramics	Polymers
316L	Alumina	Ultra high molecular
Stainless steel	Zirconia	weight polyethylene
	Carbon	Polyurethane
Co-Cr alloys	Hydroxyapatite	
Titanium		
Ti6Al4V		

Key properties

The main property required of a biomaterial is that it does not illicit an adverse reaction when placed into service.

The range of applications for biomaterials is large. The number of different biomaterials is also significant. However, in general:

1. Metallic biomaterials are used for load bearing applications and must have sufficient fatigue strength to endure the rigors of daily activity, e.g. walking, chewing etc.

2. Ceramic biomaterials are generally used for their hardness and wear resistance for applications such as articulating surfaces in joints and in teeth as well as bone bonding surfaces in implants.

3. Polymeric materials are usually used for their flexibility and stability, but have also been used for low friction articulating surfaces.

Polymer

A polymer is a large molecule (macromolecule) composed of repeating structural units typically connected by covalent chemical bonds. While polymer in popular usage suggests plastic, the term actually refers to a large class of natural and synthetic materials with a variety of properties.

Due to the extraordinary range of properties accessible in polymeric materials, they have come to play an essential and ubiquitous role in everyday life — from plastics and elastomers on the one hand to natural biopolymers such as DNA and proteins that are essential for life on the other. A simple example is polyethylene, whose repeating unit is based on ethylene (IUPAC name *ethene*) monomer. Most commonly, as in this example, the continuously linked backbone of a polymer used for the preparation of plastics consists mainly of carbon atoms. However, other structures do exist; for example, elements such as silicon form familiar materials such as silicones, examples being silly putty and waterproof plumbing sealant. The backbone of DNA is in fact based on a phosphodiester bond, and repeating units of polysaccharides (e.g. cellulose) are joined together by glycosidic bonds via oxygen atoms (Fig. 4.1).

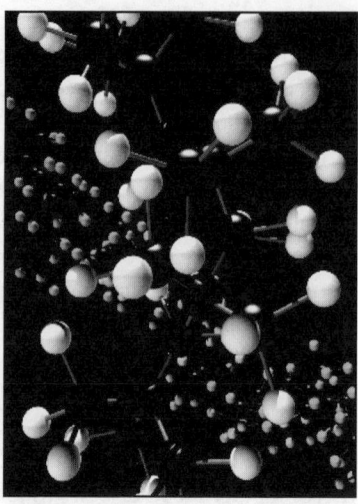

Fig. 4.1. Polymer: polyisobutylene chain.

Natural polymeric materials such as shellac, amber, and natural rubber have been in use for centuries. Biopolymers such as proteins and nucleic acids play crucial roles in biological processes. A variety of other natural polymers exist, such as cellulose, which is the main constituent of wood and paper.

The list of synthetic polymers includes synthetic rubber, Bakelite, neoprene, nylon, PVC, polystyrene, polyethylene, polypropylene, polyacrylonitrile, PVB, silicone, and many more.

MOLECULES AND TISSUE ENGINEERING

Tissue Engineering

Tissue engineering was once categorised as a subfield of biomaterials, but having grown in scope and importance it can be considered as a field in its own right. It is the use of a combination of cells, engineering and materials methods, and suitable biochemical and physio-chemical factors to improve or replace biological functions. While most definitions of tissue engineering cover a broad range of applications, in practice the term is closely associated with applications that repair or replace portions of or whole tissues (i.e. bone, cartilage, blood vessels, bladder, skin etc.). Often, the tissues involved require certain mechanical and structural properties for proper functioning. The term has also been applied to efforts to perform specific biochemical functions using cells within an artificially-created support system (e.g. an artificial pancreas, or a bioartificial liver). The term regenerative medicine is often used synonymously with tissue engineering, although those involved in regenerative medicine place more emphasis on the use of stem cells to produce tissues. A commonly applied definition of tissue engineering, as stated by Langer and Vacanti, is 'an interdisciplinary field that applies the principles of engineering and life sciences toward the development of biological substitutes that restore, maintain, or improve tissue function or a whole organ'. Tissue engineering has also been defined as 'understanding the principles of tissue growth, and applying this to produce functional replacement tissue for clinical use.' A further description goes on to say that an 'underlying supposition of tissue engineering is that the employment of natural biology of the system will allow for greater success in developing therapeutic strategies aimed at the replacement, repair, maintenance, and/or enhancement of tissue function.'

Cellular Composites

Tissues are multiphase systems of cellular composites. We can identify three main structural components: cells organised into functional units, the extracellular matrix, and scaffolding architecture.

The three-dimensional structures that characterise bioartificial tissues represent a cell mass that is greater, by several orders of magnitude, than the two-dimensional cell cultures traditionally developed by biologists. Tissue engineering also concentrates on the development of *in vitro* models that overcome the absence of an adequate extracellular matrix in conventional cell cultures. Some examples of applications of tissue engineering are given in Table 4.2.

Table 4.2. Some examples of applications in tissue engineering.

Biological system	Example of application
Blood	Hematopoietic (production of red blood cells by) stem cells culture
Cardiovascular	Endothelialised synthetic vascular grafts (angiogenesis)

(Contd ...)

Biological system	Example of application
	Regeneration of the arterial wall
	Compliant vascular prostheses
Liver and pancreas	Bioartificial pancreatic islets
	Bioartificial liver
Musculoskeletal	Cartilage reconstruction
	Bone reconstruction
Neural	Neurotransmitter-secreting cells (polymer-encapsulated)
	Neural circuits and biosensors
	Peripheral nerve regeneration
Skin	Bioartificial skin substitutes

SURFACE ANALYSIS METHODS FOR CHARACTERISING POLYMERIC BIOMATERIALS

Since the properties of the surface can impact enormously on the success or failure of a biomaterial, the application of appropriate surface analysis techniques for correlating surface properties, including chemical structure, hydrophobicity, morphology and topography, and material performance is of paramount importance. Surface analysis methods can be used for verication of an intended surface modification procedure as well as for correlating surface properties to the biological performance. They also play key roles in understanding the effects of model surfaces with systematically varied surface properties. Characterisation of biomaterials surface properties should therefore be as thorough as possible given technical and practical limitations. A combination of surface characterisation methods is usually necessary to provide the comprehensive information necessary for correlation with performance. Spectroscopic techniques such as XPS are often used in combination to broaden knowledge about the surface. The ease and rapidity with which water contact angles can be applied means that this technique is often used in combination with others. Spectroscopic methods are also frequently used in combination with the microscopic methods. The choice of surface characterisation method can be influenced by numerous factors that must be considered. In this section we have provided an overview of techniques commonly used in biomaterials, particularly polymeric biomaterials, characterisation, as well as some discussion of emerging methods that have recently come to the forefront of biomaterials research, including the applications and limitations of each.

Surface properties can have an enormous effect on the success or failure of a biomaterial device. It is widely accepted that such factors as surface preparation and the subsequent characterisation are central issues in biomaterials research. Characterisation of biomaterial surface properties should be thorough. While acknowledging that individual research groups may be limited, due to a variety of factors, in the availability of surface characterisation techniques, it must be recognised that such characterisation is essential for correlating any surface modifications with changes in biological performance. In addition, information gained may allow for tailoring future surface modifications to favour specific biological responses. The properties that are of interest in the characterisation of biomaterial surfaces include the chemical structure, the hydrophilicity or hydrophobicity, the presence of ionic groups, the morphology (i.e. the domain structure), and the topography (i.e. the surface roughness, planarity, and feature dimensions). Varying degrees of information about these properties can be obtained using different analysis methods including microscopic, spectroscopic and thermodynamic as well as other methods. Choice of the surface characterisation method used can be influenced by a plethora of considerations including the type of measurement required, the extent of the analysed surface region, the required precision and accuracy, the influence of the technique on the surface (i.e. does the probe, electron beam, ion beam, X-ray, required sample preparation, or the analysis environment induce undesirable effects on the surface of interest), the influence of the sample on the instrument, limitations imposed by the surface, as well as the ease of use and availability of equipment. In addition, a very realistic factor or constraint that may influence the choice of surface analysis techniques used is that many surface analysis facilities have become centralised, and there are significant costs associated with sample processing and preparation, the timed usage of equipment, and technician time. The aim of

this section is to provide a brief, easy to understand, synopsis of some of the specific techniques frequently used in the characterisation of biomaterial, particularly polymeric biomaterial, surfaces. In addition some discussion and reference is made to emerging methods that have recently come to the forefront of biomaterials research.

Microscopic Methods

The success of using microscopic methods to characterise biomaterial surfaces is well established. The microscopy techniques often found in the biomaterials literature include scanning electron microscopy (SEM), transmission electron spectroscopy (TEM), scanning tunneling microscopy (STM) and atomic force microscopy (AFM). More recent developments in the area of light microscopy include the optical near-field principle, and the confocal laser scanning technique.

Scanning electron microscopy and transmission electron microscopy

Scanning electron microscopy (SEM) and transmission electron microscopy (TEM) are commonly used for studying both the surface morphology of and the cellular response to biomaterials. These techniques make use of a primary beam of electrons that interact with the specimen of interest, in a vacuum environment, resulting in different types of electrons and electromagnetic waves being emitted. The secondary electrons ejected from the specimen surface are collected and displayed to provide a high-resolution micrograph.

SEM sample preparation involves fixation (if proteins, cells, or tissue are present), followed by drying, attachment to a metallic stub, and then coating with a metal prior to data collection. The thin metallic coating, usually applied by sputter coating, is typically 20 to 30 nm in thickness. Common conductive metals used include gold, platinum, or gold/palladium alloy. It should be noted that the drying and metal coating processes used in the preparation of some polymeric materials might alter surface morphology, particularly those surfaces that may undergo changes in a hydrated environment. Upon insertion of the sample into the SEM, acquisition of the micrographs can usually be done fairly quickly allowing for a large number of images to be obtained with varying magnifications. Newer SEM models are reported to resolve in the nm range with magnifications in excess of 2,00,000×. Photographic prints, or computerised image acquisition, provide a permanent record. Micrographs typically included in the biomaterial literature depict images of 10 to 300 μm in length (see Fig. 4.2). In addition to imaging the surface morphology of polymeric biomaterials, the SEM can be combined with other analysis methods such as energy dispersive X-ray analysis (EDX) to determine elemental distribution and IR and Raman spectroscopy to monitor surface modification procedures. EDX results are typically obtained from a sampling depth on the order of micrometers, thus are more representative of the bulk material rather than the surface.

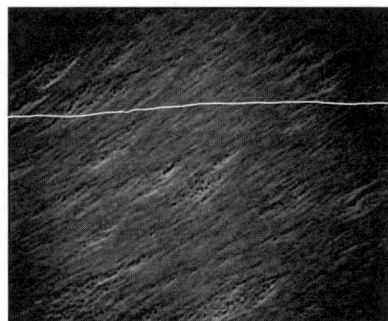

Fig. 4.2. Scanning electron micrograph of the inside polymer surface of a fibre obtained from a bleach/ formaldehyde reprocessed Gambro 21S Polyamide hemodialyser. Bar = 1 μm. SEM image was obtained using a Phillips SEM 502 microscope. Sample was air dried and sputter coated with gold prior to insertion into the SEM.

TEM sample preparation involves fixation (if proteins, cells, or tissue are present), processing, embedding and sectioning. Embedding media can include methacrylates, polyester and acrylic resins, although epoxy resins are now commonly used. Specimens are typically sectioned using a microtome and need to be very thin since electrons with an accelerating voltage of 100 kV will not penetrate specimens more than 1 μm thick. Good resolution and clarity of detail can normally be obtained with sample thicknesses on the order of 50–90 nm. A

modest TEM can resolve in the sub nm range with magnifications considerably higher than 2,00,000×. It should however be noted that the embedding and sectioning processes used in the preparation of some polymeric materials may alter the polymeric material itself or the quality of the image obtained due to factors such as drying, thickness variations, wrinkling or compression. Micrographs typically included in the biomaterial literature depict images of 5 to 300 μm in length (see Fig. 4.3).

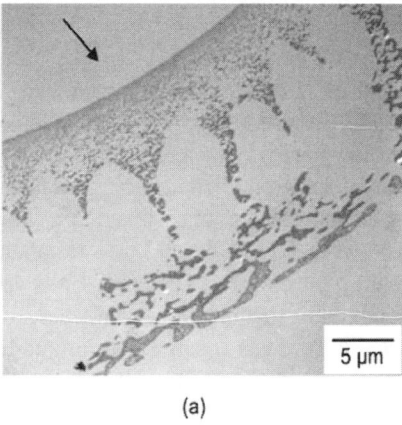

(a)

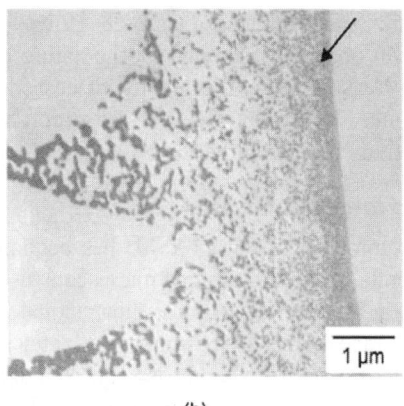

(b)

Fig. 4.3. Transmission electron micrographs of a cross section of a fibre obtained from a bleach/ formaldehyde reprocessed Gambro 21S Polyamide hemodialyser. Arrow indicates inside polymer surface of the fibre. (a) Bar = 5 μm; (b) bar = 1 μm. TEM images were obtained using a JEOL 1200EX biosystem. Fibres were embedded in epoxy and 60 nm thick cross sections of the fibre were cut.

Scanning tunneling microscopy

In scanning tunneling microscopy (STM), 3-dimensional images of surface topography of samples are obtained by monitoring the tunneling current flowing between an extremely sharp conductive probe and the sample surface. As the probe scans the surface, the magnitude of this current is inversely proportional to the probe/surface separation, with a change in the separation producing an order of magnitude change in the tunneling current. If the probe scans a raised area on the surface, the current increases. To compensate, a piezoscanner tube moves the probe tip, returning the tunneling current to its original value. Scan sizes typically range from 10 nm × 10 nm to 15 μm × 15 μm, and detect less than nm vertical changes in topography not possible with electron microscopes. This technique also has advantages over other imaging techniques, such as SEM and TEM, in that no special sample preparation procedures are required. However, the application of this method in the characterisation of polymeric biomaterials is somewhat limited in that most polymers are not sufficiently conductive to allow STM images to be generated. A way around this limitation is to coat the polymeric materials of interest with an extremely thin conductive metallic coating and then image the surface. However the resolution obtained is limited by the nature of the coating. Atomic force microscopy, discussed next, overcomes the problem of the required sample conductivity needed for STM.

Atomic force microscopy

Atomic force microscopy (AFM) has become the most common type of scanning microscopy used for polymeric biomaterials. A three-dimensional image of the surface is created by scanning a tip attached to the end of a cantilever across the surface and monitoring the minute forces of interaction between the sample surface and probe. The forces of interaction may be repulsive or attractive and this gives rise to the different modes of operation of the AFM. A very high resolution of surface topography can be obtained, with dimensions on the nanometer scale, although it should be noted that properties and dimensions of the cantilever and tip, as well as the

selected mode of operation, play an important role in determining the sensitivity and resolution of the acquired image. Unlike electron microscopes, a significant advantage of AFM is that sample topographies, as well as surfaces roughness values, can be obtained without surface treatment or coating which may damage or alter the material surface under investigation. Furthermore, AFM images can be acquired under vacuum, air, or liquid conditions. The ability to image polymeric materials within an aqueous environment is extremely useful in the biomaterials field, as it allows for the examination of the surface of biomaterials in an environment similar to one that would be found in an implant situation, thus allowing for the examination of dynamic processes such as erosion, hydration, and adsorption at interfaces. For example, it is possible to visualise individual plasma protein molecules under aqueous environments using phase imaging AFM. Although AFM is proving to be an extremely useful technique in providing a 3D visualisation of the biomaterial surfaces being studied, the time required, dependant on such factors as scan size and scan rate, to obtain quality images can be significant (i.e. in excess of 20 min/image). In addition, since typically scan sizes are small (i.e. ranging from 500 nm × 500 nm to 15 μm × 15 μm), variations in the surface may be missed (Fig. 4.4).

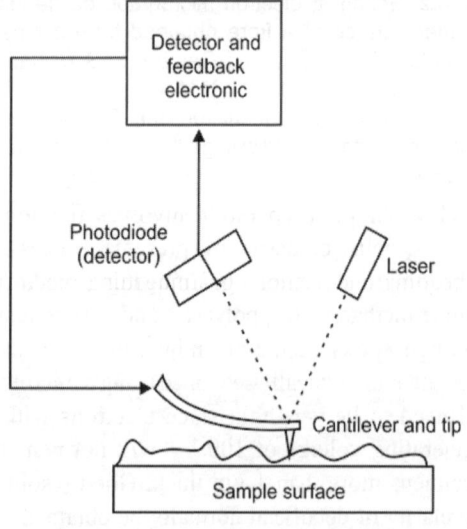

Fig. 4.4. Atomic force microscopy (AFM).

AFM—contact mode

In contact mode, the AFM tip scans across a surface at very low force and is deflected by repulsive forces acting between the tip and the surface atoms. A photodiode detector monitors the deflections of a laser light reflected from the tip of a cantilever. A feedback loop maintains constant deflection of the cantilever, by vertically moving the scanner as it scans laterally across the surface. A computer stores the information and a topographic image with potentially atomic-scale resolution is generated. The forces at the tip are very small (0.01 to 1.0 N/m in air) and metal or hard polymeric surfaces are not generally damaged. However, the lateral shear forces caused by the scanning motion may alter soft materials, thus distorting measurement data and causing damage to the sample. Obtaining images of hydrated polymeric materials in fluid may be further hampered by the fact that some hydrated polymers are softer than dried samples leading to an increase in sample deformation and damage and a reduced image quality resulting from the dragging motion of the tip.

AFM—non contact mode

In non-contact mode, attractive rather than repulsive forces are measured. The scanning tip is oscillated perpendicular to, and just above the sample surface with an amplitude typically less than 10 nm. As with contact mode, a photodiode detector monitors the deflections of the laser light reflected from the tip of a cantilever. A feedback loop maintains constant oscillation amplitude or frequency, as the scanner moves laterally. A computer stores the information and a topographic image, with a lower resolution than in contact mode, is generated. Noncontact mode may work well with hydrophobic polymers. However hydrophilic polymers or imaging in a liquid environment in non-contact mode is not typically used due to the low resolution obtained.

AFM—tapping mode

In tapping mode, the cantilever is vibrated at or near its resonance frequency, and lightly taps the sample surface with an amplitude typically ranging from 20 to 100 nm. A split photodiode detector monitors the deflections of the laser light reflected from the tip of the cantilever. A feedback loop maintains constant oscillation amplitude or frequency, as the scanner moves laterally across the surface. This mode therefore maintains the high-resolution capabilities of contact mode but is not destructive since there are no lateral frictional forces applied to the sample that can distort or damage the material. Tapping mode AFM has proved to be very successful for high-resolution studies of polymeric biomaterials allowing for characterisation of nanometer scale features not visible by other microscopic techniques (see Fig. 4.5). Tapping mode AFM images typically included in the biomaterial literature have a scan size ranging from 500 nm × 500 nm, to 15 μm × 15 μm.

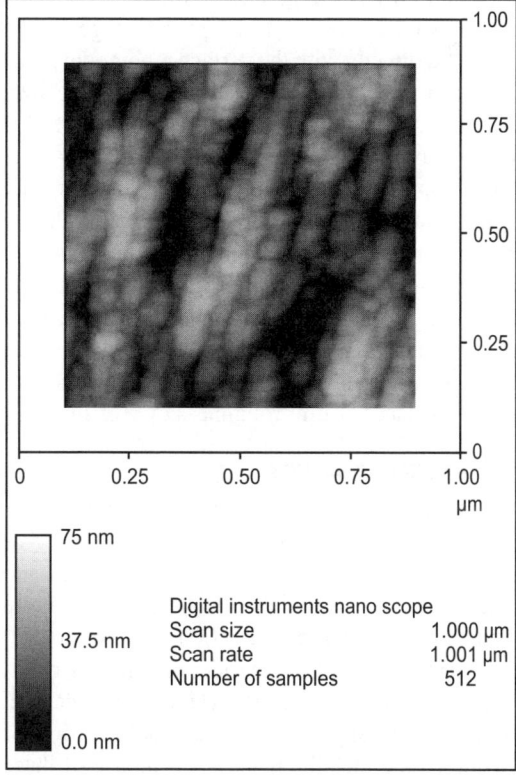

Fig. 4.5. AFM image of the inside polymer surface of a fibre obtained from a bleach/ formaldehyde reprocessed Gambro 21S polyamide hemodialyser. Scan size is 1 μm × 1 μm. AFM image was obtained using a nanoscope III scanning probe microscope operated in tapping mode in air.

AFM — phase imaging mode

The phase imaging mode can be used to map the surface composition of a sample. In this mode, the cantilever is vibrated at or near its resonance frequency, and lightly taps the sample surface. A feedback loop maintains constant oscillation amplitude, as the scanner moves laterally across the surface. A phase image shows the phase difference between oscillation of the piezoelectric crystal that drives the cantilever and oscillation of the cantilever itself as it interacts with the surface. Phase imaging can reveal fine features that are obscured by a rough surface topography. However factors such as surface hardness, elasticity, adhesive properties, and surface charge may affect the phase images obtained. Phase and tapping mode (height) images can be obtained simultaneously (see Fig. 4.6), so the position of the surface features observed in a phase image can be correlated directly with the surface topography. This mode can therefore be used to determine the size, shape and spacing of different material domains that could not otherwise be discerned from height alone. For example, phase imaging AFM can successfully detect adsorbed proteins that are not observable in conventional topographic images, since proteins imaged on surfaces with roughness near the dimensions of the protein cannot be distinguished from the material topography with conventional AFM, which is limited to imaging proteins only on smooth surfaces (1 μm^2 roughness of <0.5 nm).

AFM using coated tips

Recently the power of AFM has been coupled with appropriate biomolecules to enable the study of interactions of the surface with various proteins and lipids. While this technique has been applied more often to study specific interactions with biological systems including polysaccharides of living microbial cells, as well as extracellular ATP on living cells, it has also been applied to the characterisation of polymeric and metallic materials. The use of these techniques has added an additional dimension to AFM in addition to that used conventionally for analysis of morphology and topography of a biomaterial surface. Often a variety of characterisation techniques are used in the evaluation of biomaterial surfaces. However, it should be noted

that the use of even different microscopic techniques might give rise to a different view of the surfaces obtained. Figures 4.2, 4.3, and 4.5 show SEM, TEM and AFM images respectively of the same polyamide polymeric material.

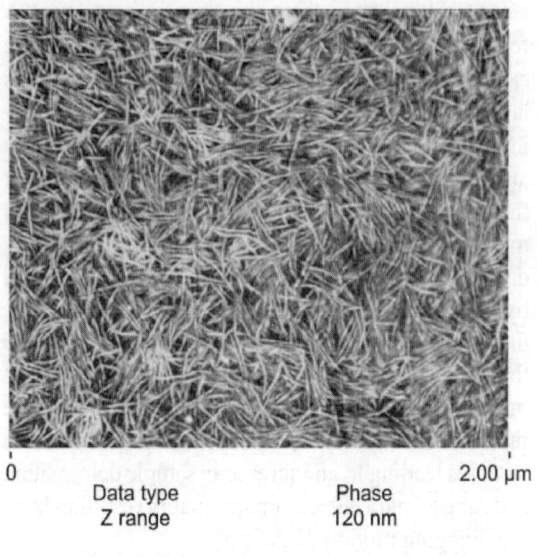

Data type	Phase
Z range	120 nm

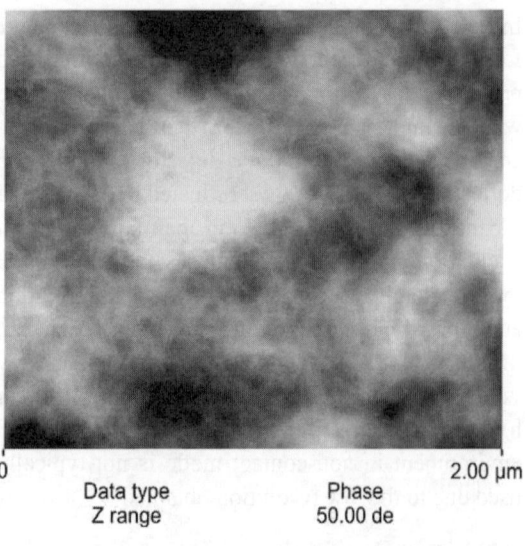

Data type	Phase
Z range	50.00 de

Fig. 4.6. AFM height and phase images of a polycarbonate urethane. Phase mode image shows a densely crystallised top layer believed to contain a high hard segment component. Images were obtained using a Multimode AFM operated in tapping mode in air.

The results obtained by SEM show a fairly smooth surface, with some very distinct porous regions. TEM results show a smooth surface, and in addition show that the bulk polymer contains a thick support layer consisting of interconnected highly porous domains. AFM results show significant surface morphology, not visible by the other techniques used. Thus, the combination of microscopic techniques used may play a valuable role in the characterisation of surface features and morphology of polymer biomaterials.

Confocal scanning microscopy

The major disadvantage with conventional light microscopy (LM) lies in illumination: because the entire specimen is illuminated, in-focus and out-of-focus information points contribute equally to the image resulting in blurring and poor contrast. There is also a sharp decline in image quality with increasing sample thickness, resulting in the need for thinly sectioned samples.

Confocal scanning light microscopy (CSLM) provides blur-free optical sectioning of a specimen by eliminating out-of-focus information through spatial filtering using a point source of light for excitation. The technique is convenient, in that no special sample preparation is required and features high-resolution images as compared to LM. Confocal microscopy is capable of resolving details at interfaces that could previously only be seen using electron microscopy of processed specimens. Image resolution in CSLM is generally given as 0.2 μm in the xy-plane (transverse plane) and about 0.6 μm in the z-plane (the in-focus optical section). The actual useful depth of CSLM is limited to approximately 100–200 μm, even with the use of near infrared illumination, which is more penetrating than visible light. The truly outstanding feature of CLSM is that two-dimensional pictures can be generated by scanning points across the focal plane of the specimen and subsequently compiled to give detailed three-dimensional images.

Three imaging modes available with confocal microscopes, each named according to the origin of the light that is imaged include confocal epitransmission with backscattered light from within the tissue, confocal reflectance, with light reflected from an opaque surface and confocal epifluorescence with light emitted by fluorescence. Confocal microscopy is sensitive to chromatic aberrations, which can be a problem in work employing white light or laser excitation of multiple fluorophores, which need to be imaged simultaneously, but which fluoresce with and are excited by different wavelengths. Despite this drawback, photobleaching and phototoxicity to the surrounding specimen is minimal. Also, the confocal image may be degraded by unwanted reflections of light from the surface of the objective lens or the specimen surface. However, this problem can be minimised using suitable immersion optics.

In the field of biomaterials, CSLM has been used in a number of applications. By conjugating a fluorophore to aqueous hydrogel solutions, CLSM in fluorescence mode has been used to investigate the bulk structure of hydrogels. In this manner, hydrogel samples may be imaged *in situ*, a distinct advantage over techniques such as SEM where critical point drying and freeze etching may alter the original gel structure. Detailed morphological characterisation of the hydrogel may be accomplished by assembling images collected at successive depth intervals from the surface into the bulk of the polymer. Pore sizes in the micrometer range and the polymer's three-dimensional structure may thus be obtained.

While there are problems with tissue accessibility in live animal work due to equipment design, real time (video rate) confocal imaging is achievable using the tandem scanning confocal microscope. Confocal microscopes also possess the ability to view individual cells, nuclei and nucleoli without staining and to view hollow organs via intraluminal endoscopy.

Spectroscopic methods

Spectroscopic methods are widely used to reveal valuable information regarding the constituent elements and chemical structure near the surface region of a sample. Two new characterisation techniques utilised in the biomaterials field are scanning transmission X-ray microscopy (STXM), and photoelectron emission microscopy (PEEM). Both techniques require synchrotron light sources and advanced instrumentation. While STXM has the advantages of not being affected by sample charging or topography, as well as the ability to image the sample in solution, the depth of sampling is full film often on the order of 100 nm. PEEM has a sampling depth of typically 5–10 nm for polymers. However, it requires ultra high vacuum, no sample charging and a sample roughness of <30 nm. Both techniques, STXM and PEEM, have a high lateral spatial resolution on the order of 50 nm, and excellent chemical sensitivity. Another section will discuss the relevance of these two emerging techniques (STXM, PEEM) in the biomaterials field. Much more commonly utilised in the surface characterisation of biomaterials, the traditional spectroscopic techniques used include:

1. Auger electron spectroscopy (AES).
2. X-ray photon spectroscopy (XPS).
3. Secondary ion mass spectrometry (SIMS).
4. Attenuated total reflection Fourier transform infrared spectroscopy (ATR-FTIR).

Auger electron spectroscopy (AES)

Auger electron spectroscopy (AES) has been used for investigating surface morphology, and in particular elemental analysis. A focused beam of electrons is used to excite Auger electrons from the surface, which are then detected and analysed. No special sample preparation is required and data collection is rapid (i.e. a few minutes) and reproducible. This technique has proven very useful in some engineering fields for elemental analysis and composition depth profiling. However, in general AES is limited in its use in the analysis of polymeric biomaterials as it is generally considered unsuitable for studying organic matter. Organic samples literally burn up in the electron beam, radically altering the chemistry and morphology of the sample being measured. Because the risk of artifact and misinterpretation is large, the use of AES for characterising organic, polymeric or biological specimens must be approached with caution (Fig. 7.7).

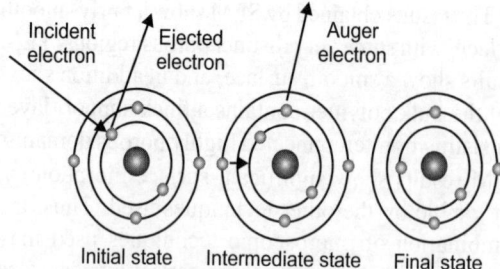

Fig. 4.7. Auger electron spectroscopy (AES).

X-ray photoelectron spectroscopy

X-ray photoelectron spectroscopy (XPS), also called ESCA (electron spectroscopy for chemical analysis) is widely used in biomaterial applications to determine the elemental composition of solid surfaces. Special sample preparation is generally not required for XPS, although surface contamination upon storage or during transport from the research laboratory to the XPS facilities may certainly have an adverse effect on the XPS results obtained. In addition, additives, such as catalysts that may be used during the polymerisation of polymeric biomaterials, or impurities can be present at the surface of the polymers and thus contribute significantly to the XPS results obtained.

The principle of XPS is based upon the emission of electrons from matter in response to irradiation of the surface by a beam of monochromatic X-rays. The kinetic energy of the emitted photoelectrons (K_E) is unique for the different elements as well as being sensitive to the chemical state of the atoms. The two energies of X-rays commonly used in experimental practice are 1253.6 eV (MgK_α) and 1486.6 eV (AlK_α). Since the emitted electrons have little ability to penetrate matter, only those electrons emitted near from the outermost 100 Å of a polymeric sample can escape from the surface and be quantified. All elements, except hydrogen and helium, can be detected by the characteristic binding energies of the electrons with a sensitivity of about 0.1 atom %. XPS survey (low resolution) scans (see Fig. 4.8a) are typically 1000 eV wide and are often used to identify, as well as quantify in terms of atomic per cent, the elements (Table 4.3) present at the biomaterial surface. High resolution scans are typically 20 eV wide and are used to obtain information about chemical shifts which can provide additional details about the chemical environment of the detected elements as well as shake-up transitions which provide details about aromatic or unsaturated structures. High resolution scans (Fig. 4.8b) are referred to as such, because typically more time is spent acquiring data over a narrower energy range as compared to a survey scan (Fig. 4.8a) resulting in a better signal to noise ratio.

Table 4.3. Oxygen Content (atomic %) of a PU control surface, and a PU surface modified with PEO, determined from an XPS survey (low resolution) scan. The expected increase in oxygen content of the PEO modified surface was observed.

Polymer	Oxygen content (%)
PU control surface (theoretical)	17
PU control surface	17.1
PU surface modified with PEO	26.2

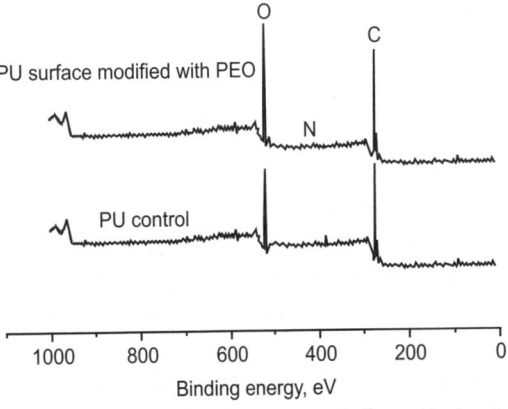

Fig. 4.8a. Survey (low resolution) XPS scans of a polyurethane (PU) surface, and a PU surface modified with polyethylene oxide (PEO). XPS signals for carbon (C), nitrogen (N) and oxygen (O) are indicated. Scans show an increase in the O peak. Table 4.3 shows the corresponding atomic % of oxygen present clearly indicating that the surface has been successfully modified with PEO. XPS spectra were obtained using a Leybold MAX200 X-ray photoelectron spectrometer, and analysed using ESCATOOLS (Surface/Interface, Mountain View, CA).

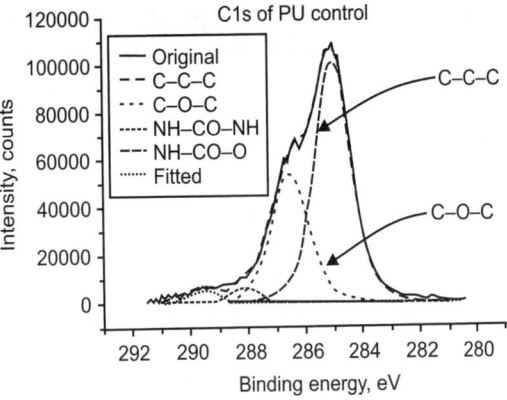

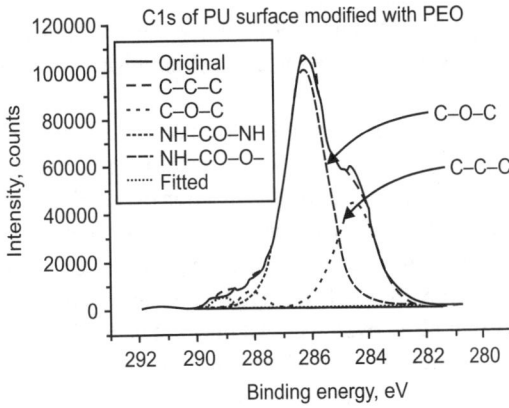

Fig. 4.8b. High resolution XPS C1s detailed spectra of a polyurethane (PU) surface, and a PU surface modified with polyethylene oxide (PEO). Representative 4 peak curve fits of the XPS C1s signal are also shown. Table 4.3 shows the corresponding Carbon Atom Bonding (%) of C—O—C determined from best fit of C1s High Resolution XPS Spectra clearly indicating that the surface has been successfully modified with PEO. XPS spectrum was obtained using a Leybold MAX200 X-ray photoelectron spectrometer, and analysed using ESCATOOLS (Surface/Interface, Mountain View, CA).

The XPS technique is highly versatile, with a sampling depth related to the inelastic mean free path of photoelectrons in the surface region, which is typically greater that 30 Å for polymeric materials, although this depends on both the photoelectron energy and on the material studied. Typically, the signal, under ultra-high vacuum, is gathered from a large sample area (i.e. ~6 mm in diameter) in order to minimise collection time, and possible damage to some polymeric materials. However, lateral resolution using a smaller sample area, in the range of square microns, has been reported. Refined instrumentation simplifies sampling handling and data collection. Well developed theory and computer programs are available to assist in the interpretation of the data obtained. XPS is considered to be a relatively non-destructive technique, although some care is needed to ensure that the X-ray does not alter the surface chemistry. Problems have been reported to occur with polymers, especially flouropolymers, with the effects being minimised by use of a monochromatic source in conjunction with an effective compensation method to avoid surface charging problems or by simply minimising the X-ray exposure to the surface and optimising spectral acquisition times.

Information about functional groups can be obtained by using derivitisation reactions. Compositional variation as a function of sample depth can be obtained by measurement of the photoelectron intensities at different emission angles, termed angle resolved XPS. Angle resolved XPS can also be used to examine an overlayer that may not be uniform, to investigate a surface where coverage is believed to be patchy, or to examine the change or transition between bulk and surface of a 'surface modified' material. To obtain elemental information several thousand angstroms into the sample, argon etching can be used in conjunction with XPS although this method is sample destructive. While the signal is typically gathered from a large sample area (i.e. 25 mm^2), it is possible, as mentioned earlier, to use XPS to determine lateral variations in surface composition and to estimate the thickness of both organic and inorganic layers. In addition, hydrated freeze dried surfaces can be examined using XPS which may be of considerable interest when characterising polymer surfaces that may reorient upon exposure to an air, vacuum or aqueous environment (Table 4.4).

There is considerable literature available on the principles of XPS, analytical procedures, instrumentation and approaches to quantitative analyses. In the study and characterisation of biomaterial surfaces, XPS is possibly the most extensively used technique. It has been used for a variety of surfaces and surface modifications, including studies of adsorption and retention of chemicals such as antibiotics and bonding agents, for the detection of immobilised proteins, understanding the chemistry of the structure, formation and stability of plasma treated surfaces, as well as for the characterisation of the steps of formation of thin coatings.

Table 4.4. Carbon atom bonding (%) of C—O—C determined from best fit of C1s high resolution XPS spectra of a PU control surface, and a PU surface modified with PEO. The expected increase in C—O—C content of the PEO modified surface was observed.

Polymer	C—O—C content (%)
PU control surface	33.5
PU surface modified with PEO	66.1

Secondary ion mass spectrometry (SIMS) and time-of-flight secondary ion mass spectrometry (ToF-SIMS)

Secondary ion mass spectrometry (SIMS) is effective for providing detailed molecular surface information and increased usage of this technique in the surface characterisation of polymeric biomaterials has been observed in recent years. Typically, no special sample preparation is required for SIMS. However as with XPS, the surface must be clean and free of any contamination that may occur upon storage or transport. Surfaces are bombarded with a focused beam of ions or atoms and the energy from the incident beam (approximately 5–25 keV) is transferred to the surface zone of the material resulting in the emission of secondary particles, some of which are ionised, at and around the impact site. These ionised particles are separated as a function of the ration of mass per electric charge and positively and negatively charged species are detected in two different acquisitions.

Low flux or static SIMS results in minimal damage to the sample and the fragments emitted are characteristic of the surface molecular structure. High flux, or dynamic SIMS results in rapid etching of the surface during analysis and can be used to monitor changes in the elemental composition with depth.

Time-of-flight SIMS (ToF-SIMS) is a very efficient method for characterising the elemental (including H and isotopes) and molecular composition of the top surface of biomaterials. Developments in the ToF-SIMS analyser have increased the capabilities of static SIMS due to significantly improved mass transmission (independent of the ion mass), mass resolution, mass range and sensitivity. In this case, the sample surface is bombarded with very short-pulsed ion beams. Between two consecutive pulses, all of the secondary ions are extracted and electrostatically accelerated into a field free drift region. Lighter ions will have higher velocities and hence will reach the detector at the end of the drift region earlier than the heavier masses. From the time of flight, the mass to charge ratio can be determined. Under static conditions, there is minimal surface damage with ToF SIMS. This technique is also associated with a high mass range, that is theoretically unlimited but has a practical limit of $m/z = 15000$. While there is a high surface sensitivity of 10^7 to 10^{11} atoms/cm^2) and mass and lateral resolutions, quantification of data is difficult and information depth can be different from the sampling depth.

SIMS can be used for the identification of all elements including hydrogen as well as atomic and molecular ions and extremely high mass fragments at very low concentrations. Dynamic SIMS permits depth profiling from one to two atomic layers (1 nm in thickness) up to 1 μm into the sample with a high mass resolution. Although the analysis destroys the surface, information generated is directly related to the initial surface. While static SIMS can be applied successfully to the analysis of both organic and inorganic surfaces, the accuracy of the information with dynamic SIMS is considerably reduced for organic and biological surfaces. These techniques can be used to obtain direct proof of covalent binding of molecules to a surface, as well as to predict other surface properties including wettability, adhesiveness, and biological reactivity. SIMS spectra can provide characteristic 'fingerprints' for biomaterial surfaces, and has been used to correlate surface chemistry with cell growth as well as for monitoring the degradation kinetics of biodegradable polymers using molecular weight distributions of the oligomeric hydrolytic reaction products. Temperature-programmed SIMS offers information on adsorption energy and thus helps to distinguish between physisorption and chemisorption phenomena. It is often used in conjunction with XPS to examine the integrity, mean thickness and chemical state of multi-layer biomaterial coatings, corroborating contact angle and XPS measurements and complementing data obtained from less surface sensitive techniques.

Infrared spectroscopy (IR) and attenuated total reflection fourier transform infrared spectroscopy (ATR-FTIR)

Infrared spectroscopy is used to obtain information about molecular structure by measuring the frequency of IR radiation needed to excite vibrations in molecular bonds. Sample preparation is minimal involving application of the polymeric material of interest, in film form, onto a crystal element. Instrumentation is relatively inexpensive, and the resulting spectra provide chemical bonding information. Infrared spectroscopy in attenuated total reflection (ATR-FTIR) couples the analytical method of infrared spectroscopy with the physical phenomena of total internal reflection (i.e. reflection and refraction of electromagnetic radiation at an interface of two media having different indices of refraction) to restrict the analysed volume on the surface region of the sample. For this technique, the incident electromagnetic waves are entirely reflected back into the initial medium. The electromagnetic field is established in the second medium as represented by an evanescent wave due to diffraction at the edges of the incident radiation at the interface. In attenuated total reflectance (ATR) sampling mode the second medium is the material to be studied, with the first medium acting as the internal reflection element. Information about the molecular structure of the material, inter — and intra — molecular interactions, crystallinity, conformation (e.g. proteins) and orientation of molecules can be obtained through analysis of the infrared spectra. Although depth profiles can be obtained using this technique, the XPS and SIMS techniques discussed earlier are considered much more surface sensitive (Fig 4.9).

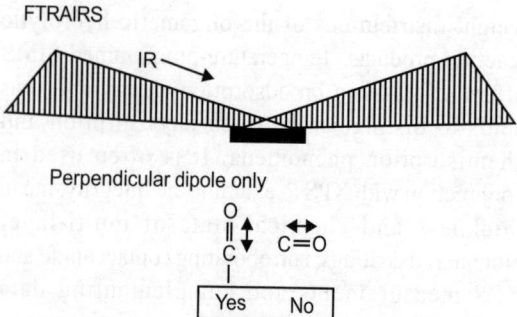

Fig. 4.9. Attenuated total reflection fourier transform infrared spectroscopy (ATR-FTIR).

Surface matrix-assisted laser desorption ionisation mass spectrometry (surface MALDI)

Surface matrix-assisted laser desorption ionisation mass spectrometry (surface-MALDI), also known as MALDI-time of flight mass spectrometry (MALDI-TOFMS) is a novel surface analytical method that is an extension of conventional MALDI-MS, offering extremely high mass resolution and very low detection limits for macromolecular analytes. Compared to traditional MALDI-MS which is used to record the molecular weights and purities of known solution-based analytes, MALDI-TOFMS can be used to analyse adsorbed multicomponent bimolecular layers directly on the biomaterial surface using the charge to mass ratio of expelled ions. Macromolecule adsorbed surfaces are coated with matrix molecules. The matrix molecules that form on the surface are subsequently irradiated by a pulsed UV laser with various wavelengths dependent on the applications for 3–15 ns, resulting in the volatilisation of surface adsorbed entities which are detected. Analysis area is a spot with a diameter of approximately 10 μm. For good mass resolution, ions of equal masses but different energies must be detected simultaneously, meaning that the time from ionisation to detection should be less than a nanosecond. Analyte ejection into the vapour phase, while not fully understood, is thought to be affected by the ability of the matrix molecules to mediate UV energy transfer to organic molecules that do not absorb in the UV wavelength range. Nicotinic acid, dihydroxybenzoic acid and sinapinic acid have been found to be suitable matrix

molecules. Due to the low pHs involved (pH < 4.5), it is however not unlikely that the matrix molecules will affect the structure of the bioactive adsorbents, resulting in crosslinking, denaturation, or degradation. It is also essential that the samples under study be pure, that the matrix be present at a 100–1000 fold excess (vol/vol) and that the layer under study be between 0.1 and 1 μm thick (Fig. 4.10).

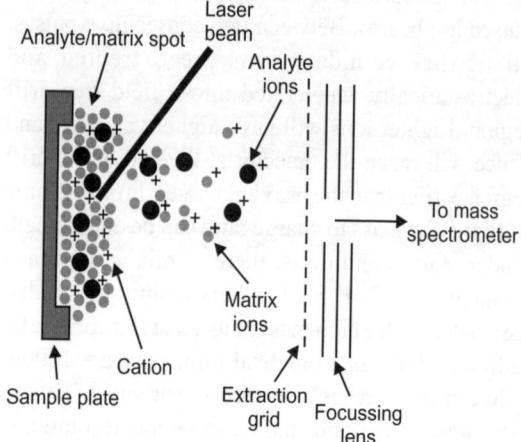

Fig. 4.10. A schematic diagram of the mechanism of MALDI.

MALDI-TOFMS has a theoretically unlimited mass detection range that is limited in practice by the fact that larger ions with higher mass are usually moving too slowly to be registered by the detector which has a limited threshold detection energy. Furthermore, while the technique has a relatively high sensitivity for low adsorbent concentrations, the mass resolving power decreases as the molecular weight of the macromolecule increases. For example, the mass resolving power of small molecules is 300–500, while molecules larger than 200 kDa have a mass resolving power of 50–100. This is clearly evident as the peaks become broader with increases in molecular weight, amplifying the error in molecular weight determination, which is dependent on finding the centre of the peak. Other limitations of MALDI-TOFMS include the requirement for vacuum operation and the ions measured can be products of side reactions between adsorbents that can decay with time. The main sources of error in this technique are time errors, where ions of equal mass reach the detector at different times and metastable ion decay during flight to the detector. At present, the technique is not quantitative and requires control experiments and parallel XPS analyses for quantification of adsorbed amounts.

This technique has been applied to a variety of systems. Polymer MALDI-TOFMS studies are extensive and the technique has been used to determine surface coupling reaction yields, and polyethylene glycol molecular weight distributions for example. The technique is said to provide very high mass resolution and thus has the ability to separate proteins that may give overlapping signals in PAGE analysis with very low detection limits and can detect physiosorbed from covalently bound proteins on synthetic polymers carrying thin layers of biological molecules. It has been successfully applied to detect molecular ions of a number of proteins adsorbed from single and complex solutions onto various synthetic biomaterials even though the adsorbed proteins are bound strongly enough to resist removal by standard aqueous rinsing protocols. However, there can exist a residence time effect. With increasing time following adsorption onto the synthetic biomaterial, some proteins are increasingly difficult to desorb and analyse by surface-MALDI-MS. This is believed to be a consequence of protein denaturation, which increases the binding strength of physiosorbed proteins. MALDI-TOFMS also allows detection of minor and major proteinaceous constituents of biofouled layers at substantially below monolayer coverage and has been used for the direct analysis of biofilms produced *in vivo* on synthetic biomaterials.

Thermodynamic Methods

Several methods can be used to obtain surface parameters related to the interfacial free energy and other thermodynamic interaction measures such as the enthalpy of adsorption or displacement. This type of analysis has been shown to be an efficient method for obtaining preliminary information on the biocompatibility of biomaterials. The major thermodynamic method used to characterise biomaterial surfaces are wetting or contact angle experiments.

Contact angle methods

Measurement of the contact angle of a liquid test droplet on a solid surface is a straightforward technique revealing surface energetic information inaccessible by the surface spectroscopies. Although, this method represents perhaps one of the earliest methods used to investigate surface structure, it still yields very useful information. Contact angle measurements at biomaterials surfaces can be carried out by several different methods including:

1. The wilhelmy plate method.
2. The sessile drop method.
3. The captive bubble method.

A drop of fluid is placed on the biomaterial surface of interest, an equilibrium position is achieved, and the contact angle determined from the tangent associated with the drop/polymer surface. Contact angles, for immobile surfaces, are believed to be sensitive to the outermost 3–10 Angstroms of a surface. Typically, in the biomaterials literature, contact angles are measured in air, utilising a goniometer, using the sessile drop method with water as the test fluid. Contact angle analysis of control and modified polymeric materials can quickly provide valuable information about the relative hydrophilicity/hydrophobicity of the surfaces. In addition, information about the hysteresis can be obtained when comparing contact angles obtained during increase, referred to as the advancing contact angle, and decrease, referred to as the receding contact angle, in the test droplet volume. Comparison of contact angle measurements obtained for control and surface modified polymeric materials can be used to confirm the successful alteration of the control surface (Fig. 4.11). Acid base contact angles can also give information about surface chemistry and underwater contact angles, using the captive bubble technique, can be used to give information about hydrated surfaces.

Typically no special procedures are required in the preparation of polymeric materials for contact angle analysis. However, the surfaces should be clean, smooth, homogeneous and not swell or dissolve in the test fluid. It should also be recognised that factors such as the choice and purity of the organic liquids and water, droplet size, and time required to obtain readings may affect the contact angle results obtained. Although the application of contact angles in evaluating polymeric biomaterial surface properties is a simple and straight forward approach, the use of this technique assumes thermodynamic equilibrium as well as a smooth, homogeneous surface which does not swell or dissolve in the test liquid. Contact angle hysteresis has been reported to occur with surfaces that are rough, chemically heterogeneous, or contaminated with surface-active agents, as well as for surfaces that reorient upon exposure to different fluids.

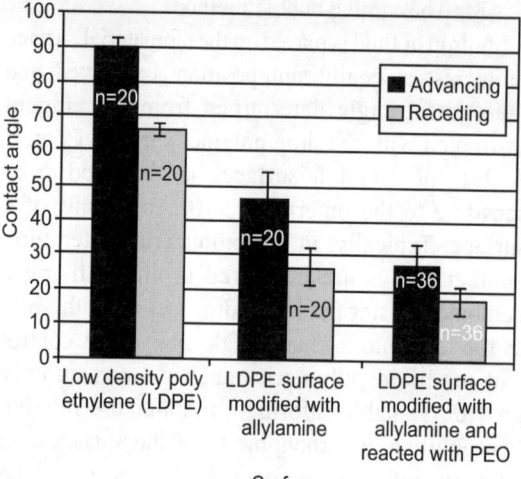

Fig. 4.11. Advancing and receding water contact angles measured by a goniometer using the sessile drop method for low density polyethylene (LDPE), LDPE surface modified with allylamine, LDPE surface modified with allylamine and reacted with polyethylene oxide (PEO). Figure clearly shows a reduction in advancing and receding contact angles due to the allylamine surface modification of the control surface, as well as a further reduction upon reaction with PEO. Surfaces were rinsed with methanol and dried prior to contact angle determination.

Other Methods

Specular neutron reflectivity

Specular neutron reflectivity (SNR) has the potential to be a powerful tool for elucidating biomaterial surface information and protein interfacial mechanisms. SNR measures the change in scattering length density at the interface between two different neutron refractive index materials. It is suited to evaluating the adsorbed protein conformation for all three interface types, and is perhaps the best technique for studying adsorption at the liquid/liquid interface. This technique offers the benefit of spatial resolution of ~1.0 nm and penetration depths for some systems of several hundred nanometers. By reflecting neutrons from the sample, it is possible to independently and simultaneously determine both the composition and concentration distribution normal to the interface in question from the resulting interference fringes as shown in Fig. 4.12. The high penetrating power of neutrons allows them to pass through a medium before reaching the interface under study. Other advantages include enhanced contrast through isotope substitution like deuterium labeling, minimal surface damage allowing for successive measurements on a single sample and neutron sensitivity to magnetic interactions. The sensitivity of neutron reflection is ~2 Å, or two methylene groups. Contrast is achieved by using the difference in the coherent scattering length densities (β) of D and H. However, the specialised nature of the equipment resulting in limited access. An additional limitation is the requirement of a large surface (20 cm^2) for thin film experiments.

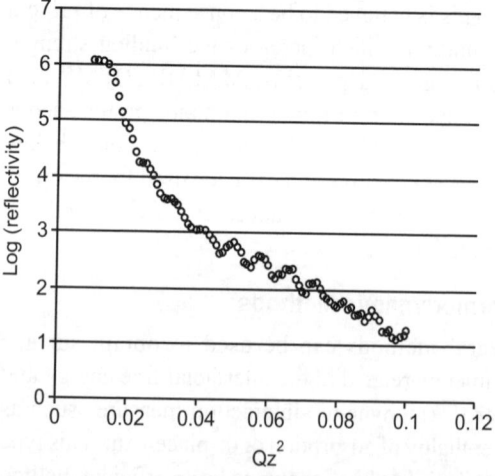

Fig. 4.12. Illustration of interference fringes for a gold coated silicon wafer, with chemisorbed PEG-thiol. This can be used to determine the thin film thickness, and composition profile both normal and parallel to the interface.

SNR has been used to identify the surface composition for complex polymer mixtures, surface and interfacial segregation, time dependant processes, liquid mixture adsorptions, surfactant (ethylene glycol) adsorption used in colloidal dispersions, copolymer adsorption at the liquid/liquid interface and protein adsorption at various interfaces. Studies have also been done on the adsorption of star and deuterated polyethylene oxide (PEO) at the solid liquid interface and lipidated PEO and peptides at the air water interface. In our lab, SNR studies have been used to understand the adsorbed film characteristics for thiolated PEG on gold-coated silicon wafers. An example of the data that can be obtained is shown in Fig. 4.12. Once analysed, these interference fringes will reveal the thickness of the adsorbed PEG layer and that change in the macromolecular density normal to the interface.

PROTEIN ADSORPTION TO BIOMATERIAL

It is now well accepted that the initial rapid adsorption of blood proteins to biomaterial surfaces is important in the long-term performance of the implant. Cells that interact with the implant will be reacting to a layer (single or multiple) of adsorbed protein. The parameters of importance in a study of protein adsorption to surfaces of biomaterial interest include total amounts of different adsorbed proteins and the conformation and orientation of these adsorbed proteins. Researchers have developed a number of techniques with which we can now address all these questions, Fourier transform infrared (FTIR) attenuated total internal reflection (ATR) techniques can be used for the study of biomaterial surfaces and events at biomaterial surfaces such as protein adsorption. FTIR spectroscopy offers higher signal-to-noise and speeds than spectrometers that use gratings and hence offers the capability of observing the critical early events when proteins interact with surfaces. Perhaps the biggest advantage of the FTIR technique over dispersive spectrometers is wavelength precision. This allows the subtraction of water, a strong infrared absorber, from the spectra of proteins in aqueous solutions.

It is known that within minutes surfaces of implants placed in the body become coated with a proteinacious layer which is a key mediator of cell adhesion. Hence, developing a surface that has the correct physico-chemical properties influences the interaction of proteins, cell and tissues. This study aimed to investigate the adsorption of selected proteins; fibrinogen and fibronectin on a series of materials with different surface modifications. Methods: 8 different materials were used in this study; carbon (2), cobalt-chrome (1), stainless steel (1), and Titanium (Ti) alloy with 4 different surface modifications, i.e. polished, glass-bead blast, aluminium blast, and hydroxyapatite (HA) coated. All sample surfaces had the same sizes which were 10 mm in diameter. After incubating all surfaces with human plasma for 1 hour at 37°C, surfaces were rinsed and adsorbed proteins were assessed by SDS-PAGE. In addition the adsorptions of fibrinogen and fibronectin (protein associated with cell adhesion) were assessed by Western-Blot analysis. Scanning Electron Microscope (SEM) was also used for surface characterisation. Results: SDS-PAGE results showed that all materials adsorbed plasma proteins in varying amounts. The relative adsorbed protein amounts were as follow; Ti alloy HA coated and aluminium blast > Ti glass-bead blast and polished > cobalt-chromium and stainless steel. Western-Blot, using specific antibodies to fibrinogen and fibronectin, indicated that their adsorption was dependent on molecular weight. Surface characterisation of the test surfaces using SEM revealed differents degree of surface topography, which may influence protein adsorption. This preliminary study showed that different surfaces finishes influenced the relative adsorption of fibrinogen and fibronectin. Although all surfaces adsorbed proteins to a certain extent, the amount and type of proteins were different. Understanding the interaction of cells with proteins in the extracellular matrix will assist in the development of optimised surfaces for the enhancement of osseointegration.

A wide range of techniques provides information on protein adsorption onto solid surfaces such as Vibrational sum frequency spectroscopy (VSFS). The interaction force between two solid surfaces can be measured as a function of distance by the surface force apparatus (SFA). Claesson employed SFA to study a wide range of proteins (globular, unordered, fibrous) and determined protein conformation, orientation, and the operative forces. Small compact globular and soft globular proteins could be distinguished by measuring their compressibility. Blomberg. used SFA to study the adsorption of lysozyme on mica as a function of protein concentration, determining the protein's adsorption orientation, ability to form multilayers, and adsorption irreversibility.

Conformation information on adsorbed protein is also available from several spectroscopic methods. Circular dichroism spectroscopy (CD), Fourier transform infrared spectroscopy (FTIR), and Raman spectroscopy all probe protein secondary structure. These techniques have been useful in demonstrating how proteins alter their structure upon adsorption. Proteins have been shown to have greater structural perturbation on hydrophobic surfaces, compared to hydrophilic surfaces using CD, FTIR, and Raman spectroscopy.

A significant amount of literature on protein adsorption is concerned with the kinetics and total mass of protein adsorbed onto a solid surface. The quartz crystal microbalance (QCM) measures the changes in resonance frequency and dissipation factor of an oscillating quartz crystal and can provide information on the adsorbed mass and temporal variations in surface viscoelastic properties. Otzen employed QCM to study the adsorption of protein S6 onto a methyl-terminated quartz surface and found that the adsorption kinetics of protein S6 depends on the equilibrium fraction of denatured protein in the bulk, rather than on the kinetics of bulk denaturation. Upon comparison with optical techniques, such as ellipsometry and optical waveguide lightmode spectroscopy (OWLS), Hook showed that QCM reports higher adsorbed mass, this being attributed to water bound to the adsorbed protein.

Proteins (also known as polypeptides) are organic compounds made of amino acids arranged in a linear chain and folded into a globular form. The amino acids in a polymer are joined together by the peptide bonds between the carboxyl and amino groups of adjacent amino acid residues. The sequence of amino acids in a protein is defined by the sequence of a gene, which is encoded in the genetic code. In general, the genetic code specifies 20 standard amino acids; however, in certain organisms the genetic code can include selenocysteine — and in certain archaea — pyrrolysine. Shortly after or even during synthesis, the residues in a protein are often chemically modified by post-translational modification, which alters the physical and chemical properties, folding, stability, activity, and ultimately, the function of the proteins. Proteins can also work together to achieve a particular function, and they often associate to form stable complexes.

Like other biological macromolecules such as polysaccharides and nucleic acids, proteins are essential parts of organisms and participate in virtually every process within cells. Many proteins are enzymes that catalyse biochemical reactions and are vital to metabolism. Proteins also have structural or mechanical functions, such as actin and myosin in muscle and the proteins in the cytoskeleton, which form a system of scaffolding that maintains cell shape. Other proteins are important in cell signaling, immune responses, cell adhesion, and the cell cycle. Proteins are also necessary in animals' diets, since animals cannot synthesise all the amino acids they need and must obtain essential amino acids from food. Through the process of digestion, animals break down ingested protein into free amino acids that are then used in metabolism.

Different amino acids combine to form polypeptides and these in turn give rise to a very high number of complex structures (proteins). The combination of polypeptides gives each protein a distinct three-dimensional shape. This spatial relationship between the amino acid chains giving rise to the structure of a protein is called conformation. On the surface of a protein molecule there are hydrophobic, charged and polar domains. The particular regions of a protein to which antibodies or cells can bind are called epitopes. The existence, arrangement, and availability of different protein epitopes is called organisation.

Protein Adsorption Fundamentals

For a single protein solution, the rate of adsorption to the substrate depends upon transport of the protein to the substrate. Four primary transport mechanisms have been identified: diffusion, thermal convection, flow convection, and combined convection-diffusion. For constant temperature and static systems, transport is exclusively by diffusion, and the net rate of adsorption can be described by Langmuir's theory of gas adsorption.

The Langmuir equation or Langmuir isotherm or Langmuir adsorption equation or Hill-Langmuir equation relates the coverage or adsorption of molecules on a solid surface to gas pressure or concentration of a medium above the solid surface at a fixed temperature. The equation was developed by Irving Langmuir in 1916. The equation is stated as:

$$\theta = \frac{\alpha \cdot P}{1 + \alpha \cdot P}$$

θ or theta is the fractional coverage of the surface, P is the gas pressure or concentration, α alpha is α constant.

The constant α is the Langmuir adsorption constant and increases with an increase in the binding energy of adsorption and with a decrease in temperature (Fig. 4.13).

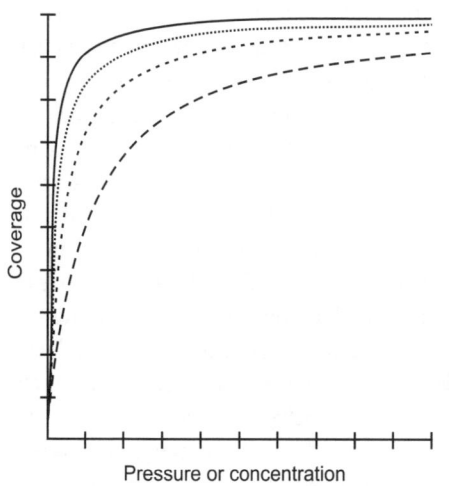

Fig. 4.13. Langmuir isotherm.

The Langmuir equation is derived starting from the equilibrium between empty surface sites (S^*),

particles (P) and filled particle sites (SP)

$$S^* + P \leftrightarrow SP$$

The equilibrium constant K is thus given by the equation:

$$K = \frac{[SP]}{[S^*][P]}$$

Because the number of filled surface sites (SP) is proportional to θ, the number of unfilled sites (S^*) is proportional to $1-\theta$, and the number of particles is proportional to the gas pressure or concentration (P), the equation can be rewritten as:

$$\alpha = \frac{\theta}{[1-\theta]P}$$

where α is a constant.

Rearranging this as follows:

$\theta = \alpha(1 - \theta)P$
$\theta = P\alpha - P\theta\alpha$
$\theta + P\theta\alpha = P\alpha$
$\theta(1 + P\alpha) = P\alpha$

leads to Langmuir equation:

$$\theta = \frac{\alpha \cdot P}{1 + \alpha \cdot P}$$

Other equations relating to adsorption exist, such as the Temkin equation or the Freundlich equation. The Langmuir equation (as a relationship between the concentration of a compound adsorbing to binding sites and the fractional occupancy of the binding sites) is equivalent to the Hill equation.

The langmuir equation is expressed here as:

$$\Gamma = \Gamma_{max} \frac{Kc}{1 + kc}$$

where,

K = Langmuir equilibrium constant.
c = aqueous concentration (or gaseous partial pressure).
Γ = amount adsorbed.
Γ_{max} = maximum amount adsorbed as c increases.

The equilibrium constant is actually given by Γ_{max}:

$$\Gamma(c = K^{-1}) = \Gamma_{max} \frac{KK^{-1}}{1 + KK^{-1}} = \frac{\Gamma_{max}}{2}$$

The Langmuir equation can be fitted to data by linear regression and nonlinear regression methods. Commonly used linear regression methods are: Lineweaver-Burk, Eadie-Hofstee, Scatchard, and Langmuir.

The double reciprocal of the Langmuir equation yields the Lineweaver-Burk equation:

$$\frac{1}{\Gamma} = \frac{1}{\Gamma_{max}} + \frac{1}{\Gamma_{max} Kc}$$

A plot of $(1/\Gamma)$ versus $(1/c)$ yields a slope = $1/(\Gamma_{max}K)$ and an intercept = $1/\Gamma_{max}$. The Lineweaver-Burk regression is very sensitive to data error and it is strongly biased toward fitting the data in the low concentration range. Another common linear form of the Langmuir equation is the Eadie-Hofstee equation:

$$\Gamma = \Gamma_{max} - \frac{\Gamma}{Kc}$$

A plot of (Γ) versus (Γ/c) yields a slope = $-1/K$ and an intercept = Γ_{max}. The Eadie-Hofstee regression has some bias toward fitting the data in the low concentration range. Another rearrangement yields the Scatchard regression:

$$\frac{\Gamma}{c} = K\Gamma_{max} - K\Gamma$$

A plot of (Γ/c) versus (Γ) yields a slope = $-K$ and an intercept = $K\Gamma_{max}$. The Scatchard regression is biased toward fitting the data in the high concentration range. Note that if you invert the x and y axes, then this regression would convert into the Eadie-Hofstee regression discussed earlier. The last linear regression commonly used is the Langmuir linear regression proposed by Langmuir himself in 1918:

$$\frac{c}{\Gamma} = \frac{c}{\Gamma_{max}} + \frac{1}{K\Gamma_{max}}$$

A plot of (c/Γ) versus (c) yields a slope = $1/\Gamma_{max}$ and an intercept = $1/(K\Gamma_{max})$. This regression is often erroneously called the Hanes-Woolf regression. The Hanes-Woolf regression was proposed in 1932 and 1957 for fitting the Michaelis-Menten equation, which is similar in form to the Langmuir equation. Nevertheless, Langmuir proposed this linear regression technique in 1918, and it should be referred to as the *Langmuir linear regression* when applied to adsorption isotherms. The Langmuir regression has very little sensitivity to data error. It has some bias toward fitting the data in the middle and high concentration range.

There are two kinds of nonlinear least squares (NLLS) regression techniques that can be used to fit the Langmuir equation to a data set. They differ only on how the goodness-of-fit is defined. In the v-NLLS regression method, the best goodness-of-fit is defined as the curve with the smallest vertical error between the fitted curve and the data. In the n-NLLS regression method, the best goodness-of-fit is defined as the curve with the smallest normal error between the fitted curve and the data. Using the vertical error is the most common form of NLLS regression criteria. Definitions based on the normal error are less common. The normal error is the error of the datum point to the nearest point on the fitted curve. It is called the normal error because the trajectory is normal (that is, perpendicular) to the curve.

Protein Adsorption Measurements

In order to understand protein adsorption, quantitative evaluation of the adsorption process must be performed, along with information on gathering the properties and characteristics of the protein molecule itself that will affect the adsorption mechanisms.

Although a set of useful information is obtained from a protein adsorption experiment, the available techniques are limited and in general do not provide all the information desired. The amount of adsorbed protein (adsorbed isotherms) is measured using XPS and ATR-IR. Adsorption as a function of time is also measured using ATR-IR and fluorescence spectroscopy. The conformation and conformational changes (denaturation) of the protein molecule can be determined using IR techniques circular dichroism (CD), and calorimetry. The thickness of the adsorbed layer is measured by ellipsometry. For studying the heterogeneity of adsorption, election microscopy and microautoradiography are used. The use of radiolabelled proteins allows direct measurement of protein adsorbed to substrate.

Differential scanning calorimetry

Differential scanning calorimetry or DSC is a thermoanalytical technique in which the difference in the amount of heat required to increase the temperature of a sample and reference are measured as a function of temperature. Both the sample and reference are maintained at nearly the same temperature throughout the experiment. Generally, the temperature program for a DSC analysis is designed such that the sample holder temperature increases linearly as a function of time. The reference sample should have a well-defined heat capacity over the range of temperatures to be scanned (Fig. 4.14).

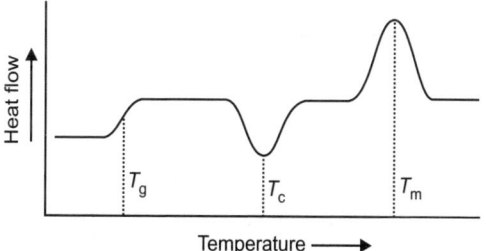

Fig. 4.14. Differential scanning calorimetry (DSC).

The main application of DSC is in studying phase transitions, such as melting, glass transitions, or exothermic decompositions. These transitions involve energy changes or heat capacity changes that can be detected by DSC with great sensitivity.

The basic principle underlying this technique is that, when the sample undergoes a physical transformation such as phase transitions, more or less heat will need to flow to it than the reference to maintain both at the same temperature. Whether less or more heat must flow to the sample depends on whether the process is exothermic or endothermic. For example, as a solid sample melts to a liquid it will require more heat flowing to the sample to increase its temperature at the same rate as the reference. This is due to the absorption of heat by the sample as it undergoes the endothermic phase transition from solid to liquid. Likewise, as the sample undergoes exothermic processes (such as crystallisation) less heat is required to raise the sample temperature. By observing the difference in heat flow between the sample and reference, differential

scanning calorimeters are able to measure the amount of heat absorbed or released during such transitions. DSC may also be used to observe more subtle phase changes, such as glass transitions. It is widely used in industrial settings as a quality control instrument due to its applicability in evaluating sample purity and for studying polymer curing.

An alternative technique, which shares much in common with DSC, is differential thermal analysis (DTA). In this technique it is the heat flow to the sample and reference that remains the same rather than the temperature. When the sample and reference are heated identically phase changes and other thermal processes cause a difference in temperature between the sample and reference. Both DSC and DTA provide similar information and modern DTA developed from the Boersma DTA, which first used one furnace with fixed thermocouples. Many modern commercial DTA are called heat flux DSC.

DSC curves

The result of a DSC experiment is a curve of heat flux versus temperature or versus time. There are two different conventions: exothermic reactions in the sample shown with a positive or negative peak; it depends on the different kind of technology used by the instrumentation to make the experiment. This curve can be used to calculate enthalpies of transitions. This is done by integrating the peak corresponding to a given transition. It can be shown that the enthalpy of transition can be expressed using the following equation:

$$\Delta H = KA$$

where ΔH is the enthalpy of transition, K is the calorimetric constant, and A is the area under the curve. The calorimetric constant will vary from instrument to instrument, and can be determined by analysing a well-characterised sample with known enthalpies of transition.

Applications

Differential scanning calorimetry can be used to measure a number of characteristic properties of a sample. Using this technique it is possible to observe fusion and crystallisation events as well as glass transition temperatures T_g. DSC can also be used to study oxidation, as well as other chemical reactions (Fig. 4.15).

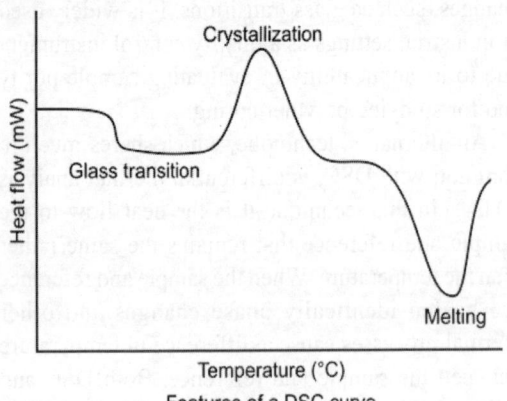

Features of a DSC curve

Fig 4.15. A schematic DSC curve demonstrating the appearance of several common features.

Glass transitions may occur as the temperature of an amorphous solid is increased. These transitions appear as a step in the baseline of the recorded DSC signal. This is due to the sample undergoing a change in heat capacity; no formal phase change occurs.

As the temperature increases, an amorphous solid will become less viscous. At some point the molecules may obtain enough freedom of motion to spontaneously arrange themselves into a crystalline form. This is known as the crystallisation temperature (T_c). This transition from amorphous solid to crystalline solid is an exothermic process, and results in a peak in the DSC signal. As the temperature increases the sample eventually reaches its melting temperature (T_m). The melting process results in an endothermic peak in the DSC curve. The ability to determine transition temperatures and enthalpies makes DSC an invaluable tool in producing phase diagrams for various chemical systems.

Circular dichroism

Circular dichroism (CD) is the differential absorption of left- and right-handed circularly polarised light. A CD spectrometer is an instrument that records this phenomenon as a function of wavelength. Modern instruments, however, can generally also record CD as a function of temperature or chemical environment, at several wavelengths. This phenomenon is exhibited in the absorption bands of an optically active molecule. CD can be used to help determine the structure of macromolecules (including the secondary structure of proteins and the handedness of DNA).

Linearly polarised light is polarised in a certain direction (that is, the magnitude of its electric field vector oscillates only in one plane, similar to a sine wave). In circularly polarised light, the electric field vector has a constant length, but rotates about its propagation direction. Hence it forms a helix in space while propagating. If this is a left-handed helix, the light is referred to as left circularly polarised, and vice versa for a right-handed helix (Fig. 4.16).

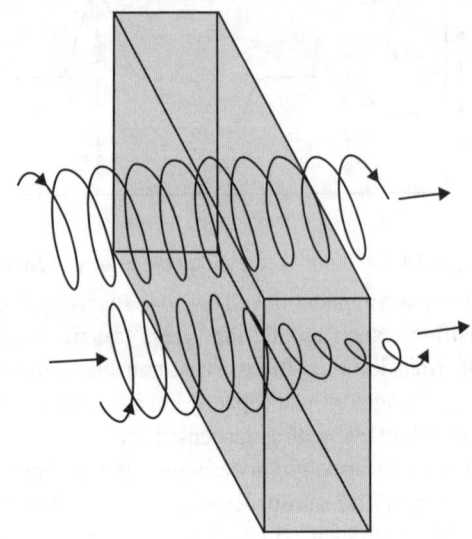

Fig. 4.16. Circular dichroism.

Total internal reflection fluorescence microscope

A total internal reflection fluorescence microscope (TIRFM) is a type of microscope with which a thin region of a specimen, usually less than 200 nm, can be observed (Fig. 4.17).

In cell and molecular biology, a large number of molecular events in cellular surfaces such as cell adhesion, binding of cells by hormones, secretion of neurotransmitters, and membrane dynamics have been studied with conventional fluorescence microscopes. However, fluorophores that are bound to the specimen surface and those in the surrounding medium exist in an equilibrium state. When these molecules are excited and detected with a conventional fluorescence microscope, the resulting fluorescence from those fluorophores bound to the surface is often overwhelmed by the background fluorescence due to the much larger population of non-bound molecules.

beneath the plasma membrane is necessarily visualised in addition to the plasma membrane during TIRF microscopy. The selective visualisation of the plasma membrane renders the features and events on the plasma membrane in living cells with high axial resolution (Fig. 4.18).

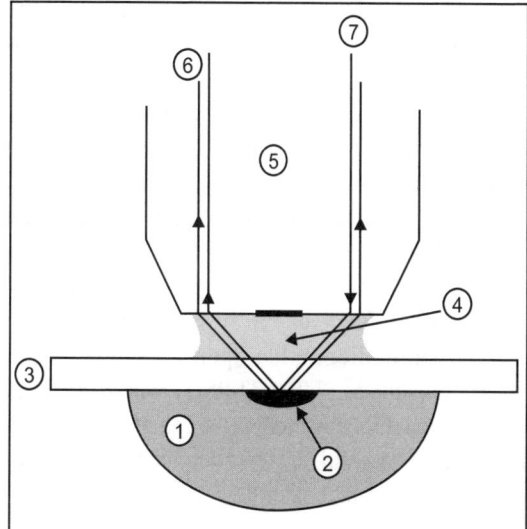

Fig. 4.17. Total internal reflection fluorescence microscope (TIRFM) diagram 1. Specimen 2. Evanescent wave range 3. Cover slip 4. Immersion oil 5. Objective 6. Emission beam (signal) 7. Excitation beam.

To solve this problem, the TIRFM was developed by Daniel Axelrod at the University of Michigan, Ann Arbor in the early 1980s. A TIRFM uses evanescent wave to selectively illuminate and excite fluorophores in a restricted region of the specimen immediately adjacent to the glass-water interface. The evanescent wave is generated only when the incident light is totally reflected at the glass-water interface. The evanescent electromagnetic field decays exponentially from the interface, and thus penetrates to a depth of only approximately 100 nm into the sample medium. Thus the TIRFM enables a selective visualisation of surface regions such as the basal plasma membrane (which are about 7.5 nm thick) of cells as shown in the figure above. Note, however, that the region visualised is at least a few hundred nanometers wide, so the cytoplasmic zone immediately

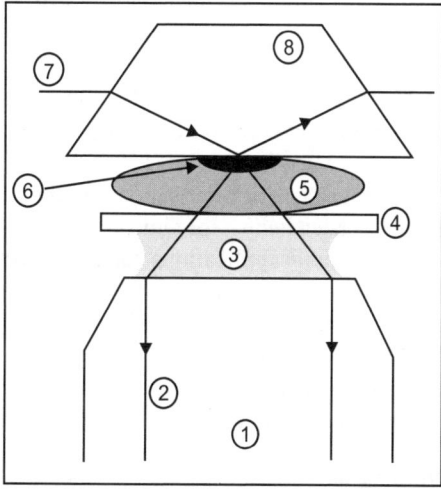

Fig. 4.18. Total internal reflection fluorescence Microscope trans- (TIRFM) diagram 1. Objective 2. Emission beam (signal) 3. Immersion oil 4. Cover slip 5. Specimen 6. Evanescent wave range 7. Excitation beam 8. Quartz prism.

TIRF can also be used to observe the fluorescence of a single molecule, making it an important tool of biophysics and quantitative biology.

Ellipsometry

Ellipsometry is a versatile and powerful optical technique for the investigation of the dielectric properties (complex refractive index or dielectric function) of thin films. It has applications in many different fields, from semiconductor physics to microelectronics and biology, from basic research to industrial applications. Ellipsometry is a very sensitive measurement technique and provides unequalled capabilities for thin film metrology. As an optical technique, spectroscopic ellipsometry is non-destructive and contactless.

Upon the analysis of the change of polarisation of light, which is reflected off a sample, ellipsometry can yield information about layers that are thinner than the wavelength of the probing light itself, even down to a single atomic layer. Ellipsometry can probe the complex refractive index or dielectric function tensor, which gives access to fundamental physical parameters and is related to a variety of sample properties, including morphology, crystal quality, chemical composition, or electrical conductivity. It is commonly used to characterise film thickness for single layers or complex multilayer stacks ranging from a few angstroms or tenths of a nanometer to several micrometers with an excellent accuracy.

The name 'ellipsometry' stems from the fact that the most general state of polarisation is elliptic. The technique has been known for almost a century, and has many standard applications today. However, ellipsometry is also becoming more interesting to researchers in other disciplines such as biology and medicine. These areas pose new challenges to the technique, such as measurements on unstable liquid surfaces and microscopic imaging.

Autoradiograph

An autoradiograph is an image on an X-ray film or nuclear emulsion produced by the pattern of decay emissions (e.g. beta particles or gamma rays) from a distribution of a radioactive substance. Alternatively, the autoradiograph can also be available as a digital image (digital autoradiography), thanks to the recent development of scintillation gas detectors or rare earth phosphorimaging systems. In biology, this technique may be used to determine the tissue localisation of a radioactive substance, either introduced into a metabolic pathway, bound to a receptor or enzyme, or hybridised to a nucleic acid. The film or emulsion is apposed to the labelled tissue section to obtain the autoradiograph (also called an autoradiogram). The auto — prefix indicates that the radioactive substance is within the sample, as distinguished from the case of historadiography or microradiography, in which the sample is X-rayed using an external source.

The use of radiolabelled ligands to determine the tissue distributions of receptors is termed either *in vivo* or *in vitro* receptor autoradiography if the ligand is administered into the circulation (with subsequent tissue removal and sectioning) or applied to the tissue sections, respectively. The ligands are generally labeled with ^{3}H (tritium) or ^{125}I. The distribution of RNA transcripts in tissue sections by the use of radiolabelled, complementary oligonucleotides or ribonucleic acids ('riboprobes') is called *in situ* hybridisation histochemistry. Radioactive precursors of DNA and RNA, ^{3}H (thymidine) and ^{3}(uridine) respectively, may be introduced to living cells to determine the timing of several phases of the cell cycle. RNA or DNA viral sequences can also be located in this fashion. These probes are usually labelled with ^{32}P, ^{33}P, or ^{35}S.

This autoradiographic approach contrasts to techniques such as PET and SPECT where the exact 3-dimensional localisation of the radiation source is provided by careful use of coincidence counting, gamma counters and other devices.

MOLECULAR SIZE

Most molecules are far too small to be seen with the naked eye, but there are exceptions. DNA, a macromolecule, can reach macroscopic sizes, as can molecules of many polymers. The smallest molecule is the diatomic hydrogen (H_2), with an overall length of roughly twice the 74 picometres (0.74 Å) bond length. Molecules commonly used as building blocks for organic synthesis have a dimension of a few Å to several dozen Å. Single molecules cannot usually be observed by light (as noted above), but small molecules and even the outlines of individual atoms may be traced in some circumstances by use of an atomic force microscope. Some of the largest molecules are macromolecules or supermolecules.

5

Haematology

INTRODUCTION

This chapter discusses various measurements and bioinstrumentations related to blood and its function in the human body.

Haematology is the branch of internal medicine, physiology, pathology, clinical laboratory work, and pediatrics that is concerned with the study of blood, the blood-forming organs, and blood diseases. Haematology includes the study of etiology, diagnosis, treatment, prognosis, and prevention of blood diseases. The laboratology work that goes into the study of blood is frequently performed by a medical technologist. Haematologists physicians also very frequently do further study in oncology—the medical treatment of cancer.

Blood diseases affect the production of blood and its components, such as blood cells, haemoglobin, blood proteins, the mechanism of coagulation, etc.

In a clinical laboratory the haematology department performs numerous different tests on blood. The most commonly performed test is the complete blood count (CBC) also called full blood count (FBC). Studies of blood coagulation is a sub-specialty of haematology; basic general coagulation tests are the prothrombin time (PT) and partial thromboplastin time (PTT). Another common haematology test in the erythrocyte sedimentation rate (ESR).

In the circulatory system, venous blood is blood returning to the heart (in veins). With one exception (the pulmonary vein) this blood is deoxygenated and high in carbon dioxide, having released oxygen and absorbed CO_2 in the tissues. It is also typically warmer than arterial blood, has a lower pH, has lower concentrations of glucose and other nutrients, and has higher concentrations of urea and other waste products. Venous blood is obtained by venipuncture (also called phlebotomy), or in small quantities by fingerprick. Most medical laboratory tests are conducted on venous blood, with the exception of arterial blood gas. Venous blood is dark red, not blue as it is often depicted in many medical diagrams. Venous blood is used during stem cell donation.

RED BLOOD CELL

Red blood cells (also referred to as erythrocytes) are the most common type of blood cell and the vertebrate organism's principal means of delivering oxygen (O_2) to the body tissues via the blood flow through the circulatory system. They take up oxygen in the lungs or gills and release it while squeezing through the body's capillaries. These cells' cytoplasm is rich in haemoglobin, an iron-containing biomolecule that can bind oxygen and is responsible for the blood's red colour.

In humans, mature red blood cells are flexible biconcave disks that lack a cell nucleus and most organelles. The cells develop in the bone marrow and circulate for about 100–120 days in the body before their components are recycled by macrophages. Each circulation takes about 20 seconds. Approximately a quarter of the cells in the human body are red blood cells.

BLOOD COMPONENTS AND PROCESSING

Blood is a specialised bodily fluid that delivers necessary substances to the body's cells—such as nutrients and oxygen — and transports waste products away from those same cells.

In vertebrates, it is composed of blood cells suspended in a liquid called blood plasma. Plasma, which comprises 55 per cent of blood fluid, is mostly water (90 per cent by volume), and contains dissolved proteins, glucose, mineral ions, hormones, carbon dioxide (plasma being the main medium for excretory product transportation), platelets and blood cells themselves. The blood cells present in blood are mainly red blood cells (also called RBCs or erythrocytes) and white blood cells, including leukocytes and platelets. The most abundant cells in vertebrate blood are red blood cells. These contain haemoglobin, an iron-containing protein, which facilitates transportation of oxygen by reversibly binding to this respiratory gas and greatly increasing its solubility in blood. In contrast, carbon dioxide is almost entirely transported extracellularly dissolved in plasma as bicarbonate ion.

Vertebrate blood is bright red when its haemoglobin is oxygenated. Some animals, such as crustaceans and mollusks, use hemocyanin to carry oxygen, instead of haemoglobin. Insects and some molluscs use a fluid called haemolymph instead of blood, the difference being that haemolymph is not contained in a closed circulatory system. In most insects, this 'blood' does not contain oxygen-carrying molecules such as haemoglobin because their bodies are small enough for their tracheal system to suffice for supplying oxygen.

Jawed vertebrates have an adaptive immune system, based largely on white blood cells. White blood cells help to resist infections and parasites. Platelets are important in the clotting of blood. Arthropods, using haemolymph, have haemocytes as part of their immune system.

Blood is circulated around the body through blood vessels by the pumping action of the heart. In animals with lungs, arterial blood carries oxygen from inhaled air to the tissues of the body, and venous blood carries carbon dioxide, a waste product of metabolism produced by cells, from the tissues to the lungs to be exhaled.

Red blood cells (RBCs), white blood cells (WBCs), and platelets are formed elements. Red blood cells, also known as erythrocytes, contain haemoglobin, which makes oxygen delivery possible by RBCs throughout the body. Erythrocytes are relatively large compared to other types of blood cells. In fact, they are the limiting factor in capillary size and must deform slightly to squeeze through. White blood cells, also known as leukocytes, help defend the body against foreign bodies. There are many different types of leukocytes, each much smaller than red blood cells. Platelets are essential for clotting.

Water is the primary unformed element, but others include proteins, carbohydrates, vitamins, hormones, enzymes, lipids, and salts. These are distributed throughout the body via the circulatory system.

When anticoagulants are used, the protein fibrinogen is present, and separation yields the straw-coloured liquid plasma. When blood is allowed to clot, the protein fibrinogen is not present, and separation yields the straw-coloured liquid serum. The basic techniques used in haematology are spectrometers, electron microscopy, phase microscopy. A centrifuge is also frequently used for separating the components of blood.

BLOOD COLLECTION

Blood Test

A blood test is a laboratory analysis performed on a blood sample that is usually extracted from a vein in the arm using a needle, or via fingerprick.

Blood tests are used to determine physiological and biochemical states, such as disease, mineral content, drug effectiveness, and organ function. Although the term blood test is used, most routine tests (except for most haematology) are done on plasma or serum, instead of blood cells.

Extraction

Venipuncture is useful as it is a relatively non-invasive way to obtain cells and extracellular fluid (plasma) from the body for analysis. Since blood flows throughout the body, acting as a medium for providing oxygen and nutrients, and drawing waste products back to the excretory systems for disposal, the state of the bloodstream affects, or is affected by, many medical conditions. For these reasons, blood tests are the most commonly performed medical tests.

Phlebotomists, laboratory technicians and nurses are those charged with patient blood extraction. However, in special circumstances, and emergency situations, paramedics and physicians sometimes extract blood. Also, respiratory therapists are trained to extract arterial blood for arterial blood gases.

Cord Blood

Umbilical cord blood is blood that remains in the placenta and in the attached umbilical cord after childbirth. Cord blood is obtained from the umbilical cord at the time of childbirth, after the cord has been detached from the newborn. Cord blood is collected because it contains stem cells, including haematopoietic cells, which can be used to treat haematopoietic and genetic disorders. Some placental blood may be returned to the neonatal circulation if the umbilical cord is not prematurely clamped. If the umbilical cord is not clamped, such as in an extended-delayed cord clamping protocol, a physiological postnatal occlusion occurs upon interaction with cold air, when the internal gelatinous substance, called Wharton's jelly, swells around the umbilical artery and veins.

Regenerative medicine is a field of medical research developing treatments to repair or re-grow specific tissue in the body. Because a person's own (autologous) cord blood stem cells can be safely infused back into that individual without being rejected by the body's immune system — and because they have unique characteristics compared to other sources of stem cells — they are an increasing focus of regenerative medicine research.

Research in this area that has the potential to revolutionise medicine is advancing rapidly and it is difficult for professional medical societies, and other resources that expectant parents turn to for information, to keep pace.

Human Iron Metabolism

Human iron metabolism is the set of chemical reactions maintaining human homeostasis of iron.

Iron is an essential element for most life on earth, including human beings. The control of this necessary but potentially toxic substance is an important part of many aspects of human health and disease. Haematologists have been especially interested in the system of iron metabolism because iron is essential to red blood cells. Most of the human body's iron is contained in red blood cells' haemoglobin, and iron deficiency anemia is the most common type of anemia.

Understanding this system is also important for understanding diseases of iron overload, like haemochromatosis. Recent discoveries in the field have shed new light on how humans control the level of iron in their bodies and created new understanding of the mechanisms of several diseases.

Factors Affecting Red Blood Cell Count

The concentration of red blood cells is a basic indicator of how well the body is able to deliver oxygen. Average values for the number of red blood cells per litre vary by sex and age.

There are many factors that can affect RBC count. Some of these include: children and adolescents, who have slightly lower counts than adults; people over 50 years of age, who have slightly lower counts than younger adults; strenuous physical activity, which increases RBC count; daily fluctuations between morning (highest count) and evening (lowest count).

Haemoglobin

Haemoglobin (also spelled haemoglobin and abbreviated Hb or Hgb) is the iron-containing oxygen-transport metalloprotein in the red blood cells of vertebrates, and the tissues of some invertebrates.

In mammals, the protein makes up about 97 per cent of the red blood cell's dry content, and around 35 per cent of the total content (including water). Haemoglobin transports oxygen from the lungs or gills to the rest of the body (i.e. the tissues) where it releases the oxygen for cell use. It also has a variety of other roles of gas transport and effect-modulation which vary from species to species, and are quite diverse in some invertebrates. For example, haemoglobin transports CO_2 back from the tissues to the lungs.

Haemoglobin has an oxygen binding capacity of between 1.36 and 1.37 ml O_2 per gram of haemoglobin, which increases the total blood oxygen capacity seventyfold.

Haemoglobin is also found in outside red blood cells and their progenitor lines. Other cells that contain haemoglobin include the A9 dopaminergic neurons in the substantia nigra, macrophages, alveolar cells, and mesangial cells in the kidney. In these tissues, haemoglobin has a non-oxygen carrying function as an antioxidant and a regulator of iron metabolism.

Haematocrit

The haematocrit (Ht or HCT) or packed cell volume (PCV) or erythrocyte volume fraction (EVF) is the proportion of blood volume that is occupied by red blood cells. It is normally about 48 per cent for men and 38 per cent for women. It is considered an integral part of a person's complete blood count results, along with haemoglobin concentration, white blood cell count, and platelet count (Fig 5.1).

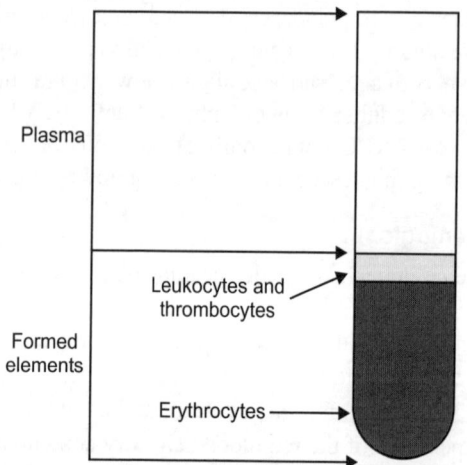

Fig. 5.1. Erythrocyte volume fraction (EVF).

In mammals, haematocrit is independent of body size.

Measurement methods

The packed cell volume (PCV) can be determined by centrifuging heparinised blood in a capillary tube (also known as a microhaematocrit tube) at 10,000 rpm for five minutes. This separates the blood into layers. The volume of packed red blood cells, divided by the total volume of the blood sample gives the PCV. Because a tube is used this can be calculated by measuring the lengths of the layers (Fig. 5.2).

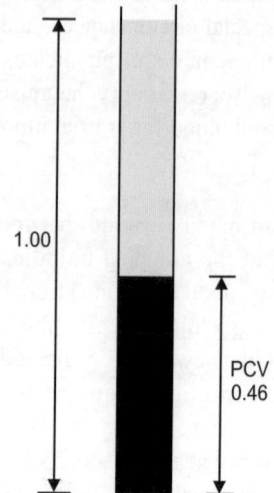

Fig. 5.2. Packed cell volume diagram.

With modern lab equipment, the haematocrit is calculated by an automated analyser and not directly measured. It is determined by multiplying the red cell count by the mean cell volume. The haematocrit is slightly more accurate as the PCV includes small amounts of blood plasma trapped between the red cells. An estimated haematocrit as a percentage may be derived by tripling the haemoglobin concentration in g/dL and dropping the units. The haemoglobin level is the measure used by blood banks.

There have been cases where the blood for testing was inadvertently drawn proximal to an intravenous line that was infusing packed red cells or fluids. In these situations, the haemoglobin level in the blood sample will not be the true level for the patient because the sample would contain a large amount of the infused material rather than what is diluted into the circulating whole blood. That is, if packed red cells are being supplied, the sample will contain a large amount of those cells and the haematocrit will be artificially very high. Conversely, if saline or other fluids are being supplied, the blood sample would be diluted and the haematocrit will be artificially low.

Elevated haematocrit

In cases of dengue fever a high haematocrit is a danger sign of an increased risk of dengue shock syndrome.

Polycythemia vera (PV), a myeloproliferative disorder in which the bone marrow produces excessive numbers of red cells, is associated with elevated haematocrit. Chronic obstructive pulmonary disease (COPD) and other pulmonary conditions associated with hypoxia may elicit an increased production of red blood cells. This increase is mediated by the increased levels of erythropoietin by the kidneys in response to hypoxia.

Professional athletes' haematocrit levels are measured as part of tests for blood doping or Erythropoietin (EPO) use; the level of haematocrit in a blood sample is compared with the long-term level for that athlete (to allow for individual variations in haematocrit level), and against an absolute permitted maximum (which is based on maximum expected levels within the population, and the haematocrit level which causes increased risk of blood clots resulting in strokes or heart attacks).

Steroid use can also increase the amount of RBC's and therefore impact the haematocrit.

If a patient is dehydrated, the haematocrit may be elevated. Repeat testing after adequate hydration therapy will usually result in a more reliable result.

Lowered haematocrit

Lowered haematocrit can imply significant haemorrhage. The mean corpuscular volume (MCV) and the red cell distribution width (RDW) can be quite helpful in evaluating a lower-than-normal haematocrit, because it can help the clinician determine whether blood loss is chronic or acute. The MCV is the size of the red cells and the RDW is a relative measure of the variation in size of the red cell population. A low haematocrit with a low MCV with a high RDW suggests a chronic iron-deficient erythropoiesis, but a normal RDW suggests a blood loss that is more acute, such as a haemorrhage.

Groups of individuals who are at risk for developing anemia include:

1. Infants who may not have adequate iron intake.

2. Children going through a rapid growth spurt, during which the iron available cannot keep up with the demands for a growing red cell mass.

3. Women in childbearing years who have an excessive need for iron because of blood loss during menstruation.

4. Pregnant women, in whom the growing fetus creates a high demand for iron.

5. Patients with chronic kidney disease, as their kidneys no longer secrete sufficient levels of the hormone erythropoietin, which stimulates red blood cell production by the bone arrow.

Red Blood Cell Indices

Red blood cell indices are blood tests that provide information about the haemoglobin content and size of red blood cells. Abnormal values indicate the presence of anemia and which type of anemia it is.

Mean corpuscular volume (MCV) is the average size of a red blood cell and is calculated by dividing the haematocrit (Hct) by the red blood cell count.

1. $MCV = \dfrac{Hct}{RBC}$.

2. Normal range: 80–100 fL.

Mean corpuscular haemoglobin (MCH) is the average amount of haemoglobin (Hb) per red blood cell and is calculated by dividing the haemoglobin by the red blood cell count.

1. $MCH = \dfrac{Hb}{RBC}$.

2. Normal range: 27–31 pg/cell.

Mean corpuscular haemoglobin concentration (MCHC) is the average concentration of haemoglobin per red blood cell and is calculated by dividing the haemoglobin by the haematocrit.

1. $MCHC = \dfrac{Hb}{Hct}$.

2. Normal range: 32–36 g/dL.

Red Blood Cell Count

Haemocytometer

The haemocytometer or haemocytometer is a device originally designed for the counting of blood cells. It is now also used to count other types of cells as well as other microscopic particles (Fig. 5.3).

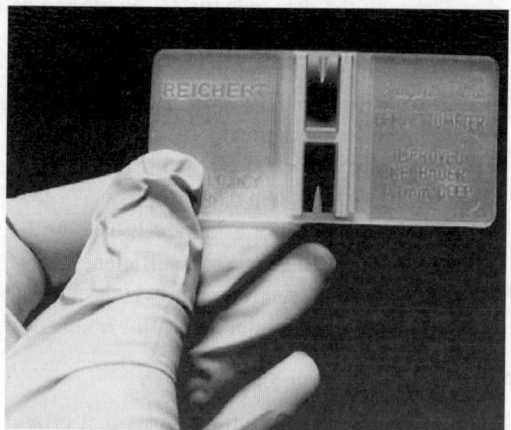

Fig. 5.3. A haemocytometer. The two semi-reflective rectangles are the counting chambers.

The haemocytometer was invented by Louis-Charles Malassez and consists of a thick glass microscope slide with a rectangular indentation that creates a chamber. This chamber is engraved with a laser-etched grid of perpendicular lines. The device is carefully crafted so that the area bounded by the lines is known, and the depth of the chamber is also known. It is therefore possible to count the number of cells or particles in a specific volume of fluid, and thereby calculate the concentration of cells in the fluid overall (Fig. 5.4).

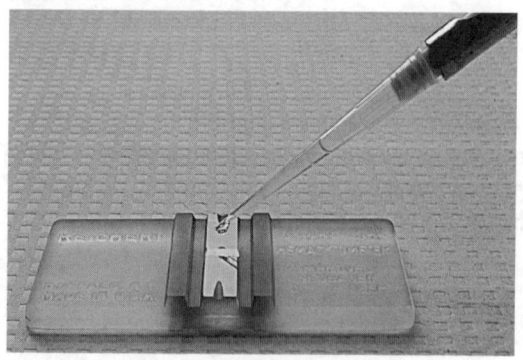

Fig. 5.4. Load a chamber.

The ruled area of the haemocytometer consists of several, large, 1×1 mm (1 mm^2) squares. These are subdivided in 3 ways; 0.25×0.25 mm (0.0625 mm^2), 0.25×0.20 mm (0.05 mm^2) and 0.20×0.20 mm

(0.04 mm^2). The central, 0.20×0.20 mm marked, 1×1 mm square is further subdivided into 0.05×0.05 mm (0.0025 mm^2) squares. The raised edges of the haemocytometer hold the coverslip 0.1 mm off the marked grid. This gives each square a defined volume (Fig 5.5 and 5.6).

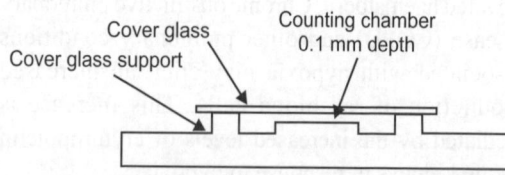

Fig. 5.5. The parts of the hemocytometer (as viewed from the side) are identified.

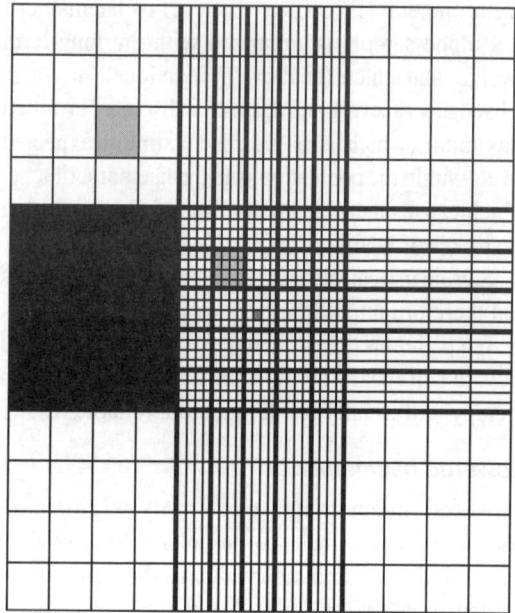

Fig. 5.6. Haemocytometer grid: Black square = 1 mm^2, 100 nl grey square = 0.0625 mm^2, 6.25 nl light grey square = 0.04 mm^2, 4 nl light black square = 0.0025 mm^2, 0.25 nl at a depth of 0.1 mm.

Dimensions	Area	Volume at 0.1 mm depth
1×1 mm	1 mm^2	100 nl
0.25×0.25 mm	0.0625 mm^2	6.25 nl
0.25×0.20 mm	0.05 mm^2	5 nl
0.20×0.20 mm	0.04 mm^2	4 nl
0.05×0.05 mm	0.0025 mm^2	0.25 nl

The cell-sized structures to be counted are those which lie between the middle of the three lines on the top and right of the square and the inner of the three lines on the bottom and left of the square.

In an improved Neubauer haemocytometer (common medium), the total number of cells per ml can be discovered by simply multiplying the total number of cells found in the haemocytometer grid (area equal to the black square in) by 10^4 (10000).

Usage

When a liquid sample containing immobilised cells is placed on the chamber, it is covered with a cover glass, and capillary action completely fills the chamber with the sample. Looking at the chamber through a microscope, the number of cells in the chamber can be determined by counting. Different kinds of cells can be counted separately as long as they are visually distinguishable. The number of cells in the chamber is used to calculate the concentration or density of the cells in the mixture from which the sample was taken: it is the number of cells in the chamber divided by the chamber's volume (the chamber's volume is known from the start), taking account of any dilutions and counting shortcuts:

Concentration of cells in original mixture =

$$\left(\frac{\text{Number of cells counted}}{\text{(Proportion of chamber counted)}} \right)$$

$$\left(\frac{\text{Volume of sample dilution}}{\text{Volume of original mixture in sample}} \right)$$

Haemocytometers are often used to count blood corpuscles, organelles within cells, blood cells in cerebrospinal fluid after performing a lumbar puncture, or other cell types in suspension. Using a hemocytometer to count bacteria results in a 'total count' as it is difficult to distinguish between living and dead organisms unless Trypan blue is used to stain the non-viable cells.

Usage tips

1. Mix the original mixture thoroughly before taking a sample. This ensures that the sample is representative, and not just an artifact of the particular region of the original mixture from which it was drawn.

2. Use an appropriate dilution of the mixture with regard to the number of cells to be counted. If the sample is not diluted enough, the cells will be too crowded and difficult to count. If it is too dilute, the sample size will not be enough to make strong inferences about the concentration in the original mixture. Naturally, a rough idea of the concentration must be known before beginning in order to guess an appropriate dilution. If the mixture is coloured, it may be helpful to memorise a particular intensity of that colour at which the mixture tends to be easy to analyse.

3. Analyse multiple chambers. By performing a redundant test on a second chamber, the results can be compared. If they differ greatly, the method of taking the sample may be unreliable (e.g. the original mixture is not mixed thoroughly). Take the average of the results for a more accurate calculation.

4. Make sure to put enough liquid on the instrument that some leaks out of the cover glass when it is placed over the chamber. Otherwise, it is uncertain whether the space under the cover glass is completely filled with liquid. This volume should be the same every time the instrument is used.

5. Do not use a paper wipe to dry the excess liquid. The same capillary action that filled the chamber will then dry it out. If using trypan blue, rinse the haemocytometer with distilled water to remove the dye and allow it to dry. Methylated spirits or alcohol (preferably ethanol) may also be used to cleanse the hemocytometer, and it is safe to use lens tissue to wipe the excess away, as long as great care is taken not to warp the hemocytometer grid. For this reason, it is not safe to autoclave (sterilise) a hemocytometer however sterilisation should not be essential.

6. Watch out for the objective lens. Remember that the haemocytometer is thicker than a

normal microscope slide. If focused too closely, the objective lens may contact the instrument. This may affect the choice of objective lens used.

7. Count across the rows or down the columns. Use the gridlines to help remember which areas' cells have already been counted.

8. There is no need to count the whole chamber. If there are lot of cells, perform a count in a section of the chamber and use the grid to determine what proportion of the chamber that is. Then extrapolate to estimate how many cells are in the chamber, and use that figure in the final calculation. This gives speed at the expense of potential accuracy; if possible, using a more appropriate dilution is better.

9. Are the lines in or out? Some cells inevitably fall on top of the outside gridlines that mark the edges of the chamber. The usual practice is to include cells overlapping the top and left lines, but not those overlapping the bottom or right lines — this has the advantage of eliminating redundant counting if adjacent regions are counted.

Biochemical analysers

Biochemical analyses are gaining in importance among various types of medical laboratory investigations in our country and abroad. Just in the last 5 years the number of biochemical anlysis conducted in clinical institutions of US and European countries have more than tripled (Fig. 5.7).

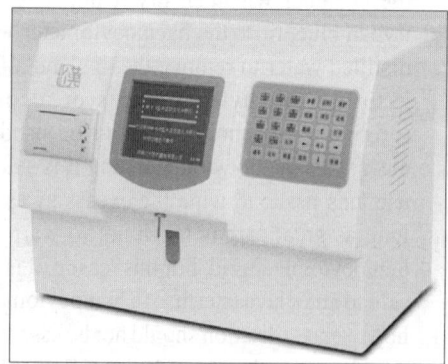

Fig. 5.7. Biochemical analysers.

Prophylactic examination of the population requires a great increase in the productivity of laboratories. This task can be realised only provided the conduction of biochemical investigations is centralised and laboratories are outfitted with modern equipment.

In order to select the most rational solution it is necessary to evaluate preliminarily the experience gained by foreign companies to the area of development of automatic biochemical analysers, since the design features and characteristics of these instruments fully reflect the requirements imposed on the equipment of modern laboratories. Such an evaluation was carired out on material covering eight types of single-channel and six types of multichannel automatic biochemical analysers used most widely abroad during the last 15 years.

In modern medical laboratory practice the conduction of the usual biochemical analyses of blood serum or plasma is based on photometric or fluorometric methods. In a general form the conduction of photometric biochemical investigations can be represented in two variants.

Variant I: The following operations are performed when investigating any component in blood serum without precipitation of proteins: (i) the blood for analysis is taken by a dry hypodermic syringe from the patient's vein, (ii) the blood is transferred to a centrifuge test tube on which the patient's code number is placed, (iii) after the blood clots, it is centrifuged and the upper layer (serum) is removed from the sediment by pipet, (iv) a certain volume of the serum is placed in a reaction vessel by pipet, and the same volume of serum or solution not containing the component to be determined is placed in the control sample, (v) reagents are added to the reaction vessel and control sample, but in the case of checking serum the specific reagent is not added to the control sample, (vi) the reaction vessel is placed and held under certain temperaute conditions, (vii) after a certain time interval required for completion of the reaction the samples are transferred to the photometric cells, (viii) the light absorption of the experimental and control samples is measured, and (ix) the readings of the control sample are subtracted from the readings of the experimental sample, and the content of the component being determined is calculated from a calibration curve.

Variant II: The following operations are performed when investigating any component in blood serum with precipitation of proteins: (i), (ii), and (iii) same as variant I, (iv) to remove proteins a certain volume of serum is introduced into the centrifuge test tube, one of the solutions precipitating proteins is added, mixed, and centriguged, (v) the upper layer is removed from the sediment by pipette and the analysisis carried out with this material according to variant I.

Fluorometric investigations of blood plasma involve the following operations: (i) the blood for investigation is taken by a dry syringe from the patient's vein, (ii) the blood is transferred to a coded centrifuge test tube to which a certain volume of anticoagulant is added preliminarily, and (iii) the blood is centrifuged, and the upper layer (plasma) is removed by pipet from the lower layer and used for the investigatios.

Coulter counter

A coulter counter is an apparatus for counting and sizing particles and cells. It is used, for example, for bacteria or prokaryotic cells and air quality particle size distributions. The counter detects change in electrical conductance of a small aperture as fluid containing cells is drawn through. Cells, being non-conducting particles, alter the effective cross-section of the conductive channel.

It was an American inventor named Wallace H. Coulter who was responsible for the theory and design of the coulter counter. He first devised the theory behind its operation in 1947 while experimenting with electronics. Coulter determined that electrical charge could be used to determine the size and number of microscopic particles in a solution. This phenomenon is now known as the coulter principle.

The coulter counter is a vital constituent of today's hospital laboratory. Its primary function being the quick and accurate analysis of complete blood counts (often referred to as CBC). The CBC is used to determine the number or proportion of white and red blood cells in the body. Previously, this procedure involved preparing a blood cell stain and manually counting each type of cell under a microscope, a process that typically took a half hour. Coulter counters have a wide variety of applications including paint, ceramics, glass, and food manufacture. They are also routinely employed for quality control.

Other cell counting technologies that employ similar systems are also used, one of these being the CASY cell counting technology. These systems have some differences but operate on similar principles.

A typical coulter counter has one or more microchannels that separate two chambers containing electrolyte solutions. When a particle flows through one of the microchannels, it results in the electrical resistance change of the liquid filled microchannel. This resistance change can be recorded as electric current or voltage pulses, which can be correlated to size, mobility, surface charge and concentration of the particles.

Due to the simple construction of these devices and the reliable sensing method, Coulter devices have found application in a broad range of particle analyses from blood cells to polymeric beads, DNA, virus particles and even metal ions. Quantitative measurements of the size and concentration of micro and nano scale particles has been accomplished using Coulter counters with reduced microchannel size so that particles pass one by one from one chamber to the other. Because this would substantially extend measurement times, multiple microchannels are used to reduce measurement times by counting particles in parallel with one another.

Dynamic light scattering

Dynamic light scattering (also known as photon correlation spectroscopy or quasi-elastic light scattering) is a technique in physics, which can be used to determine the size distribution profile of small particles in suspension (chemistry) or polymers in solution. It can also be used to probe the behaviour of complex fluids such as concentrated polymer solutions.

When light hits small particles the light scatters in all directions (Rayleigh scattering) so long as the particles are small compared to the wavelength (below 250 nm). If the light source is a laser, and thus is monochromatic and coherent, then one observes a time-dependent fluctuation in the scattering intensity. These fluctuations are due to the fact that the small molecules in solutions are undergoing Brownian motion and so the distance between the scatterers in the solution is constantly changing with time. This scattered light then undergoes either constructive or destructive interference by the surrounding particles and within this intensity fluctuation, information is contained about the time scale of movement of the scatterers.

There are several ways to derive dynamic information about particles' movement in solution by Brownian motion. One such method is dynamic light scattering, also known as quasi-elastic laser light scattering. The dynamic information of the particles is derived from an autocorrelation of the intensity trace recorded during the experiment. The second order autocorrelation curve is generated from the intensity trace as follows:

$$g^2(q;\tau) = \frac{\langle I(t)I(t+\tau)\rangle}{\langle I(t)\rangle^2}$$

where $g^2(q;\tau)$ is the autocorrelation function at a particular wave vector, q, and delay time, τ, and I is the intensity. At short time delays, the correlation is high because the particles do not have a chance to move to a great extent from the initial state that they were in. The two signals are thus essentially unchanged when compared after only a very short time interval. As the time delays become longer, the correlation starts to exponentially decay to zero, meaning that after a long time period has elapsed, there is no correlation between the scattered intensity of the initial and final states. This exponential decay is related to the motion of the particles, specifically to the diffusion coefficient. To fit the decay (i.e. the autocorrelation function), numerical methods are used, based on calculations of assumed distributions. If the sample is monodisperse then the decay is simply a single exponential. The Siegert equation relates the second order autocorrelation function with the first

order autocorrelation function $g^1(q;\tau)$ as follows:

$$g^2(q;\tau) = 1 + \beta\left[g^1(q;\tau)\right]^2$$

where the parameter β is a correction factor that depends on the geometry and alignment of the laser beam in the light scattering setup. It is roughly equal to the inverse of the number of speckle from which light is collected. The most important use of the autocorrelation function is its use for size determination.

Data analysis

Once the autocorrelation data have been generated, different mathematical approaches can be employed to determine from it. Analysis of the scattering is facilitated when particles do not interact through collisions or electrostatic forces between ions. Particle-particle collisions can be suppressed by dilution, and charge effects are reduced by the use of salts to collapse the electrical double layer.

The simplest approach is to treat the first order autocorrelation function as a single exponential decay. This is appropriate for a monodisperse population.

$$g^1(q;\tau) = \exp(-\Gamma\tau)$$

where Γ is the decay rate. The translational diffusion coefficient D_t may be derived at a single angle or at a range of angles depending on the wave vector q.

$$\Gamma = q^2 D_t$$

with

$$q = \frac{4\pi n_0}{\lambda}\sin\left(\frac{\theta}{2}\right)$$

where λ is the incident laser wavelength, n_0 is the refractive index of the sample and θ is angle at which the detector is located with respect to the sample cell.

Depending on the anisotropy and polydispersity of the system, a resulting plot of Γ/q^2 vs. q^2 may or may not show an angular dependence. Small spherical particles will show no angular dependence, hence no anisotropy. A plot of Γ/q^2 vs. q^2 will result in a horizontal line. Particles with a shape other than a sphere will show anisotropy and thus an angular dependence when plotting of Γ/q^2 vs. q^2. The intercept will be in any case the D_t.

D_t is often used to calculate the hydrodynamic radius of a sphere through the Stokes-Einstein equation. It is important to note that the size determined by dynamic light scattering is the size of a sphere that moves in the same manner as the scatterer. So, for example, if the scatterer is a random coil polymer, the determined size is not the same as the radius of gyration determined by static light scattering. It is also useful to point out that the obtained size will include any other molecules or solvent molecules that move with the particle. So, for example colloidal gold with a layer of surfactant will appear larger by dynamic light scattering (which includes the surfactant layer) than by transmission electron microscopy (which does not 'see' the layer due to poor contrast).

In most cases, samples are polydisperse. Thus, the autocorrelation function is a sum of the exponential decays corresponding to each of the species in the population.

$$g^1(q;\tau) = \sum_{i=1}^{n} G_i(\Gamma_i)\exp(-\Gamma_i\tau) = \int G(\Gamma)\exp(-\Gamma\tau)d\Gamma.$$

It is tempting to obtain data for $g^1(q;\tau)$ and attempt to invert the above to extract $G(\Gamma)$. Since $G(\Gamma)$ is proportional to the relative scattering from each species, it contains information on the distribution of sizes. However, this is known as an ill-posed problem. The methods described below (and others) have been developed to extract as much useful information as possible from an autocorrelation function.

Cumulant method

One of the most common methods is the cumulant method, from which in addition to the sum of the exponentials above, more information can be derived about the variance of the system as follows:

$$g^1(q;\tau) = \exp(-\bar{\Gamma}\tau)\left(1 + \frac{\mu_2}{2!}\tau^2 - \frac{\mu_3}{2!}\tau^3 + ...\right)$$

where $\bar{\Gamma}$ the average decay rate and $\mu_2/\bar{\Gamma}^2$ the second order polydispersity index (or an indication of the variance). A third order polydispersity index may also be derived but this is only necessary if the

particles of the system are highly polydisperse. The z-averaged translational diffusion coefficient D_z may be derived at a single angle or at a range of angles depending on the wave vector q.

$$\bar{\Gamma} = q^2 D_z$$

One must note that the cumulant method is valid for small τ and sufficiently narrow $G(\Gamma)$. One should seldom use parameters beyond μ_3, because overfitting data with many parameters in a power-series expansion will render all the parameters including $\bar{\Gamma}$ and μ_2, less precise.

The cumulant method is far less affected by experimental noise than the methods below.

Fluorescence-activated cell sorting

Fluorescence-activated cell sorting is a specialised type of flow cytometry. It provides a method for sorting a heterogeneous mixture of biological cells into two or more containers, one cell at a time, based upon the specific light scattering and fluorescent characteristics of each cell. It is a useful scientific instrument, as it provides fast, objective and quantitative recording of fluorescent signals from individual cells as well as physical separation of cells of particular interest. The acronym FACS is trademarked and owned by Becton Dickinson. While many immunologists use this term frequently for all types of sorting and non-sorting applications, it is not a generic term for flow cytometry. The first cell sorter was invented by Mack Fulwyler in 1965, using the principle of Coulter volume, a relatively difficult technique and one no longer used in modern instruments (Fig. 5.8).

The cell suspension is entrained in the centre of a narrow, rapidly flowing stream of liquid. The flow is arranged so that there is a large separation between cells relative to their diameter. A vibrating mechanism causes the stream of cells to break into individual droplets. The system is adjusted so that there is a low probability of more than one cell per droplet. Just before the stream breaks into droplets, the flow passes through a fluorescence measuring station where the fluorescent character of interest of each cell is measured. An electrical charging ring is placed just at the point where the stream breaks into droplets. A charge is placed on the ring based on the immediately-prior fluorescence intensity measurement, and the opposite charge is trapped on the droplet as it breaks from the stream.

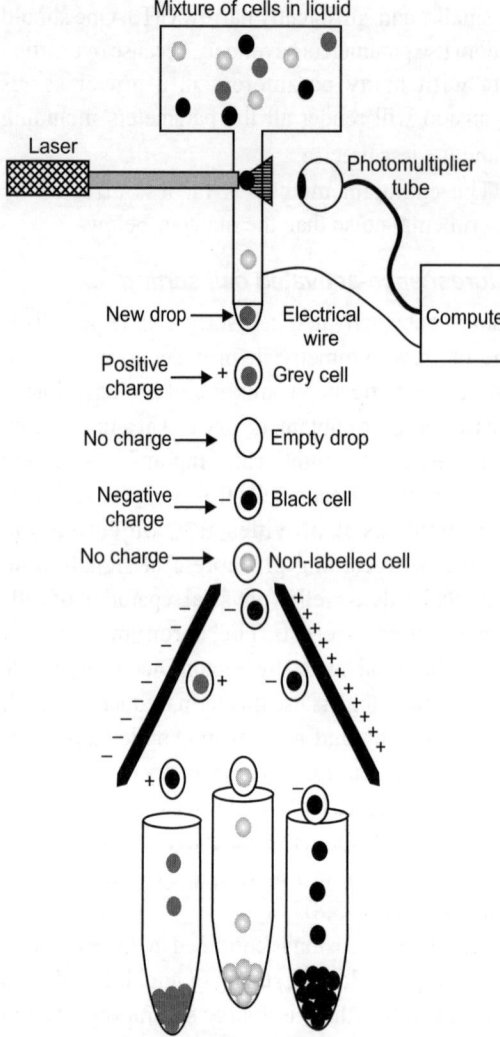

Fig. 5.8. Diagram of FACS machine.

The charged droplets then fall through an electrostatic deflection system that diverts droplets into containers based upon their charge. In some systems, the charge is applied directly to the stream, and the droplet breaking off retains charge of the same sign as the stream. The stream is then returned to neutral after the droplet breaks off.

Reticulocyte

Reticulocytes are immature red blood cells, typically composing about 1 per cent of the red cells in the human body. Reticulocytes develop and mature in the red bone marrow and then circulate for about a day in the blood stream before developing into mature red blood cells. Like mature red blood cells, reticulocytes do not have a cell nucleus. They are called reticulocytes because of a reticular (mesh-like) network of ribosomal RNA that becomes visible under a microscope with certain stains such as new methylene blue.

To accurately measure reticulocyte counts, automated counters that use lasers mark cell samples with fluorescent dye that marks RNA and DNA (such as thiazole orange or polymethine). This distinguishes reticulocytes as the middle ground of dye response to laser light, between red blood cells (which have neither RNA nor DNA) and lymphocytes (which have a large amount of DNA, unlike reticulocytes).

The specimen requirement for a reticulocyte count is EDTA anti-coagulated whole blood (lavender-top bottle if using the Vacutainer, Vacuette or Monoject systems; red-top if using the S-Monovette system).

Reticulocytes appear slightly bluer than other red cells when looked at with the normal Romanowsky stain. Reticulocytes are also slightly larger, which can be picked up as a high MCV (mean corpuscular volume) with a full blood count done by a trained medical scientist, who has specialised in haematology, or a machine.

Flowcytometry for mouse reticulocytes: one can use a cell-permeable thiazole orange dye to stain for reticulocytes' residual RNA in conjunction with DRAQ5 DNA-only dye (reticulocytes have no DNA and are thus DRAQ5 negative) and Ter119 (glycophorin-A) that is a marker of erythroid lineage. (Thiazole orange dye binds to nucleic acids of both DNA and RNA).

Interpretation

The normal range of values for reticulocytes in the blood depends on the clinical situation and the lab, but broadly speaking is 0.5 per cent to 1.5 per cent. However, if a person has anemia, their reticulocyte percentage should be higher than 'normal' if the bone marrow's ability to produce new blood cells remains intact. Thus, calculating the reticulocyte production index is an important step in understanding whether the reticulocyte count is appropriate or inappropriate to the situation. This is often a more important question than whether the percentage is in the normal range; for instance, if someone is anemic but only has a reticulocyte percentage of 1 per cent, this means that the bone marrow is likely not producing new blood cells at a rate that will correct the anemia. The number of reticulocytes is a good indicator of bone marrow activity, because it represents recent production. This means that the reticulocyte count, and the reticulocyte production index that can be calculated from it, can be used to determine whether a production problem is contributing to the anaemia, and can also be used to monitor the progress of treatment for anaemia.

When there is an increased production of red blood cells to overcome chronic or severe loss of mature red blood cells, such as in a haemolytic anaemia, people often have a markedly high number and percentage of reticulocytes. A very high number of reticulocytes in the blood can be described as reticulocytosis.

Abnormally low numbers of reticulocytes can be attributed to chemotherapy, aplastic anaemia, pernicious anaemia, bone marrow malignancies, problems of erythropoietin production, various vitamin or mineral deficiencies (B9, B12, iron), disease states (anemia of chronic disease) and other causes of anaemia due to poor RBC production.

Sickle-cell test

Sickle-cell disease, or sickle-cell anaemia (or drepanocytosis), is a genetic life-long blood disorder characterised by red blood cells that assume an abnormal, rigid, sickle shape. Sickling decreases the cells' flexibility and results in a risk of various complications. The sickling occurs because of a mutation in the haemoglobin gene. Life expectancy is shortened, with studies reporting an average life expectancy of 42 and 48 years for males and females, respectively.

Sickle-cell disease, usually presenting in childhood, occurs more commonly in people (or their descendants) from parts of tropical and sub-tropical regions where malaria is or was common. One-third of all indigenous inhabitants of Sub-saharan Africa carry the gene, because in areas where malaria is common, there is a survival value in carrying only a single sickle-cell gene (sickle cell trait). Those with only one of the two alleles of the sickle-cell disease are more resistant to malaria, since the infestation of the malaria plasmodium is halted by the sickling of the cells which it infests.

The prevalence of the disease in the United States is approximately 1 in 5,000, mostly affecting Americans of Sub-Saharan African descent, according to the National Institutes of Health. In the United States, about 1 in 500 black births have sickle-cell anemia.

Sickle test

Sickle-cell anaemia is the name of a specific form of sickle-cell disease in which there is homozygosity for the mutation that causes HbS. Sickle-cell anaemia is also referred to as 'HbSS', 'SS disease', 'haemo-globin S' or permutations thereof. In heterozygous people, who have only one sickle gene and one normal adult haemoglobin gene, it is referred to as 'HbAS' or 'sickle cell trait'. Other, rarer forms of sickle-cell disease include sickle-haemoglobin C disease (HbSC), sickle beta-plus-thalassaemia (HbS/β^+) and sickle beta-zero-thalassaemia (HbS/β^0). These other forms of sickle-cell disease are compound heterozygous states in which the person has only one copy of the mutation that causes HbS and one copy of another abnormal haemoglobin allele.

The term disease is applied, because the inherited abnormality causes a pathological condition that can lead to death and severe complications. Not all inherited variants of haemoglobin are detrimental, a concept known as genetic polymorphism.

To test for anemia, whole blood is mixed with sodium metabisulphite, a strong reducing agent that deoxygenates the haemoglobin. The sample is examined under the microscope after one hour. If sickling is present this indicates sickle cell anemia. If sickling occurs after 24 hours the sickle cell trait is present.

White blood cell

White blood cells (WBCs), or leukocytes (also spelled 'leucocytes'), are cells of the immune system defending the body against both infectious disease and foreign materials. Five different and diverse types of leukocytes exist, but they are all produced and derived from a multipotent cell in the bone marrow known as a haematopoietic stem cell. Leukocytes are found throughout the body, including the blood and lymphatic system.

The number of WBCs in the blood is often an indicator of disease. There are normally between 4×10^9 and 1.1×10^{10} white blood cells in a litre of blood, making up approximately 1 per cent of blood in a healthy adult. An increase in the number of leukocytes over the upper limits is called leukocytosis, and a decrease below the lower limit is called leukopenia. The physical properties of leukocytes, such as volume, conductivity, and granularity, may change due to activation, the presence of immature cells, or the presence of malignant leukocytes in leukemia.

The name 'white blood cell' derives from the fact that after centrifugation of a blood sample, the white cells are found in the *buffy coat*, a thin, typically white layer of nucleated cells between the sedimented red blood cells and the blood plasma. The scientific term leukocyte directly reflects this description, derived from Greek leukos (white), and kytos (cell). Blood plasma may sometimes be green if there are large amounts of neutrophils in the sample, due to the haemecontaining enzyme myeloperoxidase that they produce. There are several different types of white blood cells. They all have many things in common, but are all different. A major distinguishing feature of some leukocytes is the presence of granules; white blood cells are often characterised as granulocytes or agranulocytes.

Wedge smear and staining

The blood sample is diluted with a solution that lyses the red blood cells. A sample of blood is placed on a microscope slide using the wedge smear technique. Each type of white blood cells is stained, and the sample is examined under the microscope where each cell type is counted. The accuracy of such a technique is usually fairly good, but precision is poor.

Flow cytometry

Flow cytometry is a technique for counting and examining microscopic particles, such as cells and chromosomes, by suspending them in a stream of fluid and passing them by an electronic detection apparatus. It allows simultaneous multiparametric analysis of the physical and/or chemical characteristics of up to thousands of particles per second. Flow cytometry is routinely used in the diagnosis of health disorders, especially blood cancers, but has many other applications in both research and clinical practice. A common variation is to physically sort particles based on their properties, so as to purify populations of interest.

A beam of light (usually laser light) of a single wavelength is directed onto a hydrodynamically-focused stream of fluid. A number of detectors are aimed at the point where the stream passes through the light beam: one in line with the light beam (forward scatter or FSC) and several perpendicular to it (side scatter (SSC) and one or more fluorescent detectors). Each suspended particle from 0.2 to 150 micrometers passing through the beam scatters the light in some way, and fluorescent chemicals found in the particle or attached to the particle may be excited into emitting light at a longer wavelength than the light source. This combination of scattered and fluorescent light is picked up by the detectors, and, by analysing fluctuations in brightness at each detector (one for each fluorescent emission peak), it is then possible to derive various types of information about the physical and chemical structure of each individual particle FSC correlates with the cell volume and SSC depends on the inner complexity of the particle (i.e. shape of the nucleus, the amount and type of cytoplasmic granules or the membrane roughness). Some flow cytometers on the market have eliminated the need for fluorescence and use only light scatter for measurement. Other flow cytometers form images of each cell's fluorescence, scattered light, and transmitted light.

Flow cytometers

Modern flow cytometers are able to analyse several thousand particles every second, in 'real time,' and can actively separate and isolate particles having specified properties. A flow cytometer is similar to a microscope, except that, instead of producing an image of the cell, flow cytometry offers 'high-throughput' (for a large number of cells) automated quantification of set parameters. To analyse solid tissues, a single-cell suspension must first be prepared.

A flow cytometer has 5 main components:

1. A flow cell-liquid stream (sheath fluid), which carries and aligns the cells so that they pass single file through the light beam for sensing.
2. An optical system-commonly used are lamps (mercury, xenon); high-power water-cooled lasers (argon, krypton, dye laser); low-power air-cooled lasers (argon (488 nm), red-HeNe (633 nm), green-HeNe, HeCd (UV)); diode lasers (blue, green, red, violet) resulting in light signals.
3. A detector and Analogue-to-digital conversion (ADC) system-which generates FSC and SSC as well as fluorescence signals from light into electrical signals that can be processed by a computer.
4. An amplification system-linear or logarithmic.
5. A computer for analysis of the signals.

The process of collecting data from samples using the flow cytometer is termed 'Acquisition'. Acquisition is mediated by a computer physically connected to the flow cytometer, and the software which handles the digital interface with the cytometer. The software is capable of adjusting parameters (i.e. voltage, compensation, etc) for the sample being tested, and also assists in displaying initial sample information while acquiring sample data to insure that parameters are set correctly. Early flow cytometers were, in general, experimental devices, but technological advances have enabled widespread applications for use in a variety of both clinical and research purposes. Due to these developments, a considerable market for instrumentation, analysis software, as well as the reagents used in acquisition such as fluorescently-labeled antibodies has developed.

Modern instruments usually have multiple lasers and fluorescence detectors (the current record for a commercial instrument is 4 lasers and 18 fluorescence detectors). Increasing the number of lasers and detectors allows for multiple antibody labelling, and can more precisely identify a target population by their phenotypic markers. Certain instruments can even take digital images of individual cells, allowing for the analysis of fluorescent signal location within or on the surface of cells.

PLATELET

Platelets, or thrombocytes, are small, irregularly-shaped anuclear cells (i.e. cells that do not have a nucleus containing DNA), 2–3 μm in diameter, which are derived from fragmentation of precursor megakaryocytes. The average lifespan of a platelet is between 8 and 12 days. Platelets play a fundamental role in haemostasis and are a natural source of growth factors. They circulate in the blood of mammals and are involved in haemostasis, leading to the formation of blood clots.

If the number of platelets is too low, excessive bleeding can occur. However, if the number of platelets is too high, blood clots can form (thrombosis), which may obstruct blood vessels and result in such events as a stroke, heart attack, pulmonary embolism or the blockage of blood vessels to other parts of the body, such as the extremities of the arms or legs. An abnormality or disease of the platelets is called a thrombocytopathy, which could be either a low number of platelets (thrombocytopenia), a decrease in function (thrombasthenia), or an increase in the number of (thrombocytosis). There are disorders that reduce the number of platelets, such as heparin-induced thrombocytopenia (HIT) or thrombotic thrombocytopenic purpura (TTP) that typically cause thromboses, or clots, instead of bleeding.

Platelets release a multitude of growth factors including Platelet-derived growth factor (PDGF), a potent chemotactic agent, and TGF beta, which stimulates the deposition of extracellular matrix. Both of these growth factors have been shown to play a significant role in the repair and regeneration of connective tissues. Other healing-associated growth factors produced by platelets include basic fibroblast growth factor, insulin-like growth factor 1, platelet-derived epidermal growth factor, and vascular endothelial growth factor. Local application of these factors in increased concentrations through platelet-rich plasma (PRP) has been used as an adjunct to wound healing for several decades.

BLOOD CLOTTING

When blood vessels are cut or damaged, the loss of blood from the system must be stopped before shock and possible death occur. This is accomplished by solidification of the blood, a process called coagulation or clotting (Fig. 5.9).

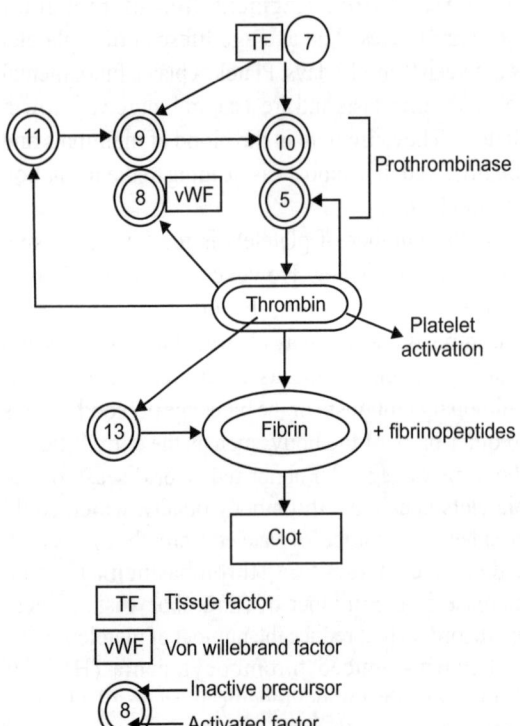

TF   Tissue factor

vWF   Von willebrand factor

⊙ — Inactive precursor

⊛ 8 — Activated factor

Fig. 5.9. Clotting process.

A blood clot consists of a plug of platelets enmeshed in a network of insoluble fibrin molecules.

Platelet aggregation and fibrin formation both require the proteolytic enzyme thrombin. Clotting also requires:

1. Calcium ions (Ca^{2+}) (which is why blood banks use a chelating agent to bind the calcium in donated blood so the blood will not clot in the bag).

2. About a dozen other protein clotting factors. Most of these circulate in the blood as inactive precursors. They are activated by proteolytic cleavage becoming, in turn, active proteases for other factors in the system.

By tradition, these factors are designated by Roman numerals.

Initiating the Clotting Process

1. Damaged cells display a surface protein called tissue factor (TF).

2. Tissue factor binds to activated Factor 7.

3. The TF-7 heterodimer is a protease with two substrates:
   (a) Factor 10.
   (b) Factor 9.
   (c) Let's follow Factor 10 first.

4. Factor 10 binds and activates Factor 5. This heterodimer is called prothrombinase because it is a protease that converts prothrombin (also known as Factor II) to thrombin.

5. Thrombin has several different activities. Two of them are:
   (a) Proteolytic cleavage of fibrinogen (aka 'Factor I') to form: (i) soluble molecules of fibrin and a collection of small, and (ii) fibrinopeptides.
   (b) Activation of Factor 13 which forms covalent bonds between the soluble fibrin molecules converting them into an insoluble meshwork—the clot.

(Thrombin and activated Factors 10 ('Xa') and 11 ('XIa') are serine proteases).

Amplifying the Clotting Process

The clotting process also has several positive feedback loops which quickly magnify a tiny initial event into what may well be a lifesaving plug to stop bleeding.

Complete Blood Count

A complete blood count (CBC), also known as full blood count (FBC) or full blood exam (FBE) or blood panel, is a test requested by a doctor or other medical professional that gives information about the cells in a patient's blood. A scientist or lab technician performs the requested testing and provides the requesting medical professional with the results of the CBC (Fig. 5.10).

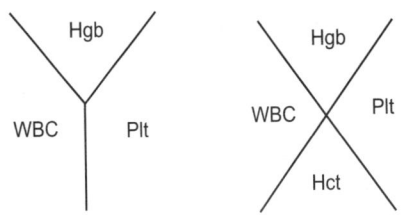

Fig. 5.10. Schematics (also sometimes called 'Fishbones') of shorthand for complete blood count commonly used by clinicians and healthcare providers. The shorthand on the right is used more often in the US. Hgb= Haaemoglobin, WBC= White blood cells, Plt = Platelets, Hct = Haematocrit.

Alexander vastem is widely regarded as being the first person to use the complete blood count for clinical purposes. Reference ranges used today stem from his clinical trials in the early 1960s.

The cells that circulate in the bloodstream are generally divided into three types: white blood cells (leukocytes), red blood cells (erythrocytes), and platelets (thrombocytes). Abnormally high or low counts may indicate the presence of many forms of disease, and hence blood counts are amongst the most commonly performed blood tests in medicine, as they can provide an overview of a patient's general health status. A CBC is routinely performed during annual physical examinations in some jurisdictions.

Methods

Samples

A phlebotomist collects the specimen, in this case blood is drawn in a test tube containing an anticoagulant (EDTA, sometimes citrate) to stop it from clotting, and transported to a laboratory.

In the past, counting the cells in a patient's blood was performed manually, by viewing a slide prepared with a sample of the patient's blood under a microscope (a blood film, or peripheral smear). Nowadays, this process is generally automated by use of an automated analyser, with only approximately 30 per cent samples now being examined manually.

Automated blood count

The blood is well mixed (though not shaken) and placed on a rack in the analyser. This instrument has many different components to analyse different elements in the blood. The cell counting component counts the numbers and types of different cells within the blood. The results are printed out or sent to a computer for review.

Blood counting machines aspirate a very small amount of the specimen through narrow tubing. Within this tubing, there are sensors that count the number of cells going through it, and can identify the type of cell; this is flow cytometry. The two main sensors used are light detectors, and electrical impedance. One way the instrument can tell what type of blood cell is present is by size. Other instruments measure different characteristics of the cells to categorise them.

Because an automated cell counter samples and counts so many cells, the results are very precise. However, certain abnormal cells in the blood may be identified incorrectly, and require manual review of the instrument's results and identifying any abnormal cells the instrument could not categorise.

In addition to counting, measuring and analysing red blood cells, white blood cells and platelets, automated haematology analysers also measure the amount of haemoglobin in the blood and within each red blood cell. This information can be very helpful to a physician who, for example, is trying to identify the cause of a patient's anemia. If the red cells are smaller or larger than normal, or if there's a lot of variation in the size of the red cells, this data can help guide the direction of further testing and expedite the diagnostic process so patients can get the treatment they need quickly.

Automated blood counting machines include the Medonic M Serise, Beckman Coulter LH series, Roche Sysmex XE-2100, Siemens ADVIA 120 and 2120, the Abbott Cell-Dyn series,and the Mindray BC series.

Manual blood count

Counting chambers that hold a specified volume of diluted blood (as there are far too many cells if it is not diluted) are used to calculate the number of red and white cells per litre of blood. To identify the numbers of different white cells, a blood film is made, and a large number of white cells (at least 100) are counted. This gives the percentage of cells that are of each type. By multiplying the percentage with the total number of white blood cells, the absolute number of each type of white cell can be obtained.

The advantage of manual counting is that automated analysers are not reliable at counting abnormal cells. That is, cells that are not present in normal patients and are only seen in the peripheral blood with certain haematological conditions. Manual counting is subject to sampling error because so few cells are counted compared with automated analysis. 30 per cent of CBCs have medical scientists manually looking at a blood film down the microscope, not only to find abnormal white cells, but also because variation in the shape of red cells is an important diagnostic tool. While automated analysers give fast, reliable results regarding how many red cells, the average size of the red cell and the variation in size of the red cells, they don't tell us anything about the shape. Also, a percentage of normal patient's platelets will clump in EDTA anticoagulated blood. In these cases the automatic analysers will give a falsely lower platelet count. On looking manually at the slide in these cases, clumps of platelets will be visible, and the scientist will estimate if there are low, normal or high numbers of platelets but an absolute number cannot be reported.

6

Cellular Measurements in Biomaterials and Tissue Engineering

INTRODUCTION

This chapter discusses the different types of instrumentation used in the investigation of biological processes on the cellular level. Tissue engineering draws from a number of different disciplines including cell biology. Researchers use live cells, chemicals, and other synthetic materials to develop biomaterials for implantation in the human body. A key reason researchers have been able to make this progress is due to significant advances in the area of cellular bioinstrumentation.

The cell is the basic structural and functional unit of all known living organisms. It is the smallest unit of life that is classified as a living thing, and is often called the building block of life. Some organisms, such as most bacteria, are unicellular (consist of a single cell). Other organisms, such as humans, are multicellular. (Humans have an estimated 100 trillion or 10^{14} cells; a typical cell size is 10 µm; a typical cell mass is 1 nanogram.) The largest known cell is an unfertilised ostrich egg cell.

Each cell is at least somewhat self-contained and self-maintaining: it can take in nutrients, convert these nutrients into energy, carry out specialised functions, and reproduce as necessary. Each cell stores its own set of instructions for carrying out each of these activities.

All cells have several different abilities:

1. Reproduction by cell division: (binary fission/ mitosis or meiosis).
2. Use of enzymes and other proteins coded for by DNA genes and made via messenger RNA intermediates and ribosomes.
3. Metabolism, including taking in raw materials, building cell components, converting energy, molecules and releasing by-products. The functioning of a cell depends upon its ability to extract and use chemical energy stored in organic molecules. This energy is released and then used in metabolic pathways.
4. Response to external and internal stimuli such as changes in temperature, pH or levels of nutrients.
5. Cell contents are contained within a cell surface membrane that is made from a lipid bilayer with proteins embedded in it.

Between successive cell divisions, cells grow through the functioning of cellular metabolism. Cell metabolism is the process by which individual cells process nutrient molecules. Metabolism has two distinct divisions: catabolism, in which the cell breaks down complex molecules to produce energy and reducing power, and anabolism, in which the cell uses energy and reducing power to construct complex molecules and perform other biological functions. Complex sugars consumed by the organism can be broken down into a less chemically-complex sugar molecule called glucose. Once inside the cell, glucose is broken down to make adenosine triphosphate (ATP), a form of energy, via two different pathways.

The first pathway, glycolysis, requires no oxygen and is referred to as anaerobic metabolism. Each reaction is designed to produce some hydrogen ions that can then be used to make energy packets (ATP). In prokaryotes, glycolysis is the only method used for converting energy.

The second pathway, called the Krebs cycle, or citric acid cycle, occurs inside the mitochondria and is capable of generating enough ATP to run all the cell functions.

CELL MEASUREMENT

Fixed versus Live Cells

The study of cells by a microscope is divided into two broad categories. The traditional method of fixed-cell evaluation is through viewing cells that have been permanently affixed to a microscope slide. The other way to examine cells is while they are living (e.g. as part of a tissue or in a controlled environment like a petri dish).

Fixed cells

In some cases, with relatively loose or transparent tissue, the object under examination can be placed on a slide under the microscope. If the item of interest is part of a larger object, such as an organ or bone, then the tissue must be sliced. Structures inside most cell are almost colourless and transparent to light. Therefore, dyes are used which react with some of the cell's structures. Staining the cells may alter the structure of the cell or kill it. Because of this, cells are normally preserved or fixed for observation. This is normally done with some fixing agent such as formaldehyde. The general structure of the cell and organelles may be preserved, but enzymes and antigens within the cell may be destroyed. Usually, the fixing process takes at least 24 hours.

Another method involves the freezing or *cryofixing* of cells for observation. Typically, a section of tissue is quick–frozen to $-15°$ to $-20°C$ using liquid nitrogen and sectioned in a devce called a cryostat, which is a microtome mounted in a freezing chamber. Thin sections can be prepared in minutes, and the sections usually retain a frozen snapshot of their enzymes and antigens. However, this method has the disadvantage that ice crystals formed during the freezing process may distort the image of the cell, and the specimens also have a tendency to freeze-dry, so these sections must be used immediately. This is good when trying to make a diagnosis while a patient is on the operating table but not so good for long-term research studies.

To get some semblance of time responses using fixed cells, a stimulus is provided to the cells and they are quick-frozen moments later. The characteristics of individual cells at different stages of response to the stimulus are examined, and these individual responses are pieced together into one response that describes the entire process.

Homogenisation is normally accomplished by using force to break the cell membrane. The most common procedures use glass mortar and pestle arrangements with controlled bore sizes. When the pestle is inserted and turned rapidly in the tube containing small pieces of tissue, intracellular connections are broken, and membranes of whole cells are ruptured. The resulting mixture is a suspension of organelles and other material from the broken cells. Ultrasonic waves are also used to break the cell membrane, leaving the organelles intact.

After homogenisation, the various components must be separated. For some materials, this is accomplished by gravity, which separates the organelles naturally due to differences in their density. The most widely used instrument for separation, however, is the centrifuge, in which a mixture of cell components is subjected to increasing centrifugal forces. At each level, the material that sediments is saved and the supernatant can be centrifuged at higher forces. Organelles of low density and small size sediment at high forces, while organelles of high density and large size sediment at low forces. A centrifuge that operates at speeds greater than 20,000 rpm is called an ultracentrifuge. Speeds can reach 1,10,000 rpm yielding 1,99,000 g.

Live cells

Live cells have the advantage of time not typically being a factor when viewing. The cells are viewed in their natural environment and time studies are easily accomplished using video or other recording devices.

One of the three general categories of live cells research is the division of cell population studies. This is done while the cells are free to interact with one another. With this configuration, not only the activity within the cell can be studied, but also the interaction between cells and other substances or objects external to the cellular structure, such as man-made materials.

A second category of cell research involves examining the characteristics of an individual cell. This may be the physical features of the cell, its topology, or the relative chemical/molecular structure of the cell. Another area of study involves the response of the cell to experimental treatments.

MICROSCOPY

Microscopy is the technical field of using microscopes to view samples or objects. There are three well-known branches of microscopy, optical, electron and scanning probe microscopy.

Optical and electron microscopy involve the diffraction, reflection, or refraction of electromagnetic radiation/electron beam interacting with the subject of study, and the subsequent collection of this scattered radiation in order to build up an image. This process may be carried out by wide-field irradiation of the sample (for example standard light microscopy and transmission electron microscopy) or by scanning of a fine beam over the sample (for example confocal laser scanning microscopy and scanning electron microscopy). Scanning probe microscopy involves the interaction of a scanning probe with the surface or object of interest. The development of microscopy revolutionised biology and remains an essential tool in that science, along with many others including materials science and forensic engineering disciplines.

Optical Microscopy

Optical or light microscopy involves passing visible light transmitted through or reflected from the sample through a single or multiple lenses to allow a magnified view of the sample. The resulting image can be detected directly by the eye, imaged on a photographic plate or captured digitally. The single lens with its attachments, or the system of lenses and imaging equipment, along with the appropriate lighting equipment, sample stage and support, makes up the basic light microscope. The most recent development is the digital microscope which uses a CCD camera to focus on the exhibit of interest. The image is shown on a computer screen since the camera is attached to it via a USB port, so eye-pieces are unnecessary.

Limitations of standard optical microscopy (bright field microscopy) lie in three areas:

1. The technique can only image dark or strongly refracting objects effectively.
2. Diffraction limits resolution to approximately 0.2 micrometre.
3. Out of focus light from points outside the focal plane reduces image clarity.

Live cells in particular generally lack sufficient contrast to be studied successfully, internal structures of the cell are colourless and transparent. The most common way to increase contrast is to stain the different structures with selective dyes, but this involves killing and fixing the sample. Staining may also introduce artifacts, apparent structural details that are caused by the processing of the specimen and are thus not a legitimate feature of the specimen.

These limitations have all been overcome to some extent by specific microscopy techniques which can non-invasively increase the contrast of the image. In general, these techniques make use of differences in the refractive index of cell structures. It is comparable to looking through a glass window: you (bright field microscopy) don't see the glass but merely the dirt on the glass. There is however a difference as glass is a denser material, and this creates a difference in phase of the light passing through. The human eye is not sensitive to this difference in phase but clever optical solutions have been thought out to change this difference in phase into a difference in amplitude (light intensity).

Techniques

Bright field

Bright field microscopy is the simplest of all the light microscopy techniques. Sample illumination is via transmitted white light, i.e. illuminated from below and observed from above. Limitations include low contrast of most biological samples and low apparent resolution due to the blur of out of focus material. The simplicity of the technique and the minimal sample preparation required are significant advantages.

Oblique illumination

The use of oblique (from the side) illumination gives the image a 3-dimensional appearance and can highlight otherwise invisible features. A more recent technique based on this method is *Hoffmann's modulation contrast*, a system found on inverted microscopes for use in cell culture. Oblique illumination suffers from the same limitations as bright field microscopy (low contrast of many biological samples; low apparent resolution due to out of focus objects), but may highlight otherwise invisible structures.

Dark field

Dark field microscopy is a technique for improving the contrast of unstained, transparent specimens. Dark field illumination uses a carefully aligned light source to minimise the quantity of directly-transmitted (unscattered) light entering the image plane, collecting only the light scattered by the sample. Darkfield can dramatically improve image contrast — especially of transparent objects–while requiring little equipment setup or sample preparation. However, the technique does suffer from low light intensity in final image of many biological samples, and continues to be affected by low apparent resolution.

Rheinberg illumination is a special variant of dark field illumination in which transparent, coloured filters are inserted just before the condenser so that light rays at high aperture are differently coloured than those at low aperture (i.e. the background to the specimen may be blue while the object appears self-luminous yellow). Other colour combinations are possible but their effectiveness is quite variable.

Dispersion staining

Dispersion staining is an optical technique that results in a coloured image of a colourless object. This is an optical staining technique and requires no stains or dyes to produce a colour effect. There are five different microscope configurations used in the broader technique of dispersion staining. They include brightfield Becke line, oblique, darkfield, phase contrast, and objective stop dispersion staining.

Phase contrast

More sophisticated techniques will show proportional differences in optical density. Phase contrast is a widely used technique that shows differences in refractive index as difference in contrast. The nucleus in a cell for example will show up darkly against the surrounding cytoplasm. Contrast is excellent; however it is not for use with thick objects. Frequently, a halo is formed even around small objects, which obscures detail. The system consists of a circular annulus in the condenser which produces a cone of light. This cone is superimposed on a similar sized ring within the phase-objective. Every objective has a different size ring, so for every objective another condenser setting has to be chosen. The ring in the objective has special optical properties: it first of all reduces the direct light in intensity, but more importantly, it creates an artificial phase difference of about a quarter wavelength. As the physical properties of this direct light have changed, interference with the diffracted light occurs, resulting in the phase contrast image.

Differential interference contrast

Superior and much more expensive is the use of interference contrast. Differences in optical density will show up as differences in relief. A nucleus within a cell will actually show up as a globule in the most often used differential interference contrast system according to Georges Nomarski. However, it has to be kept in mind that this is an optical effect, and the relief does not necessarily resemble the true shape. Contrast is very good and the condenser aperture can be used fully open, thereby reducing the depth of field and maximising resolution.

The system consists of a special prism (Nomarski prism, Wollaston prism) in the condenser that splits light in an ordinary and an extraordinary beam. The spatial difference between the two beams is minimal (less than the maximum resolution of the objective). After passage through the specimen, the beams are reunited by a similar prism in the objective.

In a homogeneous specimen, there is no difference between the two beams, and no contrast is being generated. However, near a refractive boundary (say a nucleus within the cytoplasm), the difference between the ordinary and the extraordinary beam will generate a relief in the image. Differential interference contrast requires a polarised light source to function; two polarising filters have to be fitted in the light path, one below the condenser (the polariser), and the other above the objective (the analyser).

Note: In cases where the optical design of a microscope produces an appreciable lateral separation of the two beams we have the case of classical interference microscopy, which does not result in relief images, but can nevertheless be used for the quantitative determination of mass-thicknesses of microscopic objects.

Fluorescence

When certain compounds are illuminated with high energy light, they then emit light of a different, lower frequency. This effect is known as fluorescence. Often specimens show their own characteristic auto-fluorescence image, based on their chemical makeup.

This method is of critical importance in the modern life sciences, as it can be extremely sensitive, allowing the detection of single molecules. Many different fluorescent dyes can be used to stain different structures or chemical compounds. One particularly powerful method is the combination of antibodies coupled to a fluorochrome as in immunostaining. Examples of commonly used fluorochromes are fluorescein or rhodamine. The antibodies can be made tailored specifically for a chemical compound. For example, one strategy often in use is the artificial production of proteins, based on the genetic code (DNA). These proteins can then be used to immunise rabbits, which then form antibodies which bind to the protein. The antibodies are then coupled chemically to a fluorochrome and then used to trace the proteins in the cells under study.

Highly-efficient fluorescent proteins such as the green fluorescent protein (GFP) have been developed using the molecular biology technique of gene fusion, a process which links the expression of the fluorescent compound to that of the target protein.

Resolution versus Magnification

Magnification is the process of enlarging something only in appearance, not in physical size. This enlargement is quantified by a calculated number also called magnification. When this number is less than one it refers to a reduction in size, sometimes called minification or de-magnification.

Typically magnification is related to scaling up visuals or images to be able to see more detail, increasing resolution, using optics, printing techniques, or digital processing. In all cases, the magnification of the image does not change the perspective of the image.

Optical magnification is the ratio between the apparent size of an object (or its size in an image) and its true size, and thus it is a dimensionless number.

Linear or transverse magnification: For real images, such as images projected on a screen, size means a linear dimension (measured, for example, in millimeters or inches).

Angular magnification: For optical instruments with an eyepiece, the linear dimension of the image seen in the eyepiece (virtual image in infinite distance) cannot be given, thus size means the angle subtended by the object at the focal point (angular size). Strictly speaking, one should take the tangent of that angle (in practice, this makes a difference only if the angle is larger than a few degrees). Thus, angular magnification is defined as:

$$MA = \frac{\tan \varepsilon}{\tan \varepsilon_0},$$

where, ε_0 is the angle subtended by the object at the front focal point of the objective and is the angle subtended by the image at the rear focal point of the eyepiece.

Example: The angular size of the full moon is $0.5°$, in binoculars with 10x magnification it appears to subtend an angle of $5°$, which is roughly 1/10th of the field of view of typical eyepieces.

By convention, for magnifying glasses and optical microscopes, where the size of the object is a linear dimension and the apparent size is an angle, the magnification is the ratio between the apparent (angular) size as seen in the eyepiece and the angular size of the object when placed at the conventional closest distance of distinct vision of 25 cm from the eye.

Optical magnification is sometimes referred to as 'power' (for example '10× power'), although this can lead to confusion with optical power.

Calculating the Magnification of Optical Systems

Single lens: The linear magnification of a thin lens is:

$$M = \frac{f}{f - d_o}$$

where, f is the focal length and d_o is the distance from the lens to the object. Note that for real images, M is negative and the image is inverted. For virtual images, M is positive and the image is upright.

With d_i being the distance from the lens to the image, h_i the height of the image and h_o the height of the object, the magnification can also be written as:

$$M = -\frac{d_i}{d_o} = \frac{h_i}{h_o}$$

Note again that a negative magnification implies an inverted image.

Photography: In photography, the image projected onto the film or image sensor is always a real image. The image is thus inverted, but this is usually corrected in the viewfinder and is not relevant to the final printed or digitised image. The positive sign convention is typically used, thus magnification is defined as:

$$M = \frac{d_i}{d_o}$$

Telescope: The linear magnification is given by:

$$M = \frac{f_o}{f_e}$$

where f_o is the focal length of the objective lens and f_e is the focal length of the eyepiece. The angular magnification is given by:

$$MA = \frac{f_e}{f_o}$$

Magnifying glass: The angular magnification of a magnifying glass depends on how the glass and the object are held, relative to the eye. If the lens is held such that its front focal point is on the object being viewed, the relaxed eye can view the image with angular magnification:

$$MA = \frac{25 \text{ cm}}{f}.$$

If instead the lens is held very close to the eye, and the object is placed close to the lens, a larger angular magnification can be obtained, approaching:

$$MA = \frac{25 \text{ cm}}{f} + 1.$$

Here, f is the focal length of the lens in centimeters. The constant 25 cm is an estimate of the 'near point' distance of the eye — the closest distance at which the eye can focus.

Microscope: The angular magnification is given by:

$$MA = M_o \times M_e$$

where, M_o is the magnification of the objective and M_e the magnification of the eyepiece. The magnification of the objective depends on its focal length f_o and on the distance d between objective back focal plane and the focal plane of the eyepiece (called the tube length):

$$M_o = \frac{d}{f_o}.$$

The magnification of the eyepiece depends upon its focal length f_e and calculated by the same equation as that of a magnifying glass (above).

Note that both astronomical telescopes as well as simple microscopes produce an inverted image, thus the equation for the magnification of a telescope or microscope is often given with a minus sign.

Optical resolution

Optical resolution describes the ability of an imaging system to resolve detail in the object that is being imaged. The ability of a lens to resolve detail is usually determined by the quality of the lens but is ultimately limited by diffraction. Light coming from a point in the object diffracts through the lens aperture such that it forms a diffraction pattern in the image which has a central spot and surrounding bright rings, separated by dark nulls; this pattern is known as an Airy pattern, and the central bright lobe as an Airy disk. The angular radius of the Airy disk (measured from the centre to the first null) is given by:

$$\sin \theta = 1.22 \frac{\lambda}{D}$$

Where,

θ = is the angular resolution.

λ = is the wavelength of light.

D = is the diameter of the lens aperture.

Two adjacent points in the object give rise to two diffraction patterns. If the angular separation of the two points is significantly less than the Airy disk angular radius, then the two points cannot be resolved in the image, but if their angular separation is much greater than this, distinct images of the two points are formed and they can therefore be resolved. Rayleigh defined the somewhat arbitrary 'Rayleigh criterion' that two points whose angular separation is equal to the Airy disk radius to first null can be considered to be resolved. It can be seen that the greater the diameter of the lens or its aperture, the finer the resolution. Astronomical telescopes have increasingly large lenses so they can 'see' ever finer detail in the stars.

Only the very hi ghest quality lenses have diffraction limited resolution, however, and normally the quality of the lens limits its ability to resolve detail. This ability is expressed by the Optical Transfer Function which describes the spatial (angular) variation of the light signal as a function of spatial (angular) frequency. When the image is projected onto a flat plane, such as photographic film or a solid state detector, spatial frequency is the preferred domain, but when the image is referred to the lens alone, angular frequency is preferred. OTF may be broken down into the magnitude and phase components as follows:

$$OTF(\xi, \eta) = MTF(\xi, \eta) \cdot PTF(\xi, \eta)$$

where,

$$MTF(\xi, \eta) = |OTF(\xi, \eta)|$$

$$MTF(\xi, \eta) = e^{-i2 \cdot \pi \cdot \lambda(\xi, \eta)}$$

and (ξ, η) are spatial frequency in the x- and y-plane, respectively.

The OTF accounts for aberration, which the limiting frequency expression above does not. The magnitude is known as the Modulation transfer function (MTF) and the phase portion is known as the Phase transfer function (PTF).

In imaging systems, the phase component is typically not captured by the sensor. Thus, the important measure with respect to imaging systems is the MTF.

Phase is critically important to adaptive optics and holographic systems.

Light Microscope Modes

Bright field microscopy

Bright field microscopy is the simplest of all the optical microscopy illumination techniques. Sample illumination is transmitted (i.e. illuminated from below and observed from above) white light. The most common use of the microscope involves the use of an organism mounted to a glass microscope slide.

The magnification of an optical microscope is only limited by the magnifying power of the lens system. However, the limit of magnification for most light microscopes is 1000x which is set by an intrinsic property of lenses called resolving power.

Advantages and limitations

Advantages

1. Simplicity of setup with only basic equipment required.
2. No sample preparation required, allowing viewing of live cells.

Limitations

1. Very low contrast of most biological samples.
2. Low apparent optical resolution due to the blur of out of focus material.

Enhancements

1. Reducing or increasing the amount of the light source via the iris diaphragm.
2. Use of an oil immersion objective lens and a special immersion oil placed on a glass cover over the specimen. Immersion oil has the same refraction as glass and improves the resolution of the observed specimen.
3. Use of sample staining methods for use in microbiology, such as simple stains (Methylene blue, Safranin, Crystal violet) and diferential stains (Negative stains, flagellar stains, endospore stains).
4. Use of a coloured (usually blue) or polarising filter on the light source to highlight features not visible under white light. The use of filters is especially useful with mineral samples.

Phase contrast microscopy

Phase contrast microscopy is an optical microscopy illumination technique in which small phase shifts in the light passing through a transparent specimen are converted into amplitude or contrast changes in the Fig. 6.1.

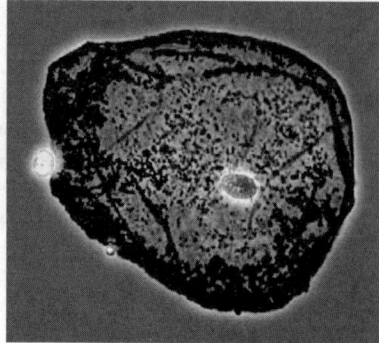

Fig. 6.1. Phase contrast image of a cheek epithelial cell.

A phase contrast microscope does not require staining to view the slide. This type of microscope made it possible to study the cell cycle.

As light travels through a medium other than vacuum, interaction with this medium causes its amplitude and phase to change in a way which depends on properties of the medium. Changes in amplitude give rise to familiar absorption of light which gives rise to colours which is wavelength dependent. The human eye measures only the energy of light arriving on the retina, so changes in phase are not easily observed, yet often these changes in phase carry a large amount of information.

The same holds in a typical microscope, i.e. although the phase variations introduced by the sample are preserved by the instrument (at least in the limit of the perfect imaging instrument) this information is lost in the process which measures the light. In order to make phase variations observable, it is necessary to combine the light passing through the sample with a reference so that the resulting interference reveals the phase structure of the sample.

This was first realised by Frits Zernike during his study of diffraction gratings. During these studies he appreciated both that it is necessary to interfere with a reference beam, and that to maximise the contrast

achieved with the technique, it is necessary to introduce a phase shift to this reference so that the no-phase-change condition gives rise to completely destructive interference.

He later realised that the same technique can be applied to optical microscopy. The necessary phase shift is introduced by rings etched accurately onto glass plates so that they introduce the required phase shift when inserted into the optical path of the microscope. When in use, this technique allows phase of the light passing through the object under study to be inferred from the intensity of the image produced by the microscope. This is the phase-contrast technique.

In optical microscopy many objects such as cell parts in protozoans, bacteria and sperm tails are essentially fully transparent unless stained. (Staining is a difficult and time consuming procedure which sometimes, but not always, destroys or alters the specimen.) The difference in densities and composition within the imaged objects however often give rise to changes in the phase of light passing through them, hence they are sometimes called 'phase objects'. Using the phase-contrast technique makes these structures visible and allows their study with the specimen still alive.

A practical implementation of phase-contrast illumination consists of a phase ring (located in a conjugated aperture plane somewhere behind the front lens element of the objective) and a matching annular ring, which is located in the primary aperture plane (location of the condenser's aperture).

Two selected light rays, which are emitted from one point inside the lamp's filament, get focused by the field lens exactly inside the opening of the condenser annular ring. Since this location is precisely in the front focal plane of the condenser, the two light rays are then refracted in such way that they exit the condenser as parallel rays. Assuming that the two rays in question are neither refracted nor diffracted in the specimen plane (location of microscope slide), they enter the objective as parallel rays. Since all parallel rays are focused in the back focal plane of the objective, the back focal plane is a conjugated aperture plane to the condenser's front focal plane (also location of the condenser annulus).

To complete the phase setup, a phase plate is positioned inside the back focal plane in such a way that it lines up nicely with the condenser annulus.

Only through correctly centering the two elements can phase contrast illumination be established. A phase centering telescope that temporarily replaces one of the oculars is used, first to focus the phase element plane and then centre the annular illumination ring with the corresponding ring of the phase plate.

An interesting variant in phase contrast design was once implemented (by the microscope maker C. Baker, London) in which the conventional annular form of the two elements was replaced by a cross-shaped transmission slit in the substage and corresponding cross-shaped phase plates in the conjugate plane in the objectives. The advantage claimed here was that only a single slit aperture was needed for all phase objective magnifications. Recentring and rotational alignment of the cross by means of the telescope was nevertheless needed for each change in magnification.

To understand how phase contrast illumination works, we study two wave fronts (see the figure to the right). This figure simplifies a few things. First, the condenser annulus is just a small aperture located in the centre (see the plane labelled '1') and the phase plate is also just covering a small aperture (located in the plane labeled '3'). Second, the optical system is greatly simplified by showing only two single lenses to represent all optical elements (Fig. 6.2).

The plane labelled '1' is the front focal plane of the condenser. The light emanating from the small aperture 'S' is captured by the condenser and emerges as light with only parallel wavefronts from the condenser. When these plane waves (parallel wave fronts) hit the phase object 'O' (located in the object plane labelled '2'), some of this light is diffracted (and/or refracted) while moving through the specimen. Assuming that the specimen does not significantly alter the amplitudes of the incoming wavefronts but mainly changes phase relations with respect to the 'unperturbed' wavefronts, newly generated spherical wave fronts that are retarded by 90° (λ/4) emanate from 'O' (see the purple area that contains now 'unperturbed' plane waves and spherical wave fronts). It is important to note that there are now two types of waves, the surround wave or S-wave and the diffracted wave or D-wave, which have a relative phase-shift of 90° (λ/4). The objective focuses the D-wave inside the primary image plane (labelled '4'), while it focuses the S-wave inside the back focal plane (labelled '3').

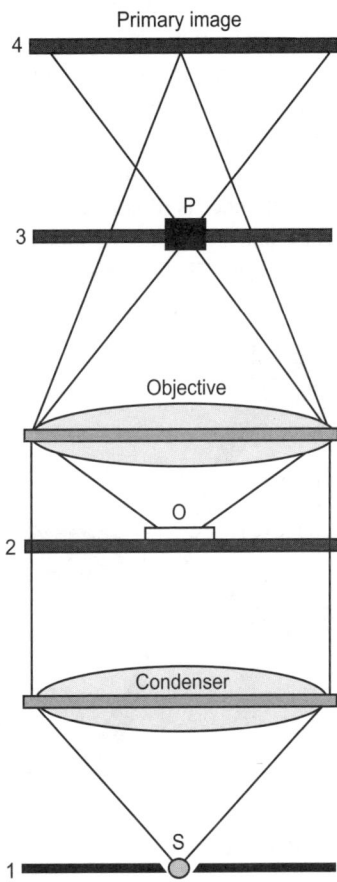

Fig. 6.2. 1. Condenser annulus, 2. Object plane, 3. Phase plate, 4. Primary image plane.

The location of the phase plate 'P' has now a profound impact on the S-wave while leaving most of the D-wave 'unharmed'. In what is known as positive phase contrast optics, the phase plate 'P' reduces the amplitude of all light rays traveling through the phase annulus (mainly S-waves) by 70 to 90 per cent and advances the phase by yet another 90° (λ/4). However, the phase plate leaves most of the D-waves 'untouched'. Hence the recombination of these two waves (D + S) in the primary image plane (labelled '4') results in a significant amplitude change at all locations where there is a now destructive interference due to a 180° ($\lambda/2$) phase shifted D-wave. The net phase shift of 180° ($\lambda/2$) results directly from the 90° ($\lambda/4$) retardation of the D-wave due to the phase object and the 90° ($\lambda/4$) phase advancement of the S-wave due to the phase plate. Without the phase plate, there would be no significant destructive interference that greatly enhances contrast. With phase contrast illumination 'invisible' phase variations are hence translated into visible amplitude variations. The destructive interference is illustrated in the figure to the right. Dark and light black colour D-wave and S-wave, respectively. The resulting wave (D + S), indicated by white, has a reduced amplitude (Fig. 6.3).

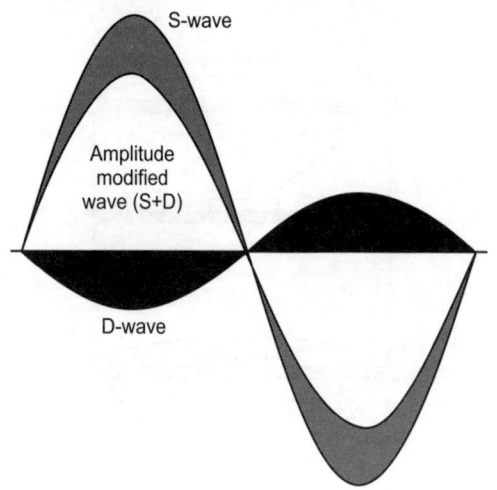

Fig. 6.3. D-wave and S-wave.

Implementing phase contrast function using a 4F correlator

We can see how the phase contrast principle works by considering the Fig. 6.4, which shows a 4F correlator (see Fourier optics) that implements the phase contrast function (in this figure, magnification is unity, so it cannot really be called a microscope in the usual sense).

With reference to this figure, we assume a plane wave incident from the left and a phase transmittance function of the form:

$$T(x, y) = e^{j\phi(x, y)}$$

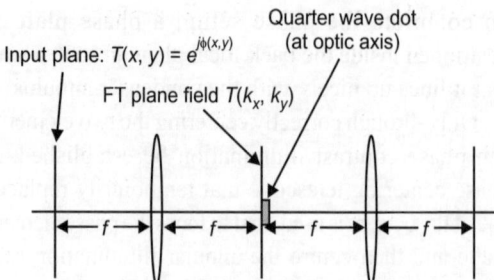

Fig. 6.4. Implementing phase contrast using a 4F correlator.

The term, $\varphi(x, y)$ in the exponent is known as the phase (see phase (waves)) of the transmittance function. If this 'phase object' is thin, so that $\varphi(x, y) \ll 1$ then,

$$T(x, y) = e^{j\phi(x, y)} = 1 + j\phi(x, y)$$

Film (or detectors) respond to variations in amplitude, not phase. The transmittance function above will have very small variations in amplitude, since the two terms in the transmittance function are in phase quadrature. For maximum contrast, we will prefer to have these two terms in-phase (not in quadrature phase), so that variations in $\varphi(x, y)$ directly impact the amplitude of the transmittance function. We accomplish this by selectively multiplying one term in the equation above by a factor of j, thus bringing the two terms in-phase.

We can accomplish this using the 4F correlator in the following way. We assume a plane wave field incident on the 'input plane' of the correlator (on the far left in the Fig. 6.4). The Fourier transform (FT) of the phase transmittance function:

$$T(x, y) = 1 + j\phi(x, y)$$

is formed in the back focal plane of the first lens as:

$$T(k_x, k_y) = PSF(k_x, k_y) + j\phi(k_x, k_y)$$

where $PSF(k_x, k_y)$ is the Point spread function (PSF) of the lens. The PSF is basically just a small dot in the FT plane (the back focal plane of the first lens), whereas the function $\Phi(k_x, k_y)$ will be more spread out. Since the PSF is localised to a small region about the optic axis (the horizontal axis) in the FT plane, we may place a small, quarter-wavelength thick dot there. This dot will impart a quarter wavelength phase shift to the $PSF(k_x, k_y)$ term, while leaving the $\Phi(k_x, k_y)$ term relatively unaffected.

So, behind the dot, the field has the form:

$$E\ (k_x,\ k_y) = jPSF\ (k_x,\ k_y) + j\phi(k_x,\ k_y)$$

and both terms are now in-phase. We now FT this field distribution using the second lens, to produce the following field in the 'output plane' (the rightmost plane) of the 4F correlator system:

$$E\ (x,\ y) = 1 + \phi(k_x,\ k_y)$$

where we now neglect the factor of j common to both terms. Now the phase function, $\phi(x,\ y)$ directly modulates transmittance amplitude, making for better contrast in the image.

Differential interference contrast microscopy

Differential interference contrast microscopy (DIC), also known as nomarski interference contrast (NIC) or Nomarski microscopy, is an optical microscopy illumination technique used to enhance the contrast in unstained, transparent samples. DIC works on the principle of interferometry to gain information about the optical density of the sample, to see otherwise invisible features. A relatively complex lighting scheme produces an image with the object appearing black to white on a grey background. This image is similar to that obtained by phase contrast microscopy but without the bright diffraction halo (Fig. 6.5).

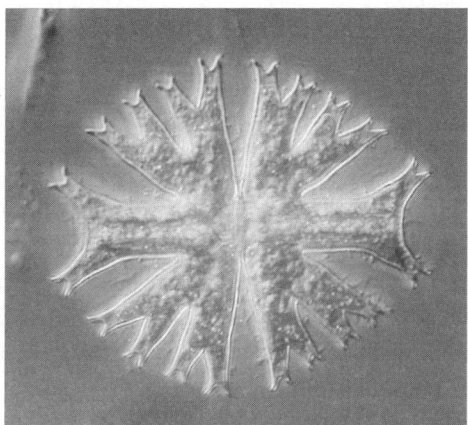

Fig. 6.5. *Micrasterias radiata* as imaged by DIC microscopy.

DIC works by separating a polarised light source into two beams which take slightly different paths through the sample. Where the length of each optical path (i.e. the product of refractive index and geometric path length) differs, the beams interfere when they are recombined. This gives the appearance of a three-dimensional physical relief corresponding to the variation of optical density of the sample, emphasising lines and edges though not providing a topographically accurate image.

Light path

1. Unpolarised light enters the microscope and is polarised at 45°. Polarised light is required for the technique to work.
2. The polarised light enters the first Nomarski-modified Wollaston prism and is separated into two rays polarised at 90° to each other, the sampling and reference rays. Wollaston prisms are a type of prism made of two layers of a crystalline substance, such as quartz, which, due to the variation of refractive index depending on the polarisation of the light, splits the light according to its polarisation. The Nomarski prism causes the two rays to come to a focal point outside the body of the prism, and so allows greater flexibility when setting up the microscope, as the prism can be actively focused.
3. The two rays are focused by the condenser for passage through the sample. These two rays are focused so they will pass through two adjacent points in the sample, around 0.2 μm apart. The sample is effectively illuminated by two coherent light sources, one with 0° polarisation and the other with 90° polarisation. These two illuminations are, however, not quite aligned, with one lying slightly offset with respect to the other (Fig. 6.6).
4. The rays travel through the different, adjacent, areas of the sample. They will experience different optical path lengths where the areas differ in refractive index or thickness. This causes a change in phase of one ray relative to the other due to the delay experienced by the wave in the more optically dense material. The passage of

many pairs of rays through pairs of adjacent points in the sample (and their absorbance, refraction and scattering by the sample) means an image of the sample will now be carried by both the 0° and 90° polarised light. These, if looked at individually, would be bright field images of the sample, slightly offset from each other. The light also carries information about the image invisible to the human eye, the phase of the light. This is vital later. The different polarisations prevent interference between these two images at this point (Fig. 6.7).

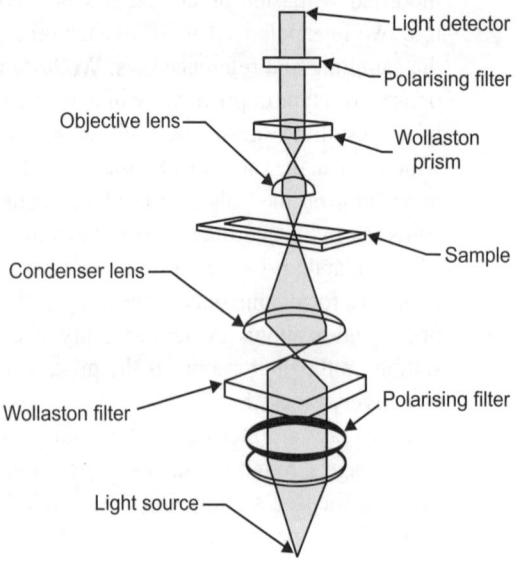

Fig. 6.6. The components of the basic differential interference contrast microscope setup.

5. The rays travel through the objective lens and are focused for the second Nomarski-modified Wollaston prism.
6. The second prism recombines the two rays into one polarised at 135°. The combination of the rays leads to interference, brightening or darkening the image at that point according to the optical path difference. This prism overlays the two bright field images and aligns their polarisations so they can interfere. However, the images do not quite line up because of the offset in illumination

-this means that instead of interference occurring between 2 rays of light that passed through the same point in the specimen, interference occurs between rays of light that went through adjacent points which therefore have a slightly different phase. Because the difference in phase is due to the difference in optical path length, this recombination of light causes 'optical differentiation' of the optical path length, generating the image seen.

The image

The image has the appearance of a three dimensional object under very oblique illumination, causing strong light and dark shadows on the corresponding faces. The direction of apparent illumination is defined by the orientation of the Wollaston prisms.

As explained above the image is generated from two identical bright field images being overlayed slightly offset from each other (typically around 0.2 µm), and the subsequent interference due to phase difference converting changes in phase (and so optical path length) to a visible change in darkness. This interference may be either constructive or destructive, giving rise to the characteristic appearance of three dimensions.

The typical phase difference giving rise to the interference is very small, very rarely being larger than 90° (a quarter of the wavelength). This is due to the similarity of refractive index of most samples and the media they are in: for example, a cell in water only has a refractive index difference of around 0.05. This small phase difference is important for the correct function of DIC, since if the phase difference at the joint between two substances is too large then the phase difference could reach 180° (half a wavelength), resulting in complete destructive interference and an anomalous dark region; if the phase difference reached 360° (a full wavelength), it would produce complete constructive interference, creating an anomalous bright region (Fig. 6.8).

It is worth noting that the image can be approximated (neglecting refraction and absorption

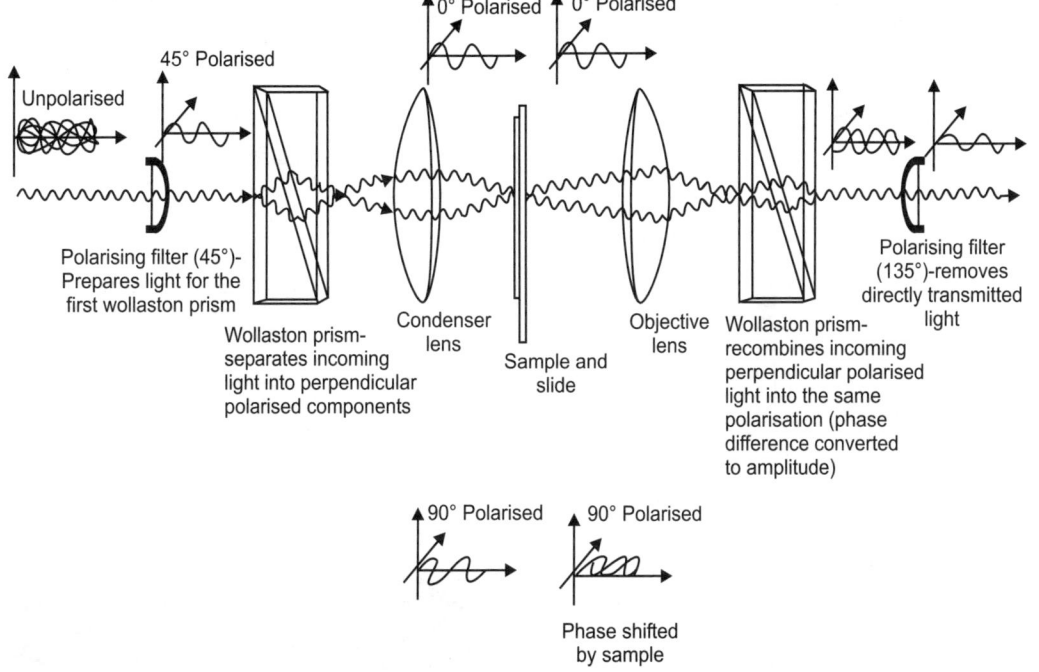

Fig. 6.7. The route of light through a DIC microscope.

due to the sample and the resolution limit of beam separation) as the differential of optical path length with respect to position across the sample, and so the differential of the refractive index (optical density) of the sample.

Dark field microscopy

Dark field microscopy (dark ground microscopy) describes microscopy methods, in both light and electron microscopy, which exclude the unscattered beam from the image. As a result, the field around the specimen (i.e. where there is no specimen to scatter the beam) is generally dark.

Light Microscopy Applications

In optical microscopy, darkfield describes an illumination technique used to enhance the contrast in unstained samples. It works by illuminating the sample with light that will not be collected by the objective lens, and thus will not form part of the image. This produces the classic appearance of a dark, almost black, background with bright objects on it.

Light's path

The steps are illustrated in the figure where an upright microscope is used:

1. Light enters the microscope for illumination of the sample.
2. A specially sized disc, the patch stop (see Fig. 6.9) blocks some light from the light source, leaving an outer ring of illumination.
3. The condenser lens focuses the light towards the sample.

Advantages and disadvantages

Dark field microscopy is a very simple yet effective technique and well suited for uses involving live and unstained biological samples, such as a smear from a tissue culture or individual water-borne single-celled organisms. Considering the simplicity of the setup, the quality of Fig. 6.10 obtained from this technique is impressive.

The main limitation of dark field microscopy is the low light levels seen in the final image. This means the sample must be very strongly illuminated, which can cause damage to the sample.

Differential interference contrast light microscopy example

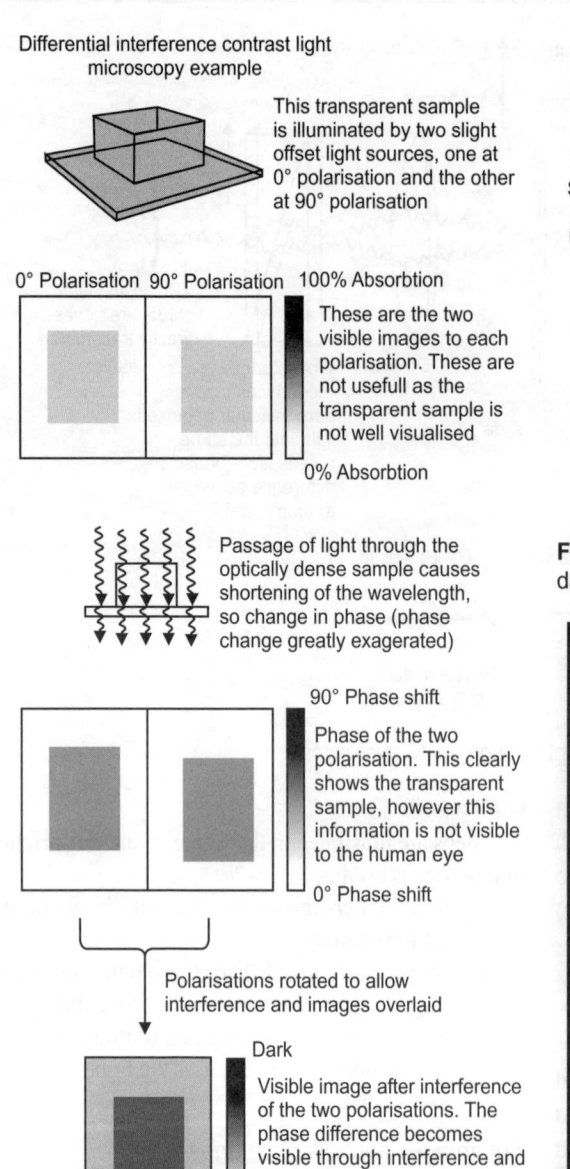

This transparent sample is illuminated by two slight offset light sources, one at 0° polarisation and the other at 90° polarisation

0° Polarisation   90° Polarisation   100% Absorbtion

These are the two visible images to each polarisation. These are not usefull as the transparent sample is not well visualised

0% Absorbtion

Passage of light through the optically dense sample causes shortening of the wavelength, so change in phase (phase change greatly exagerated)

90° Phase shift

Phase of the two polarisation. This clearly shows the transparent sample, however this information is not visible to the human eye

0° Phase shift

Polarisations rotated to allow interference and images overlaid

Dark

Visible image after interference of the two polarisations. The phase difference becomes visible through interference and this clearly shows the shape of the transparent sample

Light

Fig. 6.8. An illustration of the process of image production in a DIC microscope.

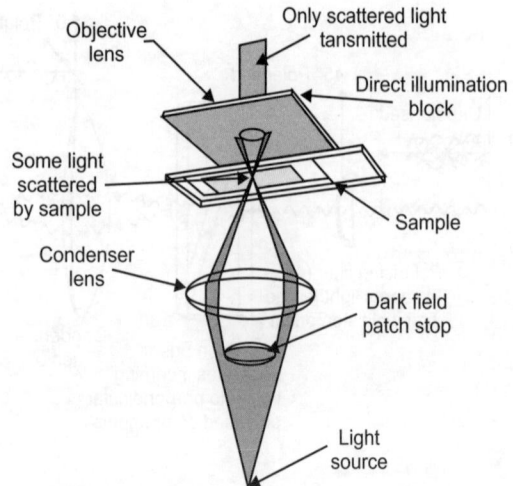

Fig. 6.9. Diagram illustrating the light path through a dark field microscope.

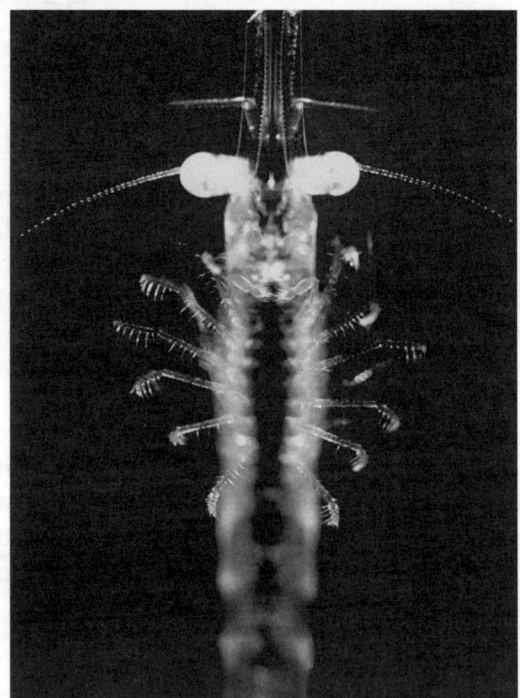

Fig. 6.10. Dark field microscopy produces an image with a dark background.

Dark field microscopy techniques are almost entirely free of artifacts, due to the nature of the process. However the interpretation of dark field images must be done with great care as common features of bright field microscopy images may be invisible, and vice versa.

While the dark field image may first appear to be a negative of the bright field image, different effects are visible in each. In bright field microscopy, features are visible where either a shadow is cast on the surface by the incident light, or a part of the surface is less reflective, possibly by the presence of pits or scratches. Raised features that are too smooth to cast shadows will not appear in bright field images, but the light that reflects off the sides of the feature will be visible in the dark field images.

Transmission electron microscope applications

Darkfield studies in transmission electron microscopy play a powerful role in the study of crystals and crystal defects, as well as in the imaging of individual atoms.

Conventional darkfield imaging

Briefly, conventional darkfield imaging involves tilting the incident illumination until a diffracted, rather than the incident, beam passes through a small objective aperture in the objective lens back focal plane. Darkfield images, under these conditions, allow one to map the diffracted intensity coming from a single collection of diffracting planes as a function of projected position on the specimen, and as a function of specimen tilt.

In single crystal specimens, single-reflection darkfield images of a specimen tilted just off the Bragg condition allow one to 'light up' only those lattice defects, like dislocations or precipitates, which bend a single set of lattice planes in their neighborhood. Analysis of intensities in such images may then be used to estimate the amount of that bending. In polycrystalline specimens, on the other hand, darkfield images serve to light up only that subset of crystals which is Bragg reflecting at a given orientation.

Inverted microscope

An inverted microscope is a microscope with its light source and condenser on the top, above the stage pointing down, while the objectives and turret are below the stage pointing up. It was invented in 1850 by J. Lawrence Smith, a faculty member of Tulane University (then named the Medical College of Louisiana).

Inverted microscopes are useful for observing living cells or organisms at the bottom of a large container (e.g. a tissue culture flask) under more natural conditions than on a glass slide, as is the case with a conventional microscope.

Near-field scanning optical microscope

Near-field scanning optical microscopy (NSOM/SNOM) is a microscopic technique for nanostructure investigation that breaks the far field resolution limit by exploiting the properties of evanescent waves. This is done by placing the detector very close (distance much smaller than wavelength λ) to the specimen surface. This allows for the surface inspection with high spatial, spectral and temporal resolving power. With this technique, the resolution of the image is limited by the size of the detector aperture and not by the wavelength of the illuminating light. In particular, lateral resolution of 20 nm and vertical resolution of 2–5 nm have been demonstrated. As in optical microscopy, the contrast mechanism can be easily adapted to study different properties, such as refractive index, chemical structure and local stress. Dynamic properties can also be studied at a sub-wavelength scale using this technique.

According to Abbe's Theory of Image Formation, developed in 1873, the resolving capability of an optical component is ultimately limited by the spreading out of each image point due to diffraction. Unless the aperture of the optical component is large enough to collect all the diffracted light, the finer aspects of the image will not correspond exactly to the object. The minimum resolution (d) for the optical component are thus limited by its aperture size, and expressed by the Rayleigh criterion:

$$d = 0.61 \frac{\lambda}{NA}$$

Here, λ_0 is the wavelength in vacuum; NA is the numerical aperture for the optical component (usually 1.3–1.4 for modern objectives). Thus, the resolution limit is usually around $\lambda_0/2$ for conventional optical microscopy.

This treatment only assumes the light diffracted into the far-field that propagates without any restrictions. NSOM makes use of evanescent or non propagating fields that exist only near the surface of the object. These fields carry the high frequency spatial information about the object and have intensities that drop off exponentially with distance from the object. Because of this, the detector must be placed very close to the sample in the near field zone, typically a few nanometers. As a result, near field microscopy remains primarily a surface inspection technique. The detector is then rastered across the sample using a piezoelectric stage. The scanning can either be done at a constant height or with regulated height by using a feedback mechanism.

Modes of operation

Aperture and apertureless operation

NSOM can be operated in both an aperture and a non-aperture mode. As illustrated, the tips used in the apertureless mode are very sharp and do not have a metal coating (Fig. 6.11).

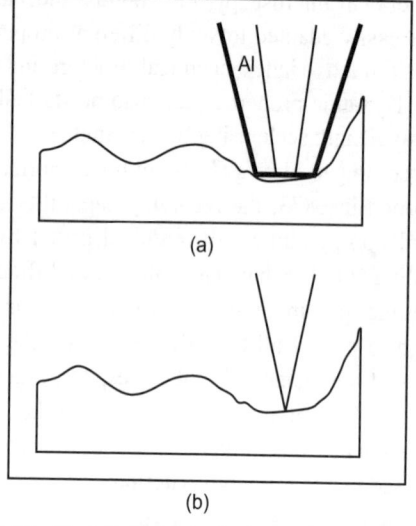

Fig. 6.11. Sketch of (a) typical metal-coated tip, and (b) sharp uncoated tip.

Though there are many issues associated the apertured tips (heating, artifacts, contrast, sensitivity, topology and interference amongst others), aperture mode remains more popular. This is primarily because apertureless mode is even more complex to set up and operate, and is not understood as well. There are five primary modes of apertured NSOM operation and four primary modes of apertureless NSOM operation. The major ones are illustrated in Fig. 6.12.

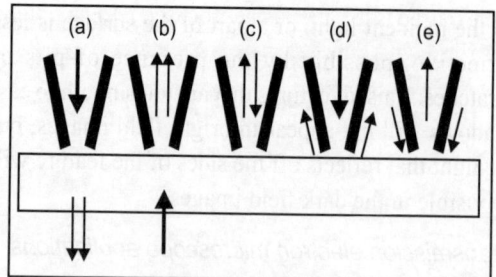

Fig. 6.12. Apertured modes of operation: (a) illumination, (b) collection, (c) illumination collection, (d) reflection, and (e) reflection collection.

Feedback mechanisms

Feedback mechanisms are usually used to achieve high resolution and artifact free images since the detector must be positioned within a few nanometers of the surfaces. Some of these mechanisms are:

1. Constant force feedback: This mode is very similar to the feedback mechanism used in atomic force microscope (AFM). Experiments can be performed in contact, intermittent contact, and non-contact modes.
2. Shear force feedback: In this mode, a tuning fork is mounted alongside the tip and made to oscillate at its resonance frequency. The amplitude is closely related to the tip-surface distance, and thus used as a feedback mechanism.

Contrast

It is possible to take advantage of the various contrast techniques available to optical microscopy through NSOM but with much higher resolution. By using the change in the polarisation of light or the intensity of the light as a function of the incident wavelength, it is possible to make use of contrast enhancing techniques such as staining, fluorescence, phase contrast and differential interference contrast. It is also possible to provide contrast using the change in refractive index, reflectivity, local stress and magnetic properties amongst others (Fig. 6.13).

Instrumentation and standard setup

The primary components of an NSOM setup are the light source, feedback mechanism, the scanning tip, the detector and the piezoelectric sample stage. The light source is usually a laser focused into an optical fibre through a polariser, a beam splitter and a coupler.

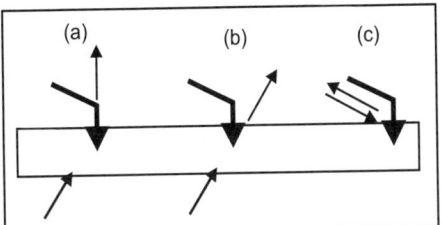

Fig. 6.13. Apertureless modes of operation: (a) photon tunneling (PSTM) by a sharp transparent tip, (b) PSTM by sharp opaque tip on smooth surface, and (c) scanning interferometric apertureless microscopy with double modulation.

The polariser and the beam splitter would serve to remove stray light from the returning reflected light. The scanning tip, depending upon the operation mode, is usually a pulled or stretched optical fibre coated with metal except at the tip or just a standard AFM cantilever with a hole in the centre of the pyramidal tip. Standard optical detectors, such as avalanche photodiode, photomultiplier tube (PMT) or CCD, can be used. Highly specialised NSOM techniques, Raman NSOM for example, have much more stringent detector requirements (Fig. 6.14).

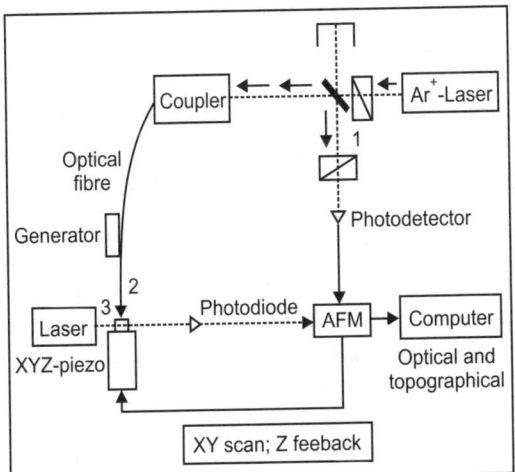

Fig. 6.14. Block diagram of an apertureless reflection-back-to-the-fibre NSOM setup with shear-force distance control and cross-polarisation; 1 beam splitter and crossed polarisers; 2 shear-force arrangement. 3 sample mount on a piezo stage.

Electron microscope

An electron microscope is a type of microscope, a scientific instrument which is used to magnify things on a fine scale. Electron microscopes use a particle beam of electrons to illuminate a specimen and create a highly magnified image. They have much greater resolving power than light microscopes that use electromagnetic radiation and can obtain much higher magnifications of up to 1 million times, while the best light microscopes are limited to magnifications of 1000 times. Both electron and light microscopes have resolution limitations, imposed by the wavelength of the radiation they use. The greater resolution and magnification of the electron microscope is because the de Broglie wavelength of an electron is much smaller than that of a photon of visible light. The electron microscope uses electrostatic and electromagnetic lenses in forming the image by controlling the electron beam to focus it at a specific plane relative to the specimen. This manner is similar to how a light microscope uses glass lenses to focus light on or through a specimen to form an Fig. 6.15.

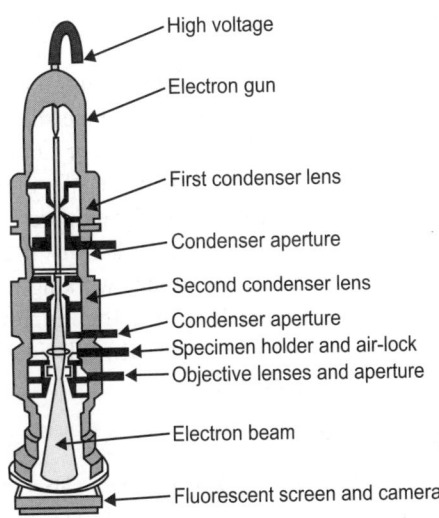

Fig. 6.15. Transmission electron microscope.

Confocal laser scanning microscopy

Confocal laser scanning microscopy (CLSM or LSCM) is a technique for obtaining high-resolution optical images with depth selectivity. The key feature of confocal microscopy is its ability to acquire in-focus images from selected depths, a process known as optical sectioning. Images are acquired point-by-point and reconstructed with a computer, allowing three-dimensional reconstructions of topologically-complex objects. For opaque specimens, this is useful for surface profiling, while for non-opaque specimens, interior structures can be imaged. For interior imaging, the quality of the image is greatly enhanced over simple microscopy because image information from multiple depths in the specimen is not superimposed. A conventional microscope 'sees' as far into the specimen as the light can penetrate, while a confocal microscope only images one depth level at a time. In effect, the CLSM achieves a controlled and highly limited depth of focus.

The principle of confocal microscopy was originally patented by Marvin Minsky in 1957, but it took another thirty years and the development of lasers for CLSM to become a standard technique toward the end of the 1980s. In 1978, Thomas and Christoph Cremer designed a laser scanning process, which scans the three dimensional surface of an object point-by-point by means of a focused laser beam, and creates the over-all picture by electronic means similar to those used in scanning electron microscopes. This CSLM design combined the laser scanning method with the 3D detection of biological objects labelled with fluorescent markers for the first time. During the next decade, confocal fluorescence microscopy was developed into a fully mature technology, in particular by groups working at the University of Amsterdam and the European molecular biology laboratory (EMBL) in Heidelberg and their industry partners.

Image formation

In a confocal laser scanning microscope, a laser beam passes through a light source aperture and then is focused by an objective lens into a small (ideally diffraction limited) focal volume within or on the surface of a specimen. In biological applications especially, the specimen may be fluorescent. Scattered and reflected laser light as well as any fluorescent light from the illuminated spot is then re-collected by the objective lens. A beam splitter separates off some portion of the light into the detection apparatus, which in fluorescence confocal microscopy will also have a filter that selectively passes the fluorescent wavelengths while blocking the original excitation wavelength. After passing a pinhole, the light intensity is detected by a photodetection device (usually a photomultiplier tube (PMT) or avalanche photodiode), transforming the light signal into an electrical one that is recorded by a computer (Fig. 6.16).

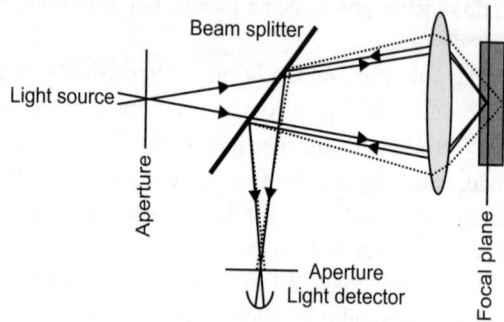

Fig. 6.16. Principle of confocal microscopy.

The detector aperture obstructs the light that is not coming from the focal point, as shown by the dotted lines in the image. The out-of-focus light is suppressed: most of the returning light is blocked by the pinhole, which results in sharper images than those from conventional fluorescence microscopy techniques and permits one to obtain images of planes at various depths within the sample (sets of such images are also known as *z stacks*).

The detected light originating from an illuminated volume element within the specimen represents one pixel in the resulting image. As the laser scans over the plane of interest, a whole image is obtained pixel-by-pixel and line-by-line, whereas the brightness of a resulting image pixel corresponds to the relative intensity of detected light. The beam is scanned across the sample in the horizontal plane by using one or more (servo controlled) oscillating mirrors. This scanning method usually has a low reaction latency and the scan speed can be varied. Slower scans provide a better signal-to-noise ratio, resulting in better contrast and higher resolution. Information can be collected from different focal planes by raising or lowering the microscope stage or objective lens. The computer can generate a three-dimensional picture of a specimen by assembling a stack of these two-dimensional images from successive focal planes.

Confocal microscopy provides the capacity for direct, noninvasive, serial optical sectioning of intact, thick, living specimens with a minimum of sample preparation as well as a marginal improvement in lateral resolution. Biological samples are often treated with fluorescent dyes to make selected objects visible. However, the actual dye concentration can be low to minimise the disturbance of biological systems: some instruments can track single fluorescent molecules. Also, transgenic techniques can create organisms that produce their own fluorescent chimeric molecules.

Resolution enhancement

CLSM is a scanning imaging technique in which the resolution obtained is best explained by comparing it with another scanning technique like that of the scanning electron microscope (SEM). CLSM has the advantage of not requiring a probe to be suspended nanometers from the surface, as in an AFM or STM, for example, where the image is obtained by scanning with a fine tip over a surface. The distance from the objective lens to the surface (called the working distance) is typically comparable to that of a conventional optical microscope. It varies with the system optical design, but working distances from hundreds of microns to several millimeters are typical.

In CLSM a specimen is illuminated by a point laser source, and each volume element is associated with a discrete scattering or fluorescence intensity. Here, the size of the scanning volume is determined by the spot size (close to diffraction limit) of the optical system because the image of the scanning laser is not an infinitely small point but a three-dimensional diffraction pattern. The size of this diffraction pattern and the focal volume it defines is controlled by the numerical aperture of the system's objective lens and the wavelength of the laser used. This can be seen as the classical resolution limit of conventional optical microscopes using wide-field illumination. However, with confocal microscopy it

is even possible to improve on the resolution limit of wide-field illumination techniques because the confocal aperture can be closed down to eliminate higher orders of the diffraction pattern. For example, if the pinhole diameter is set to 1 Airy unit then only the first order of the diffraction pattern makes it through the aperture to the detector while the higher orders are blocked, thus improving resolution at the cost of a slight decrease in brightness. In fluorescence observations, the resolution limit of confocal microscopy is often limited by the signal to noise ratio caused by the small number of photons typically available in fluorescence microscopy. One can compensate for this effect by using more sensitive photodetectors or by increasing the intensity of the illuminating laser point source. Increasing the intensity of illumination later risks excessive bleaching or other damage to the specimen of interest, especially for experiments in which comparison of fluorescence brightness is required.

CLSM is widely-used in numerous biological science disciplines, from cell biology and genetics to microbiology and developmental biology.

Clinically, CLSM is used in the evaluation of various eye diseases, and is particularly useful for imaging, qualitative analysis, and quantification of endothelial cells of the cornea. It is used for localising and identifying the presence of filamentary fungal elements in the corneal stroma in cases of keratomycosis, enabling rapid diagnosis and thereby early institution of definitive therapy. Research into CLSM techniques for endoscopic procedures is also showing promise. In the pharmaceutical industry, it was recommended to follow the manufacturing process of thin film pharmaceutical forms, to control the quality and uniformity of the drug distribution. CLSM is also used as the data retrieval mechanism in some 3D optical data storage systems and has helped determine the age of the Magdalen papyrus.

Two-photon excitation microscopy

Two-photon excitation microscopy is a fluorescence imaging technique that allows imaging living tissue up to a depth of one millimeter. The two-photon excitation microscope is a special variant of the multiphoton fluorescence microscope. Two-photon excitation can be a superior alternative to confocal microscopy due to its deeper tissue penetration, efficient light detection and reduced phototoxicity (Fig. 6.17).

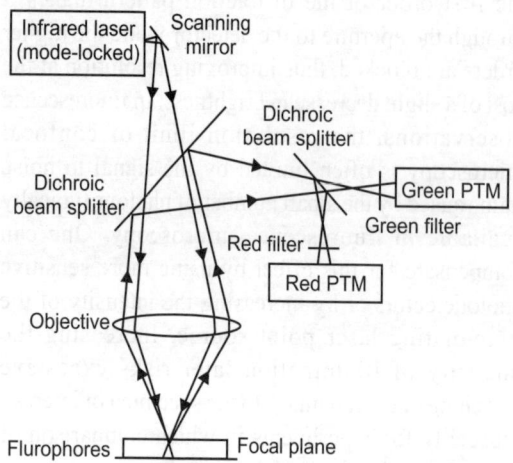

Fig. 6.17. A diagram of a two-photon microscope.

Two-photon excitation employs a concept first described by Maria Goeppert-Mayer (1906–1972) in her 1931 doctoral dissertation, and first observed in 1962 in cesium vapour using laser excitation by Isaac Abella.

The concept of two-photon excitation is based on the idea that two photons of low energy can excite a fluorophore in a quantum event, resulting in the emission of a fluorescence photon, typically at a higher energy than either of the two excitatory photons. The probability of the near-simultaneous absorption of two photons is extremely low. Therefore a high flux of excitation photons is typically required, usually a femtosecond laser.

Two-photon microscopy was pioneered by Winfried Denk in the lab of Watt W. Webb at Cornell University. He combined the idea of two-photon absorption with the use of a laser scanner. In two-photon excitation microscopy an infrared laser beam is focused through an objective lens. The Ti-sapphire laser normally used has a pulse width of approximately 100 femtoseconds and a repetition rate of about 80 MHz, allowing the high photon density and flux required for two photons absorption and is tunable across a wide range of wavelengths.

The most commonly used fluorophores have excitation spectra in the 400–500 nm range, whereas the laser used to excite the fluorophores lies in the ~700–1000 nm (infrared) range. If the fluorophore absorbs two infrared photons simultaneously, it will absorb enough energy to be raised into the excited state. The fluorophore will then emit a single photon with a wavelength that depends on the type of fluorophore used (typically in the visible spectrum). Because two photons need to be absorbed to excite a fluorophore, the probability for fluorescent emission from the fluorophores increases quadratically with the excitation intensity. Therefore, much more two-photon fluorescence is generated where the laser beam is tightly focused than where it is more diffuse. Effectively, excitation is restricted to the tiny focal volume (~1 femtoliter), resulting in a high degree of rejection of out-of-focus objects. This *localisation of excitation* is the key advantage compared to single-photon excitation microscopes, which need to employ additional elements such as pinholes to reject out-of-focus fluorescence. The fluorescence from the sample is then collected by a high-sensitivity detector, such as a photomultiplier tube. This observed light intensity becomes one pixel in the eventual image; the focal point is scanned throughout a desired region of the sample to form all the pixels of the image.

The use of infrared light to excite fluorophores in light-scattering tissue has added benefits. Longer wavelengths are scattered to a lesser degree than shorter ones, which is a benefit to high-resolution imaging. In addition, these lower-energy photons are less likely to cause damage outside the focal volume. Compared to a confocal microscope, photon detection is much more effective since even scattered photons contribute to the usable signal. There are several caveats to using two-photon microscopy. The pulsed lasers needed for two-photon excitation are much more expensive then the constant wave (CW) lasers used in confocal microscopy. The two-photon absorption spectrum of a molecule may vary significantly from its one-photon counterpart. For very thin objects such as isolated cells, single-photon (confocal) microscopes can produce images with higher optical resolution due to their shorter excitation wavelengths. In scattering tissue, on the other hand, the superior optical sectioning and light detection capabilities of the two-photon microscope result in better performance.

Image Processing

In electrical engineering and computer science, image processing is any form of signal processing for which the input is an image, such as photographs or frames of video; the output of image processing can be either an image or a set of characteristics or parameters related to the image. Most image-processing techniques involve treating the image as a two-dimensional signal and applying standard signal-processing techniques to it.

Image processing usually refers to digital image processing, but optical and analog image processing are also possible.

Among many other image processing operations are:

1. Euclidean geometry transformations such as enlargement, reduction, and rotation.
2. Colour corrections such as brightness and contrast adjustments, colour mapping, colour balancing, quantisation, or colour translation to a different colour space.
3. Digital compositing or optical compositing (combination of two or more images). Used in film-making to make a 'matte'.
4. Interpolation, demosaicing, and recovery of a full image from a raw image format using a Bayer filter pattern.
5. Image registration, the alignment of two or more images.
6. Image differencing and morphing.
7. Image recognition, for example, extract the text from the image using optical character recognition or checkbox and bubble values using optical mark recognition.
8. Image segmentation.
9. High dynamic range imaging by combining multiple images.
10. Geometric hashing for 2-D object recognition with affine invariance.

Applications: (i) computer vision, (ii) augmented reality, (iii) face detection, (iv) feature detection, (v) lane departure warning system, (vi) non-photorealistic rendering, (vii) medical image processing, (viii) microscope image processing, (ix) morphological image processing, and (x) remote sensing.

Computational photography

Computational imaging refers to any image formation method that involves a digital computer. Computational photography refers broadly to computational imaging techniques that enhance or extend the capabilities of digital photography. The output of these techniques is an ordinary photograph, but one that could not have been taken by a traditional camera.

The term was first used by Steve Mann, and possibly others, to describe their own research. Its current definition, which stems from a 2004 course at Stanford University and a 2005 symposium at MIT (see links below), has evolved to cover a number of subject areas in computer graphics, computer vision, and applied optics. These areas are given below, organised according to a taxonomy proposed by Shree Nayar. Within each area is a list of techniques, and for each technique one or two representative papers or books are cited. Deliberately omitted from the taxonomy are image processing (see also digital image processing) techniques applied to traditionally captured images in order to produce better images. Examples of such techniques are image scaling, dynamic range compression (i.e. tone mapping), colour management, image completion (a.k.a. inpainting or hole filling), image compression, digital watermarking, and artistic image effects. Also omitted are techniques that produce range data, volume data, 3D models, 4D light fields, 4D, 6D, or 8D BRDFs, or other high-dimensional image-based representations.

Computational illumination in a structured fashion, then processing the captured images, to create new images. The applications include image-based relighting, image enhancement, image deblurring, geometry/material recovery and so forth.

Cellular tomography

Cellular tomography involves examining the cellular structures in all three dimensions to generate an accurate three-dimensional map of the interior of the cell. It enables researchers to analyse molecular structures in relation to the cellular architecture, the cytoskeleton and the cell organelles. Most proteins do not function as individual entities, but in coordination or dependence with other proteins. The knowledge of the three-dimensional organisation is essential to understand protein function at the cellular level.

Cellular tomography using transmission electron microscopy (TEM) is the only available technology to chart the inside of a cell and is therefore an essential technology in the cell biologists' tool box.

Video Enhanced Differential Interference Contrast Microscopy

Video enhanced differential interference contrast microscopy (VEDICM) permits an immediate, rapid characterisation of association colloid aggregates and other colloidal aggregates by direct visualisation on a television screen. Particles with sizes down to 500 A, their dynamics, fusion and slow flocculation can be directly pictured, recorded and analysed in real time, freezeframe, slow motion or time lapse. It is precisely in the distance regime, 500–10,000 A, joining micellar chemistry to the field of biological structures, that classical techniques do have most difficulty. In this domain surfactant aggregates-vesicles, liposomes, microemulsions, microtubules-can exhibit an astonishing dynamic structural diversity and distribution of structures. These are highly sensitive to pH, salt, temperature, and surfactant concentration in ways which are partially understood at a theoretical level, but not formerly easily accessible.

Transmission Electron Microscopy

Transmission electron microscopy (TEM) is a microscopy technique whereby a beam of electrons is transmitted through an ultra thin specimen, interacting with the specimen as it passes through. An image is formed from the interaction of the electrons transmitted through the specimen; the image is magnified and focused onto an imaging device, such as a fluorescent screen, on a layer of photographic film, or to be detected by a sensor such as a CCD camera (Fig. 6.18).

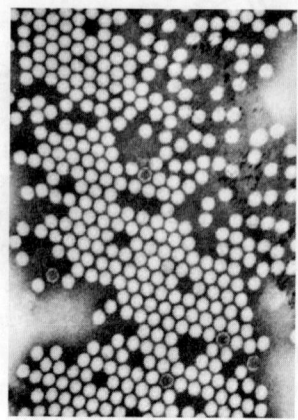

Fig. 6.18. A TEM image of the polio virus. The polio virus is 30 nm in size.

TEMs are capable of imaging at a significantly higher resolution than light microscopes, owing to the small de Broglie wavelength of electrons. This enables the instrument's user to examine fine detail — even as small as a single column of atoms, which is tens of thousands times smaller than the smallest resolvable object in a light microscope. TEM forms a major analysis method in a range of scientific fields, in both physical and biological sciences. TEMs find application in cancer research, virology, materials science as well as pollution and semiconductor research.

At smaller magnifications TEM image contrast is due to absorption of electrons in the material, due to the thickness and composition of the material. At higher magnifications complex wave interactions modulate the intensity of the image, requiring expert analysis of observed images. Alternate modes of use allow for the TEM to observe modulations in chemical identity, crystal orientation, electronic structure and sample induced electron phase shift as well as the regular absorption based imaging.

The Scanning electron microscope (SEM) is also useful in cellular analysis because of its ability to show cell surface detail at resolutions in the 3 to 10 nm range and its ability to show 3-D structure as shown in Fig. 6.19. The 3-D structure is obtained through the process of secondary emission ion scanning. As the electron beam of the scanning microscope scans the surface of an object, it can be designed to etch or wear away the outermost atomic layer. The particles are analysed with each scan of the electron beam. Thus, the outer layer is analysed on the first scan, and subsequently lower layers analysed with each additional scan. The data from each layer are then analysed and reconstructed to produce a 3-D atomic image of the object. Since electron are relatively small, the etching is sometimes enhanced by bombarding the surface with ions rather than electrons.

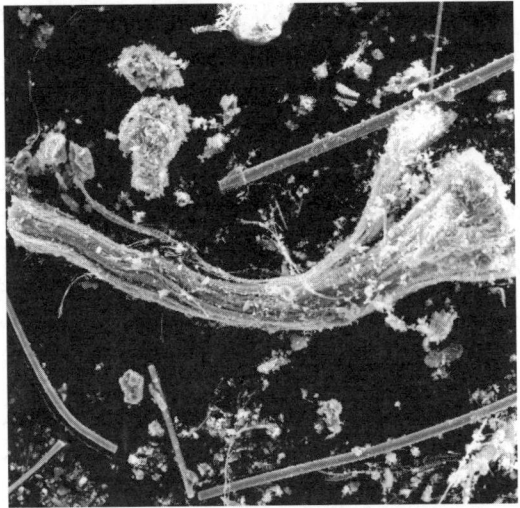

Fig. 6.19. A SEM image of stressed liver cells.

CELL ADHESION

Cellular adhesion is the binding of a cell to a surface, extracellular matrix or another cell using cell adhesion molecules such as selectins, integrins, and cadherins.

Cell adhesion molecules involved in the process are first hydrolysed by extracellular enzymes.

Eukaryotic protozoans express multiple adhesion molecules. An example of a pathogenic protozoan is the malarial parasite (*Plasmodium falciparum*), which uses one adhesion molecule called the circumsporozoite protein to bind to liver cells, and another adhesion molecule called the merozoite surface protein to bind red blood cells. In human cells, which have many

different types of adhesion molecules, the major classes are named integrins, Ig superfamily members, cadherins, and selectins. Each of these adhesion molecules has a different function and recognises different ligands. Defects in cell adhesion are usually attributable to defects in expression of adhesion molecules.

Prokaryotes have adhesion molecules usually termed 'adhesins'. Adhesins may occur on pili (fimbriae), flagellae, or the cell surface. Adhesion of bacteria is the first step in colonisation and regulates tropism (tissue- or cell-specific interactions).

Viruses also have adhesion molecules required for viral binding to host cells. For example, influenza virus has a hemagglutinin on its surface that is required for recognition of the sugar sialic acid on host cell surface molecules. HIV has an adhesion molecule termed gp120 that binds to its ligand CD4, which is expressed on lymphocytes.

Interferometry

Interferometry is the technique of diagnosing the properties of two or more waves by studying the pattern of interference created by their superposition. The instrument used to interfere the waves together is called an interferometer. Interferometry is an important investigative technique in the fields of astronomy, fibre optics, engineering metrology, optical metrology, oceanography, seismology, quantum mechanics, nuclear and particle physics, plasma physics, and remote sensing.

Interferometry makes use of the principle of superposition to combine separate waves together in a way that will cause the result of their combination to have some meaningful property that is diagnostic of the original state of the waves. This works because when two waves with the same frequency combine, the resulting pattern is determined by the phase difference between the two waves—waves that are in phase will undergo constructive interference while waves that are out of phase will undergo destructive interference. Most interferometers use light or some other form of electromagnetic wave (Fig. 6.20).

Typically a single incoming beam of light will be split into two identical beams by a grating or a partial mirror. Each of these beams will travel a different route, called a path, until they are recombined before arriving at a detector. The path difference, the difference in the distance traveled by each beam, creates a phase difference between them. It is this introduced phase difference that creates the interference pattern between the initially identical waves. If a single beam has been split along two paths then the phase difference is diagnostic of anything that changes the phase along the paths. This could be a physical change in the path length itself or a change in the refractive index along the path.

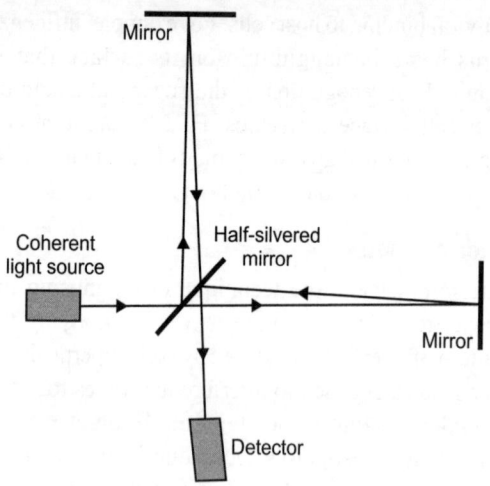

Fig. 6.20. The light path through a Michelson interferometer.

CELL MIGRATION

Cell migration is a central process in the development and maintenance of multicellular organisms. Tissue formation during embryonic development, wound healing and immune responses all require the orchestrated movement of cells in particular directions to specific locations. Errors during this process have serious consequences, including mental retardation, vascular disease, tumor formation and metastasis. An understanding of the mechanism by which cells migrate may lead to the development of novel therapeutic strategies for controlling, for example, invasive tumour cells. Cells often migrate in response to, and towards, specific external signals, a process called chemotaxis.

The migration of single mammalian cells is usually viewed in the microscope as the cells move randomly on a glass slide. As the actual movement is very slow — usually a few micrometers/minute — time-lapse films are taken so that a speeded up movie can be viewed. This shows that, although the shape of a moving cell varies considerably, its leading front has a characteristic behaviour. This region of the cell is highly active, sometimes spreading forwards quickly, sometimes retracting, sometimes ruffling or bubbling. It is generally accepted that the leading front is the main motor which pulls the cell forward.

There is still great uncertainty of how cell migration really works. However, because the locomotion of all mammalian cells (except sperm) has several common features, the underlying processes are believed to be similar. The two main constant features are: (i) the behaviour of the leading front and (ii) the observation that any debris on the dorsal surface of the cell moves backwards on the cell's surface towards its trailing end. The latter feature is most easily observed when aggregates of a surface molecule are cross-linked with a fluorescent antibody or when small beads become artificially bound to the front of the cell.

Besides mammalian cells, many other eukaryotic cells appear to move in a similar way. One of the most valuable model creatures for studying locomotion and chemotaxis is the amoeba Dictyostelium discoideum because they move more quickly than most mammalian cells grown in the lab and they chemotax towards cyclic AMP. In addition, they have a haploid genome which assists understanding the role of a particular gene product in movement.

Molecular Processes at the Front

There are two main theories for how the cell advances its front edge: the cytoskeletal model and membrane flow model. It is possible that both underlying processes contribute to cell extension.

Cytoskeletal model

Experimentally it is found that the cell's front is a site of rapid actin polymerisation: soluble actin monomers polymerise there to form filaments. This has led to the view that it is the formation of these actin filaments which pushes the leading front forward and is the main motile force for advancing the cell's front. In addition, cytoskeletal elements are able to interact extensively and intimately with a cell's plasma membrane (Fig. 6.21a).

Membrane flow model

Studies have also shown that the front is the site at which membrane is returned to the cell surface from internal membrane pools at the end of the endocytic cycle. This has led to the view that extension of the leading edge occurs primarily by addition of membrane at the front of the cell. If so, the actin filaments which form at the front might stabilise the added membrane so that a structured extension, or lamella, is formed rather than the cell blowing bubbles (or 'blebs') at its front. For a cell to move, it is necessary to bring a fresh supply of feet — those molecules, called integrins, which attach a cell to the surface on which it is crawling — to the front. It is likely that these feet are endocyosed towards the rear of the cell and brought to the cell's front by exocytosis, to be reused to form new attachments to the substrate (Fig. 6.21b).

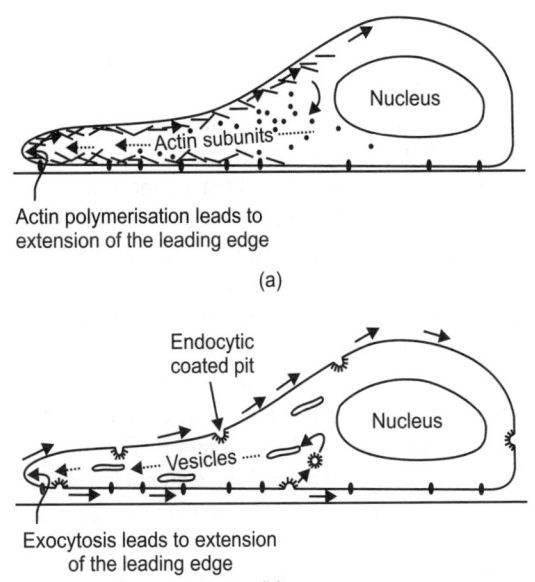

Actin polymerisation leads to extension of the leading edge

(a)

Exocytosis leads to extension of the leading edge

(b)

Fig. 6.21. Two different models for how cells move, (a) cytoskeletal model,(b) membrane flow model.

CELL UPTAKE

Cell uptake is the study of the various types and amounts of biological molecules in the cell. Cell capacitance has been used as an index of secretion in cells. The capacitance of the cell membrane can be measured using techniques similar to the voltage clamp. Fluorescent microscopy is commonly used since fluorescent probes are now available to measure pH, sodium, magnesium, potassium, calcium, and chloride ions.

Nanovid Microscopy

Nanovid microscopy, from 'nanometer video-enhanced microscopy', is a microscopic technique aimed at visualising colloidal gold particles of 20–40 nm diameter (nanogold, immunogold) as dynamic markers at the light microscopic level. The nanogold particles as such are smaller than the diffraction limit of light, but can be visualised by using Video-enhanced differential interference contrast (VEDIC). The technique is based on the use of contrast enhancement by video techniques and digital image processing. Nanovid microscopy, by combining small colloidal gold probes with Video-enhanced quantitative microscopy, allows for studying the intracellular dynamics of specific proteins in living cells.

Electroporation

Electroporation, or electropermeabilisation, is a significant increase in the electrical conductivity and permeability of the cell plasma membrane caused by an externally applied electrical field. It is usually used in molecular biology as a way of introducing some substance into a cell, such as loading it with a molecular probe, a drug that can change the cell's function, or a piece of coding DNA (Fig. 6.22).

Electroporation is a dynamic phenomenon that depends on the local transmembrane voltage at each cell membrane point. It is generally accepted that for a given pulse duration and shape, a specific transmembrane voltage threshold exists for the manifestation of the electroporation phenomenon (from 0.5 V to 1 V). This leads to the definition of an electric field magnitude threshold for electroporation

(E_{th}). That is, only the cells within areas where $E \geq E_{th}$ are electroporated. If a second threshold (E_{ir}) is reached or surpassed, electroporation will compromise the viability of the cells, i.e. irreversible electroporation.

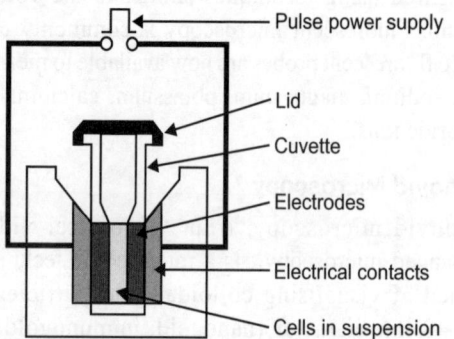

Fig. 6.22. Diagram of the major components of an electroporator with cuvette loaded.

In molecular biology, the process of electroporation is often used for the transformation of bacteria, yeast, and plant protoplasts. In addition to the lipid membranes, bacteria also have cell walls which are different from the lipid membranes and are made of peptidoglycan and its derivatives. However, the walls are naturally porous and only act as stiff shells that protect bacteria from severe environmental impacts. If bacteria and plasmids are mixed together, the plasmids can be transferred into the cell after electroporation. Several hundred volts across a distance of several millimeters are typically used in this process. Afterwards, the cells have to be handled carefully until they have had a chance to divide producing new cells that contain reproduced plasmids. This process is approximately ten times as effective as chemical transformation.

This procedure is also highly efficient for the introduction of foreign genes in tissue culture cells, especially mammalian cells. For example, it is used in the process of producing knockout mice, as well as in tumor treatment, gene therapy, and cell-based therapy. The process of introducing foreign DNAs into eukaryotic cells is known as transfection.

Electroporation is done with electroporators, appliances which create an electro-magnetic field in the cell solution. The cell suspension is pipetted into a glass or plastic cuvette which has two aluminum electrodes on its sides Fig. 6.23.

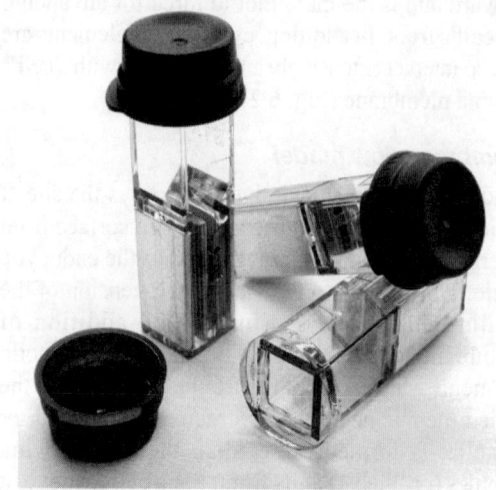

Fig. 6.23. Cuvettes for electroporation. These are plastic with aluminium electrodes and a black lid. They hold a maximum of 400 µl.

For bacterial electroporation, typically a suspension of around 50 microliters is used. Prior to electroporation it is mixed with the plasmid to be transformed. The mixture is pipetted into the cuvette, the voltage and capacitance is set and the cuvette inserted into the electroporator. Immediately after electroporation, one milliliter of liquid medium is added to the bacteria (in the cuvette or in an eppendorf tube), and the tube is incubated at the bacteria's optimal temperature for an hour or more to allow recovery of the cells and expression of antibiotic resistance, followed by spreading on agar plates.

The success of the elecroporation depends greatly on the purity of the plasmid solution, especially on its salt content. Solutions with high salt concentrations might cause an electrical discharge (known as arcing), which often reduces the viability of the bacteria.

For a further detailed investigation of the process more attention should be paid to the output impedance of the porator device and the input impedance of the cells suspension (e.g. salt content). As the process needs direct electrical contact between the electrodes and the suspension, and is inoperable with isolated electrodes, obviously the process involves certain electrolytic effects, due to small currents and not only fields.

Benchtop electroporators are generally used as common lab equipments, residing atop a central bench or hood. They offer the advantage of electroporating multiple samples at the same time. They can also be set to different operating parameters depending on whether the cell has a cell-wall or not. Unlike them, the handheld electroporators are cordless, rechargeable and use disposable pipectrodes, which combine elements of both cuvettes and pipettes. It's operating parameters are pre-set to the optimal parameters for transforming either bacteria or mammalian cells.

Both types of electoporators have been used on a wide range of cells-including *E. coli* (for transformation) and mammalian cells such as neurons, astrocytes, neuroglia, lymphocytes, monocytes, fibroblasts, epithelial and endothelial cells from humans, mice, rats and monkeys (for transfection).

A higher voltage of electroporation was found in pigs to irreversibly destroy target cells within a narrow range while leaving neighboring cells unnaffected, and thus represents a promising new treatment for cancer, heart disease and other disease states that require removal of tissue.

Electroporation can also be used to help deliver drugs or genes into the cell by applying of short and intense electric pulses that transiently permeabilise cell membrane, thus allowing transport of molecules otherwise not transported through a cellular membrane. This proceedure is referred to as electrochemotherapy when the molecules to be transported is a chemotherapeutic agent or 'gene electrotransfer' when the molecule to be transported is DNA.

SECRETION

Secretion is the process of elaborating, releasing, and oozing chemicals from a cell, a secreted chemical substance or amount of substance. In contrast to excretion, the substance may have a certain function, rather than being a waste product.

Secretion in bacterial species means the transport or translocation of effector molecules for example proteins, enzymes or toxins (such as cholera toxin in pathogenic bacteria for example *Vibrio cholerae*) from across the interior (cytoplasm or cytosol) of a bacterial cell to its exterior. Secretion is a very important mechanism in bacterial functioning and operation in their natural surrounding environment for adaptation and survival.

Eukaryotic cells, including human cells, have a highly evolved process of secretion. Proteins targeted for the outside are synthesised by ribosomes docked to the rough endoplasmic reticulum (ER). As they are synthesised, these proteins translocate into the ER lumen, where they are glycosylated and where molecular chaperones aid protein folding. Misfolded proteins are usually identified here and retrotranslocated by ER-associated degradation to the cytosol, where they are degraded by a proteasome. The vesicles containing the properly-folded proteins then enter the Golgi apparatus.

In the Golgi apparatus, the glycosylation of the proteins is modified and further posttranslational modifications, including cleavage and functionalisation, may occur. The proteins are then moved into secretory vesicles which travel along the cytoskeleton to the edge of the cell. More modification can occur in the secretory vesicles (for example insulin is cleaved from proinsulin in the secretory vesicles).

Eventually, there is vesicle fusion with the cell membrane at a structure called the porosome, in a process called exocytosis, dumping its contents out of the cell's environment.

Strict biochemical control is maintained over this sequence by usage of a pH gradient: the pH of the cytosol is 7.4, the ER's pH is 7.0, and the *cis*-golgi has a pH of 6.5. Secretory vesicles have pHs ranging between 5.0 and 6.0; some secretory vesicles evolve into lysosomes, which have a pH of 4.8.

Nonclassical Secretion

There are many proteins like FGF1 (aFGF), FGF2 (bFGF), interleukin1 (IL1) etc. which do not have a signal sequence. They do not use the classical ER-golgi pathway. These are secreted through various nonclassical pathways.

Secretion in Human Tissues

Many human cell types have the ability to be secretory cells. They have a well developed endoplasmic reticulum and Golgi apparatus to fulfill their function. Tissues in humans that produce secretions include the gastrointestinal tract which secretes digestive enzymes and gastric acid, and the lung which secretes surfactants.

Secretion is not unique to eukaryotes alone, it is present in bacteria and archaea as well. ATP binding cassette (ABC) type transporters are common to all the three domains of life. The Sec system is also another conserved secretion system which is homologous to the translocon in the eukaryotic endoplasmic reticulum consisting of Sec 61 translocon complex in yeast and Sec Y-E-G complex in bacteria. Secretion via the Sec pathway generally requires the presence of an N-terminal signal peptide on the secreted protein. Gram negative bacteria have two membranes, thus making secretion topologically more complex.

Atomic Force Microscope

The atomic force microscope (AFM) or scanning force microscope (SFM) is a very high-resolution type of scanning probe microscopy, with demonstrated resolution of fractions of a nanometer, more than 1000 times better than the optical diffraction limit. The AFM is one of the foremost tools for imaging, measuring, and manipulating matter at the nanoscale. The information is gathered by 'feeling' the surface with a mechanical probe. Piezoelectric elements that facilitate tiny but accurate and precise movements on (electronic) command enable the very precise scanning (Fig. 6.24).

The AFM consists of a cantilever with a sharp tip (probe) at its end that is used to scan the specimen surface. The cantilever is typically silicon or silicon nitride with a tip radius of curvature on the order of nanometers. When the tip is brought into proximity of a sample surface, forces between the tip and the sample lead to a deflection of the cantilever according to Hooke's law. Depending on the situation, forces that are measured in AFM include mechanical contact force, van der Waals forces, capillary forces, chemical bonding, electrostatic forces, magnetic forces, Casimir forces, solvation forces, etc. As well as force, additional quantities may simultaneously be measured

through the use of specialised types of probe. Typically, the deflection is measured using a laser spot reflected from the top surface of the cantilever into an array of photodiodes. Other methods that are used include optical interferometry, capacitive sensing or piezoresistive AFM cantilevers. These cantilevers are fabricated with piezoresistive elements that act as a strain gauge. Using a Wheatstone bridge, strain in the AFM cantilever due to deflection can be measured, but this method is not as sensitive as laser deflection or interferometry.

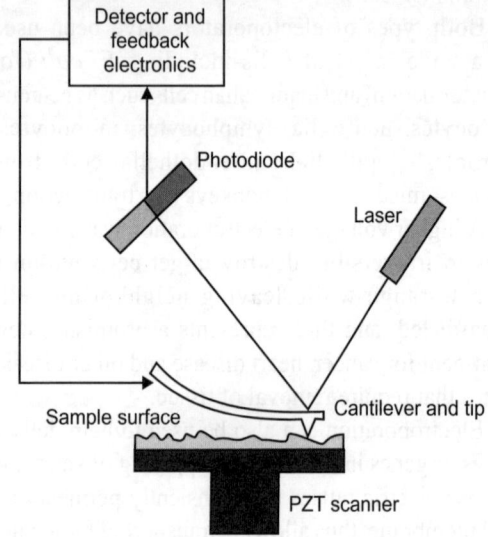

Fig. 6.24. Block diagram of atomic force microscope.

If the tip was scanned at a constant height, a risk would exist that the tip collides with the surface, causing damage. Hence, in most cases a feedback mechanism is employed to adjust the tip-to-sample distance to maintain a constant force between the tip and the sample. Traditionally, the sample is mounted on a piezoelectric tube, that can move the sample in the z direction for maintaining a constant force, and the x and y directions for scanning the sample. Alternatively a 'tripod' configuration of three piezo crystals may be employed, with each responsible for scanning in the x, y and z directions. This eliminates some of the distortion effects seen with a tube scanner. In newer designs, the tip is mounted on a vertical piezo scanner while the sample is being scanned in

X and Y using another piezo block. The resulting map of the area $s = f(x, y)$ represents the topography of the sample. The AFM can be operated in a number of modes, depending on the application. In general, possible imaging modes are divided into static (also called contact) modes and a variety of dynamic (or non-contact) modes where the cantilever is vibrated.

Imaging modes

The primary modes of operation are static (contact) mode and dynamic mode. In the static mode operation, the static tip deflection is used as a feedback signal. Because the measurement of a static signal is prone to noise and drift, low stiffness cantilevers are used to boost the deflection signal. However, close to the surface of the sample, attractive forces can be quite strong, causing the tip to 'snap-in' to the surface. Thus static mode AFM is almost always done in contact where the overall force is repulsive. Consequently, this technique is typically called 'contact mode'. In contact mode, the force between the tip and the surface is kept constant during scanning by maintaining a constant deflection.

In the dynamic mode, the cantilever is externally oscillated at or close to its fundamental resonance frequency or a harmonic. The oscillation amplitude, phase and resonance frequency are modified by tip-sample interaction forces; these changes in oscillation with respect to the external reference oscillation provide information about the sample's characteristics. Schemes for dynamic mode operation include frequency modulation and the more common amplitude modulation. In frequency modulation, changes in the oscillation frequency provide information about tip-sample interactions. Frequency can be measured with very high sensitivity and thus the frequency modulation mode allows for the use of very stiff cantilevers. Stiff cantilevers provide stability very close to the surface and, as a result, this technique was the first AFM technique to provide true atomic resolution in ultra-high vacuum conditions.

Fluorescence Lifetime Imaging Microscopy

Fluorescence lifetime imaging microscopy or FLIM is a powerful tool for producing an image based on the differences in the exponential decay rate of the fluorescence from a fluorescent sample. It can be used as an imaging technique in confocal microscopy, Two-photon excitation microscopy, and multiphoton tomography.

The lifetime of the fluorophore signal, rather than its intensity, is used to create the image in FLIM. This has the advantage of minimising the effect of photon scattering in thick layers of sample.

A fluorophore which is excited by a photon will drop to the ground state with a certain probability based on the decay rates through a number of different (radiative and/or nonradiative) decay pathways. To observe fluorescence, one of these pathways must be by spontaneous emission of a photon. In the ensemble description, the fluorescence emitted will decay with time according to

$$F(t) = F_0 e^{-t/\tau}$$

where,

$$\frac{1}{\tau} = \sum_f wfik_j.$$

In the above, t is time, τ is the fluorescence lifetime, F_0 is the initial fluorescence at $t = 0$, and k_i are the rates for each decay pathway, at least one of which must be the fluorescence decay rate k_f. More importantly, the lifetime, τ, is independent of the initial intensity of the emitted light. This can be utilised for making non-intensity based measurements in chemical sensing.

Measurement and processing

Fluorescence lifetime imaging yields images with the intensity of each pixel determined by τ, which allows one to view contrast between materials with different fluorescence decay rates (even if those materials fluoresce at the exact same wavelength), and also produces images which show changes in other decay pathways, such as in FRET imaging.

Pulsed illumination

Fluorescence lifetimes can be determined in the time domain by using a pulsed source. Time-correlated single photon counting (TCSPC) is usually employed because variations in source intensity and photoelectron amplitudes are ignored, the time resolution can be upwards of 4 ps, and the data obeys Poisson statistics (useful in determining goodness of fit during reconvolution).

When a population of fluorophores is excited by an ultrashort or delta pulse of light, the time-resolved fluorescence will decay exponentially as described above. However, if the excitation pulse or detection response is wide, the measured fluorescence, $M(t)$, will not be purely exponential. The instrumental response function, $IRF(t)$ will be convolved or blended with the decay function, $F(t)$.

$$M(t) = IRF(t) \otimes F(t)$$

The decay function (and corresponding lifetimes) cannot be recovered by direct deconvolution using Fourier transforms because division by zero will produce errors and noise will be amplified. However, the instrumental response of the source, detector, and electronics can be measured, usually from scattered excitation light. The IRF can then be convolved with a trial decay function to produce a calculated fluorescence, which can be compared to the measured fluorescence. The parameters for the trial decay function can be varied until the calculated and measured fluorescence curves fit well. This process is known as reconvolution or reiterative convolution, and can be performed quickly by several software packages.

Phase modulation

Alternatively, fluorescence lifetimes can be determined in the frequency domain by a phase-modulated method. The intensity of a continuous wave source is modulated at high frequency, by an acousto-optic modulator for example, which will modulate the fluorescence. Since the excited state has a lifetime, the fluorescence will be delayed with respect to the excitation signal, and the lifetime can be determined from the phase shift. Also, y-components to the excitation and fluorescence sine waves will be modulated, and lifetime can be determined from the modulation ratio of these y-components. Hence, 2 values for the lifetime can be determined from the phase-modulation method.

FLIM has primarily been used in biology as a method to detect photosensitisers in cells and tumors as well as FRET in instances where ratiometric imaging is difficult. In cell culture, it has been used

to study EGF receptor signaling and ErbB1 receptor trafficking. FLIM imaging is particularly useful in neurons, where light scattering by brain tissue is problematic for ratiometric imaging.

Fluorescence Recovery After Photobleaching

Fluorescence recovery after photobleaching (FRAP) denotes an optical technique capable of quantifying the two dimensional lateral diffusion of a molecularly thin film containing fluorescently labelled probes, or to examine single cells. This technique is very useful in biological studies of cell membrane diffusion and protein binding. In addition, surface deposition of a fluorescing phospholipid bilayer (or monolayer) allows the characterisation of hydrophilic (or hydrophobic) surfaces in terms of surface structure and free energy. Similar, though less well known, techniques have been developed to investigate the 3-dimensional diffusion and binding of molecules inside the cell; they are also referred to as FRAP (Fig. 6.25).

Experimental setup

The basic apparatus comprises an optical microscope, a light source and some fluorescent probe. Fluorescent emission is contingent upon absorption of a specific optical wavelength or colour which restricts the choice of lamps. Most commonly, a broad spectrum mercury or xenon source is used in conjunction with a colour filter. The technique begins by saving a background image of the sample before photobleaching. Next, the light source is focused onto a small patch of the viewable area either by switching to a higher magnification microscope objective or with laser light of the appropriate wavelength. The fluorophores in this region receive high intensity illumination which causes their fluorescence lifetime to quickly elapse (limited to roughly 10^5 photons before extinction). Now the image in the microscope is that of a uniformly fluorescent field with a noticeable dark spot. As Brownian motion proceeds, the still-fluorescing probes will diffuse throughout the sample and replace the non-fluorescent probes in the bleached region. This diffusion proceeds in an ordered fashion, analytically determinable from the diffusion equation. Assuming a Gaussian profile for the bleaching beam, the diffusion constant D can be simply calculated from:

$$D = \frac{w^2}{4t_{1/2}}$$

where w is the width of the beam and $t_{1/2}$ is the time required for the bleach spot to recover half of its initial integrated intensity.

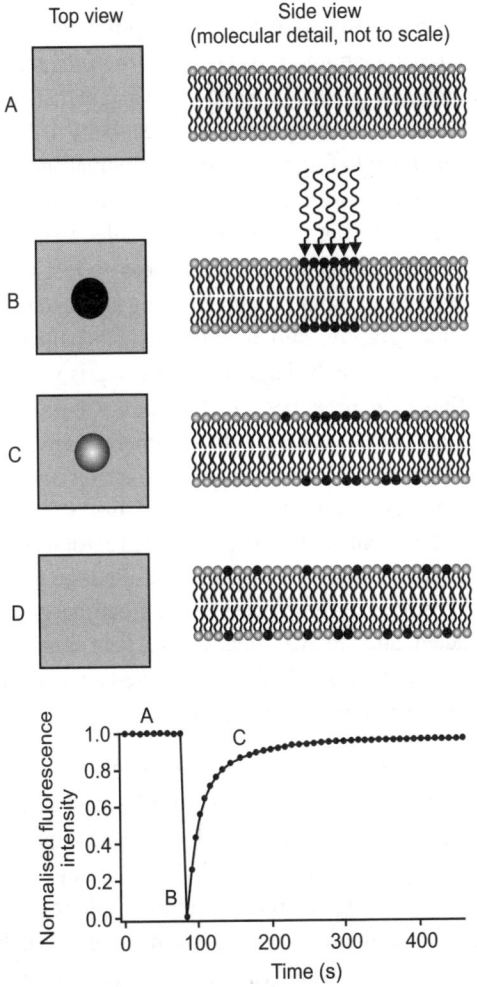

Fig. 6.25. Principle of FRAP (A) The bilayer is uniformly labelled with a fluorescent tag (B) This label is selectively photobleached by a small (~30 micrometre) fast light pulse (C) The intensity within this bleached area is monitored as the bleached dye diffuses out and new dye diffuses in (D) Eventually uniform intensity is restored.

Applications

Supported lipid bilayers

Originally, the FRAP technique was intended for use as a mean to characterise the mobility of individual lipid molecules within a cell membrane. While providing great utility in this role, current research leans more toward investigation of artificial lipid membranes. Supported by hydrophilic or hydrophobic substrates (to produce lipid bilayers or monolayers respectively) and incorporating membrane proteins, these biomimetic structures are potentially useful as analytical devices for determining the identity of unknown substances, understanding cellular transduction, and identifying ligand binding sites.

Protein binding

This technique is commonly used in conjunction with green fluorescent protein (GFP) fusion proteins, where the studied protein is fused to a GFP. When excited by a specific wavelength of light, the protein will fluoresce. When the protein that is being studied is produced with the GFP, then the fluorescence can be tracked. Photodestroying the GFP, and then watching the repopulation into the bleached area can reveal information about protein interaction partners, organelle continuity and protein trafficking.

If after some time the fluorescence doesn't reach the initial level anymore, then some part of the fluorescence is caused by an immobile fraction (that cannot be replenished by diffusion). Similarly, if the fluorescent proteins bind to static cell receptors, the rate of recovery will be retarded by a factor related to the association and disassociation coefficients of binding. This observation has most recently been exploited to investigate protein binding.

FRAP can also be used to monitor proteins outside the membrane. After the protein of interest is made fluorescent, generally by expression as a GFP fusion protein, a confocal microscope is used to photobleach and monitor a region of the cytoplasm, mitotic spindle, nucleus, or another cellular structure. The mean fluorescence in the region can then be plotted versus time since the photobleaching, and the resulting curve can yield kinetic coefficients for the protein's binding reactions and/or the protein's diffusion coefficient in the medium where it is being monitored. The analysis is most simple when the curve is dominated by only the diffusional or only the binding components.

CELLULAR DIFFERENTIATION

In developmental biology, cellular differentiation is the process by which a less specialised cell becomes a more specialised cell type. Differentiation occurs numerous times during the development of a multicellular organism as the organism changes from a single zygote to a complex system of tissues and cell types. Differentiation is a common process in adults as well: adult stem cells divide and create fully-differentiated daughter cells during tissue repair and during normal cell turnover. Differentiation dramatically changes a cell's size, shape, membrane potential, metabolic activity, and responsiveness to signals. These changes are largely due to highly-controlled modifications in gene expression. With a few exceptions, cellular differentiation almost never involves a change in the DNA sequence itself. Thus, different cells can have very different physical characteristics despite having the same genome (Fig. 6.26).

A cell that is able to differentiate into many cell types is known as *pluripotent*. Such cells are called stem cells in animals and meristematic cells in higher plants. A cell that is able to differentiate into all cell types is known as *totipotent*. In mammals, only the zygote and early embryonic cells are totipotent, while in plants many differentiated cells can become totipotent with simple laboratory techniques. In cytopathology, the level of cellular differentiation is used as a measure of cancer progression. 'Grade' is a marker of how differentiated a cell in a tumor is.

Fluorescent *in situ* Hybridisation

FISH (fluorescence *in situ* hybridisation) is a cytogenetic technique used to detect and localise the presence or absence of specific DNA sequences on chromosomes. FISH uses fluorescent probes that bind to only those parts of the chromosome with which they show a high degree of sequence similarity.

Fluorescence microscopy can be used to find out where the fluorescent probe bound to the chromosomes. FISH is often used for finding specific features in DNA for use in genetic counseling, medicine, and species identification. FISH can also be used to detect and localise specific mRNAs within tissue samples. In this context, it can help define the spatial-temporal patterns of gene expression within cells and tissues.

Probes are often derived from fragments of DNA that were isolated, purified, and amplified for use in the Human Genome Project. The size of the human genome is so large, compared to the length that could be sequenced directly, that it was necessary to divide the genome into fragments. (In the eventual analysis, these fragments were put into order by digesting a copy of each fragment into still smaller fragments using sequence-specific endonucleases, measuring the size of each small fragment using size-exclusion chromatography, and using that information to determine where the large fragments overlapped one another.) To preserve the fragments with their individual DNA sequences, the fragments were added into a system of continually replicating bacteria populations. Clonal populations of bacteria, each population maintaining a single artificial chromosome, are stored in various laboratories around the world. The artificial chromosomes (BAC) can be grown, extracted, and labelled, in any lab. These fragments are on the order of 100 thousand base-pairs, and are the basis for most FISH probes.

Preparation and hybridisation process

First, a probe is constructed. The probe must be large enough to hybridise specifically with its target but not so large as to impede the hybridisation process. The probe is tagged directly with fluorophores, with targets for antibodies or with biotin. Tagging can be done in various ways, such as nick translation, or PCR using tagged nucleotides.

Then, an interphase or metaphase chromosome preparation is produced. The chromosomes are firmly attached to a substrate, usually glass. Repetitive DNA sequences must be blocked by adding short fragments

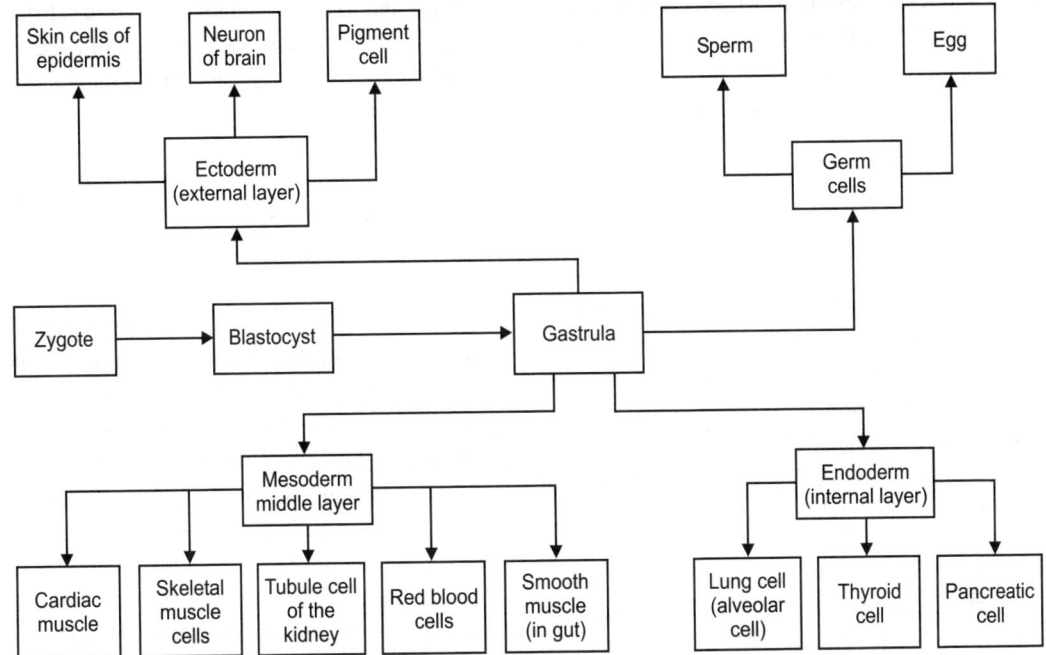

Fig. 6.26. In the centre of the diagram the early steps in the development of a mammal. On the top and bottom are some of the fully-differentiated cell types that will eventually form in the adult.

of DNA to the sample. The probe is then applied to the chromosome DNA and incubated for approximately 12 hours while hybridising. Several wash steps remove all unhybridised or partially-hybridised probes. The results are then visualised and quantified using a microscope that is capable of exciting the dye and recording images.

If the fluorescent signal is weak, amplification of the signal may be necessary in order to exceed the detection threshold of the microscope. Fluorescent signal strength depends on many factors such as probe labelling efficiency, the type of probe, and the type of dye. Fluorescently-tagged antibodies or streptavidin are bound to the dye molecule. These secondary components are selected so that they have a strong signal. FISH experiments designed to detect or localise gene expression within cells and tissues rely on the use of a reporter gene, such as one expressing green fluorescent protein, to provide the fluorescence signal.

Fibre FISH

In an alternative technique to interphase or metaphase preparations, fibre FISH, interphase chromosomes are attached to a slide in such a way that they are stretched out in a straight line, rather than being tightly coiled, as in conventional FISH, or adopting a random conformation, as in interphase FISH. This is accomplished by applying mechanical shear along the length of the slide, either to cells that have been fixed to the slide and then lysed, or to a solution of purified DNA. A technique known as chromosome combing is increasingly used for this purpose. The extended conformation of the chromosomes allows dramatically higher resolution-even down to a few kilobases. The preparation of fibre FISH samples, although conceptually simple, is a rather skilled art, and only specialised laboratories use the technique routinely.

Variations on probes and analysis

FISH is a very general technique. The differences between the various FISH techniques are usually due to variations in the sequence and labelling of the probes; and how they are used in combination. These few modifications make possible all FISH techniques.

Probe size is important because longer probes hybridise more specifically than shorter probes. The overlap defines the resolution of detectable features. For example, if the goal of an experiment is to detect the breakpoint of a translocation, then the overlap of the probes — the degree to which one DNA sequence is contained in the adjacent probes — defines the minimum window in which the breakpoint may be detected.

The mixture of probe sequences determines the type of feature the probe can detect. Probes that hybridise along an entire chromosome are used to count the number of a certain chromosome, show translocations, or identify extra-chromosomal fragments of chromatin. This is often called 'whole-chromosome painting.' If every possible probe is used, every chromosome, (the whole genome) would be marked fluorescently, which would not be particularly useful for determining features of individual sequences. However, a mixture of smaller probes can be created that is specific to a particular region (locus) of DNA; these mixtures are used to detect deletion mutations. When combined with a specific colour, a locus-specific probe mixture is used to detect very specific translocations. Special locus-specific probe mixtures are often used to count chromosomes, by binding to the centromeric regions of chromosomes, which are unique enough to identify each chromosome.

Radioactive tracer

A radioactive tracer, also called a radioactive label, is a substance containing a radioisotope (which is an isotope that has an unstable nucleus and that stabilises itself by spontaneously emitting energy and particles). Tracers can be used to measure the speed of chemical processes and to track the movement of a substance through a natural system such as a cell or a tissue.

Radioactive tracers are substances that contain a radioactive atom to allow easier detection and measurement. (Radioactivity is the property possessed by some elements of spontaneously emitting energy in the form of particles or waves by disintegration of their atomic nuclei.) For example, it is possible to make a molecule of water in which one of the two hydrogen atoms is a radioactive tritium (hydrogen-3) atom. This molecule behaves in almost the same way as a normal molecule of water. The main difference between the tracer molecule containing tritium and the normal molecule is that the tracer molecule continually gives off radiation that can be detected with a Geiger counter or some other type of radiation detection instrument.

One application for the tracer molecule described above would be to monitor plant growth by watering plants with it. The plants would take up the water and use it in leaves, roots, stems, flowers, and other parts in the same way it does with normal water. In this case, however, it would be possible to find out how fast the water moves into any one part of the plant. One would simply pass a Geiger counter over the plant at regular intervals and see where the water has gone.

In medicine tracers are applied, such as Technetium-99 in autoradiography and nuclear medicine, including single photon emission computed tomography (SPECT), positron emission tomography (PET) and scintigraphy. It has a basic isotope requirement during its isotopic reactions.

7

Nervous System

INTRODUCTION

The nervous system is an organ system containing a network of specialised cells called neurons that coordinate the actions of an animal and transmit signals between different parts of its body. In most animals the nervous system consists of two parts, central and peripheral. The central nervous system contains the brain and spinal cord. The peripheral nervous system consists of sensory neurons, clusters of neurons called ganglia, and nerves connecting them to each other and to the central nervous system. These regions are all interconnected by means of complex neural pathways. The enteric nervous system, a subsystem of the peripheral nervous system, has the capacity, even when severed from the rest of the nervous system through its primary connection by the vagus nerve, to function independently in controlling the gastrointestinal system.

CELL POTENTIAL

The nervous system is comprised of neuron cells, the conducting elements of the nervous system responsible for transferring information across the body. Only these and muscle cells are able to generate potentials, and therefore are called excitable cells. Neurons contain special ion channels that allow the cell to change its membrane potential in response to stimuli the cell receives.

Resting Potential

Relatively static membrane potential of quiescent cells is called resting membrane potential (or resting voltage), as opposed to the specific dynamic electro-

chemical phenomenona called action potential and graded membrane potential.

Apart from the latter two, which occur in excitable cells (neurons, muscles, and some secretory cells in glands), membrane voltage in the majority of not-excitable cells can also undergo changes in response to environmental or intracellular stimuli. In principle, there is no difference between resting membrane potential and dynamic voltage changes like action potential from biophysical point of view: all these phenomena are caused by specific changes in membrane permeabilities for potassium, sodium, calcium, and chloride, which in turn result from concerted changes in functional activity of various ion channels, ion transporters, and exchangers. Conventionally, resting membrane potential can be defined as a relatively stable, ground, value of transmembrane voltage in animal and plant cells.

Any voltage is a difference in electric potential between two points—for example, the separation of positive and negative electric charges on opposite sides of a resistive barrier. The typical resting membrane potential of a cell arises from the separation of potassium ions from intracellular, relatively immobile anions across the membrane of the cell. Because the membrane permeability for potassium is much higher than that for other ions (disregarding voltage-gated channels at this stage), and because of the strong chemical gradient for potassium, potassium ions flow from the cytosol into the extracellular space carrying out positive charge, until their movement is balanced by build-up of negative charge on the inner surface of the membrane. Again, because of the high relative permeability for potassium, the resulting membrane potential is almost always close to the potassium reversal potential. But in order for this process to occur, a concentration gradient of potassium ions must first be set up. This work is done by the ion pumps/transporters and/or exchangers and generally is powered by ATP.

In the case of the resting membrane potential across an animal cell's plasma membrane, potassium (and sodium) gradients are established by the Na^+/K^+-ATPase (sodium-potassium pump) which transports 2 potassium ions inside and 3 sodium ions outside at the cost of 1 ATP molecule. In other cases, for example, a membrane potential may be established by acidification of the inside of a membranous compartment (such as the proton pump that generates membrane potential across synaptic vesicle membranes).

The resting membrane potential is not an equilibrium potential as it relies on the constant expenditure of energy (for ionic pumps as mentioned above) for its maintenance. It is a dynamic diffusion potential that takes mechanism into account—wholly unlike the equilibrium potential, which is true no matter the nature of the system under consideration. The resting membrane potential is dominated by the ionic species in the system that has the greatest conductance across the membrane. For most cells this is potassium. As potassium is also the ion with the most negative equilibrium potential, usually the resting potential can be no more negative than the potassium equilibrium potential. The resting potential can be calculated with the Goldman-Hodgkin-Katz voltage equation using the concentrations of ions as for the equilibrium potential while also including the relative permeabilities, or conductances, of each ionic species. Under normal conditions, it is safe to assume that only potassium, sodium (Na^+) and chloride (Cl^-) ions play large roles for the resting potential:

$$E_m = \frac{RT}{F} \ln \left(\frac{P_{Na^+}[Na^+]_o + P_{K^+}[K^+]_o + P_{Cl^-}[Cl^-]_i}{P_{Na^+}[Na^+]_i + P_{K^+}[K^+]_i + P_{Cl^-}[Cl^-]_o} \right)$$

This equation resembles the Nernst equation, but has a term for each permeant ion. Also, z has been inserted into the equation, causing the intracellular and extracellular concentrations of Cl^- to be reversed

relative to K^+ and Na^+, as chloride's negative charge is handled by inverting the fraction inside the logarithmic term. E_m is the membrane potential, measured in volts R, T, and F are as above P_X is the relative permeability of ion X in arbitrary units (e.g. siemens for electrical conductance) $[X]_Y$ is the concentration of ion X in compartment Y as above. Another way to view the membrane potential is using the Millman equation:

$$E_m = \frac{P_{K^+} E_{eq,\,K^+} + P_{Na^+} E_{eq,\,Na^+} + P_{Cl^-} E_{eq,\,Cl^-}}{P_{K^+} + P_{Na^+} + P_{Cl^-}}$$

or reformulated

$$E_m = \frac{P_{K^+}}{P_{tot}} E_{eq,\,K^+} + \frac{P_{Na^+}}{P_{tot}} E_{eq,\,Na^+} + \frac{P_{Cl^-}}{P_{tot}} E_{eq,\,Cl^-}$$

where, P_{tot} is the combined permeability of all ionic species, again in arbitrary units. The latter equation portrays the resting membrane potential as a weighted average of the reversal potentials of the system, where the weights are the relative permeabilites across the membranes (P_X/P_{tot}). During the action potential, these weights change. If the permeabilities of Na^+ and Cl^- are zero, the membrane potential reduces to the Nernst potential for K^+ (as $P_K^+ = P_{tot}$). Normally, under resting conditions P_{Na+} and P_{Cl-} are not zero, but they are much smaller than P_{K+}, which renders E_m close to $E_{eq,K+}$. Medical conditions such as hyperkalemia in which blood serum potassium (which governs $[K^+]_o$) is changed are very dangerous since they offset $E_{eq,K+}$, thus affecting E_m. This may cause arrhythmias and cardiac arrest. The use of a bolus injection of potassium chloride in executions by lethal injection stops the heart by shifting the resting potential to a more positive value, which depolarises and contracts the cardiac cells permanently, not allowing the heart to repolarise and thus enter diastole to be refilled with blood.

Measuring resting potentials

In some cells, the membrane potential is always changing (such as cardiac pacemaker cells). For such cells there is never any rest and the resting potential is a theoretical concept. Other cells with little in the way of membrane transport functions that change with time have a resting membrane potential that can be measured by inserting an electrode into the cell. Transmembrane potentials can also be measured optically with dyes that change their optical properties according to the membrane potential.

Action Potential

An action potential (or nerve impulse) is a transient alteration of the transmembrane voltage (or membrane potential) across an excitable membrane in an excitable cell (such as a neuron or myocyte) generated by the activity of voltage-gated ion channels embedded in the membrane. The best known action potentials are pulse-like waves of voltage that travel along the axons of neurons (Fig. 7.1).

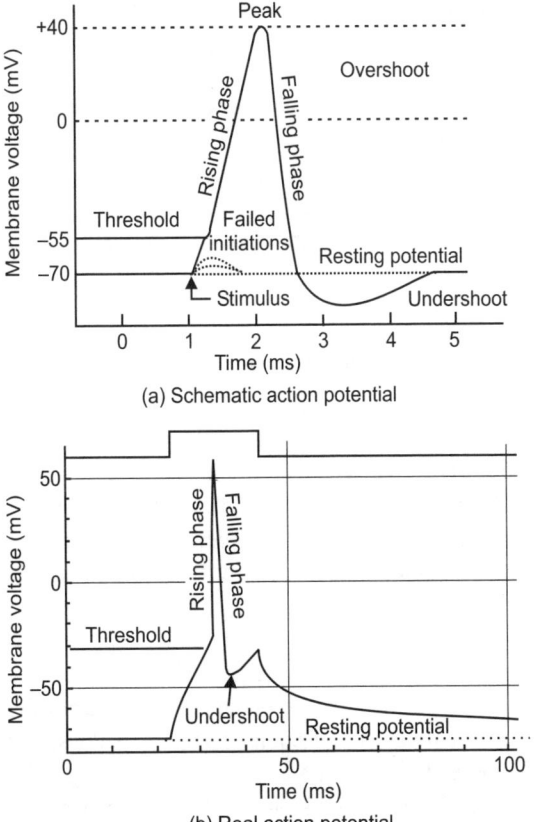

(a) Schematic action potential

(b) Real action potential

Fig. 7.1. (a) View of an idealised action potential shows its various phases as the action potential passes a point on a cell membrane. (b) Recordings of action potentials are often distorted compared to the schematic view because of variations in electrophysiological techniques used to make the recording.

A typical action potential is initiated at the axon hillock when the membrane is depolarised sufficiently (i.e. when its voltage is increased sufficiently). As the membrane potential is increased, sodium ion channels open, allowing the entry of sodium ions into the cell. This is followed by the opening of potassium ion channels that permit the exit of potassium ions from the cell. The inward flow of sodium ions increases the concentration of positively-charged cations in the cell and causes depolarisation, where the potential of the cell is higher than the cell's resting potential. The sodium channels close at the peak of the action potential, while potassium continues to leave the cell. The efflux of potassium ions decreases the membrane potential or hyperpolarises the cell. For small voltage increases from rest, the potassium current exceeds the sodium current and the voltage returns to its normal resting value, typically –70 mV. However, if the voltage increases past a critical threshold, typically 15 mV higher than the resting value, the sodium current dominates. This results in a runaway condition whereby the positive feedback from the sodium current activates even more sodium channels. Thus, the cell 'fires', producing an action potential.

Currents produced by the opening of voltage-gated channels in the course of an action potential are typically significantly larger than the initial stimulating current. Thus the amplitude, duration, and shape of the action potential are largely determined by the properties of the excitable membrane and not the amplitude or duration of the stimulus. This all-or-nothing property of action potential sets it apart from graded potentials such as receptor potentials, electrotonic potentials, and synaptic potentials, which do scale with the magnitude of the stimulus. A variety of action potential types exist in many cell types and cell compartments as determined by the types of voltage-gated channels, leak channels, channel distributions, ionic concentrations, membrane capacitance, temperature, and other factors.

The principal ions involved in an action potential are sodium and potassium cations; sodium ions enter the cell, and potassium ions leave, restoring equilibrium. Relatively few ions need to cross the membrane for the membrane voltage to change drastically. The ions exchanged during an action potential, therefore, make a negligible change in the interior and exterior ionic concentrations. The few ions that do cross are pumped out again by the continual action of the sodium–potassium pump, which, with other ion transporters, maintains the normal ratio of ion concentrations across the membrane. Calcium cations and chloride anions are involved in a few types of action potentials, such as the cardiac action potential and the action potential in the single-celled alga *Acetabularia*, respectively.

Although action potentials are generated locally on patches of excitable membrane, the resulting currents can trigger action potentials on neighbouring stretches of membrane, precipitating a domino-like propagation. In contrast to passive spread of electric potentials (electrotonic potential), action potentials are generated anew along excitable stretches of membrane and propagate without decay.

BRAIN, EEG AND EVOKED POTENTIALS

Brain

The brain is the centre of the nervous system in all vertebrate, and most invertebrate, animals. Some primitive animals such as jellyfish and starfish have a decentralised nervous system without a brain, while sponges lack any nervous system at all. In vertebrates, the brain is located in the head, protected by the skull and close to the primary sensory apparatus of vision, hearing, balance, taste, and smell.

Brains can be extremely complex. The cerebral cortex of the human brain contains roughly 15–33 billion neurons depending on gender and age, linked with up to 10,000 synaptic connections each. Each cubic millimeter of cerebral cortex contains roughly one billion synapses. These neurons communicate with one another by means of long protoplasmic fibres called axons, which carry trains of signal pulses called action potentials to distant parts of the brain or body and target them to specific recipient cells.

The brain controls the other organ systems of the body, either by activating muscles or by causing secretion of chemicals such as hormones. This centralised control allows rapid and coordinated responses to changes in the environment. Some basic types of responsiveness are possible without a brain: even single-celled organisms may be capable of extracting information from the environment and acting in response to it. Sponges, which lack a central nervous system, are capable of coordinated body contractions and even locomotion. In vertebrates, the spinal cord by itself contains neural circuitry capable of generating reflex responses as well as simple motor patterns such as swimming or walking. However, sophisticated control of behaviour on the basis of complex sensory input requires the information-integrating capabilities of a centralised brain.

Despite rapid scientific progress, much about how brains work remains a mystery. The operations of individual neurons and synapses are now understood in considerable detail, but the way they cooperate in ensembles of thousands or millions has been very difficult to decipher. Methods of observation such as EEG recording and functional brain imaging tell us that brain operations are highly organised, but these methods do not have the resolution to reveal the activity of individual neurons.

Electroencephalography

Electroencephalography (EEG) is the recording of electrical activity along the scalp produced by the firing of neurons within the brain. In clinical contexts, EEG refers to the recording of the brain's spontaneous electrical activity over a short period of time, usually 20–40 minutes, as recorded from multiple electrodes placed on the scalp. In neurology, the main diagnostic application of EEG is in the case of epilepsy, as epileptic activity can create clear abnormalities on a standard EEG study. A secondary clinical use of EEG is in the diagnosis of coma, encephalopathies, and brain death.

EEG used to be a first-line method for the diagnosis of tumours, stroke and other focal brain disorders, but this use has decreased with the advent of anatomical imaging techniques such as MRI and CT.

Derivatives of the EEG technique include evoked potentials (EP), which involves averaging the EEG activity time-locked to the presentation of a stimulus of some sort (visual, somatosensory, or auditory). Event-related potentials refer to averaged EEG responses that are time-locked to more complex processing of stimuli; this technique is used in cognitive science, cognitive psychology, and psychophysiological research.

Source of EEG activity

The electrical activity of the brain can be described in spatial scales from the currents within a single dendritic spine to the relatively gross potentials that the EEG records from the scalp, much the same way that the economics can be studied from the level of a single individual's personal finances to the macroeconomics of nations. Neurons, or nerve cells, are electrically active cells which are primarily responsible for carrying out the brain's functions. Neurons create action potentials, which are discrete electrical signals that travel down axons and cause the release of chemical neurotransmitters at the synapse, which is an area of near contact between two neurons. This neurotransmitter then activates a receptor in the dendrite or body of the neuron that is on the other side of the synapse, the postsynaptic neuron. The neurotransmitter, when combined with the receptor, typically causes an electrical current within the dendrite or body of the postsynaptic neuron. Thousands of postsynaptic currents from a single neuron's dendrites and body then sum up to cause the neuron to generate an action potential (or not). This neuron then synapses on other neurons, and so on.

EEG reflects correlated synaptic activity caused by postsynaptic potentials of cortical neurons. The ionic currents involved in the generation of fast action potentials may not contribute greatly to the averaged field potentials representing the EEG. More specifically, the scalp electrical potentials that produce EEG are generally thought to be caused by the extracellular ionic currents caused by dendritic electrical activity, whereas the fields producing magnetoencephalographic signals are associated with intracellular ionic currents.

The electric potentials generated by single neurons are far too small to be picked by EEG or MEG. EEG activity therefore always reflects the summation of the synchronous activity of thousands or millions of neurons that have similar spatial orientation, radial to the scalp. Currents that are tangential to the scalp are not picked up by the EEG. The EEG therefore benefits from the parallel, radial arrangement of apical dendrites in the cortex. Because voltage fields fall off with the fourth power of the radius, activity from deep sources is more difficult to detect than currents near the skull.

Scalp EEG activity shows oscillations at a variety of frequencies. Several of these oscillations have characteristic frequency ranges, spatial distributions and are associated with different states of brain functioning (e.g. waking and the various sleep stages). These oscillations represent synchronised activity over a network of neurons. The neuronal networks underlying some of these oscillations are understood (e.g. the thalamocortical resonance underlying sleep spindles), while many others are not (e.g. the system that generates the posterior basic rhythm). Research that measures both EEG and neuron spiking finds the relationship between the two is complex with the power of surface EEG only in two bands that of gamma and delta relating to neuron spike activity.

Clinical use

A routine clinical EEG recording typically lasts 20–30 minutes (plus preparation time) and usually involves recording from 25 scalp electrodes. Routine EEG is typically used in the following clinical circumstances:

1. To distinguish epileptic seizures from other types of spells, such as psychogenic non-epileptic seizures, syncope (fainting), subcortical movement disorders and migraine variants.
2. To differentiate 'organic' encephalopathy or delirium from primary psychiatric syndromes such as catatonia.
3. To serve as an adjunct test of brain death.
4. To prognosticate, in certain instances, in patients with coma.

5. To determine whether to wean anti-epileptic medications.

At times, a routine EEG is not sufficient, particularly when it is necessary to record a patient while he/she is having a seizure. In this case, the patient may be admitted to the hospital for days or even weeks, while EEG is constantly being recorded (along with time-synchronised video and audio recording). A recording of an actual seizure (i.e. an ictal recording, rather than an inter-ictal recording of a possibly epileptic patient at some period between seizures) can give significantly better information about whether or not a spell is an epileptic seizure and the focus in the brain from which the seizure activity emanates.

Epilepsy monitoring is typically done:

1. To distinguish epileptic seizures from other types of spells, such as psychogenic non-epileptic seizures, syncope (fainting), subcortical movement disorders and migraine variants.
2. To characterise seizures for the purposes of treatment.
3. To localise the region of brain from which a seizure originates for work-up of possible seizure surgery.

Additionally, EEG may be used to monitor certain procedures:

1. To monitor the depth of anaesthesia.
2. As an indirect indicator of cerebral perfusion in carotid endarterectomy.
3. To monitor amobarbital effect during the Wada test.

EEG can also be used in intensive care units for brain function monitoring:

1. To monitor for nonconvulsive seizures/non-convulsive status epilepticus
2. To monitor the effect of sedative/anaesthesia in patients in medically induced coma (for treatment of refractory seizures or increased intracranial pressure).
3. To monitor for secondary brain damage in conditions such as subarachnoid haemorrhage (currently a research method).

If a patient with epilepsy is being considered for respective surgery, it is often necessary to localise the focus (source) of the epileptic brain activity with a resolution greater than what is provided by scalp EEG. This is because the cerebrospinal fluid, skull and scalp smear the electrical potentials recorded by scalp EEG. In these cases, neurosurgeons typically implant strips and grids of electrodes (or penetrating depth electrodes) under the dura mater, through either a craniotomy or a burr hole. The recording of these signals is referred to as electrocorticography (ECoG), subdural EEG (sdEEG) or intracranial EEG (icEEG)—all terms for the same thing. The signal recorded from ECoG is on a different scale of activity than the brain activity recorded from scalp EEG. Low voltage, high frequency components that cannot be seen easily (or at all) in scalp EEG can be seen clearly in ECoG. Further, smaller electrodes (which cover a smaller parcel of brain surface) allow even lower voltage, faster components of brain activity to be seen. Some clinical sites record from penetrating microelectrodes. EEG, and its derivative, ERPs, are used extensively in neuroscience, cognitive science, cognitive psychology, and psychophysiological research. Many techniques used in research contexts are not standardised sufficiently to be used in the clinical context (Fig. 7.2).

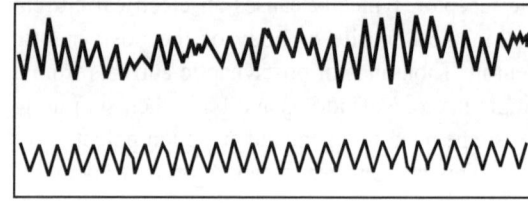

Fig. 7.2. An early EEG recording, obtained by Hans Berger in 1924. The upper tracing is EEG, and the lower is a 10 Hz timing signal.

Block Diagram Description of Electroencephalograph

The basic block diagram of an EEG machine with both analog and digital components is shown in Fig. 7.3.

Montages

A pattern of electrodes on the head and the channels they are connected to is called a montage. Montages

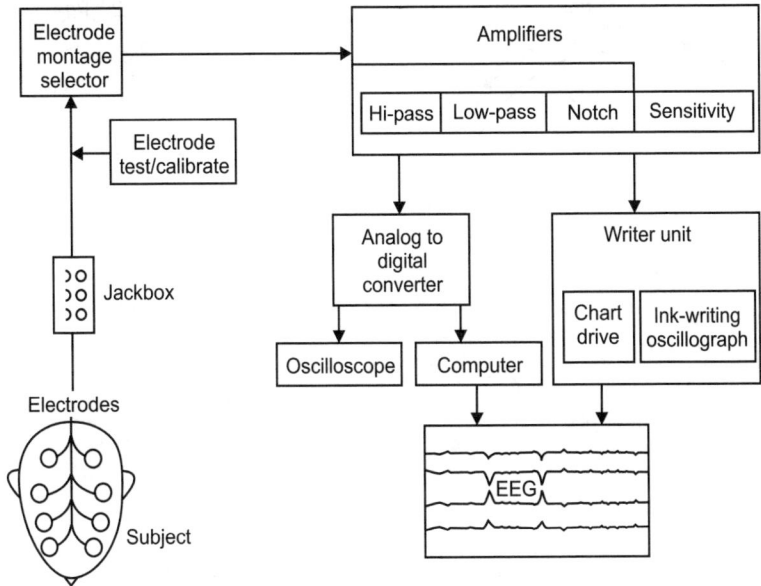

Fig. 7.3. Schematic diagram of an EEG machine.

are always symmetrical. The reference electrode is generally placed on a nonactive site such as the forehead or earlobe.

EEG electrodes are arranged on the scalp according to a standard known as the 10/20 system, adopted by the American EEG Society. Traditionally, there are 21 electrode locations in the 10/20 system. This system involves placement of electrodes at distances of 10 and 20 per cent of measured coronal, sagittal and circumferential arcs between landmarks on the cranium (Fig. 7.4). Electrodes are identified according to their position on the head; Fp for frontal-polar, F for frontal, C for central, P for parietal, T for temporal and 0 for occipital. Odd numbers refer to electrodes on the left side of the head and even numbers represent those on the right while Z denotes midline electrodes. One electrode is labelled isoground and placed at a relatively neutral site on the head, usually the midline forehead. A new montage convention has recently been introduced in which electrodes are spaced at 5 per cent distances along the cranium. These electrodes are called closely spaced electrodes and have their own naming convention (Fig. 7.5).

Electrode montage selector

EEG signals are transmitted from the electrodes to the head box, which is labelled according to the 10–20 system, and then to the montage selector. The montage selector on analog EEG machine is a large panel containing switches that allow the user to select which electrode pair will have signals subtracted from each other to create an array of channels of output called a montage. Each channel is created in the form of the input from one electrode minus the input from a second electrode.

Montages are either bipolar (made by the subtraction of signals from adjacent electrode pairs) or referential (made by subtracting the potential of a common reference electrode from each electrode on the head). In order to minimise noise, a separate reference is often chosen for each side of the head, e.g. the ipsilateral ear. Bipolar and referential montages contain the same basic information that is transformable into either format by simple substration as long as all the electrodes, including reference, are included in both montages and linked to one common reference. Many modern digital EEG machines record information referentially, allowing easy

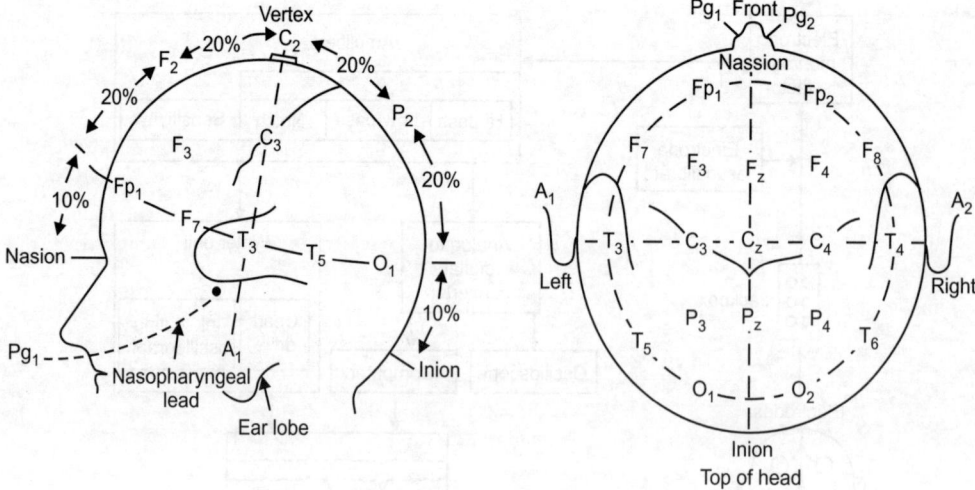

Fig. 7.4. 10–20 system of placement of electrodes.

conversion to several different bipolar montages. The advantage of recording EEG in several montages is that each montage displays different spatial characteristics of the same data.

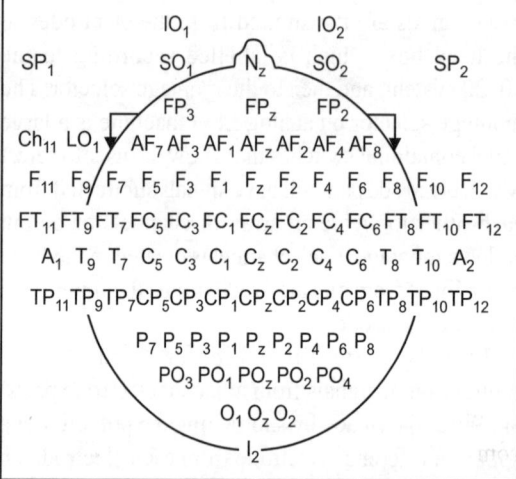

Fig. 7.5. Pictorial representation of closely spaced electrodes.

Preamplifier

Every channel has an individual, multistage, AC coupled, very sensitive amplifier with differential input and adjustable gain in a wide range. Its frequency response can be selected by single-stage passive filters. A calibrating signal is used for controlling and documenting the sensitivity of the amplifier channels. This supplies a voltage step of adequate amplitude to the input of the channels. A typical value of the calibration signal is 50 uV/cm.

The preamplifier used in electroencephalographs must have high gain and low noise characteristics because the EEG potentials are small in amplitude. In addition, the amplifier must have very high common-mode rejection to minimise stray interference signals from power lines and other electrical equipments. The amplifier must be free from drift so as to prevent the slow movement of the recording pen from its centre position as a result of changes in temperature, etc.

EEG amplifiers must have high gain in the presence of unbalanced source resistances and DC skin potentials at least up to 100 mV. Noise performance is crucial in EEG work because skin electrodes couple brain waves of only a few microvolts to the amplifier. Each individual EEG signal should be preferably amplified at the bedside. Therefore, a specially designed connector box, which can be mounted near the patient, is generally employed with EEG machines. This ensures the avoidance of cable or switching artefacts. The use of electrode amplifiers at the site also eliminates undesirable crosstalk effects of the individual electrode potentials. The connector box also carries a circuit arrangement for measuring the skin contact impedance of electrodes with AC. Thus, poor electrode-to-skin contacts above a predetermined level can be easily spotted out.

Sensitivity control

The overall sensitivity of an EEG machine is the gain of the amplifier multiplied by the sensitivity of the writer. Thus, if the writer sensitivity is 1 cm/V, the amplifier must have an overall gain of 20,000 for a 50 μV signal. The various stages are capacitor coupled. An EEG machine has two types of gain controls. One is continuously variable and it is used to equalise the sensitivities of all channels. The other control operates in steps and is meant to increase or reduce the sensitivity of a channel by known amounts. This control is usually calibrated in decibels. The gain of amplifiers is normally set so that signals of about 200 μV deflect the pens over their full linear range. Artefacts, several times greater than this, can cause excessive deflections of the pen by charging the coupling capacitors to large voltages. This will make the system unusable over a period depending upon the value of the coupling capacitors. To overcome this problem, most modern EEG machines have de-blocking circuits similar to those used in ECG machines.

Filters

Just like in an ECG when recorded by surface electrodes, an EEG may also contain muscle artefacts due to contraction of the scalp and neck muscles, which overlie the brain and skull. The artefacts are large and sharp, in contrast to the ECG, causing great difficulty in both clinical and automated EEG interpretation. The most effective way to eliminate muscle artefact is to advise the subject to relax, but it is not always successful. These artefacts are generally removed using low-pass filters. This filter on an EEG machine has several selectable positions, which are usually labelled in terms of a time constant. A typical set of time constant values for the low-frequency control are 0.03, 0.1, 0.3 and 1.0 s. These time constants correspond to 3 dB points at frequencies of 5.3, 1.6, 0.53 and 0.16 Hz.

The upper cutoff frequency can be controlled by the high frequency filter. Several values can be selected, typical of them being 15, 30, 70 and 300 Hz.

Some EEG machines have a notch filter sharply tuned at 50 Hz so as to eliminate mains frequency interference. These however have the undesirable property of 'ringing', i.e. they produce a damped oscillatory response to a square wave calibration waveform or a muscle potential. The use of notch filters should preferably be restricted to exceptional circumstances when all other methods of eliminating interference have been found to be ineffective.

The high frequency response of an EEG machine will be the resultant of the response of the amplifier and the writing part. However, the figure mentioned on the high frequency filter control of most EEG machines generally refers to the amplifier. The typical frequency range of standard EEG machines is from 0.1 Hz to 70 Hz, though newer machines allow the detection and filtering of frequencies up to several hundred Hertz. This may be of importance in some intracranial recordings.

Noise

EEG amplifiers are selected for minimum noise level, which is expressed in terms of an equivalent input voltage. Two microvolts is often stated as the acceptable figure for EEG recording. Noise contains components at all frequencies and because of this, the recorded noise increases with the bandwidth of the system. It is therefore important to restrict the bandwidth to that required for faithful reproduction of the signal. Noise level should be specified as peak-to-peak value as it is seen on the record rather than rms value, which could be misleading.

Writing part

The writing part of an EEG machine is usually of the ink type direct writing recorder. The best types of pen motors used in EEG machines have a frequency response of about 90 Hz. Most of the machines have a response lower than this, and some of them have it even as low as 45 Hz. The ink jet recording system, which gives a response up to 1000 Hz, is useful for some special applications.

Paper drive

This is provided by a synchronous motor. An accurate and stable paper drive mechanism is necessary and it is normal practice to have several paper speeds available for selection. Speeds of 15, 30 and 60 mm/s are essential. Some machines also provide speed values outside this range. A time scale is usually registered on the record by one or two time marker pens, which make a mark once per second. Timing pulses are preferably generated independently of the paper drive mechanism in order to avoid difference in timing marks due to changes in paper speed.

Channels

An electroencephalogram is recorded simultaneously from an array of many electrodes. The record can be made from bipolar or monopolar leads. The electrodes are connected to separate amplifiers and writing systems. Commercial EEG machines have up to 32 channels, although 8 or 16 channels are more common.

Microprocessors are now employed in most of the commercially available EEG machines. These machines permit customer programmable montage selection; for example, up to eight electrode combinations can be selected with a keyboard switch. In fact, any desired combination of electrodes can be selected with push buttons and can be memorised. These machines also include a video monitor screen to display the selected pattern (montage) as well as the position of scalp sites with electrode-to-skin contact. Individual channel control settings for gain and filter positions can be displayed on the video monitor for immediate review. Therefore, a setting can be changed by a simple push button operation while looking at the display.

Modern EEG machines are mostly PC based; with a pentium processor, 16-MB RAM, atleast a 2 GB hard disk, cache memory and a 4 GB DAT tape drive. The system can store up to 40 hours of EEG. The EEG is displayed on a 43 cm colour monitor with a resolution of 1280 × 1024 pixels. The user interface is through an ASCII keyboard and the output is available in the hard copy form through a laser printer.

Computerised Analysis of EEG

Assessment of the frequency and amplitude of the EEG is crucial for rapid and accurate interpretation. This involves the need for constant analysis of the EEG signal by a skilled technician and the acquisition of volumes of recording paper. Therefore, modern machines make use of computerised EEG signal processing to extract and present the frequency and amplitude information in simple, visually enhanced formats that are directly useful to the clinician.

Frequency analysis

It takes the raw EEG waves, mathematically analyses them and breaks them into their component frequencies. The most popular method of doing this is called the Fast-Fourier Transform or FFT.

Fast-Fourier Transformation of the digitised EEG waveform is a mathematical transformation of a complex waveform (having varying frequency and amplitude content) into simpler, more uniform waveforms (such as different sine waves of varying amplitudes). In this method, the EEG signal is converted into a simplified waveform called a spectrum. It is then separated into frequency bands at intervals of 0.5 Hz over a range of 1 to 32 Hz. The redistribution of electrical activity in the brain among certain frequency bands or the predominance of one band over the others correlates with specific physiologic and pathologic conditions [Fig. 7.6(a)]. The spectral analysis transforms the analog EEG signal recorded on the time axis into a signal displayed on the frequency axis.

Amplitude analysis

Changes in the EEG amplitude can indicate clinical changes. The amplitude changes result in changes in the power of the resulting frequency spectrum. As the amplitude increases, so does the power. The most common number reflecting EEG amplitude is the total power of the EEG spectrum. Due to the microvolt amplitude of the EEG, power is either in nanowatts or picowatts. The power spectrum is calculated by squaring the amplitudes of the individual frequency components. The powers of the individual frequency bands are also commonly used

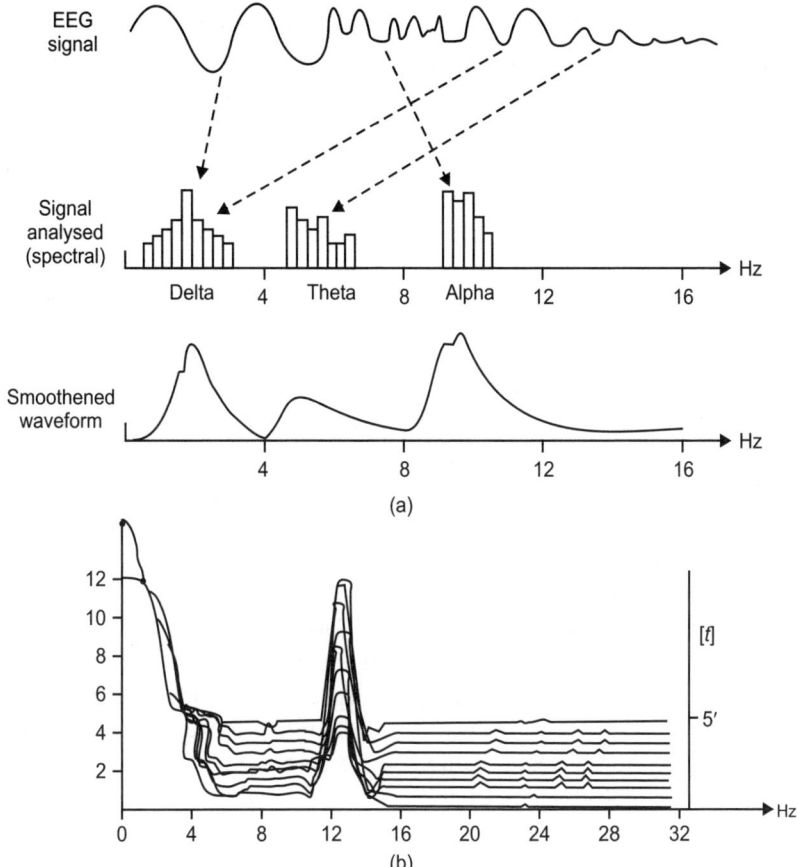

EEG signal

Signal analysed (spectral)

Delta   4   Theta   8   Alpha   12   16   Hz

Smoothened waveform

4   8   12   16   Hz

(a)

(b)

Fig. 7.6. (a) Typical ECG waveform broken down into frequency components, (b) mathematical and display techniques used to generate the compressed spectral array format.

and expressed as an absolute or a percentage of the total power. For example, 25 per cent. Alpha would indicate that 25 per cent of the total power is derived from the amplitudes of the Alpha waves.

Several different display formats have been developed for visually enhancing the computer processed information. These are:

Compressed spectral array (CSA)

In this format, a series of computer-smoothed spectral arrays are stacked vertically, usually at two second intervals, with the most recent EEG event at the bottom and the oldest at the top. Peaks appear at frequencies, which contain more power or make larger contributions to the total power spectrum.

Since the origin of the plots shifts vertically with time, this produces a pseudo three-dimensional graph [Fig. 7.6(b)]. With this method; it is easy to pick up changes in frequency and amplitude of each sample over a longer period of time as it compresses a large amount of data into a compact, easy to read trend.

Dot-density modulated spectral array (DSA)

It is another method for displaying the power spectra. This format displays a power spectrum as a line of variable intensities and/or densities with successive epochs again stacked vertically as in the CSA plots. Areas of greatest density represent frequencies, which make the greatest contribution to the EEG power spectrum. An advantage of the DSA format is that no data is hidden by the peaks as in the CSA display. DSA displays could be in the form of gray or colour-scaled densities.

Evoked Potential

An evoked potential (or evoked response) is an electrical potential recorded from the nervous system of a human or other animal following presentation of a stimulus, as distinct from spontaneous potentials as detected by electroencephalography (EEG) or electromyography (EMG).

Evoked potential amplitudes tend to be low, ranging from less than a microvolt to several microvolts, compared to tens of microvolts for EEG, millivolts for EMG, and often close to a volt for ECG. To resolve these low-amplitude potentials against the background of ongoing EEG, ECG, EMG and other biological signals and ambient noise, signal averaging is usually required. The signal is time-locked to the stimulus and most of the noise occurs randomly, allowing the noise to be averaged out with averaging of repeated responses.

Signals can be recorded from cerebral cortex, brain stem, spinal cord and peripheral nerves. Usually the term 'evoked potential' is reserved for responses involving either recording from, or stimulation of, central nervous system structures. Thus evoked compound motor action potentials (CMAP) or sensory nerve action potentials (SNAP) as used in nerve conduction studies (NCS) are generally not thought of as evoked potentials, though they do meet the above definition.

Sensory Evoked Potentials

Sensory evoked potentials (SEP) are recorded from the central nervous system following stimulation of sense organs (for example, visual evoked potentials elicited by a flashing light or changing pattern on a monitor; auditory evoked potentials by a click or tone stimulus presented through earphones) or by tactile or somatosensory evoked potential (SSEP) elicited by tactile or electrical stimulation of a sensory or mixed nerve in the periphery. They have been widely used in clinical diagnostic medicine since the 1970s, and also in intraoperative neurophysiology

monitoring (IONM), also known as surgical neurophysiology.

There are three kinds of evoked potentials in widespread clinical use since the 1970s: auditory evoked potentials, usually recorded from the scalp but originating at brainstem level (ABR, BAER, BSER, BAEP, BSEP); visual evoked potentials, and somatosensory evoked potentials, which are elicited by electrical stimulation of peripheral nerve.

Steady-state evoked potential

An evoked potential is the electrical response of the brain to a sensory stimulus. Regan constructed an analogue Fourier series analyser to record harmonics of the evoked potential to flickering (sinusoidally modulated) light but, rather than integrating the sine and cosine products, fed them to a two-pen recorder via low-pass filters.

This allowed him to demonstrate that the brain attained a steady-state regime in which the amplitude and phase of the harmonics (frequency components) of the response were approximately constant over time. By analogy with the steady-state response of a resonant circuit that follows the initial transient response he defined an idealised steady-state evoked potential (SSEP) as a form of response to repetitive sensory stimulation in which the constituent frequency components of the response remain constant with time in both amplitude and phase. Although this definition implies a series of identical temporal waveforms, it is more helpful to define the SSEP in terms of the frequency components that are an alternative description of the time-domain waveform, because different frequency components can have quite different properties.

For example, the properties of the high-frequency flicker SSEP (whose peak amplitude is near 40–50 Hz) correspond to the properties of the subsequently discovered magnocellular neurons the retina of the macaque monkey, while the properties of the medium-frequency flicker SSEP (whose amplitude peak is near 15–20 Hz) correspond to the properties of parvocellular neurons. Since a SSEP can be completely described in terms of the amplitude and phase of each frequency component it can be quantified more unequivocally than an averaged transient evoked potential.

It is sometimes said that SSEPs are elicited only by stimuli of high repetition frequency, but this is not generally correct. In principle, a sinusoidally modulated stimulus can elicit a SSEP even when its repetition frequency is low. Because of the high-frequency rolloff of the SSEP, high frequency stimulation can produce a near-sinusoidal SSEP waveform, but this is not germane to the definition of a SSEP. By using zoom-FFT to record SSEPs at the theoretical limit of spectral resolution ΔF (where ΔF in Hz is the reciprocal of the recording duration in seconds). Regan and Regan discovered that the amplitude and phase variability of the SSEP can be sufficiently small that the bandwidth of the SSEP's constituent frequency components can be at the theoretical limit of spectral resolution up to at least a 500 second recording duration (0.002 Hz in this case). Repetitive sensory stimulation elicits a steady-state magnetic brain response that can be analysed in the same way as the SSEP.

Simultaneous stimulation technique

This technique allows several (e.g. four) SSEPs to be recorded simultaneously from any given location on the scalp. Different sites of stimulation or different stimuli can be tagged with slightly different frequencies that are virtually identical to the brain, but easily separated by Fourier series analysers. For example, when two unpatterned lights are modulated at slightly different frequencies (F1 and F2) and superimposed, multiple nonlinear cross-modulation components of frequency (mF1 $\pm$ nF2) are created in the SSEP, where m and n are integers. These components allow nonlinear processing in the brain to be investigated. By frequency-tagging two superimposed gratings, spatial frequency and orientation tuning properties of the brain mechanisms that process spatial form can be isolated and studied. Stimuli of different sensory modalities can also be tagged. For example, a visual stimulus was flickered at Fv Hz and a simultaneously-presented auditory tone was amplitude modulated at Fa Hz. The existence of a (2Fv + 2Fa) component in the evoked

magnetic brain response demonstrated an audiovisual convergence area in the human brain, and the distribution of this response over the head allowed this brain area to be localised. More recently, frequency tagging has been extended from studies of sensory processing to studies of selective attention and of consciousness.

Sweep technique

The sweep technique is a hybrid frequency domain/ time domain technique. A plot of, for example, response amplitude versus the check size of a stimulus checker-board pattern plot can be obtained in 10 seconds, far faster than when time-domain averaging is used to record an evoked potential for each of several check sizes. In the original demonstration of the technique the sine and cosine products were fed through low-pass filters (as when recording a SSEP) while viewing a pattern of fine checks whose black and white squares exchanged place six times per second. Then the size of the squares was progressively increased so as to give a plot of evoked potential amplitude versus check size (hence sweep). Subsequent authors have implemented the sweep technique by using computer software to increment the spatial frequency of a grating in a series of small steps and to compute a time-domain average for each discrete spatial frequency. A single sweep may be adequate or it may be necessary to average the graphs obtained in several sweeps with the averager triggered by the sweep cycle. Averaging 16 sweeps can improve the signal-to-noise ratio of the graph by a factor of four. The sweep technique has proved useful in measuring rapidly-adapting visual processes and also for recording from babies, where recording duration is necessarily short. Norcia and Tyler have used the technique to document the development of visual acuity and contrast sensitivity through the first years of life. They have emphasised that, in diagnosing abnormal visual development, the more precise the developmental norms, the more sharply can the abnormal be distinguished from the normal, and to that end have documented normal visual development in a large group of infants. For many years the sweep technique has been used in paediatric ophthalmology (electrodiagnosis) clinics Worldwide.

Evoked potential feedback

This technique allows the SSEP to directly control the stimulus that elicits the SSEP without the conscious intervention of the experimental subject. For example, the running average of the SSEP can be arranged to increase the luminance of a checkerboard stimulus if the amplitude of the SSEP falls below some predetermined value, and to decrease luminance if it rises above this value. The amplitude of the SSEP then hovers about this predetermined value. Now the wavelength (colour) of the stimulus is progressively changed. The resulting plot of stimulus luminance versus wavelength is a plot of the spectral sensitivity of the visual system.

Visual evoked potential

Visual evoked potential (VEP) is caused by sensory stimulation of a subject's visual field and is observed using electroencephalography. Commonly used visual stimuli are flashing lights, or checker-boards on a video screen that flicker between black on white to white on black (invert contrast).

Visual evoked potentials are very useful in detecting blindness in patients that cannot communicate, such as babies or animals. If repeated stimulation of the visual field causes no changes in EEG potentials, then the subject's brain is probably not receiving any signals from his/her eyes.

Other applications include the diagnosis of optic neuritis, which causes the signal to be delayed. Such a delay is also a classic finding in Multiple Sclerosis. Visual evoked potentials are furthermore used in the investigation of basic functions of visual perception. VEPs are also sometimes used to determine if someone is fraudulently alleging blindness.

The term 'visual evoked potential' is used interchangeably with 'visually evoked potential'. It usually refers to responses recorded from the occipital cortex. Sometimes, the term 'visual evoked cortical potential' (VECP) is used to distinguish the VEP from retinal or subcortical potentials.

Brainstem auditory evoked potentials

Brainstem auditory evoked potentials (BAEPs) are very small electrical voltage potentials which are recorded in response to an auditory stimulus from electrodes placed on the scalp. They reflect neuronal activity in the auditory nerve, cochlear nucleus, superior olive and inferior colliculus of the brainstem. They typically have a response latency of no more than six milliseconds with an amplitude of approximately one millivolt. Due to their small amplitude 500 or more repetitions of the auditory stimulus are required in order to average out the random background electrical activity. Although it is possible to obtain a BSEP to a pure tone stimulus in the hearing range a more effective auditory stimulus contains a range of frequencies in the form of a short sharp click.

X-RAY COMPUTED TOMOGRAPHY

Computed tomography (CT) is a medical imaging method employing tomography created by computer processing. Digital geometry processing is used to generate a three-dimensional image of the inside of an object from a large series of two-dimensional X-ray images taken around a single axis of rotation. Figure 7.7 shows a multi-slice CT scanner.

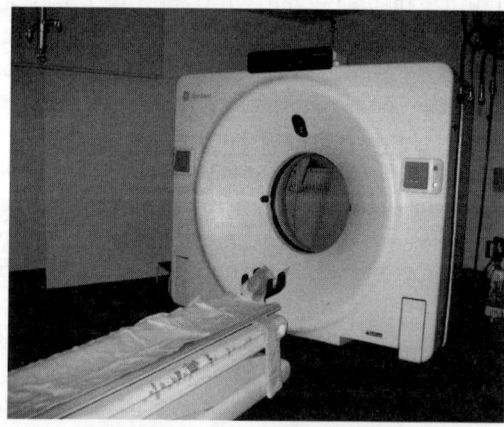

Fig. 7.7. A multi-slice CT scanner.

CT produces a volume of data which can be manipulated, through a process known as windowing, in order to demonstrate various bodily structures based on their ability to block the X-ray/Röntgen beam. Although historically the images generated were in the axial or transverse plane, orthogonal to the long axis of the body, modern scanners allow this volume of data to be reformatted in various planes or even as volumetric (3D) representations of structures. Although most common in medicine, CT is also used in other fields, such as nondestructive materials testing. Another example is the DigiMorph project at the University of Texas at Austin which uses a CT scanner to study biological and paleontological specimens.

Computed tomography differs from conventional X-ray techniques in that the pictures displayed are not photographs but are reconstructed from a large number of absorption profiles taken at regular angular intervals around a slice, with each profile being made up from a parallel set of absorption values through the object.

System Components

All computer tomography systems consist of the following four major subsystems:

1. Scanning system: This takes suitable readings for a picture to be reconstructed, and includes X-ray source and detectors.
2. Processing unit: This converts these readings into intelligible picture information.
3. Viewing part: It presents this information in visual form and includes other manipulative aids to assist diagnosis.
4. Storage unit: This enables the information to be stored for subsequent analysis.

Scanning system

The purpose of the scanning system is to acquire enough information to reconstruct a picture for an accurate diagnosis. A sufficient number of independent readings must be taken to allow picture reconstruction with the required spatial resolution and density discrimination for diagnostic purposes. The readings are taken in the form of 'profiles'.

When a plane parallel X-ray beam is passing through a required section, a profile is defined as the intensity of the emergent beam plotted along a line perpendicular to the X-ray beam. The profile represents a plot of the total absorption along each of the parallel X-ray beams. It thus follows that the higher the number of profiles obtained the better is the resulting picture. In practice, 180 such profiles at 1° intervals are normally needed to construct a diagnostically useful picture. There are several designs of scanning gantry commercially available from various manufacturers. They use different mechanical configurations.

Processing system

Data acquisition system: Although good detector properties are a prerequisite for obtaining optimal image quality, the measuring electronics must have a large dynamic range to back up the detector. The dynamic range defines the ratio of the smallest, just detectable signal to the largest signal without causing saturation. The dynamic range in a typical situation is 1:4,00,000. This implies that with such systems, an optimal image will always be obtained irrespective of whether the patient is obese or thin, or whether we are concerned with bones or soft tissues.

A typical data acquisition system is shown in Fig. 7.8. It consists of precision preamplifiers, current to voltage convertor, analog integrators, multiplexers and analog-to-digital convertors. Data transfer rates of the order of 10 Mbytes/s are required in some scanners.

This can be accomplished with a direct connection for systems having a fixed detector array. The third generation slip ring systems make use of optical transmitters on the rotating gantry to send data to fixed optical receivers. Figure 7.9 illustrates a typical computer system employed in a CT scanner.

Viewing system

In most of the CT systems, the final picture is available on a television types picture tube. The picture is constructed by a number of elements in a square matrix wherein each element has a value representative of the absorption value of the point in the body which it represents. This technique facilitates a much larger dynamic range than the eye can possibly have. The absorption values are displayed on a linear scale corresponding to air through tissue to dense bone, etc. Several values have been assigned to the two terminal points of the scale. For example, in some cases like the original EMI scale, air is assigned the value of –500, water the value of 0 and bones, that of +500. In the CT scanners that are presently being manufactured, the picture points are divided into 2000 steps. The resolution of the scale thus obtained is 1 promille difference in absorption related to the attenuation value for water.

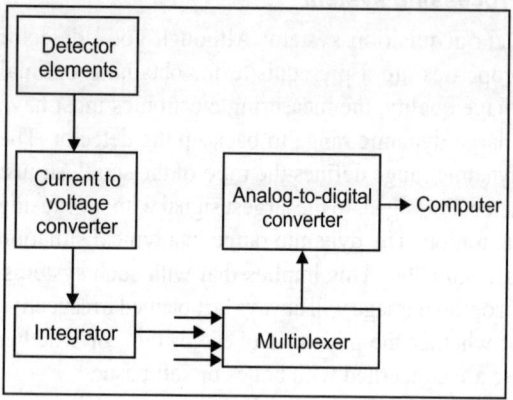

Fig. 7.8. Data acquisition system in a CT scanner.

In order to facilitate image display, it would be better if the scale could be expanded within this range. For this purpose, recourse is made to the selection of an image window. The information content of this window is spread over the representable range of colour or gray scale. As long as the original image data of the CT scan is present in the image reconstruction store of the image computer or in the image display memory of the monitor, the image window of interest can be varied in two parameters, namely window level and window width. These two parameters can be varied at will within the range of the absorption values.

Windowing is a powerful aspect of CT and shows the underlying mathematical nature of the displayed picture. This helps in defining the region of interest from where various calculations can be performed on the enclosed elements. The commonly used calculations are of the area, mean value and standard deviation which may well show an identifiable difference between healthy and diseased tissue. It is also possible to subtract one picture from another to demonstrate differences that have occurred during treatment.

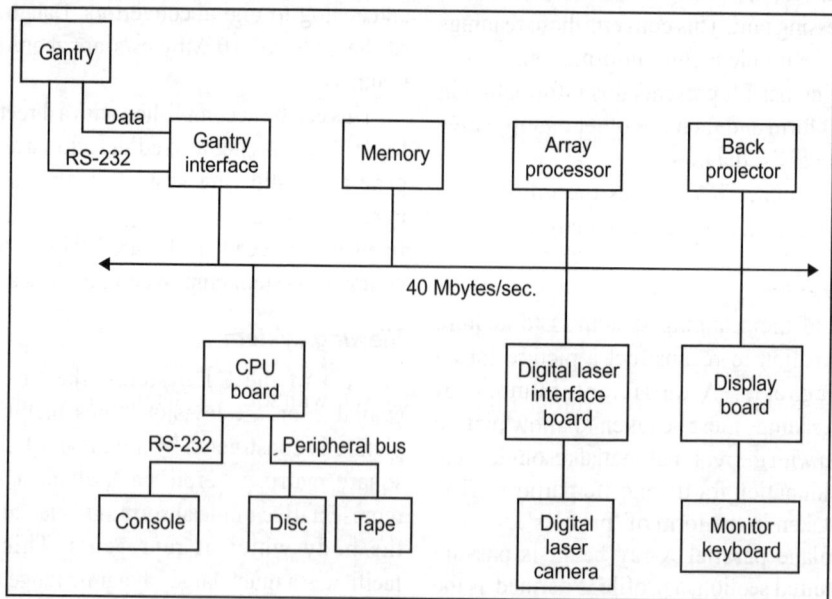

Fig. 7.9. Typical computer system organisation for a CT. The system makes use of motorola family 68000, 16 bit microprocessors.

Storing and documentation

For subsequent processing or evaluation of a CT picture, various methods of storage are used. The picture is stored in the digital form so that the evaluation is convenient on a computer-assisted programme. For this purpose, the data carriers generally employed are magnetic disc, magnetic tape and floppy disc. Most manufacturers of CT units use the magnetic tape or floppy disc. The floppy disc provides a medium-range storage. The capacity of a bilaterally coated disc is around 20 pictures, having a matrix of 256×256 and depth of information of 10 bits. Floppy discs offer advantages such as ease of handling, low maintenance costs of the drive mechanism, the considerably short access time and the possibility of patient-related storage of the data carrier. For long-term storage, magnetic tapes are preferred. They are inexpensive and extremely reliable, but retrieval of the image is time-consuming and they are sensitive to environmental influences.

Magnetic Resonance Imaging

Magnetic resonance imaging (MRI), or nuclear magnetic resonance imaging (NMRI), is primarily a medical imaging technique most commonly used in radiology to visualise detailed internal structure and limited function of the body. MRI provides much greater contrast between the different soft tissues of the body than computed tomography (CT) does, making it especially useful in neurological (brain), musculoskeletal, cardiovascular, and oncological (cancer) imaging. Unlike CT, it uses no ionising radiation, but uses a powerful magnetic field to align the nuclear magnetisation of (usually) hydrogen atoms in water in the body. Radio frequency (RF) fields are used to systematically alter the alignment of this magnetisation, causing the hydrogen nuclei to produce a rotating magnetic field detectable by the scanner. This signal can be manipulated by additional magnetic fields to build up enough information to construct an image of the body.

Magnetic resonance imaging was developed from knowledge gained in the study of nuclear magnetic resonance. In its early years the technique was referred to as nuclear magnetic resonance imaging (NMRI). However, as the word nuclear was associated in the public mind with ionising radiation exposure it is generally now referred to simply as MRI. Scientists still use the term NMRI when discussing non-medical devices operating on the same principles. The term magnetic resonance tomography (MRT) is also sometimes used.

The body is largely composed of water molecules which each contain two hydrogen nuclei or protons. When a person goes inside the powerful magnetic field of the scanner, the magnetic moments of these protons align with the direction of the field.

A radio frequency electromagnetic field is then briefly turned on, causing the protons to alter their alignment relative to the field. When this field is turned off the protons return to the original magnetisation alignment. These alignment changes create a signal which can be detected by the scanner. The frequency at which the protons resonate depends on the strength of the magnetic field. The position of protons in the body can be determined by applying additional magnetic fields during the scan which allows an image of the body to be built up. These are created by turning gradients coils on and off which creates the knocking sounds heard during an MR scan.

Diseased tissue, such as tumours, can be detected because the protons in different tissues return to their equilibrium state at different rates. By changing the parameters on the scanner this effect is used to create contrast between different types of body tissue.

Contrast agents may be injected intravenously to enhance the appearance of blood vessels, tumours or inflammation. Contrast agents may also be directly injected into a joint in the case of arthrograms, MR images of joints. Unlike CT, MRI uses no ionising radiation and is generally a very safe procedure. Patients with some metal implants, cochlear implants, and cardiac pacemakers are prevented from having an MRI scan due to effects of the strong magnetic field and powerful radio frequency pulses.

MRI is used to image every part of the body, and is particularly useful for neurological conditions, for disorders of the muscles and joints, for evaluating tumours, and for showing abnormalities in the heart and blood vessels.

Physics principles

Nuclear magnetism

Subatomic particles have the quantum mechanical property of spin. Certain nuclei such as ^1H (protons), ^2H, ^3He, ^{23}Na or ^{31}P, have a non–zero spin and therefore a magnetic moment. In the case of the so-called spin-$^1/_2$ nuclei, such as ^1H, there are two spin states, sometimes referred to as 'up' and 'down'. Nuclei such as ^{12}C have no unpaired neutrons or protons, and no net spin; however, the isotope ^{13}C does.

When these spins are placed in a strong external magnetic field they process around an axis along the direction of the field. Protons align in two energy 'eigenstates' (the 'Zeeman effect'): one low-energy and one high-energy, which are separated by a very small splitting energy.

Multinuclear imaging

Hydrogen is the most frequently imaged nucleus in MRI because it is present in biological tissues in great abundance. However, any nucleus which has a net nuclear spin could potentially be imaged with MRI. Such nuclei include helium-3, carbon-13, fluorine-19, oxygen-17, sodium-23, phosphorus-31 and xenon-129. ^{23}Na and ^{31}P are naturally abundant in the body, so can be imaged directly. Gaseous isotopes such as ^3He or ^{129}Xe must be hyperpolarised and then inhaled as their nuclear density is too low to yield a useful signal under normal conditions. ^{17}O, ^{13}C and ^{19}F can be administered in sufficient quantities in liquid form (e.g. ^{17}O-water, ^{13}C-glucose solutions or perfluorocarbons) that hyperpolarisation is not a necessity. Multinuclear imaging is primarily a research technique at present. However, potential applications include functional imaging and imaging of organs poorly seen on ^1H MRI (e.g. lungs and bones) or as alternative contrast agents. Inhaled hyperpolarised ^3He can be used to image the distribution of air spaces within the lungs. Injectable solutions containing ^{13}C or stabilised bubbles of hyperpolarised ^{129}Xe have been studied as contrast agents for angiography and perfusion imaging. ^{31}P can potentially provide information on bone density and structure, as well as functional imaging of the brain.

Susceptibility weighted imaging (SWI)

Susceptibility weighted imaging (SWI), is a new type of contrast in MRI different from spin density, T_1, or T_2 imaging. This method exploits the susceptibility differences between tissues and uses a fully velocity compensated, three dimensional, RF spoiled, high-resolution, 3D gradient echo scan. This special data acquisition and image processing produces an enhanced contrast magnitude image very sensitive to venous blood, haemorrhage and iron storage. It is used to enhance the detection and diagnosis of tumours, vascular and neurovascular diseases (stroke and haemorrhage, multiple sclerosis, Alzheimer's), and also detects traumatic brain injuries that may not be diagnosed using other methods.

Other specialised MRI techniques

MRI is a new and active field of research and new methods and variants are often published when they are able to get better results in specific fields. Examples of these recent improvements are T_2-weighted turbo spin-echo (T_2 TSE MRI), double inversion recovery MRI (DIR-MRI) or phase-sensitive inversion recovery MRI (PSIR-MRI), all of them able to improve imaging of the brain lesions. Another example is MP-RAGE (magnetisation-prepared rapid acquisition with gradient echo), which improves images of multiple sclerosis cortical lesions.

Portable instruments

Portable magnetic resonance instruments are available for use in education and field research. Using the principles of Earth's field NMR, they have no powerful polarising magnet, so that such instruments can be small and inexpensive. Some can be used for both EFNMR spectroscopy and MRI imaging. The low strength of the Earth's field results in poor signal to noise ratios, requiring long scan times to capture spectroscopic data or build up MRI images.

Basic NMR Components

The basic components of an NMR imaging system are shown in Fig. 7.10. These are:

1. A magnet, which provides it strong uniform, steady, magnet field B_0.
2. An RF transmitter, which delivers radio-frequency magnetic field to the sample.

3. A gradient system, which produces time-varying magnetic fields of controlled spatial nonuniformity.

4. A detection system, which yields the output signal.

5. An imager system, including the computer, which reconstructs and displays the images.

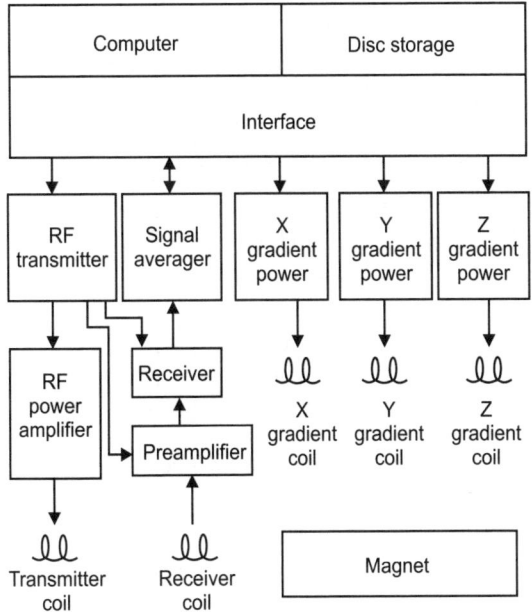

Fig. 7.10. Subsystems of a typical NMR imaging system

The imaging sequencing in the system is provided by a computer. Functions such as gates and envelopes for the NMR pulses, blanking for the pre-amplifier and RF power amplifier and voltage waveforms for the gradient magnetic fields are all under software control. The computer also performs the various data processing tasks including the Fourier transformation, image reconstruction, data filtering, image display and storage. Therefore, the computer must have sufficient memory and speed to handle large image arrays and data processing, in addition to interfacing facilities.

Magnet

In magnetic resonance tomography, the base field must be extremely uniform in space and constant in time as its purpose is to align the nuclear magnets

parallel to each other in the volume to be examined. Also, the signal-to-noise ratio increases approximately linearly with the magnetic field strength of the basic field, therefore, it must be as large as possible. Four factors characterise the performance of the magnets used in MR systems; viz. field strength, temporal stability, homogeneity and boresize. The effect of the magnetic field strength has been elaborated earlier. The temporal stability is important since instabilities of the field adversely affect resolution. The gross nonhomogeneities result in image distortion while the bore diameter limits the size of the dimension of the specimen that can be imaged.

Such a magnetic field can be produced by means of four different ways, viz. permanent magnets, electromagnets, resistive magnets and super-conducting magnets.

In case of the permanent magnet, the patient is placed in the gap between a pair of permanently magnetised pole faces. Permanent magnet materials normally used in MRI scanners include high carbon iron alloys such as alnico or neodymium iron (alloy of neodymium, boron and iron) and ceramics such as barium ferrite.

Although permanent magnets have the advantages of producing a relatively small fringing field and do not require power supplies, they tend to be very heavy (up to 100 tons) and produce relatively low fields of the order of 0.3 T or less.

Electromagnets make use of soft magnetic materials such as pole faces which become magnetised only when electric current is passed through the coils wound around them. Electromagnets obviously require external electrical power supply.

On cost considerations, the earlier NMR imaging systems were equipped with resistive magnets. Resistive magnets make use of large current-carrying coils of aluminium strips or copper tubes. In these magnets, the electrical power requirement increases proportionately to the square of the field strength which becomes prohibitively high as the field strength increases. Moreover, the total power in the coils is converted into heat which must be dissipated by liquid cooling. For instance, at 0.2 T, the power requirement is nearly 70 kW and a substantial increase of field strength above 0.2 T in resistive magnets is thus technically limited. At present, resistive magnets are seldom used except for very low field strength applications, generally limited to 0.02 to 0.06 T.

Most of the modern NMR machines utilise superconductive magnets. These magnets utilise the property of certain materials, which lose their electrical resistance fully below a specific temperature. The commonly used superconducting material is Nb Ti (Niobium Titanium) alloy for which the transition temperature lies at 9 K (–264°C). In order to prevent superconductivity from being destroyed by an external magnetic field or the current passing through the conductors, these conductors must be cooled down to temperatures significantly below this point, at least to half of the transition temperature. Therefore, superconductive magnet coils are cooled with liquid helium which boils at a temperature of 4.2 K (–269°C). The helium container with its superconductive windings is enclosed in a vacuum to keep the evaporation rate low. Internal shields cooled with liquid nitrogen prevent heating due to radiated heat passing through the vacuum vessel.

In a superconducting magnet, connection to a current supply is only necessary for energising up to the required field strength. After this, the coils are short-circuited and require no further electrical energy. The magnetic field is temporarily stable. Due to evaporation of the liquid helium and liquid nitrogen, the monthly topping of helium and weekly topping of nitrogen is necessary. The evaporation rate in the earlier scanners was about 0.5 1/hr for liquid helium and 2 1/hr for liquid nitrogen. At present, many magnets now make use of cryogenic refrigerators that reduce or eliminate the need for refilling the liquid helium reservoir. Figure 7.11 shows a schematic diagram of the superconducting magnet. Because of their capability to achieving very strong and stable magnetic field strengths without any continuous power consumption, superconducting magnets have become the most widely used and preferred source of the main magnetic fields for MRI scanners.

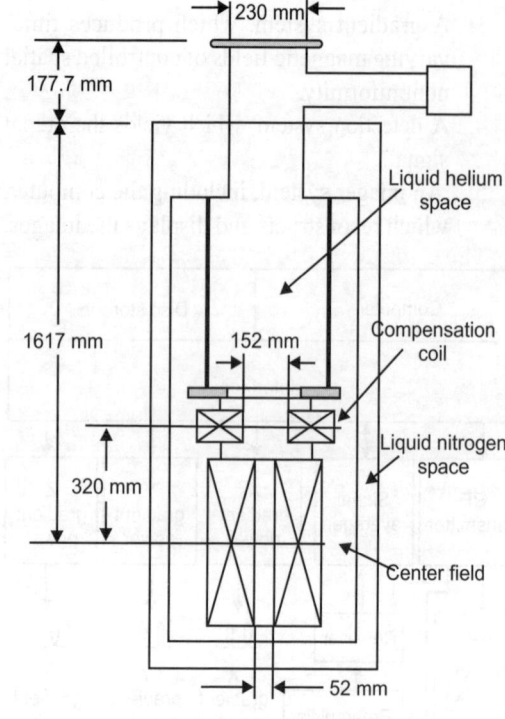

Fig. 7.11. Schematic drawing of the superconducting magnet.

Superconductive magnetic resonance magnets with an open internal diameter of 1 m, as is desirable for whole body examinations, are now produced for field strengths of upto 2 T. In a typical 1.5 T magnetic field, the current required by the superconducting coils is of the order of 200 amp. The diameter of the coils is about 1.3 m and total length of the wire could be 65 kms. The magnet is operated in the persistent mode, i.e. once the current is established, the terminals may be connected together, and a constant persistent current will flow indefinitely so long as the temperature of the coils is maintained below the superconducting transition temperature.

Besides the indisputable advantages which high magnetic field strengths have on image quality, it also implies increased technical complexity, both in the installation of magnetic resonance equipment as the well as the radio-frequency technology required. The spread of the critical fringe field of a magnet is proportional to the cube root of its field strength. If with a 0.2 T magnet, the ten-fold strength of the earths field is exceeded at about 6 m distance from the centre, then at 2 T, this fringe field strength occurs at 13 m. This can seriously affect the function of nearby clinical equipment such as image intensifiers and monitors.

A field strength of 0.5 T means that a nuclear resonance frequency of 21.3 MHz is required for protons and a field strength of 2 T means that 85.2 MHz is needed. At these higher frequencies, the usual saddle-shaped antenna coils used for lower frequencies can no longer be applied, because the conductors' self-capacity is too large and travelling wave effects play a significant role. Also, the conductor length is comparable with the quarter wavelength of the radio-frequency field.

The NMR imaging systems usually incorporate magnets with a maximum flux density of 0.5 T to 1.5 T. In the system of international units (SI units), the 'Tesla' (T) is the unit of magnetic flux density. In some countries, the unit 'Gauss' (G) is also used. For conversion 1 T = 10,000 G = 10 kG. The image quality of NMR scans depends upon the uniformity of the static magnetic field and on its stability over a long period of time. The uniformity of this magnet must be at least 20 ppm within the scanning region and stability at a level of 2 ppm during short periods and under 10 ppm over long periods.

RF transmitter system

In order to activate the nuclei so that they emit a useful signal, energy must be transmitted into the sample. This is what the transmitter does. The system consists of an RF transmitter, RF power amplifier and RF transmitting coils. The RF transmitter consists of an RF crystal oscillator at the Larmor frequency. The RF voltage is gated with the pulse envelopes from the computer interface to generate RF pulses that excite the resonance. These pulses are amplified to levels varying from 100 W to several kW depending on the imaging method and are fed to the transmitter coil. The higher power levels are necessary for the large sample volumes encountered in whole body experiments.

The RF coils can be either a single coil serving as both transmitter and receiver or two separate coils that are electrically orthogonal. The latter configuration has the advantage of reduced pulse breakthrough into the receiver during the pulse. In both cases, all coils generate RF fields orthogonal to the direction of the main magnetic field. Saddle-and solenoidal-shaped RF coils are typical geometries for the RF coils.

The coils are tuned to the NMR frequency and are usually isolated from the remainder of the system by enclosure in an RF shielding cage. For magnetic fields in the range of 0.05 to 2 T used for imaging of the human body, the resonant frequencies fall in the radio-frequency band. For example, in a field of 1 T, ^{1}H resonates at 42.57 MHz, ^{19}F at 40.05 MHz, ^{31}P at 17.24 MHz and ^{13}C at 10.71 MHz. Usually, the resonance is extremely sharp. Widths in the range of 10 Hz are typical of biological systems.

Detection system

The function of the detection system (receiver) is to detect the nuclear magnetisation and generate an output signal for processing by the computer.

SINGLE PHOTON EMISSION COMPUTED TOMOGRAPHY

Single photon emission computed tomography (SPECT, or less commonly, SPET) is a nuclear medicine tomographic imaging technique using gamma rays. It is very similar to conventional nuclear medicine planar imaging using a gamma camera. However, it is able to provide true 3D information. This information is typically presented as cross-sectional slices through the patient, but can be freely reformatted or manipulated as required.

The basic technique requires injection of a gamma-emitting radioisotope (also called radio-nuclide) into the bloodsteam of the patient. Occasionally the radioisotope is a simple soluble dissolved ion, such as a radioisotope of gallium(III), which happens to also have chemical properties which allow it to be concentrated in ways of medical interest for disease detection. However, most of the time in SPECT, a marker radioisotope, which is of interest only for its radioactive properties, has been attached to a special radioligand, which is of interest for its chemical binding properties to certain types of tissues. This marriage allows the combination of ligand and radioisotope (the radiopharmaceutical) to be carried and bound to a place of interest in the body, which then (due to the gamma-emission of the isotope) allows the ligand concentration to be seen by a gamma-camera.

In the same way that a plain X-ray is a 2-dimensional (2-D) view of a 3-dimensional structure, the image obtained by a gamma camera is a 2-D view of 3-D distribution of a radionuclide.

SPECT imaging is performed by using a gamma camera to acquire multiple 2-D images (also called projections), from multiple angles. A computer is then used to apply a tomographic reconstruction algorithm to the multiple projections, yielding a 3-D dataset. This dataset may then be manipulated to show thin slices along any chosen axis of the body, similar to those obtained from other tomographic techniques, such as MRI, CT, and PET.

SPECT is similar to PET in its use of radioactive tracer material and detection of gamma rays. In contrast with PET, however, the tracer used in SPECT emits gamma radiation that is measured directly, whereas PET tracer emits positrons which annihilate with electrons up to a few millimeters away, causing two gamma photons to be emitted in opposite directions. A PET scanner detects these emissions 'coincident' in time, which provides more radiation event localisation information and thus higher resolution images than SPECT (which has about 1 cm resolution). SPECT scans, however, are significantly less expensive than PET scans, in part because they are able to use longer-lived more easily-obtained radioisotopes than PET.

NUCLEAR MEDICAL IMAGING SYSTEMS

In nuclear medical diagnostics, the imaging of organ functions is carried out non-invasively. In contrast to other imaging diagnostic modalities (ultrasound, X-ray, MRI), the nuclear medical examination approach is primarily function-oriented. In this case, vital processes such as blood circulation, metabolism and vitality of organs and tumours can be displayed as functional images.

The clinical use of radio-nuclide imaging depends on obtaining a suitable distribution of the radio-nuclide in the patient. The radio-nuclide is labelled to a compound which will be taken up or metabolised in some way by the human tissue to be studied. The patient receives the material, usually by intravenous injection, and after a suitable delay, which may be minutes or hours, to allow uptake in the target tissues and clearance from the blood, imaging can commence. In this way useful static images, each taking 2–10 minutes, can be produced of the bone, brain, thyroid, lung, etc. Dynamic studies can be performed with the gamma camera, starting at the moment of injection and capturing frames of the data either photographically or digitally, at times ranging from minutes down to fractions of a second. Numerical analysis of such data can produce useful information on organ function, blood flow, clearance rates, etc.

Tecnetium-99 m (Tc-99 m) has proven to be the most important imaging radio-nuclide used to examine the brain, liver, lungs, bones, thyroid, kidney and heart. It combines the advantages of optimum radiation properties (emission of exclusively gamma radiation with suitable energy, short half-life of six hours) and general availability as a generator nuclide. However, Tc-99 m cannot be coupled with all required biologically active substances, so that with this radio-nuclide the spectrum of radio-pharmaceuticals for examinations of the organ metabolism is limited. For example, Iodine-123 labelled substances, which are used in many clinical examinations, therefore represent an important supplement to technetium studies.

Radiation Detectors

Depending upon the radiation emitted by the radio isotope of the radiopharmaceutical, a suitable detector is selected and operated under optimum conditions. Several methods are available for detection and measurement of radiation from radio-nuclides, The choice of a particular method depends upon the nature of the radiation and the energy of the particle involved.

If the radiation falls on a photographic plate, it would cause darkening when developed after exposure. The photographic method is useful for measuring the total exposure to radiation of workers, who are provided with film badges. Better methods are available for an exact measurement of the activity, These methods are the use of: (i) ionisation chamber, (ii) Geiger Muller counter, (iii) proportional counter, (iv) semiconductor detectors, and (vi) solid state detectors.

Pulse Height Analyser

In radioactivity measurements, the individual particles are detected as single electrical impulses in the detectors. Also, various types of detectors can be set up to operate in a region in which the particular particle produces an electrical impulse with the height proportional to the energy of the particle. The measurement of pulse height is thus a useful tool for energy determination. In order to sort out the pulses of different amplitudes and to count them, electronic circuits are employed. The instrument which accomplishes this is called a 'pulse height analyser'. These analysers are either single or multiple-channel instruments.

Uptake Monitoring Equipment

The clinical use of a radio-nuclie in medical investigations depends on obtaining a suitable distribution of the radio-nuclide in the patient. This is achieved by administering a suitable chemical substance tagged with a radio-nuclide, emitting gamma radiations. The biological system under investigation selectively assimilates the administered dose to carry out its function. Since the gamma ray gets transmitted through the body tissues, an external monitoring system can be used to detect them and provide the measurement of the chemical substance. The fraction of the chemical present in the organ at any time would indicate the functional status or what is called the uptake of the organ. The most suited gamma energy range for uptake monitoring studies is from 100 keV to 500 keV.

Radioisotope Rectilinear Scanner

The distribution of radioactive material within an organ or part of the body is studied by using radioisotope rectilinear scanners. The scanner is a moving detector imaging system with a block diagram shown in Fig. 7.12. Heart of the system is the detector-collimator assembly. The detector is usually a three or five inch diameter NaI crystal, situated behind a focusing collimator. This is so mounted that it can travel in a regular scanning pattern back and forth across the area of interest, so that detected and amplified signals can be plotted to give a picture or contour map of radioactivity within the organ. Usually, the detector-collimator assembly, the photo-multiplier and the pre-amplifier are housed in a single unit, which is attached to a motor-driven device. This device defines the lateral and longitudinal limits of the scan.

A single probe scanner makes use of one detector that scans the area of interest. There are dual probe scanners that have two synchronously moving, axially opposite detectors with the patient between the two detectors. The scanning can be linear or one-dimensional. In the whole body counting applications, the detector is moved continuously over the body and the counts are integrated over the entire scan. The recording may be done either by a photographic recorder or by dot recorders. In a photographic recorder, the light flashes can be photo-graphed on a film, from the face of a cathode ray tube. The dot recorder is most commonly used. It produces a map of the distribution of activity within the area of interest by recording dots or slit-like marks on paper. The dot recording mechanism consists of an electrically heated stylus to bum a small spot on a sheet of electrically conducting paper, each time a pulse passes through the stylus. The pulses to the stylus are delivered from the pulse height analyser after scaling down the counts by an adjustable scaling factor from 1 to 256. A scaling factor of 16, for example, would mean that for every 16 counts arriving at the input of the scaling circuit from the pulse height analyser, one dot appears on the paper. This reduction in counting rate is necessary, because extremely high counting rates will drive the stylus wild. A count-rate metre is also incorporated to display or record the average count rate.

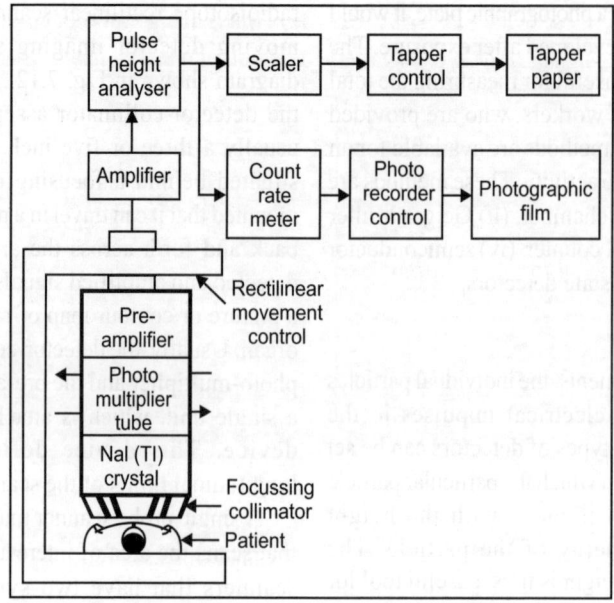

Fig. 7.12. Block diagram of a typical rectilinear scanner.

Gamma Camera

A gamma camera, also called a scintillation camera or Anger camera, is a device used to image gamma radiation emitting radioisotopes, a technique known as scintigraphy.

The applications of scintigraphy include early drug development and nuclear medical imaging to view and analyse images of the human body or the distribution of medically injected, inhaled, or ingested radionuclides emitting gamma rays. Figure 7.13 shows gamma camera.

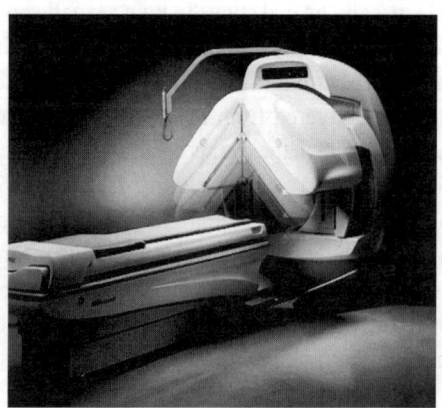

Fig. 7.13. Gama camera.

A gamma camera consists of one or more flat crystal planes (or detectors) optically coupled to an array of photomultiplier tubes, the assembly is known as a 'head', mounted on a gantry. The gantry is connected to a computer system that both controls the operation of the camera as well as acquisition and storage of acquired images.

The system accumulates events, or counts, of gamma photons that are absorbed by the crystal in the camera. Usually a large flat crystal of sodium iodide with thallium doping in a light-sealed housing is used. The highly efficient capture method of this combination for detecting gamma rays was discovered by noted physicist Robert Hofstadter. Figure 7.14 shows diagrammatic cross section of a gamma camera detector.

The crystal scintillates in response to incident gamma radiation. When a gamma photon leaves the patient (who has been injected with a radioactive pharmaceutical), it knocks an electron loose from an iodine atom in the crystal, and a faint flash of light is produced when the dislocated electron again finds a minimal energy state. The initial phenomenon of the excited electron is similar to the photoelectric effect and (particularly with gamma rays) the Compton effect.

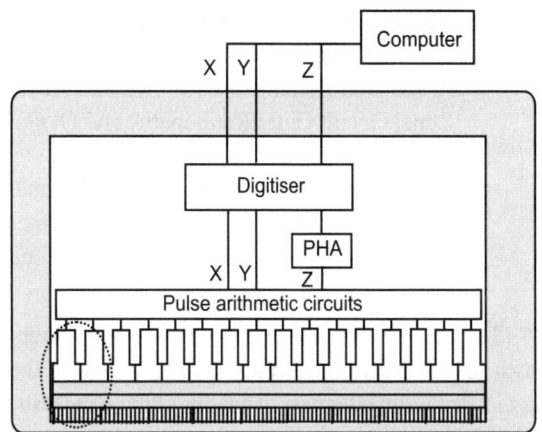

Fig. 7.14. Diagrammatic cross-section of a gamma camera detector.

After the flash of light is produced, it is detected. Photomultiplier tubes (PMTs) behind the crystal detect the fluorescent flashes (events) and a computer sums the counts. The computer reconstructs and displays a two dimensional image of the relative spatial count density on a monitor.

This reconstructed image reflects the distribution and relative concentration of radioactive tracer elements present in the organs and tissues imaged.

Positron Emission Tomography

Positron emission tomography (PET) is a nuclear medicine imaging technique which produces a three-dimensional image or picture of functional processes in the body. The system detects pairs of gamma rays emitted indirectly by a positron-emitting radionuclide (tracer), which is introduced into the body on a biologically active molecule. Images of tracer concentration in 3-dimensional or 4-dimensional space within the body are then reconstructed by computer analysis. In modern scanners, this reconstruction is often accomplished with the aid of a CT X-ray scan performed on the patient during the same session, in the same machine.

If the biologically active molecule chosen for PET is FDG, an analogue of glucose, the concentrations of tracer imaged then give tissue metabolic activity, in terms of regional glucose uptake. Although use of this tracer results in the most common type of PET scan, other tracer molecules are used in PET to image the tissue concentration of many other types of molecules of interest.

EYE, ERG, EOG AND VISUAL FIELD

Electroretinography

Electroretinography measures the electrical responses of various cell types in the retina, including the photoreceptors (rods and cones), inner retinal cells (bipolar and amacrine cells), and the ganglion cells. Electrodes are usually placed on the cornea and the skin near the eye, although it is possible to record the ERG from skin electrodes (Fig. 7.15).

During a recording, the patient's eyes are exposed to standardised stimuli and the resulting signal is displayed showing the time course of the signal's amplitude (voltage). Signals are very small, and typically are measured in microvolts or nanovolts. The ERG is composed of electrical potentials contributed by different cell types within the retina, and the stimulus conditions (flash or pattern stimulus, whether a background light is present, and the colours of the stimulus and background) can elicit stronger response from certain components.

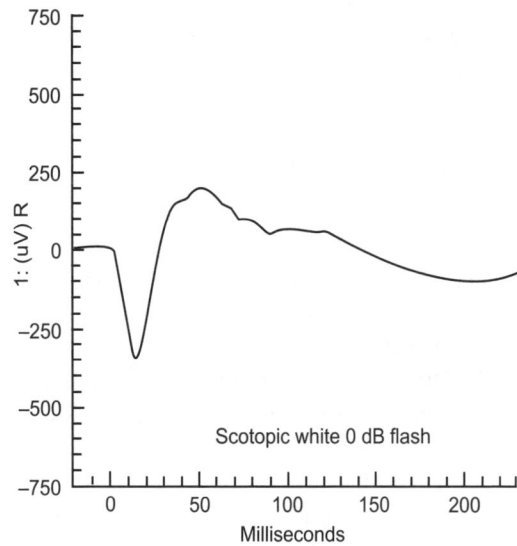

Fig. 7.15. Maximal response ERG waveform from a dark adapted eye.

If a flash ERG is performed on a dark-adapted eye, the response is primarily from the rod system and flash ERGs performed on a light adapted eye will reflect the activity of the cone system. To sufficiently bright flashes, the ERG will contain an a-wave (initial negative deflection) followed by a b-wave (positive deflection). The leading edge of the a-wave is produced by the photoreceptors, while the remainder of the wave is produced by a mixture of cells including photoreceptors, bipolar, amacrine, and Muller cells. The pattern ERG, evoked by an alternating checker-board stimulus, primarily reflects activity of retinal ganglion cells.

Clinically used mainly by ophthalmologists and optometrists, the electroretinogram (ERG) is used for the diagnosis of various retinal diseases. Inherited retinal degenerations in which the ERG can be useful include:

1. Retinitis pigmentosa and related hereditary degenerations.
2. Retinitis punctata albescens.
3. Leber's congenital amaurosis.
4. Choroideremia.
5. Gyrate atrophy of the retina and choroid.
6. Goldman-Favre syndrome.
7. Congenital stationary night blindness— normal a-wave indicates normal photo- receptors; absent b-wave indicates abnormality in the bipolar cell region.
8. X-linked juvenile retinoschisis
9. Achromatopsia.
10. Cone dystrophy.
11. Disorders mimicking retinitis pigmentosa.
12. Usher syndrome.

Other ocular disorders in which the standard ERG provides useful information include:

1. Diabetic retinopathy.
2. Other ischemic retinopathies including central retinal vein occlusion (CRVO), branch vein occlusion (BVO), and sickle cell retinopathy.
3. Toxic retinopathies, including those caused by Plaquenil and Vigabatrin. The ERG is also used to monitor retinal toxicity in many drug trials.

4. Autoimmune retinopathies such as Cancer Associated Retinopathy (CAR), Melanoma Associated Retinopathy (MAR), and Acute Zonal Occult Outer Retinopathy (AZOOR).
5. Retinal detachment.
6. Assessment of retinal function after trauma, especially in vitreous haemorrhage and other conditions where the fundus cannot be visualised.

The ERG is also used extensively in eye research, as it provides information about the function of the retina that is not otherwise available. Other ERG tests, such as the Photopic Negative Response (PhNR) and pattern ERG (PERG) may be useful in assessing retinal ganglion cell function in diseases like glaucoma. The multifocal ERG is used to record separate responses for different retinal locations.

Electrooculography

Electrooculography (EOG) is a technique for measuring the resting potential of the retina. The resulting signal is called the electrooculogram. The main applications are in ophthalmological diagnosis and in recording eye movements. Unlike the electroretinogram, the EOG does not represent the response to individual visual stimuli. Eye movement measurements: Usually, pairs of electrodes are placed either above and below the eye or to the left and right of the eye. If the eye is moved from the centre position towards one electrode, this electrode 'sees' the positive side of the retina and the opposite electrode 'sees' the negative side of the retina. Consequently, a potential difference occurs between the electrodes. Assuming that the resting potential is constant, the recorded potential is a measure for the eye position.

Ophthalmological diagnosis: The EOG is used to assess the function of the pigment epithelium. During dark adaptation, the resting potential decreases slightly and reaches a minimum (dark trough) after several minutes. When the light is switched on, a substantial increase of the resting potential occurs (light peak), which drops off after a few minutes when the retina adapts to the light. The ratio of the voltages (i.e. light peak divided by dark trough) is known as the Arden ratio. In practice, the measurement is similar to the eye movement recordings. The patient is asked to switch the eye position repeatedly between two points (usually to the left and right of the centre). Since these positions are constant, a change in the recorded potential originates from a change in the resting potential.

Application in entertainment

Electrooculography was used by Robert Zemeckis and Jerome Chen, the visual effects supervisor in the movie Beowulf during the enhanced performance capture to correctly capture and animate the eye movements of the actors. It was an improvement from The Polar Express.

Also use in the Neural Impulse Actuator, from OCZ Technology, a computer device helping gamers to increase their playing speed.

Visual Field

The term visual field is sometimes used as a synonym to field of view, though they do not designate the same thing. The visual field is the 'spatial array of visual sensations available to observation in introspectionist psychological experiments', while 'field of view' 'refers to the physical objects and light sources in the external world that impinge the retina'. In other words, field of view is everything that (at a given time) causes light to fall onto the retina. This input is processed by the visual system, which computes the visual field as the output.

The term is often used in optometry and ophthalmology, where a visual field test is used to determine whether the visual field is affected by diseases that cause local scotoma or a more extensive loss of vision or a reduction in sensitivity (threshold).

The normal human visual field extends to approximately 60° (degrees) nasally (toward the nose, or inward) in each eye, to 100° temporally (away from the nose, or outwards), and approximately 60° above and 75 below the horizontal meridian. In the United Kingdom, the minimum field requirement for driving is 60° either side of the vertical meridian, and 20° above and below horizontal. The macula corresponds to the central 13° of the visual field; the fovea to the central 3°.

Measuring the visual field

The visual field is measured by perimetry. This may be kinetic, where points of light are moved inwards until the observer sees them, or static, where points of light are flashed onto a white screen and the observer is asked to press a button if he or she sees it. The most common perimeter used is the automated Humphrey field analyser.

Another method is to use a campimeter, a small device designed to measure the visual field.

Patterns testing the central 24° or 30° of the visual field, are most commonly used. Most perimeters are also capable of testing the full field of vision.

Visual field loss

Visual field loss may occur due to disease or disorders of the eye, optic nerve, or brain. Classically, there are four types of visual field defects:

1. Altitudinal field defects, loss of vision above or below the horizontal—associated with ocular abnormalities.
2. Bitemporal hemianopia, loss of vision at the sides.
3. Central scotoma, loss of central vision.
4. Homonymous hemianopia, loss at one side in both eyes—defect behind optic chiasm.

In humans, confrontational testing and other forms of perimetry are used to detect and measure visual field loss. Different neurological difficulties cause characteristic forms of visual disturbances, including hemianopsias, quadrantanopsia, and others.

Intraocular pressure

Intraocular pressure (IOP) can be measured by Tonometry devices designed to measure the outflow (and resistance to outflow) of the aqueous humour from the eye. Diaton Tonometry can measure IOP though the Eyelid

Ophthalmoscopy

Ophthalmoscopic examination may include visually magnified inspection of the internal eye structures and also assessment of the quality of the eye's red reflex.

Ophthalmoscopy allows the one to look directly at the retina and other tissue at the back of the eye.

This is best done after the pupil has been dilated with eye drops. A limited view can be obtained through an undilated pupil, in which case best results are obtained with the room darkened and the patient looking towards the far corner.

The appearance of the optic disc and retinal vasculature are the main focus of examination during ophthalmoscopy. Anomalies in the appearance of these internal ocular structures may indicate eye disease or condition.

A red reflex can be seen when looking at a patient's pupil through a direct ophthalmoscope. This part of the examination is done from a distance of about 50 cm and is usually symmetrical between the two eyes. An opacity may indicate a cataract.

Slit-lamp

Close inspection of the anterior eye structures and ocular adnexa are often done with a slit lamp machine. A small beam of light that can be varied in width, height, incident angle, orientation and colour, is passed over the eye. Often, this light beam is narrowed into a vertical 'slit', during slit-lamp examination. The examiner views the illuminated ocular structures, through an optical system that magnifies the image of the eye.

This allows inspection of all the ocular media, from cornea to vitreous, plus magnified view of eyelids, and other external ocular related structures. Fluorescein staining before slit lamp examination may reveal corneal abrasions or herpes simplex infection. The binocular slit-lamp examination provides stereoscopic magnified view of the eye structures in striking detail, enabling exact anatomical diagnoses to be made for a variety of eye conditions.

Amsler grid

The Amsler grid, is a grid of horizontal and vertical lines used to monitor a person's central visual field. The grid was developed by Marc Amsler, a Swiss ophthalmologist. It is a diagnostic tool that aids in the detection of visual disturbances caused by changes in the retina, particularly the macula (e.g. macular degeneration, Epiretinal membrane), as well as the optic nerve and the visual pathway to the brain (Fig. 7.16).

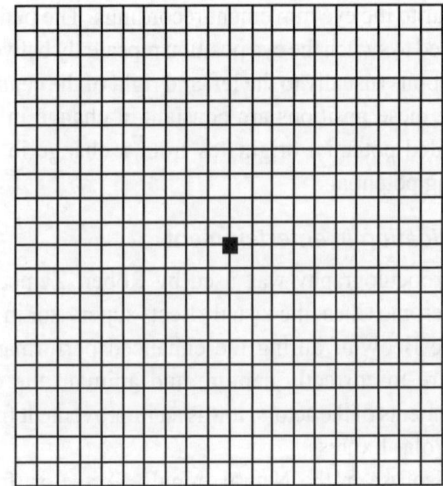

Fig. 7.16. An Amsler grid, as seen by a person with normal vision.

In the test, the person looks with each eye separately at the small dot in the centre of the grid. Patients with macular disease may see wavy lines or some lines may be missing. Amsler grids can be obtained from an ophthal-mologist or optometrist and may be used to test one's vision at home.

The original Amsler grid was black and white. A colour version with a blue and yellow grid is more sensitive and can be used to test for a wide variety of visual pathway abnormalities, including those associated with the retina, the optic nerve, and the pituitary gland (Fig. 7.17).

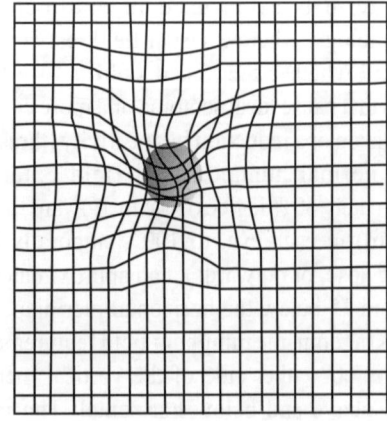

Fig. 7.17. An Amsler grid, as it might be viewed by a person with age related macular degeneration.

Ophthalmoscopy

Ophthalmoscopy is a test that allows a health professional to see inside the fundus of the eye and other structures using an Opthalmoscope. It is done as part of an eye examination and may be done as part of a routine physical examination. The invention of the opthalmoscope in 1850 by Hermann Von Helmholtz revoulutionised opthalmology.

It is of two major types: (i) direct ophthalmoscopy, and (ii) indirect ophthalmoscopy (Table 7.1).

Ophthalmoscope

The ophthalmoscope (or funduscope) is an instrument used to examine the eye. Its use is crucial in determining the health of the retina and the vitreous humour (Fig. 7.18).

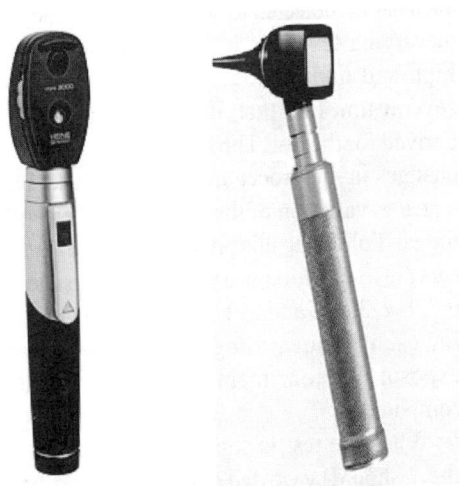

Fig. 7.18. Ophthalmoscope (left) and otoscope combination.

In patients with headaches, the finding of swollen optic discs, or papilledema, on ophthalmoscopy is a key sign, as this indicates raised intracranial pressure (ICP) which could be due to hydrocephalus, benign intracranial hypertension (aka pseudotumour cerebri) or brain tumour, amongst other conditions. Cupped optic discs are seen in glaucoma.

In patients with diabetes mellitus, regular ophthalmoscopic eye examinations (once every 6 months to 1 year) are important to screen for diabetic retinopathy as visual loss due to diabetes can be prevented by retinal laser treatment if retinopathy is spotted early.

In arterial hypertension, hypertensive changes of the retina closely mimic those in the brain, and may predict cerebrovascular accidents (strokes).

EAR AND AUDIOMETRY

Ear

The ear is the organ that detects sound. The vertebrate ear shows a common biology from fish to humans, with variations in structure according to order and species. It not only acts as a receiver for sound, but also plays a major role in the sense of balance and body position. The ear is part of the auditory system. Figure 7.19 shows human ear.

The word 'ear' may be used correctly to describe the entire organ or just the visible portion. In most animals, the visible ear is a flap of tissue that is also called the pinna and is the first of many steps in hearing. In people, the pinna is often called the

Table 7.1. Two major types of ophthalmoscopy.

Features	Direct ophthalmoscopy	Indirect ophthalmoscopy
Condensing Lens	Not Required	Required
Examination Distance	As close to patient's eye as possible	At an arm's length
Image	Virtual, Erect	Real, inverted
Illumination	Not so bright; so not useful in hazy media	Bright; so useful for hazy media
Area of field in focus	About 2 disc diopters	About 8 disc diopters
Stereopsis	Absent	Present
Accessible fundus view	Slightly beyond equator	Up to Ora serrata, i.e. peripheral retina
Examination through hazy media	Not possible	Possible

auricle. Vertebrates have a pair of ears, placed symmetrically on opposite sides of the face. This arrangement aids in the ability to localise sound sources.

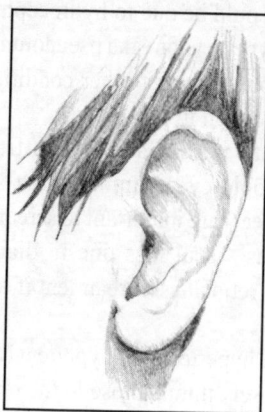

Fig. 7.19. Human ear.

Audiometry

Audiometry is the testing of hearing ability. Typically, audiometric tests determine a subject's hearing levels with the help of an audiometer, but may also measure ability to discriminate between different sound intensities, recognise pitch, or distinguished speech from background noise. Acoustic reflex and otoacoustic emissions may also be measured. Results of audiometric tests are used to diagnose hearing loss or diseases of the ear, and often make use of an Audiogram.

The most commonly used assessment of hearing is the determination of the threshold of audibility, i.e. the level of sound required to be just audible. This level can vary for an individual over a range of up to 5 dB from day to day and from determination to determination, but it provides an additional and useful tool in monitoring the potential ill effects of exposure to noise. Before carrying out a hearing test, it is important to obtain information about the person's past medical history, not only concerning the ears but also other conditions which may have a bearing on possible hearing loss detected by an audiometric test. The hearing loss is usually bilateral, but variations in each ear have been observed. Wax in the ear can also cause hearing loss, so the ear should be examined to see if syringing is needed; also to determine if the eardrum has suffered any damage which may reduce the ability of sound to be transported to the cochlea. The audiometric test can be carried out using automatic or manual audiometers, but the essential test procedure is the same.

The subject is asked to remove anything which might upset the test results, e.g. spectacles, earrings, hearing aids.

Instructions are given about the test procedure and the subject is required to indicate whether he/she can just hear or cannot hear a certain sound (the sound level may be increased from a very low level or reduced from a high level).

Earphones are fitted carefully over the ears and the test is then carried out on each ear.

Firstly, a threshold test is undertaken in which each ear is subjected to sound at a frequency of 1 kHz at varying levels of intensity ranging from low to high and high to low. The procedure is repeated several times so that an average threshold can be derived for the test. Thresholds can vary due to slight changes in the procedures adopted in setting up the test, e.g. variation of the position of the earphone on the ear. Following this pre-check, both of the subject's ears are tested through a range of frequencies (usually 0.5, 1, 2, 3, 4, 6 and 8 kHz) and hearing loss recorded for each frequency, again via a series of sound exposures. From them an average result can be computed.

When the test is completed, a second threshold check should be carried out to see that no errors have crept in during the test. Both threshold checks should agree within a maximum of 10 dB. If they do not, a re-test must be performed. The accuracy of audiometry can be affected by four main factors:

Technical limitations - how accurately can either the frequency or the hearing level be determined?

Learning effect — the first ear tested sometimes appears worse than the second one since the individual becomes more proficient at detecting the threshold.

Headphone fit — some of the variation in threshold measurement has been attributed to differences in the location of the headphones, which in turn affect the detection of the threshold.

Background noise — audiometric tests should be carried out in a soundproof chamber to eliminate external sounds from influencing the test.

A further complication of audiometric testing is that it is subjective and relies on the cooperation of the subject. If the subject is unable or unwilling to co-operate with the test then unrepresentative results will be obtained.

The technique described above enables a comparison the threshold of hearing of the individual undergoing audiometry with a reference value at a range of octave band frequencies (125, 250, 500, 1000, 2000, 4000, 8000 Hz). From this data a pictorial representation, an audiogram, of hearing loss at various frequencies is produced.

Pure tone audiometry

Pure tone audiometry (PTA) is the key hearing test used to identify hearing threshold levels of an individual, enabling determination of the degree, type and configuration of a hearing loss. Thus, providing the basis for diagnosis and management. PTA is a subjective, behavioural measurement of hearing threshold, as it relies on patient response to pure tone stimuli. Therefore, PTA is used on adults and children old enough to cooperate with the test procedure. As with most clinical tests, calibration of the test environment, the equipment and the stimuli to ISO standards is needed before testing proceeds. PTA only measures thresholds, rather than other aspects of hearing such as sound localisation. However, there are benefits of using PTA over other forms of hearing test, such as click auditory brainstem response. PTA provides ear specific thresholds, and uses frequency specific pure tones to give place specific responses, so that the configuration of a hearing loss can be identified. As PTA uses both air and bone conduction audiometry, the type of loss can also be identified via the air-bone gap. Although PTA has many clinical benefits, it is not perfect at identifying all losses, such as 'dead regions'. This raises the question of whether or not audiograms accurately predict someone's perceived degree of disability. Figure 7.20 showing schematic diagram of the human ear.

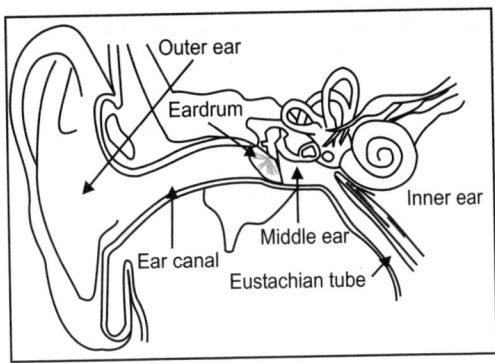

Fig. 7.20. Schematic diagram of the human ear.

Otoscope

An Otoscope or auriscope is a medical device which is used to look into the ears. Health care providers use otoscopes to screen for illness during regular check-ups and also to investigate when a symptom involves the ears. With an otoscope, it is possible to see the outer ear and middle ear.

Otoscopes consist of a handle and a head. The head contains an electric light source and a low power magnifying lens. The front end of the otoscope has an attachment for disposable plastic ear speculums. The examiner first straightens the ear canal by pulling on the pinna and then inserts the ear speculum side of the otoscope into the external ear. The examiner can then look through a lens on the rear of the instrument and see inside the ear canal. Many models have a detachable sliding rear window which allows the examiner to insert instruments through the otoscope into the ear canal, such as for removing earwax (cerumen). Most models also have an insertion point for a bulb capable of pushing air through the speculum which is called pneumatic otoscope. This puff of air allows an examiner to test the mobility of the tympanic membrane.

Many otoscopes used in doctors offices are wall-mounted, while others are portable. Wall-mounted otoscopes are attached by a flexible power cord to a base, which serves to hold the otoscope when it's not in use and also serves as a source of electric power, being plugged into an electric outlet. Portable models are powered by batteries in the handle; these batteries are usually rechargeable and can be recharged from a base unit. Otoscopes are often sold with ophthalmoscopes as a diagnostic set.

Diseases which may be diagnosed by an otoscope include otitis media and otitis externa, infection of the middle and outer parts of the ear, respectively.

Otoscopes are also frequently used for examining patients' noses (avoiding the need for a separate nasal speculum) and (with the speculum removed) upper throats.

MUSCLE

Muscle is the contractile tissue of animals and is derived from the mesodermal layer of embryonic germ cells. Muscle cells contain contractile filaments that move past each other and change the size of the cell. They are classified as skeletal, cardiac, or smooth muscles. Their function is to produce force and cause motion. Muscles can cause either locomotion of the organism itself or movement of internal organs. Cardiac and smooth muscle contraction occurs without conscious thought and is necessary for survival. Examples are the contraction of the heart and peristalsis which pushes food through the digestive system. Voluntary contraction of the skeletal muscles is used to move the body and can be finely controlled.

Examples are movements of the eye, or gross movements like the quadriceps muscle of the thigh. There are two broad types of voluntary muscle fibres: slow twitch and fast twitch. Slow twitch fibres contract for long periods of time but with little force while fast twitch fibres contract quickly and powerfully but fatigue very rapidly. A top-down view of skeletal muscle is shown in Fig. 7.21.

Muscles are predominately powered by the oxidation of fats and carbohydrates, but anaerobic chemical reactions are also used, particularly by fast twitch fibres. These chemical reactions produce adenosine triphosphate (ATP) molecules which are used to power the movement of the myosin heads.

Electromyography

Electromyography (EMG) is a technique for evaluating and recording the electrical activity produced by skeletal muscles. EMG is performed

using an instrument called an electromyograph, to produce a record called an electromyogram. An electromyograph detects the electrical potential generated by muscle cells when these cells are electrically or neurologically activated. The signals can be analysed to detect medical abnormalities, activation level, recruitment order or to analyse the biomechanics of human or animal movement.

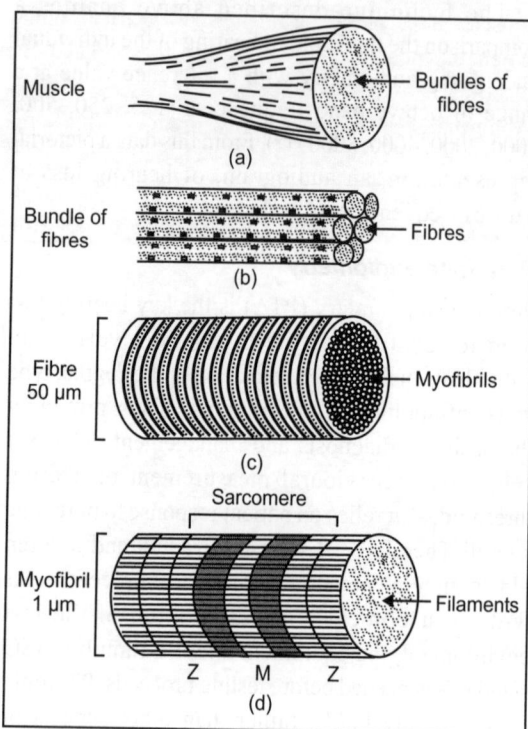

Fig. 7.21. A top-down view of skeletal muscle.

The electrical source is the muscle membrane potential of about -90 mV. Measured EMG potentials range between less than 50 μV and up to 20 to 30 mV, depending on the muscle under observation.

Typical repetition rate of muscle motor unit firing is about 7–20 Hz, depending on the size of the muscle (eye muscles versus seat (gluteal) muscles), previous axonal damage and other factors. Damage to motor units can be expected at ranges between 450 and 780 mV.

Procedure

There are two kinds of EMG in widespread use: surface EMG and intramuscular (needle and fine-wire) EMG. To perform intramuscular EMG, a needle electrode or a needle containing two fine-wire electrodes is inserted through the skin into the muscle tissue. A trained professional (most often a physiatrist, neurologist, or chiropractor) observes the electrical activity while inserting the electrode. The insertional activity provides valuable information about the state of the muscle and its innervating nerve. Normal muscles at rest make certain, normal electrical sounds when the needle is inserted into them. Then the electrical activity when the muscle is at rest is studied. Abnormal spontaneous activity might indicate some nerve and/or muscle damage. Then the patient is asked to contract the muscle smoothly. The shape, size and frequency of the resulting motor unit potentials is judged. Then the electrode is retracted a few millimeters, and again the activity is analysed until at least 10–20 units have been collected. Each electrode track gives only a very local picture of the activity of the whole muscle. Because skeletal muscles differ in the inner structure, the electrode has to be placed at various locations to obtain an accurate study.

Intramuscular EMG may be considered too invasive or unnecessary in some cases. Instead, a surface electrode may be used to monitor the general picture of muscle activation, as opposed to the activity of only a few fibres as observed using a intramuscular EMG. This technique is used in a number of settings; for example, in the physiotherapy clinic, muscle activation is monitored using surface EMG and patients have an auditory or visual stimulus to help them know when they are activating the muscle (biofeedback).

A motor unit is defined as one motor neuron and all of the muscle fibres it innervates. When a motor unit fires, the impulse (called an action potential) is carried down the motor neuron to the muscle. The area where the nerve contacts the muscle is called the neuromuscular junction, or the motor end plate. After the action potential is transmitted across the neuromuscular junction, an action potential is elicited in all of the innervated muscle fibres of that particular motor unit. The sum of all this electrical activity is known as a motor unit action potential (MUAP). This electrophysiologic activity from multiple motor units is the signal typically evaluated during an EMG. The composition of the motor unit, the number of muscle fibres per motor unit, the metabolic type of muscle fibres and many other factors affect the shape of the motor unit potentials in the myogram.

Nerve conduction testing is also often done at the same time as an EMG to diagnose neurological diseases. Some patients can find the procedure somewhat painful, whereas others experience only a small amount of discomfort when the needle is inserted. The muscle or muscles being tested may be slightly sore for a day or two after the procedure.

Normal results

Muscle tissue at rest is normally electrically inactive. After the electrical activity caused by the irritation of needle insertion subsides, the electromyograph should detect no abnormal spontaneous activity (i.e. a muscle at rest should be electrically silent, with the exception of the area of the neuromuscular junction, which is, under normal circumstances, very spontaneously active). When the muscle is voluntarily contracted, action potentials begin to appear. As the strength of the muscle contraction is increased, more and more muscle fibres produce action potentials. When the muscle is fully contracted, there should appear a disorderly group of action potentials of varying rates and amplitudes (a complete recruitment and interference pattern).

Abnormal results

EMG is used to diagnose two general categories of disease: neuropathies and myopathies.

Neuropathic disease has the following defining EMG characteristics:

1. An action potential amplitude that is twice normal due to the increased number of fibres per motor unit because of reinnervation of denervated fibres.
2. An increase in duration of the action potential.

3. A decrease in the number of motor units in the muscle (as found using motor unit number estimation techniques).

Myopathic disease has these defining EMG characteristics:

1. A decrease in duration of the action potential.
2. A reduction in the area to amplitude ratio of the action potential.
3. A decrease in the number of motor units in the muscle (in extremely severe cases only).

Because of the individuality of each patient and disease, some of these characteristics may not appear in every case. EMG signals are used in many clinical and biomedical applications. EMG is used as a diagnostics tool for identifying neuromuscular diseases, assessing low-back pain, kinesiology, and disorders of motor control. EMG signals are also used as a control signal for prosthetic devices such as prosthetic hands, arms, and lower limbs.

8

Heart and Circulation

INTRODUCTION

Cardiovascular disease or cardiovascular diseases is the class of diseases that involve the heart or blood vessels (arteries and veins). While the term technically refers to any disease that affects the cardiovascular system (as used in MeSH), it is usually used to refer to those related to atherosclerosis (arterial disease). These conditions have similar causes, mechanisms, and treatments. In practice, cardiovascular disease is treated by cardiologists, thoracic surgeons, vascular surgeons, neurologists, and interventional radiologists, depending on the organ system that is being treated. There is considerable overlap in the specialities, and it is common for certain procedures to be performed by different types of specialists in different hospitals.

By the time that heart problems are detected, the underlying cause (atherosclerosis) is usually quite advanced, having progressed for decades. There is therefore increased emphasis on preventing atherosclerosis by modifying risk factors, such as healthy eating, exercise and avoidance of smoking.

CARDIAC ANATOMY AND PHYSIOLOGY

The human heart is a hollow muscular organ, nearly the size of a closed fist, that weighs approximately 300 grams in the adult male and 250 grams in the adult female. Weight and size varies depending on age, sex, height, nutritional status, and epicardial fat. The heart lies within the central area of the thoracic cavity, in the mediastinal space, with two thirds of it extending to the left of midline. The heart is an inverted cone-shaped organ that tilts forward and to the left within the thoracic cavity. The apex of the cone lies inferiorly and the great vessels (i.e. superior vena cava, inferior vena cava) enter the base of the cone superiorly. The apex lies between the fifth and sixth ribs when one is lying down and between the sixth and seventh ribs when one is sitting or standing.

Pericardium. The heart is enclosed in a double-walled, fibroserous, inelastic sac called the pericardium. The outer fibrous layer of the pericardium is attached to the great vessels, the sternum, and diaphragm. This fibrous layer of the pericardium is very resistant to distention and helps to prevent dilation of the heart. The inner serous layer consists of a visceral and parietal portion. The visceral portion, also known as the epicardium, covers the entire heart and great vessels and folds over to form the parietal pericardium. The parietal portion also lines the fibrous pericardium.

The pericardial cavity is a potential space between the parietal and visceral pericardium. It normally contains 30 to 50 ml of serous fluid that acts as a lubricant to decrease friction as the heart contracts and relaxes. The pericardial cavity can hold up to one litre of fluid in some chronic diseases without compromising the heart. If the buildup of fluid occurs gradually, the pericardium can stretch without affecting the heart. If the fluid accumulates rapidly, however, even small amounts (i.e. 50 ml to 100 ml) can cause compression of the heart (i.e. cardiac tamponade).

The pressure of a cardiac effusion can equal diastolic pressure within the heart chambers and interfere with filling. The right atrium and ventricle are affected first because the pressure in these chambers is lower than the pressure on the left side of the heart. Disruption in cardiac filling occurs first in the right atria and leads to increased venous pressure and systemic congestion. Signs of right heart failure are distention of the jugular veins, edema, and hepatomegaly. Decreased atrial filling leads to inadequate filling, reduced cardiac output, and potential circulatory collapse. Pulsus paradoxus, in which arterial blood pressure during expiration exceeds arterial pressure during inspiration by more than 10 mm Hg, is a key indicator of cardiac tamponade. Normally, inspiration has little effect on cardiac flow or volume. A 'water bottle' cardiac silhouette on a chest X-ray, dyspnea on exertion, dull chest pain, and muffled heart sounds are other signs of cardiac tamponade.

The parietal pericardium is innervated by the phrenic nerve, which contains pain fibres; however, the visceral pericardium is insensitive to pain. The fibrous pericardium anchors the heart to the great veins and arteries at its base. It anchors the heart to the sternum anteriorly and to the diaphragm inferiorly. The pericardium receives its blood supply through branches of the internal thoracic arteries and phrenic arteries. Venous drainage is through the azygous and pericardiophrenic veins.

Layers of the heart. The heart wall consists of three layers. The outermost layer of the heart, the epicardium, also known as the visceral pericardium, consists of epithelial cells that form a serous membrane that covers the entire heart. The innermost layer of the heart is known as the endocardium. It is a serous membrane that lines the inner surface of the heart, its valves, and the chordae tendineae, which are the cords that connect the free edges of the atrioventricular valves with the papillary muscles. The papillary muscles are muscle eminences on the walls of the ventricles. The endocardium is continuous with the intima (e.g. the inner lining of arteries).

The middle layer of the heart is the muscular layer known as the myocardium. It is responsible for the major pumping action of the ventricles. The myocardial cells have an intrinsic ability to contract in the absence of stimuli (i.e. automaticity) and in a rhythmic manner (i.e. rhythmicity), and to transmit nerve impulses (i.e. conductivity). The myocardium does not undergo mitotic activity and cannot replace injured cells.

Heart chambers: The heart has four chambers, two atria and two ventricles. It is helpful to look at each chamber in the order in which blood flows within the heart: right atrium to the right ventricle, from the lungs into the left atrium, and finally into the left ventricle.

Right atrium. The right atrium has a thin muscle wall. It receives deoxygenated (i.e. venous) blood from the head and upper extremities via the superior vena cava, from the trunk and lower extremities via the inferior vena cava, and from the coronary sinus, which drains blood from the myocardium. The coronary sinus empties into the right atrium just above the tricuspid valve. Most blood flow into the right atrium occurs during inspiration when right atrium pressure drops below that in the inferior and superior venae cavae, causing the blood to flow from an area of higher to lower pressure. There are no true valves in the venae cavae; thus, when right atrium pressure rises, congestion occurs in the systemic circulation. Normal filling pressure for the fight atrium ranges from 0 to 8 mm Hg.

Right ventricle: The right ventricle may be divided into the body of the right ventricle (i.e. an inflow region consisting of the tricuspid valve, the chordae tendineae, the papillary muscle, and a heavily trabeculated myocardium), and the infundibulum, a smooth outflow region. The inflow and outflow portions of the fight ventricle are separated by four muscular bands: the infundibulum septum, the parietal band, the septal band, and the moderator band. The infundibulum septum and parietal band make up the crista supraventricularis, blood flows around the crista supraventricularis and is mixed by passing through the strands of the trabeculae carnae.

The right ventricle receives blood from the right atrium through the tricuspid valve and ejects it through the pulmonic valve into the pulmonary artery where it travels to the lungs. The resistance of the pulmonary circulation is approximately one tenth that of the systemic circulation. In addition, the vascular pathways of the lungs offer very low resistance to ejection pressure; therefore, very little pressure is needed to pump blood to the lungs. Normal systolic pressure in the right ventricle ranges from 15 to 28 mm Hg and end-diastolic pressure is 0 to 8 mm Hg. The fight ventricle generates less than one fourth the stroke work of the left ventricle.

Left atrium. The left atrium receives oxygenated (i.e. arterial) blood from the lungs through the right and left inferior and superior pulmonary veins. The wall of the left atrium is slightly thicker than that of the right atrium and breathing does not affect its filling. Normal filling pressure ranges from 4 to 12 mm Hg.

Left ventricle: The left ventricle has a thick muscular wall. It receives blood from the left atrium through the mitral valve and ejects it through the aortic valve to the systemic circulation via the aorta. Pressure in the left ventricle is high. Normal systolic pressure is 90 to 140 mm Hg and normal end-diastolic pressure is 4 to 12 mm Hg. The ventricular septum, a thick muscular area that becomes membranous as it nears the atrioventricular (AV) valves, separates the right and left ventricles. It houses electrical conduction tissue and provides stability for the ventricles during contraction.

The primary function of the heart is to pump blood through blood vessels to the body's cells. Imagine a simple machine like a water pump working for perhaps 70 or more years without attention and without stopping. Impossible? Yet this is exactly what the heart can do in our bodies. The heart is really a muscular bag surrounding four hollow compartments, with a thin wall of muscle separating the left hand side from the right hand side. The muscles in the heart are very strong because they have to work harder than any of the other muscles in our body, pushing the blood to our head and feet continuously.

The blood flow around our body is called our circulation. The heart connects the two major portions of the circulation's continuous circuit, the systemic circulation and the pulmonary circulation. The blood vessels in the pulmonary circulation carry the blood through the lungs to pick up oxygen and get rid of carbon dioxide, while the blood vessels in the systemic circulation carry the blood throughout the rest of our body (Fig. 8.1).

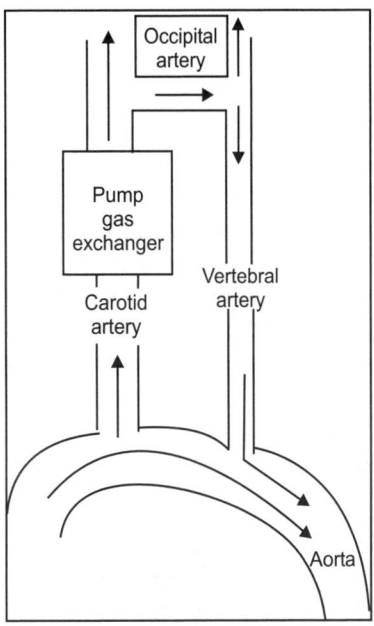

Fig. 8.1. Representation of the circulation.

The heart actually has two separate sides, one designed to pump deoxygenated blood into the pulmonary circulation where the blood becomes oxygenated, and one designed to pump the oxygenated blood into the systemic circulation where the blood flows throughout the body (Fig. 8.2). Each side of the heart has two chambers or compartments. The top chamber on each side is called the atrium. The right atrium receives incoming deoxygenated blood from the body and the left atrium receives incoming oxygenated blood from the lungs. The thin-walled atrium on each side bulges as it fills with blood, and as the lower heart muscle relaxes, the atrium contracts and squeezes the blood into a second chamber, the thick muscular ventricle. The ventricle is the pumping chamber that, with each muscular contraction, pushes the blood forcefully out and into the lungs (right ventricle) and the rest of the body (left ventricle).

The atrium and ventricle on each side of the heart are separated by tissue flaps called valves. The structure of these valves prevents blood from flowing backward into the atrium as the ventricle squeezes blood out. The valve on the right side, between the atrium and the ventricle, is called the tricuspid valve. The valve on the left side, between the atrium and the ventricle, is called the bicuspid or mitral valve. There are two other important valves that help to keep the blood rowing in the proper direction. These two valves are located at the two points where blood exits the heart. The pulmonary valve is located between the right ventricle and the pulmonary artery that carries the deoxygenated blood from the heart to the lungs, and the aortic valve is located between the left ventricle and the aorta, the major artery that carries the oxygenated blood from the heart to the rest of the body.

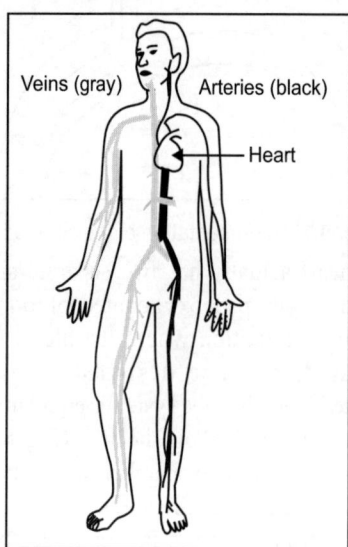

Fig. 8.2. The cardiovascular system.

The arteries are the blood vessels that transport blood out of the heart under high pressure to the tissues. The arterioles are the last small branch of the arterial system through which blood is released into the capillaries. The capillaries are very small, thin-walled blood vessels where the exchange of gases, nutrients, and waste takes place between the cells and the blood. Blood flows with almost no resistance in the larger blood vessels, but in the arterioles and capillaries, considerable resistance to flow does occur because these vessels are so small

in diameter that the blood must squeeze all its contents through them. The venules collect blood from the capillaries and gradually feed into progressively larger veins. The veins transport the blood from the tissues back to the heart. The walls of the veins are thin and very elastic and can fold or expand to act as a reservoir for extra blood, if required by the needs of the body.

Heart Valve

In anatomy, the heart valves maintain the unidirectional flow of blood in the heart by opening and closing depending on the difference in pressure on each side. They are mechanically similar to reed valves.

There are four valves in the heart (not counting the valve of the coronary sinus, and the valve of the inferior vena cava) (Fig. 8.3):

1. The two atrioventricular (AV) valves between the atria and the ventricles.
2. The two semilunar (SL) valves, in the arteries leaving the heart.

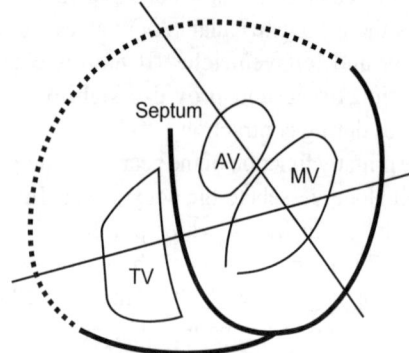

Fig. 8.3. Explanation of the echocardiogram. MV: Mitral valve, TV: Tricuspid valve, AV: Aortic valve, Septum: Interventricular septum. Continuous lines demarcate septum and free wall seen in echocardiogram, dotted line is a suggestion of where the free wall of the right ventricle should be.

Atrioventricular valves

These are small valves that prevent backflow from the ventricles into the atria during systole. They are anchored to the wall of the ventricle by chordae tendineae, which prevent the valve from inverting.

The chordae tendineae are attached to papillary muscles that cause tension to better hold the valve. Together, the papillary muscles and the chordae tendineae are known as the subvalvular apparatus. The function of the subvalvular apparatus is to keep the valves from prolapsing into the atria when they close. The subvalvular apparatus have no effect on the opening and closure of the valves, however. This is caused entirely by the pressure gradient across the valve. The closure of the AV valves is heard as the first heart sound (S1).

Bicuspid valve

Also known as the mitral valve contains two flaps. The bicuspid valve gets its name from the resemblance to a bishop's mitre (a type of hat). It allows the blood to flow from the left atrium into the left ventricle. It is on the left side of the heart and has two cusps.

A common complication of rheumatic fever is thickening and stenosis of the mitral valve.

Tricuspid valve

The tricuspid valve is the three flapped valve on the right side of the heart, between the right atrium and the right ventricle which stops the backflow of blood between the two. It has three cusps.

Semilunar valves

These are located at the base of both the pulmonary trunk (pulmonary artery) and the aorta, the two arteries taking blood out of the ventricles. These valves permit blood to be forced into the arteries, but prevent backflow of blood from the arteries into the ventricles. These valves do not have chordae tendineae, and are more similar to valves in veins than atrioventricular valves.

Aortic valve

The aortic valve lies between the left ventricle and the aorta. The aortic valve has three cusps. During ventricular systole, pressure rises in the left ventricle. When the pressure in the left ventricle rises above the pressure in the aorta, the aortic valve opens, allowing blood to exit the left ventricle into the aorta. When ventricular systole ends, pressure in the left ventricle rapidly drops. When the pressure in the left ventricle decreases, the aortic pressure forces the aortic valve to close. The closure of the aortic valve contributes the A2 component of the second heart sound (S2).

The most common congenital abnormality of the heart is the bicuspid aortic valve. In this condition, instead of three cusps, the aortic valve has two cusps. This condition is often undiagnosed until the person develops calcific aortic stenosis. Aortic stenosis occurs in this condition usually in patients in their 40s or 50s, an average of over 10 years earlier than in people with normal aortic valves.

Pulmonary valve

The pulmonary valve (sometimes referred to as the pulmonic valve) is the semilunar valve of the heart that lies between the right ventricle and the pulmonary artery and has three cusps. Similar to the aortic valve, the pulmonary valve opens in ventricular systole, when the pressure in the right ventricle rises above the pressure in the pulmonary artery. At the end of ventricular systole, when the pressure in the right ventricle falls rapidly, the pressure in the pulmonary artery will close the pulmonary valve.

The closure of the pulmonary valve contributes the P2 component of the second heart sound (S2). The right heart is a low-pressure system, so the P2 component of the second heart sound is usually softer than the A2 component of the second heart sound. However, it is physiologically normal in some young people to hear both components separated during inhalation.

Cardiac Cycle

Cardiac cycle is the term referring to all or any of the events related to the flow or blood pressure that occurs from the beginning of one heartbeat to the beginning of the next. The frequency of the cardiac cycle is the heart rate. Every single 'beat' of the heart involves five major stages: First, 'late diastole' which is when the semilunar valves close, the AV valves open and the whole heart is relaxed. Second, 'Atrial systole' when atria is contracting, AV valves open and blood flows from atrium to the ventricle. Third, 'isovolumic ventricular contraction' it is when the ventricles begin to contract, AV valves close, as well as the semilunar valves and there is no change in volume. Fourth, 'ventricular ejection', Ventricles are empty, they are still contracting and the semilunar valves are open. The fifth stage is: 'Isovolumic ventricular relaxation', Pressure decreases, no blood is entering the ventricles, ventricles stop contracting and begin to relax, semilunars are shut because blood in the aorta is pushing them shut. Throughout the cardiac cycle, the blood pressure increases and decreases. The cardiac cycle (Fig. 8.4) is coordinated by a series of electrical impulses that are produced by specialised heart cells found within the sino-atrial node and the atrioventricular node. The cardiac muscle is composed of myocytes which initiate their own contraction without help of external nerves (with the exception of modifying the heart rate due to metabolic demand). Under normal circumstances, each cycle takes approximately one second.

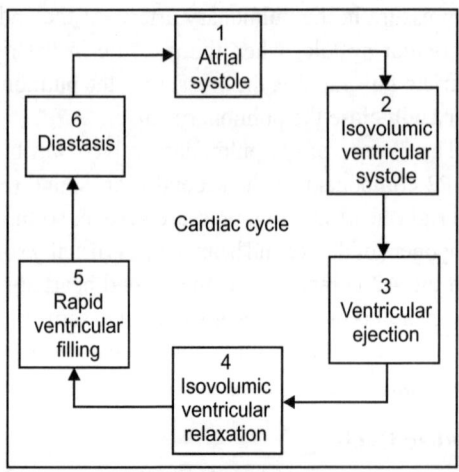

Fig. 8.4. Cardiac cycle.

Atrial systole

Atrial systole is the contraction of the heart muscle (myocardia) of the left and right atria. Normally, both atria contract at the same time. The term systole is synonymous with contraction (movement or shortening) of a muscle. Electrical systole is the electrical activity that stimulates the myocardium of the chambers of the heart to make them contract. This is soon followed by Mechanical systole, which is the

mechanical contraction of the heart. As the atria contract, the blood pressure in each atrium increases, forcing additional blood into the ventricles. The additional flow of blood is called atrial kick.

70 per cent of the blood flows passively down to the ventricles, so the atria do not have to contract a great amount.

Atrial kick is absent if there is loss of normal electrical conduction in the heart, such as during atrial fibrillation, atrial flutter, and complete heart block. Atrial kick is also different in character depending on the condition of the heart, such as stiff heart, which is found in patients with diastolic dysfunction.

Detection of atrial systole

Electrical systole of the atria begins with the onset of the P wave on the ECG. The wave of bipolarisation (or depolarisation) that stimulates both atria to contract at the same time is due to sinoatrial node which is located on the upper wall of the right atrium. 30 per cent of the ventricles are filled during this phase.

Ventricular systole

Ventricular systole is the contraction of the muscles (myocardia) of the left and right ventricles (Fig. 8.5).

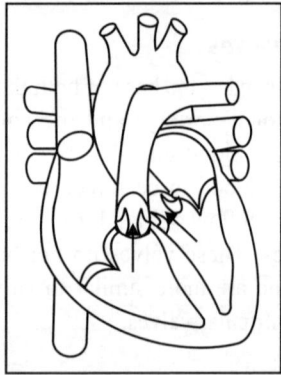

Fig. 8.5. Ventricular systole.

At the later part of the ejection phase, although the ventricular pressure falls below the aortic pressure, the aortic valve remains patent because of the inertial energy of the ejected blood.

The graph of aortic pressure throughout the cardiac cycle displays a small dip which coincides with the aortic valve closure. The dip in the graph is immediately followed by a brief rise then gradual decline. The small rise in the graph is known as the 'dicrotic notch' or 'incisure', and represents a transient increase in aortic pressure. Just as the ventricles enter into diastole, the brief reversal of flow from the aorta back into the left ventricle causes the aortic valves to shut. This results in the slight increase in aortic pressure caused by the elastic recoil of the semilunar valves and aorta.

Electrocardiography

Electrocardiography (ECG or EKG) is a transthoracic interpretation of the electrical activity of the heart over time captured and externally recorded by skin electrodes. It is a noninvasive recording produced by an electrocardiographic device. Figure 8.6 shows the image showing a patient conneted to the 10 electrodes necessary for a 12-lead ECG.

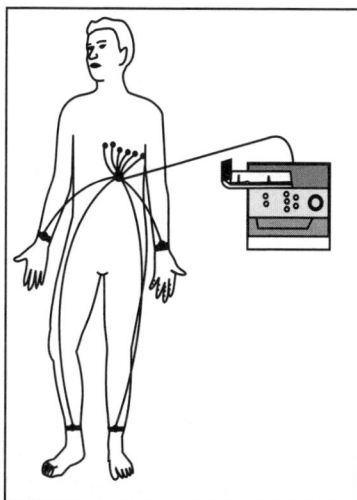

Fig. 8.6. The image showing a patient conneted to the 10 electrodes necessary for a 12-lead ECG.

Electrical impulses in the heart originate in the sinoatrial node and travel through the intimate conducting system to the heart muscle. The impulses stimulate the myocardial muscle fibres to contract and thus induce systole. The electrical waves can be measured at electrodes placed at specific points on the skin. Electrodes on different sides of the heart measure the activity of different parts of the heart muscle. An ECG displays the voltage between pairs of these electrodes, and the muscle activity that they measure, from different directions, can also be understood as vectors.

This display indicates the overall rhythm of the heart and weaknesses in different parts of the heart muscle. It is the best way to measure and diagnose abnormal rhythms of the heart, particularly abnormal rhythms caused by damage to the conductive tissue that carries electrical signals, or abnormal rhythms caused by electrolyte imbalances. In a myocardial infarction (MI), the ECG can identify if the heart muscle has been damaged in specific areas, though not all areas of the heart are covered. The ECG cannot reliably measure the pumping ability of the heart, for which ultrasound-based (echocardiography) or nuclear medicine tests are used.

Strain Gauge

A strain gauge is a device used to measure the strain of an object. The most common type of strain gauge consists of an insulating flexible backing which supports a metallic foil pattern (Fig. 8.7).

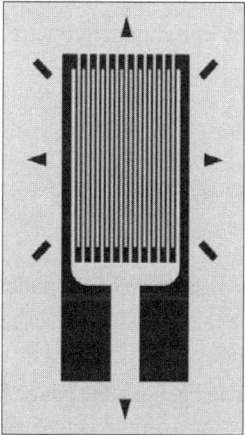

Fig. 8.7. Typical foil strain gauge. The gauge is far more sensitive to strain in the vertical direction than in the horizontal direction. The markings outside the active area help to align the gauge during installation.

The gauge is attached to the object by a suitable adhesive, such as cyanoacrylate. As the object is deformed, the foil is deformed, causing its electrical resistance to change. This resistance change, usually measured using a Wheatstone bridge, is related to the strain by the quantity known as the gauge factor.

Physical operation

A strain gauge takes advantage of the physical property of electrical conductance and its dependence on not merely the electrical conductivity of a conductor, which is a property of its material, but also the conductor's geometry. When an electrical conductor is stretched within the limits of its elasticity such that it does not break or permanently deform, it will become narrower and longer, changes that increase its electrical resistance end-to-end. Conversely, when a conductor is compressed such that it does not buckle, it will broaden and shorten, changes that decrease its electrical resistance end-to-end. From the measured electrical resistance of the strain gauge, the amount of applied stress may be inferred. A typical strain gauge arranges a long, thin conductive strip in a zig-zag pattern of parallel lines such that a small amount of stress in the direction of the orientation of the parallel lines results in a multiplicatively larger strain over the effective length of the conductor—and hence a multiplicatively larger change in resistance—than would be observed with a single straight-line conductive wire.

Gauge factor

The gauge factor GF is defined as:

$$GF = \frac{\Delta R / R_G}{\varepsilon}$$

where,

R_G is the resistance of the undeformed gauge.
ΔR is the change in resistance caused by strain.
ε is strain.

For metallic foil gauges, the gauge factor is usually a little over 2. For a single active gauge and three dummy resistors, the output v from the bridge is:

$$v = \frac{BV \cdot GF \cdot \varepsilon}{4}$$

where,

BV is the bridge excitation voltage.

Foil gauges typically have active areas of about 2–10 mm^2 in size. With careful installation, the correct gauge, and the correct adhesive, strains up to at least 10 per cent can be measured.

Gauges in practice

Foil strain gauges are used in many situations. Different applications place different requirements on the gauge. In most cases the orientation of the strain gauge is significant. Figure 8.8 shows visualisation of the working concept behind the strain gauge on a beam under exaggerated bending.

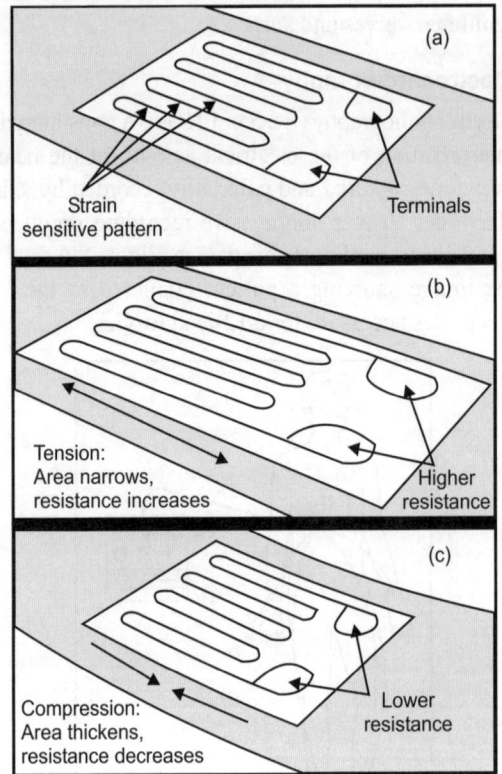

Fig. 8.8. Visualisation of the working concept behind the strain gauge on a beam under exaggerated bending.

Gauges attached to a load cell would normally be expected to remain stable over a period of years, if not decades; while those used to measure response in a dynamic experiment may only need to remain attached to the object for a few days, be energised for less than an hour, and operate for less than a second.

Strain gauge based technology is utilised commonly in the manufacture of pressure sensors. The gauges used in pressure sensors themselves are commonly made from silicon, polysilicon, metal film, thick film, and bonded foil.

Variations in temperature

Variations in temperature will cause a multitude of effects. The object will change in size by thermal expansion, which will be detected as a strain by the gauge. Resistance of the gauge will change, and resistance of the connecting wires will change.

Most strain gauges are made from a constantan alloy. Various constantan alloys and Karma alloys have been designed so that the temperature effects on the resistance of the strain gauge itself cancel out the resistance change of the gauge due to the thermal expansion of the object under test. Because different materials have different amounts of thermal expansion, self-temperature compensation (STC) requires selecting a particular alloy matched to the material of the object under test.

Even with strain gauges that are not self-temperature-compensated (such as isoelastic alloy), use of a Wheatstone bridge arrangement allows compensating for temperature changes in the specimen under test and the strain gauge. To do this in a Wheatstone bridge made of four gauges, two gauges are attached to the specimen, and two are left unattached, unstrained, and at the same temperature as the specimen and the attached gauges. (Murphy's Law was originally coined in response to a set of gauges being incorrectly wired into a Wheatstone bridge.)

Temperature effects on the lead wires can be cancelled by using a '3-wire bridge' or a '4-wire Ohm circuit' (also called a '4-wire Kelvin connection').

Other gauge types

For measurements of small strain, semiconductor strain gauges, so called piezoresistors, are often preferred over foil gauges. A semiconductor gauge usually has a larger gauge factor than a foil gauge. Semiconductor gauges tend to be more expensive, more sensitive to temperature changes, and are more fragile than foil gauges.

In biological measurements, especially blood flow/tissue swelling, a variant called mercury-in-rubber strain gauge is used. This kind of strain gauge consists of a small amount of liquid mercury enclosed in a small rubber tube, which is applied around e.g. a toe or leg. Swelling of the body part results in stretching of the tube, making it both longer and thinner, which increases electrical resistance.

Fibre optic sensing can be employed to measure strain along an optical fibre. Measurements can be distributed along the fibre, or taken at predetermined points on the fibre.

Capacitive strain gauges use a variable capacitor to indicate the level of mechanical deformation.

Catheter

In medicine, a catheter is a tube that can be inserted into a body cavity, duct, or vessel. Catheters thereby allow drainage, injection of fluids, or access by surgical instruments. The process of inserting a catheter is catheterisation. In most uses, a catheter is a thin, flexible tube (soft catheter), though in some uses, it is a larger, solid (hard) catheter. A catheter left inside the body, either temporarily or permanently, may be referred to as an indwelling catheter. A permanently inserted catheter may be referred to as a permcath (Fig. 8.9).

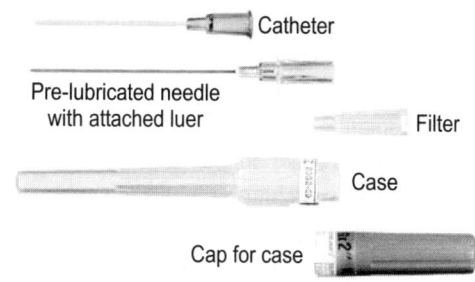

Fig. 8.9. Catheter disassembled.

Uses

Placement of a catheter into a particular part of the body may allow:

1. Draining urine from the urinary bladder as in urinary catheterisation, e.g. the Foley catheter or even when the urethra is damaged as in suprapubic catheterisation.
2. Drainage of urine from the kidney by percutaneous nephrostomy.
3. Drainage of fluid collections, e.g. an abdominal abscess.
4. Administration of intravenous fluids, medication or parenteral nutrition with a peripheral venous catheter.

5. Angioplasty, angiography, balloon septostomy, balloon sinuplasty, catheter ablation. Often the Seldinger technique is used.
6. Direct measurement of blood pressure in an artery or vein.
7. Direct measurement of intracranial pressure.
8. Administration of anaesthetic medication into the epidural space, the subarachnoid space, or around a major nerve bundle such as the brachial plexus.
9. Subcutaneous administration of insulin or other medications, with the use of an infusion set and insulin pump.
10. A central venous catheter is a conduit for giving drugs or fluids into a large-bore catheter positioned either in a vein near the heart or just inside the atrium.
11. A Swan-Ganz catheter is a special type of catheter placed into the pulmonary artery for measuring pressures in the heart.
12. An umbilical line is a catheter used in neonatal intensive care units (NICU) providing quick access to the central circulation of premature infants.
13. A Touhy borst adapter is a medical device used for attaching catheters to various other devices.
14. A Quinton catheter is a double or triple lumen, external catheter used for haemodialysis.

CARDIAC OUTPUT

Cardiac output (Q) is the volume of blood being pumped by the heart, in particular by a ventricle in a minute. This is measured in $dm^3 \, min^{-1}$ (1 dm^3 equals 1000 cm^3 or 1 litre). An average cardiac output would be 5 $L \cdot min^{-1}$ for a human male and 4.5 $L \cdot min^{-1}$ for a female.

Clinical Uses

The function of the heart is to transport the blood to deliver oxygen, nutrients and chemicals to the cells of the body to ensure their survival and proper function and to remove the cellular wastes. Q indicates how well the heart is performing this

function. Q is regulated principally by the demand for oxygen by the cells of the body. If the cells are working hard, with a high metabolic oxygen demand then the Q is raised to increase the supply of oxygen to the cells, while at rest when the cellular demand is low, the Q is said to be baseline. Q is regulated not only by the heart as it pumps, but also by the function of the vessels of the body as they actively relax and contract thereby increasing and decreasing the resistance to flow.

When Q increases in a healthy but untrained individual, most of the increase can be attributed to an increase in HR. Change of posture, increased sympathetic nervous system activity, and decreased parasympathetic nervous system activity can also increase cardiac output. HR can vary by a factor of approximately 3, between 60 and 180 beats per minute, while stroke volume (SV) can vary between 70 and 120 ml, a factor of only 1.7.

A parameter related to SV is Ejection fraction (EF). EF is the fraction of blood ejected by the left ventricle (LV) during the contraction or ejection phase of the cardiac cycle or Systole. Prior to the start of Systole, the LV is filled with blood to the capacity known as end diastolic volume (EDV) during the filling phase or diastole. During systole, the LV contracts and ejects blood until it reaches its minimum capacity known as end systolic volume (ESV), it does not empty completely. Clearly the EF is dependent on the ventricular EDV which may vary with ventricular disease associated with ventricular dilatation. Even with LV dilatation and impaired contraction the Q may remain constant due to an increase in EDV.

Stroke volume (SV) = EDV − ESV
Ejection fraction (EF) = (SV/EDV) × 100%
Cardiac output (Q) = SV × HR
Cardiac index (CI) = Q/body surface area (BSA)
= SV × HR/BSA

HR is heart rate, expressed as BPM (beats per minute).

BSA is body surface area in square metres.

Diseases of the cardiovascular system are often associated with changes in Q, particularly the pandemic diseases of hypertension and heart failure. Cardiovascular disease can be associated with increased Q as occurs during infection and sepsis, or decreased Q, as in cardiomyopathy and heart failure. The ability to accurately measure Q is important in clinical medicine as it provides for improved diagnosis of abnormalities, and can be used to guide appropriate management. Q measurement, if it were accurate and noninvasive, would be adopted as part of every clinical examination from general observations to the intensive care ward, and would be as common as simple blood pressure measurements are now. Such practice, if it were adopted, may revolutionise the treatment of many cardiovascular diseases including hypertension and heart failure. This is the reason why Q measurement is now an important research and clinical focus in cardiovascular medicine.

Measuring Cardiac Output

Circulation is critical and variable function of human physiology and disease. An accurate and noninvasive measurement of Q is the holy grail of cardiovascular assessment. This would allow continuous monitoring of central circulation and provide improved insights into normal physiology, pathophysiology and treatments for disease.

Invasive methods are well accepted, but there is increasing evidence that these methods are neither accurate nor effective in guiding therapy, so there is an increasing focus on development of noninvasive methods.

There are a number of clinical methods for measurement of Q ranging from direct intracardiac catheterisation to noninvasive measurement of the arterial pulse. Each method has unique strengths and weaknesses and relative comparison is limited by the absence of a widely accepted 'gold standard' measurement. Q can also be affected significantly by the phase of respiration; intrathoracic pressure changes influence diastolic filling. This is especially important during mechanical ventilation where Q can vary by up to 50 per cent across a single respiratory cycle, Q should therefore be measured at evenly spaced points over a single cycle or averaged over several cycles.

Fick Principle

The Fick principle was first described by Adolf Eugen Fick in 1870 and assumes that the rate at which oxygen is consumed is a function of the rate of blood flows and the rate of oxygen pick up by the red blood cells.

The Fick principle involves calculating the oxygen consumed over a given period of time from measurement of the oxygen concentration of the venous blood and the arterial blood. Q can be calculated from these measurements:

1. V_{O_2} consumption per minute using a spirometer (with the subject re-breathing air) and a CO_2 absorber.
2. The oxygen content of blood taken from the pulmonary artery (representing mixed venous blood).
3. The oxygen content of blood from a cannula in a peripheral artery (representing arterial blood).

From these values, we know that:

$$VO_2 = (Q \times C_A) - (Q \times C_V)$$

where,

C_A = Oxygen content of arterial blood
C_V = Oxygen content of venous blood.

This allows us to say

$$Q = (VO_2/[C_A - C_V]) \times 100$$

and therefore calculate Q. While considered to be the most accurate method for Q measurement, Fick is invasive, requires time for the sample analysis, and accurate oxygen consumption samples are difficult to acquire. There have also been modifications to the Fick method where respiratory oxygen content is measured as part of a closed system and the consumed oxygen calculated using an assumed oxygen consumption index which is then used to calculate Q. Other modifications use inert gas as tracers and measure the change in inspired and expired gas concentrations to calculate Q.

Additionally, the calculation of the arterial and venous oxygen content of the blood is a straightforward process. Almost all oxygen in the blood is bound to haemoglobin molecules in the red blood cells. Measuring the content of haemoglobin in the blood and the percentage of saturation of haemoglobin (the oxygen saturation of the blood) is a simple process and is readily available to physicians. Using the fact that each gram of haemoglobin can carry 1.36 ml of O_2, the oxygen content of the blood (either arterial or venous) can be estimated by the following formula:

Oxygen content of blood = [haemoglobin] (g/dl) × 1.36 (ml O_2/g of haemoglobin × saturation of blood (%) + 0.0032 × partial pressure of oxygen (torr)

Dilution Methods

This method was initially described using an indicator dye and assumes that the rate at which the indicator is diluted reflects the Q. The method measures the concentration of a dye at different points in the circulation, usually from an intravenous injection and then at a downstream sampling site, usually in a systemic artery. More specifically, the Q is equal to the quantity of indicator dye injected divided by the area under the dilution curve measured downstream (the Stewart–Hamilton equation):

$$\text{Cardiac output} = \frac{\text{Quantity of indicator}}{\int_0^\infty \text{Concentration of indicator} \cdot dt}$$

The trapezoid rule is often used as an approximation of this integral.

Ultrasound Dilution Method

Ultrasound dilution method used extensively to measure flow and volumes with extracorporeal circuits condition such as ECMO and Hemodialysis, and now it has adapted to Intensive Care Units (ICU) settings as COstatus™ (Transonic System Inc. Ithaca, NY).

COstatus™ uses body temperature normal saline (NS) as an indicator to measure cardiac output, plus a group of important haemodynamic Blood Volumes (BV) variables, such as total end-diastole volume (TEDV), central blood volume (CBV) and active circulation volume (ACVI).

COstatus™ technology is based on ultrasound indicator dilution. Blood ultrasound velocity (1560–1585 m/s) is a function of total blood protein concentration (sums of proteins in plasma and in red blood red cells), temperature etc. Injection of body temperature normal saline (ultrasound velocity of saline is 1533 m/sec) into a unique AV loop decreases blood ultrasound velocity, and produce dilution curves.

COstatus™ establishes an extracorporeal circulation through its unique AV loop with two preexisting arterial and central venous lines in ICU patients. When the saline indicator is injected into the A-V loop, it is detected by the venous clamp-on sensor on the AV loop before it enters the patient's right heart atrium. After the indicator traverses the heart and lung, the concentration curve in the arterial line is recorded and displayed on the COstatus™ HCM101 monitor. Cardiac output is calculated from the area of the concentration curve by the classic Stewart-Hamilton equation. It is a noninvasive procedure only by connection the AV loop and two lines of a patient. There lacks general methods to measure cardiac output in pediatric ICU patients, COstatus™ has been demonstrated to be a safe and reproducible tool.

Pulmonary artery thermodilution (Trans-right-heart thermodilution)

The indicator method was further developed with replacement of the indicator dye by heated or cooled fluid and temperature change measured at different sites in the circulation rather than dye concentration; this method is known as thermodilution. The pulmonary artery catheter (PAC), also known as the Swan-Ganz catheter, provides direct access to the right heart for thermodilution measurements.

The PAC is balloon tipped and is inflated, which helps 'sail' the catheter balloon through the right ventricle to occlude a smaller branch of the pulmonary artery system. The balloon is deflated. The PAC thermodilution method involves injection of a small amount (10 ml) of cold glucose at a known temperature into the pulmonary artery and measuring the temperature a known distance away (6–10 cm) using the same catheter.

The Q can be calculated from the measured temperature curve (The thermodilution curve). High

Q will change the temperature rapidly, and low Q will change the temperature slowly. Usually three or four repeated measures are averaged to improve accuracy. However it is complex to perform and there are many sources of inaccuracy in the method. Modern catheters are fitted with a heating filament which intermittently heats and measures the thermodilution curve providing serial Q measurement. However, these take an average of measurements made over 2–9 minutes, depending on the stability of the circulation, and thus do not provide continuous monitoring.

PAC use is complicated by arrhythmias, infection, pulmonary artery rupture, and right heart valve damage. Recent studies in patients with critical illness, sepsis, acute respiratory failure and heart failure suggest use of the PAC does not improve patient outcomes. PAC use is in decline as clinicians move to less invasive technologies for monitoring haemodynamics.

Doppler ultrasound method

This method uses ultrasound and the Doppler effect to measure Q. The blood velocity through the heart causes a 'Doppler shift' in the frequency of the returning ultrasound waves. This Doppler shift can then be used to calculate flow velocity and volume and effectively Q using the following equations:

$$Q = SV \times HR$$
$$SV = vti \times CSA$$

where,

CSA = valve orifice cross sectional area; use pr^2

r = valve radius.

vti = the velocity time integral of the trace of the Doppler flow profile.

Doppler ultrasound is noninvasive, accurate and inexpensive and is a routine part of clinical ultrasound with high levels of reliability and reproducibility having been in clinical use since the 1960s.

Echocardiography

Echocardiography uses a conventional ultrasound machine and a combined two dimensional (2D) and Doppler approach to measure Q. 2D measurement of the diameter (d) of the aortic annulus allows calculation of the flow CSA (cross-sectional area) which is then multiplied by the vti of the Doppler flow profile across the aortic valve to determine the flow volume or SV. Multiplying SV by HR produces Q. Echocardiographic measurement of flow volume is clinically well established and of proven accuracy but requires training and skill, and may be time consuming to perform effectively. The 2D measurement of the aortic valve diameter is challenging and associated with significant error, while measurement of the pulmonary valve to calculate right sided Q is even more difficult.

Transcutaneous doppler: USCOM

An ultrasonic cardiac output monitor (USCOM) uses continuous wave doppler (CW) to measure the Doppler flow profile vti, as in echocardiography, but uses anthropometry to calculate aortic and pulmonary valve diameters so both the right and left sided Q can be measured. Real time Automatic tracing of the Doppler flow profile allows for beat to beat right and left sided Q measurement. This single method has been used in neonates, children and adults for low and high Q measurement.

Transoesophageal doppler: TOD

Transoesophageal doppler (TOD), also known as esophageal doppler monitor (EDM), supports a CW sensor on the end of a probe which can be introduced via the mouth or nose and positioned in the oesophagus so the doppler beam aligns with the descending thoracic aorta (DTA) at a known angle. Because the transducer is close to the blood flow the signal is clear, however correct alignment may be difficult to maintain, especially during patient movement. This method has good validation, particularly for measuring changes in blood flow. As it only measures DTA flow and not true Q, it may be potentially influenced by disproportionate changes in blood flow between upper and lower body though this does not appear to be problematic in most clinical situations. This method generally requires patient sedation and is accepted for use in both adults and children.

Pulse pressure methods

Pulse pressure (PP) methods measure the pressure in an artery over time to derive a waveform and use this information to calculate cardiac performance. The problem is that any measure from the artery includes the changes in pressure associated with changes in arterial function (compliance, impedance, etc.).

Physiologic or therapeutic changes in vessel diameter are assumed to reflect changes in Q. Put simply, PP methods measure the combined performance of the heart and the vessels thus limiting the application of PP methods for measurement of Q. This can be partially compensated for by intermittent calibration of the waveform to another Q measurement method and then monitoring the PP waveform. Ideally, the PP waveform should be calibrated on a beat to beat basis.

There are invasive and noninvasive methods of measuring PP:

Noninvasive PP–sphygmomanometry and tonometry

The sphygmomanometer or cuff blood pressure device was introduced to clinical practice in 1903 allowing noninvasive measurements of blood pressure and providing the common PP waveform values of peak systolic and diastolic pressure which can be used to calculate mean arterial pressure (MAP). The pressure in the arteries, measured by sphygmomanometry, is often used as a guide to the function of the heart. Put simply, the pressure in the heart is conducted to the arteries, so the arterial pressure approximately reflects the function of the heart or the Q.

1. The pressure in the heart rises as blood is forced into the aorta
2. The more stretched the aorta, the greater the pulse pressure (PP).
3. In healthy young subjects, each additional 2 ml of blood results in a 1 mmHg rise in pressure

Therefore:

$SV = 2$ ml × Pulse pressure

$Q = 2$ ml × Pulse pressure × HR

By resting a more sophisticated pressure sensing device, a tonometer, against the skin surface and sensing the pulsatile artery, continuous PP wave forms can be acquired noninvasively and analysis made of these pressure signals. Unfortunately the heart and vessels can function independently and sometimes paradoxically so that changes in the PP may both reflect and mask changes in Q. So these measures represent combined cardiac and vascular function only. Another similar system that uses the arterial pulse is the pressure recording analytical method (PRAM).

Invasive PP

Invasive PP involves inserting a manometer (pressure sensor) into an artery, usually the radial or femoral artery and continuously measuring the PP waveform. This is usually done by connecting the catheter to a signal processing and display device. The PP waveform can then be analysed to provide measurements of cardiovascular performance. Changes in vascular function, the position of the catheter tip, or damping of the pressure waveform signal will all affect the accuracy of the readings. Invasive PP measurements can be calibrated or uncalibrated.

Calibrated PP–PiCCO, LiDCO

PiCCO (PULSION Medical Systems AG, Munich, Germany) and PulseCO (LiDCO Ltd, London, England) generate continuous Q by analysis of the arterial PP waveform. In both cases, an independent technique is required to provide calibration of the continuous Q analysis, as arterial PP analysis cannot account for unmeasured variables such as the changing compliance of the vascular bed. Recalibration is recommended after changes in patient position, therapy or condition. In the case of PiCCO, transpulmonary thermodilution is used as the calibrating technique. Transpulmonary thermodilution uses the Stewart-Hamilton principle, but measures temperatures changes from central venous line to a central arterial line (i.e. femoral or axillary) arterial line. The Q derived from this cold-saline thermodilution is used to calibrate the arterial PP contour, which can then provide continuous Q monitoring. The PiCCO algorithm is dependent on blood pressure waveform morphology (i.e.

mathematical analysis of the PP waveform) and calculates continuous Q as described by Wesseling and co-workers. Transpulmonary thermodilution spans right heart, pulmonary circulation and left heart; this allows further mathematical analysis of the thermodilution curve, giving measurements of cardiac filling volumes (GEDV), intrathoracic blood volume, and extravascular lung water. While transpulmonary thermodilution allows for less invasive Q calibration, the method is also less accurate than PA thermodilution and still requires a central venous and arterial line with the attendant infection risks.

In the case of LiDCO, the independent calibration technique is lithium dilution, again using the Stewart-Hamilton principle. Lithium dilution uses a peripheral vein to a peripheral arterial line; however, it does not provide information on cardiac filling volumes and extravascular lung water. Calibration measurements cannot be performed too frequently, and can be subject to error in the presence of certain muscle relaxants. The PulseCO algorithm used by LiDCO is based on pulse power derivation and is not dependent on waveform morphology.

Uncalibrated PP—FloTrac

This technology involves inserting a manometer tipped arterial catheter into the mid flow portion of an artery, usually radial or femoral, and then by time domain sampling converts the arterial PP to Q. While this method involves one less line than the calibrated PP Q systems, it remains uncalibrated and so is only measuring arterial PP invasively. While it estimates upstream Q, any independent changes in Q and SVR cannot be detected by this method. However, SVR can be computed if there is a central line in place and those values are slaved into the monitor. Its accuracy and ability to follow trends is however open to question as many studies show poor agreement against comparator techniques.

Uncalibrated, pre-estimed demographic data-free — PRAM

Pressure recording analytical method (PRAM), exclusively available in MostCare device (Vytech, Padova, Italy) estimates Q just from the analysis of the pressure wave profile, mininvasively obtained from an arterial catheter (choice of radial or femoral access); thanks to Physic Perturbation theory application to the physiology issue, all the elements determining Q can be simultaneously and beat-to-beat taken in consideration. Uniquely sampled at 1000 Hz, the detected pressure curve is so precise to be effectively submitted to an equally sophisticated analysis; the result is the calculation of the real (relative to the patient under examination) and actual (beat-to-beat) Stroke Volume; no constant value of impedance, deriving from an external calibration neither form pre-estimated in *vivo*/in *vitro* data are needed.

PRAM has been validated against the considered gold standard methods in stable condition and in various hemodynamic states; it can be used to monitor pediatric and mechanically supported patients.

A part to generally monitored haemodynamic values and to fluid responsiveness parameters, an exclusive reference is also provided by PRAM: cardiac cycle efficiency (CCE). Expressed by a pure number ranging from 1 (the best) and -1 (the worse) it indicates the overall heart-vascular response coupling; the ratio between the heart performed and consumed energy, represented as CCE 'stress index', can be of paramount importance in understanding patient present and next future course.

Impedance cardiography

Impedance cardiography (ICG) is a method which calculates Q from the measurement of changes in impedance across the chest over the cardiac cycle. Lower impedance indicates greater the intrathoracic fluid volume, and as the only fluid volume which changes beat to beat within the thorax is the blood, the change in impedance can be used to calculate the SV and, combined with HR, the Q. This technique has progressed clinically (often called BioZ, i.e. biologic impedance, as promoted by the leading manufacturer in the US) and allows noninvasive estimations of Q and total peripheral resistance using only 4 paired skin electrodes.

While the method is desirably noninvasive and inexpensive, it has not achieved the reliability and reproducibility required of a useful clinical tool, and the evolution of algorithms to convert impedance signals to Q across a variety of outputs and in a variety of diseases continues.

Electrical cardiometry

Electrical cardiometry is a noninvasive method similar to Impedance cardiography, in the fact that both methods measure thoracic electrical bioimpedance (TEB). The underlying model is what differs, being that Electrical Cardiometry attributes the steep increase of TEB beat to beat to the change in orientation of red blood cells. Four standard ECG electrodes are required for measurement of cardiac output. Electrical cardiometry is a method trademarked by Cardiotronic, Inc., and shows promising results in a wide range or patients (is currently US market approved for use in adults, pediatrics, and neonates). Electrical Cardiometry monitors have shown promise in postoperative cardiac surgical patients (both hemodynamicially stable and unstable).

Magnetic resonance imaging

Velocity encoded phase contrast magnetic resonance imaging (MRI) is the most accurate technique for measuring flow in large vessels in mammals. MRI flow measurements have been shown to be highly accurate compared to measurements with a beaker and timer and less variable than both the Fick principle and thermodilution.

Velocity encoded MRI is based on detection of changes in the phase of proton precession. These changes are proportional to the velocity of the movement of those protons through a magnetic field with a known gradient. When using velocity encoded MRI, the result of the MRI scan is two sets of images for each time point in the cardiac cycle. One is an anatomical image and the other is an image where the signal intensity in each pixel is directly proportional to the through-plane velocity. The average velocity in a vessel, i.e. the aorta or the pulmonary artery, is hence quantified by measuring the average signal intensity of the pixels in the cross section of the vessel, and then multiplying by a known constant. The flow is calculated by multiplying the mean velocity by the cross-sectional area of the vessel. This flow data can be used to graph flow versus time. The area under the flow versus time curve for one cardiac cycle is the stroke volume. The length of the cardiac cycle is known and determines heart rate, and thereby Q can be calculated as the product of stroke volume and heart rate. MRI is typically used to quantify the flow over one cardiac cycle as the average of several heart beats, but it is also possible quantify the stroke volume in real time on a beat-for-beat basis.

While MRI is an important research tool for accurately measuring Q, it is currently not clinically used for haemodynamic monitoring in the emergency or intensive care setting. Cardiac output measurement by MRI is currently routinely used as a part of clinical cardiac MRI examinations.

CARDIAC OUTPUT AND VASCULAR RESISTANCE

The vascular beds are a dynamic and connected part of the circulatory system against which the heart must pump to transport the blood, Q is influenced by the resistance of the vascular bed against which the heart is pumping. For the right heart this is the pulmonary vascular bed, creating pulmonary vascular resistance (PVR), while for the systemic circulation this is the systemic vascular bed, creating systemic vascular resistance (SVR). The vessels actively change diameter under the influence of physiology or therapy, vasoconstrictors decrease vessel diameter and increase resistance, while vasodilators increase vessel diameter and decrease resistance. Put simply, increasing resistance decreases Q; conversely, decreased resistance increases Q.

This can be explained mathematically:

1. By simplifying Darcy's Law, we get the equation that:

   Flow = Pressure/Resistance

2. When applied to the circulatory system, we get:

   $Q = (MAP - RAP)/TPR$

   where, MAP = mean Aortic (or Arterial) blood pressure in mmHg.

RAP = Mean right atrial pressure in mmHg .
TPR = Total peripheral resistance in dynes-sec-cm-5.

Direct Fick

The direct Fick method is a method of measuring cardiac output using the Fick principle. It divides the oxygen intake by the difference in oxygen content of aortic blood and mixed venous blood. It has been criticised as inaccurate by some because its invasive nature alters cardiac dynamics.

Radionuclide Angiography

A multi gated acquisition scan (MUGA scan) is a nuclear medicine test to evaluate the function of the heart ventricles. It is also called Radionuclide Angiography, and also Gated Blood Pool Imaging. It provides a movie-like image (also known as a cine image) of the beating heart, and allows the doctor to determine the health of the heart's major pumping chambers. The advantages of MUGA is that it is more accurate than an echocardiogram. MUGA is typically ordered for the following patients:

1. With known or suspected coronary artery disease, to diagnose the disease and predict outcomes.
2. With lesions in their heart valves.
3. With congestive heart failure.
4. Who have undergone percutaneous transluminal coronary angioplasty, coronary artery bypass graft surgery, or medical therapy, to assess the efficacy of the treatment
5. With low cardiac output after open-heart surgery.
6. Who are undergoing cardiotoxic drug agents such as in chemotherapy, e.g. with doxorubicin or immunotherapy (herceptin).
7. Who have had a cardiac transplant.

Procedure

At a high level, the MUGA test involves the introduction of a radioactive marker into the bloodstream of the patient. The patient is subsequently scanned to determine the circulation dynamics of the marker, and hence the blood.

The introduction of the radioactive marker can either take place *in vivo* or *in vitro*. In the *in vivo* method, stannous (tin) ions are injected into the patient's bloodstream. A subsequent intravenous injection of the radioactive substance, technetium-99 m-pertechnetate, labels the red blood cells *in vivo*. With an administered activity of about 800 MBq, the effective radiation dose is about 8 mSv to 12 mSv. In the *in vitro* method, some of the patient's blood is drawn and the stannous ions (in the form of stannous chloride) are injected into the drawn blood. The technetium is subsequently added to the mixture as in the *in vivo* method. In both cases, the stannous chloride dilutes the Technetium and prevents it from leaking out of the red blood cells during the procedure. The patient is placed under a gamma camera, which detects the low-level 140 keV gamma radiation being given off by technetium-99 m. As the gamma camera images are acquired, the patient's heart beat is used to 'gate' the acquisition. The final result is a series of images of the heart (usually sixteen), one at each stage of the cardiac cycle.

Depending on the objectives of the test, the doctor may decide to perform either a resting or a stress MUGA. During the resting MUGA, the patient lies stationary, whereas during a stress MUGA, the patient is asked to exercise during the scan. The stress MUGA measures the heart performance during exercise and is usually performed to assess the impact of a suspected coronary artery disease. In some rare cases, a nitroglycerine MUGA may be performed, where nitroglycerine (a vasodilator) is administered prior to the scan.

The resulting images show the blood pool in the chambers of the heart and the images can be analysed on a computer to calculate the ejection fraction of the heart together with other useful clinical parameters. This scan gives an accurate and reproducible means of measuring and monitoring the ejection fraction of the left ventricle, which is one of the most important metrics in assessing heart performance.

Results

Normal results

In normal subjects, the left ventricular ejection fraction (LVEF) should be about 60 per cent (range,

50–80 per cent). There should be no area of abnormal wall motion (hypokinesis or dyskinesis). Abnormalities in cardiac function may be manifested as a decrease in LVEF and/or the presence of abnormalities in global and regional wall motion. For normal subjects, peak filling rates should be between 2.4 and 3.6 end diastolic volume (EDV) per second, and the time to peak filling rate should be 135–212 msec.

Abnormal results

An uneven distribution of technetium in the heart indicates that the patient has coronary artery disease, a cardiomyopathy, or blood shunting within the heart. Abnormalities in a resting MUGA usually indicate a heart attack, while those that occur during exercise usually indicate ischemia. In a stress MUGA, patients with coronary artery disease may exhibit a decrease in ejection fraction. For a patient that has had a heart attack, or is suspected of having another disease that affects the heart muscle, this scan can help pinpoint the position in the heart that has sustained damage as well as assess the degree of damage. MUGA scans are also used to evaluate heart function prior to and while receiving certain chemotherapies (e.g. doxorubicin (Adriamycin)) or immunotherapy (specifically, herceptin) that have a known effect on heart function.

Echocardiography

An echocardiogram, often referred to in the medical community as a cardiac ECHO or simply an ECHO, is a sonogram of the heart (it is not abbreviated as ECG, which in medicine usually refers to an electrocardiogram). Also known as a cardiac ultrasound, it uses standard ultrasound techniques to image two-dimensional slices of the heart. The latest ultrasound systems now employ 3D real-time imaging.

In addition to creating two-dimensional pictures of the cardiovascular system, an echocardiogram can also produce accurate assessment of the velocity of blood and cardiac tissue at any arbitrary point using pulsed or continuous wave doppler ultrasound. This allows assessment of cardiac valve areas and function, any abnormal communications between the left and right side of the heart, any leaking of blood through the valves (valvular regurgitation), and calculation of the cardiac output as well as the ejection fraction.

Echocardiography was an early medical application of ultrasound. Echocardiography was also the first application of intravenous contrast-enhanced ultrasound. This technique injects gas-filled microbubbles into the venous system to improve tissue and blood delineation. Contrast is also currently being evaluated for its effectiveness in evaluating myocardial perfusion. It can also be used with Doppler ultrasound to improve flow-related measurements.

Echocardiography is either performed by cardiac sonographers or doctors trained in cardiology. Echocardiography is used to diagnose cardiovascular diseases. In fact, it is one of the most widely used diagnostic tests for heart disease. It can provide a wealth of helpful information, including the size and shape of the heart, its pumping capacity and the location and extent of any damage to its tissues. It is especially useful for assessing diseases of the heart valves. It not only allows doctors to evaluate the heart valves, but it can detect abnormalities in the pattern of blood flow, such as the backward flow of blood through partly closed heart valves, known as regurgitation. By assessing the motion of the heart wall, echocardiography can help detect the presence and assess the severity of coronary artery disease, as well as help determine whether any chest pain is related to heart disease. Echocardiography can also help detect hypertrophic cardiomyopathy.

The biggest advantage to echocardiography is that it is noninvasive (does not involve breaking the skin or entering body cavities) and has no known risks or side effects.

Transthoracic echocardiogram

A standard echocardiogram is also known as a transthoracic echocardiogram (TTE), or cardiac ultrasound. In this case, the echocardiography transducer (or probe) is placed on the chest wall (or thorax) of the subject, and images are taken through the chest wall. This is a noninvasive, highly accurate and quick assessment of the overall health of the heart.

Transoesophageal echocardiogram

This is an alternative way to perform an echocardiogram. A specialised probe containing an ultrasound transducer at its tip is passed into the patient's oesophagus. This allows image and Doppler evaluation which can be recorded. This is known as a transoesophageal echocardiogram, or TOE (TEE in the United States).

3-Dimensional echocardiography

3-D echocardiography is now possible, using an ultrasound probe with an array of transducers and an appropriate processing system. This enables detailed anatomical assessment of cardiac pathology, particularly valvular defects, and cardiomyopathies. The ability to slice the virtual heart in infinite planes in an anatomically appropriate manner and to reconstruct 3-dimensional images of anatomic structures make 3D echocardiography unique for the understanding of the congenitally malformed heart.

M-mode echocardiography

M-mode echocardiography provides a one-dimensional moving image of the heart. The waves indicate structure in the heart, such as the valves, chambers and walls.

Doppler echocardiography

Doppler echocardiography is a procedure which uses ultrasound technology to examine the heart. An echocardiogram uses high frequency sound waves to create an image of the heart while the use of doppler technology allows determination the speed and direction of blood flow by utilising the doppler effect.

An echocardiogram can, within certain limits, produce accurate assessment of the direction of blood flow and the velocity of blood and cardiac tissue at any arbitrary point using the Doppler effect. One of the limitations is that the ultrasound beam should be as parallel to the blood flow as possible. Velocity measurements allow assessment of cardiac valve areas and function, any abnormal communications between the left and right side of the heart, any leaking of blood through the valves (valvular regurgitation), and calculation of the cardiac output. Contrast-enhanced ultrasound using gas-filled microbubble contrast media can be used to improve velocity or other flow-related medical measurements.

Although 'doppler' has become synonymous with 'velocity measurement' in medical imaging, in many cases it is not the frequency shift (doppler shift) of the received signal that is measured, but the phase shift (when the received signal arrives).

This procedure is frequently used to examine children's hearts for heart disease because there is no age or size requirement.

Two dimensional echocardiography

In the past decade, M-mode echocardiography has become one of the most important investigations for the evaluation of the cardiovascular system. The major reasons for the phenomenal growth in popularity of M-mode echocardiography are: (i) it is entirely noninvasive and therefore non-harmful to the individual, (ii) it can be easily performed at the bedside and is thus applicable to those who are critically ill, as well as to those who are physically well, and (ii) it is repeatable and reproducible. However, since M-mode echocardiography can produce only a one dimensional (ice-pick) view of the heart, it is limited in its ability to provide information regarding the spatial orientation of the different cardiac structures. The second major disadvantage of M-mode echocardiography is that the various cardiac structures are displayed in an unfamiliar format which bears no resemblance to the actual anatomical structures.

It is clear that the image which is obtained does not at all resemble anatomically the mitral valve, and is thus unrecognisable to those who are untrained in M-mode echocardiography. Two dimensional or cross sectional echocardiography however overcomes both these major disadvantages of M-mode echocardiography. By enabling a wide portion of the heart to be imaged simultaneously, the spatial orientation of the different cardiac structures are clearly defined. The images that are reproduced resemble the actual cardiac anatomy and can be easily recognised even by the uninitiated.

Two dimensional echocardiography first began in the late 1960's and in the early 1970's. However, significant development in this technique was seen only in the past few years. Currently, there are three different methods of doing two-dimensional echocardiography. They are: (i) mechanical sector scanning, (ii) multielement linear array (multi scan), and (iii) electronic sector scanner or phased array systems.

Technique of examination

We are currently employing a commercially available mechanical sector scanner (ATL Mark IV) as shown in Fig. 8.10 is used. The patients are examined supine or turned slightly towards the left. Cross section views of the heart are obtained by first placing the transducer over the left parasternal region in the praecordium. The long axis view of the heart is initially obtained by appropriate manipulation of the transducer (Fig. 8.11). The short axis of the heart is then obtained by rotating the transducer 90°. By angling the transducer interiorly and superiorly, various structures of the heart can be imaged in the short axis (Figs 8.12 and 8.13).

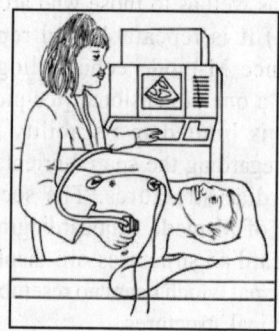

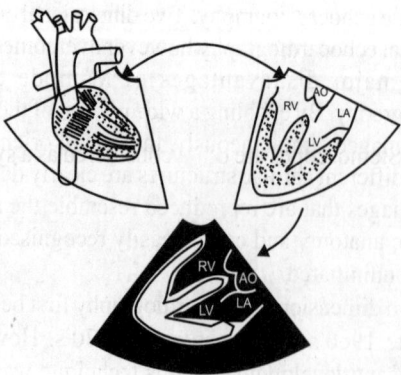

Fig. 8.10. Technique of two-dimensional examination of the heart.

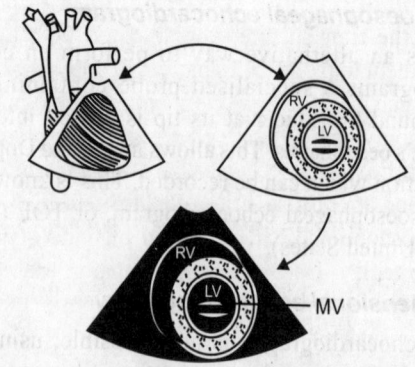

Fig. 8.12. Short axis view of heart at level of mitral valve.

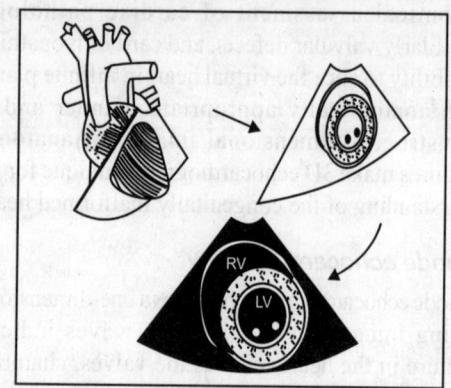

Fig. 8.13. Short axis view of heart at level of papillary muscle.

Another very useful view is the apical four chamber view obtained by positioning the transducer at the apex of the heart (Fig. 8.14).

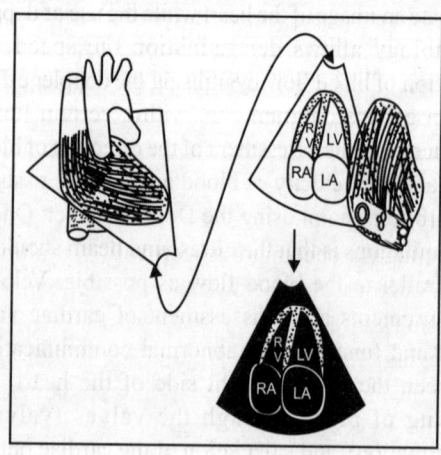

Fig. 8.11. Long axis view of heart.

Fig. 8.14. Apical 4 chamber view of heart.

If the transducer is then rotated 90°, a view equivalent to the angiographic right anterior oblique view can be obtained. Two other useful but less commonly employed views are the subxiphoid and the suprasternal views. The images which are obtained are displayed in a real time fashion on an oscilloscope and can be stored on video-tape for future replay. This form of presentation enables the actual movement of the various structures of the heart to be visualised in real time and is quite dramatic. Still photographs of single frames of the videotape can be taken from the tape. This sector scanner also has the capability of recording a simultaneous M mode echogram along any selected line in the sector arc.

Heart sounds

The heart sounds are the noises (sound) generated by the beating heart and the resultant flow of blood through it. This is also called a heartbeat. In cardiac auscultation, an examiner uses a stethoscope to listen for these sounds, which provide important information about the condition of the heart.

In healthy adults, there are two normal heart sounds often described as a lub and a dub (or dup), that occur in sequence with each heart beat. These are the first heart sound (S_1) and second heart sound (S_2), produced by the closing of the AV valves and semilunar valves respectively. In addition to these normal sounds, a variety of other sounds may be present including heart murmurs, adventitious sounds, and gallop rhythms S_3 and S_4 (Fig. 8.15).

Heart murmurs are generated by turbulent flow of blood, which may occur inside or outside the heart. Murmurs may be physiological (benign) or pathological (abnormal).

Abnormal murmurs can be caused by stenosis restricting the opening of a heart valve, resulting in turbulence as blood flows through it. Abnormal murmurs may also occur with valvular insufficiency (or regurgitation), which allows backflow of blood when the incompetent valve closes with only partial effectiveness. Different murmurs are audible in different parts of the cardiac cycle, depending on the cause of the murmur.

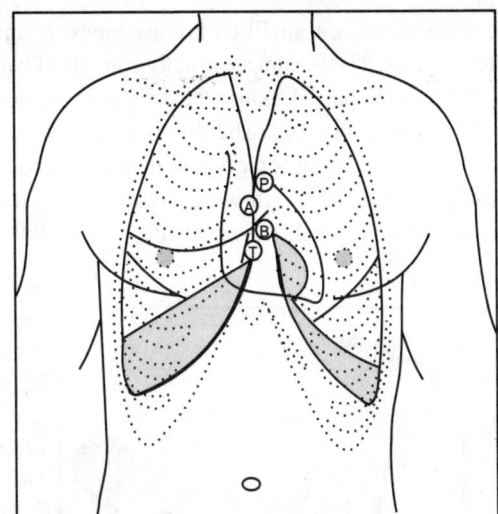

Fig. 8.15. Front of thorax, showing surface relations of bones, lungs, pleura, and heart. Heart valves are labelled with 'B', 'T', 'A', and 'P'. First heart sound: caused by atrioventricular valves - Bicuspid/Mitral (B) and Tricuspid (T). Second heart sound caused by semilunar valves — Aortic (A) and Pulmonary/Pulmonic (P).

Normal heart sounds are associated with heart valves closing, causing changes in blood flow.

Stethoscope

The stethoscope is an acoustic medical device for auscultation, or listening to the internal sounds of an animal body. It is often used to listen to lung and heart sounds. It is also used to listen to intestines and blood flow in arteries and veins. Less commonly, 'mechanic's stethoscopes' are used to listen to internal sounds made by machines, such as diagnosing a malfunctioning automobile engine by listening to the sounds of its internal parts. Stethoscopes can also be used to check scientific vacuum chambers for leaks, and for various other small-scale acoustic monitoring tasks. Stethoscopes are often considered as a symbol of the doctor's profession, as doctors are often seen or depicted with a stethoscope hanging around their neck (Fig. 18.16).

Types of stethoscopes

Acoustic

Acoustic stethoscopes (Fig. 8.17) are familiar to most people, and operate on the transmission of sound from the chest piece, via air-filled hollow tubes, to the listener's ears. The chestpiece usually consists of two sides that can be placed against the patient for sensing sound—a diaphragm (plastic disc) or bell (hollow cup). If the diaphragm is placed on the patient, body sounds vibrate the diaphragm, creating acoustic pressure waves which travel up the tubing to the listener's ears.

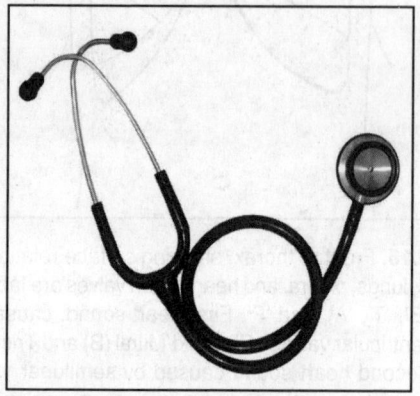

Fig. 8.16. Modern stethoscope.

If the bell is placed on the patient, the vibrations of the skin directly produce acoustic pressure waves travelling up to the listener's ears. The bell transmits low frequency sounds, while the diaphragm transmits higher frequency sounds.

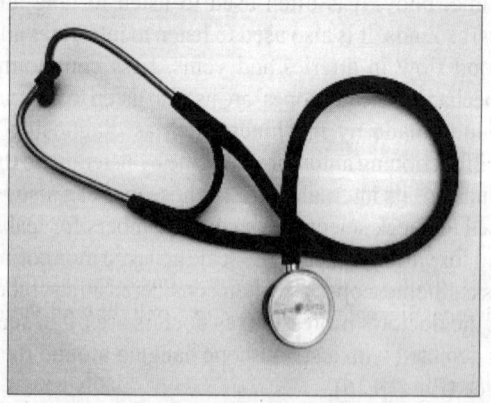

Fig. 8.17. Acoustic stethoscope.

This 2-sided stethoscope was invented by Rappaport and Sprague in the early part of the 20th century. One problem with acoustic stethoscopes was that the sound level is extremely low. This problem was surmounted in 1999 with the invention of the stratified continuous (inner) lumen, and the kinetic acoustic mechanism in 2002. Acoustic stethoscopes are the most commonly used. A recent independent review evaluated 12 common acoustic stethoscopes on the basis of loudness, clarity, and ergonomics. They did acoustic laboratory testing and recorded heart sounds on volunteers. The results are listed by brand and model.

Electronic

An electronic stethoscope (or stethophone) overcomes the low sound levels by electronically amplifying body sounds. However, amplification of stethoscope contact artifacts, and component cutoffs (frequency response thresholds of electronic stethoscope microphones, pre-amps, amps, and speakers) limit electronically amplified stethoscopes' overall utility by amplifying mid-range sounds, while simultaneously attenuating high- and low- frequency range sounds. Currently, a number of companies offer electronic stethoscopes.

Electronic stethoscopes require conversion of acoustic sound waves to electrical signals which can then be amplified and processed for optimal listening. Unlike acoustic stethoscopes, which are all based on the same physics, transducers in electronic stethoscopes vary widely. The simplest and least effective method of sound detection is achieved by placing a microphone in the chestpiece. This method suffers from ambient noise interference and has fallen out of favour. Another method, used in Welch-Allyn's Meditron stethoscope, comprises placement of a piezoelectric crystal at the head of a metal shaft, the bottom of the shaft making contact with a diaphragm. 3M also uses a piezoelectric crystal placed within foam behind a thick rubber-like diaphragm. Thinklabs' Rhythm 32 inventor, Clive Smith uses an Electromagnetic Diaphragm with a conductive inner surface to form a capacitive sensor. This diaphragm responds to sound waves identically to a conventional acoustic stethoscope, with changes in an electric field replacing changes in air pressure. This preserves the sound of an acoustic stethoscope with the benefits of amplification.

Because the sounds are transmitted electronically, an electronic stethoscope can be a wireless device, can be a recording device, and can provide noise reduction, signal enhancement, and both visual and audio output. Around 2001, Stethographics introduced PC-based software which enabled a phonocardiograph, graphic representation of cardiologic and pulmonologic sounds to be generated, and interpreted according to related algorithms. All of these features are helpful for purposes of telemedicine (remote diagnosis) and teaching.

Recording stethoscopes

Some electronic stethoscopes feature direct audio output that can be used with an external recording device, such as a laptop or MP3 recorder. The same connection can be used to listen to the previously-recorded auscultation through the stethoscope headphones, allowing for more detailed study for general research as well as evaluation and consultation regarding a particular patient's condition and telemedicine, or remote diagnosis.

Fetal stethoscope

A fetal stethoscope or fetoscope is an acoustic stethoscope shaped like a listening trumpet. It is placed against the abdomen of a pregnant woman to listen to the heart sounds of the fetus. The fetal stethoscope is also known as a Pinard's stethoscope or a pinard, after French obstetrician Adolphe Pinard.

Maintenance

The flexible vinyl, rubber, and plastic parts of stethoscopes should be kept away from solvents, including alcohol and soap. Solvents can have detrimental effects, including accelerating the natural ageing process by dissolving the plasticisers that keep these parts flexible and looking new. In addition, when they are manufactured stethoscopes with two-sided chestpieces are lubricated where the chestpiece rotates around the stem and need to be re-lubricated periodically, just like any other machine.

If these moving parts are not lubricated, they grind together and ruin the fine tolerances required for the proper acoustic performance of the stethoscope. Cleaning the stethoscope will also remove lubricants, making periodic lubrication essential. Most lubricants must be kept away from rubber, vinyl, and plastic parts. Only products that have been tested to be safe and effective for cleaning stethoscopes and similar medical instruments should be used.

Microphone

A microphone is an acoustic-to-electric transducer or sensor that converts sound into an electrical signal. Microphones are used in many applications such as telephones, tape recorders, karaoke systems, hearing aids, motion picture production, live and recorded audio engineering, FRS radios, megaphones, in radio and television broadcasting and in computers for recording voice, speech recognition, VoIP, and for non-acoustic purposes such as ultrasonic checking or knock sensors (Fig. 8.18).

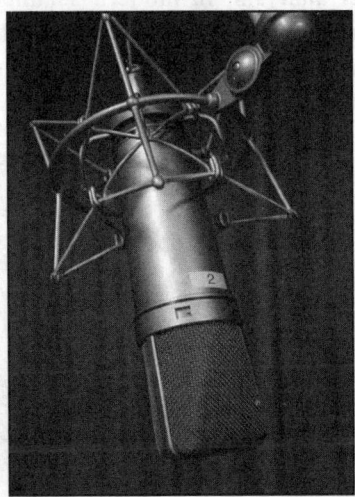

Fig. 8.18. Condenser microphone.

Most microphones today use electromagnetic induction (dynamic microphone), capacitance change, piezoelectric generation, or light modulation to produce the signal from mechanical vibration.

MYOCARDIAL VIABILITY

Knowledge about myocardial viability is very important for the management of patients with ischemic cardiomyopathy, as only viable myocardial segments will benefit from revascularisation. Several diagnostic approaches exist to assess myocardial viability though evaluation of wall thickness or myocardial contraction, perfusion or metabolism. To answer these questions several modalities may be used: cardiac molecular imaging, cardiovascular MR, echocardiography or cardiovascular CT.

Positron Emission Tomography

Positron emission tomography (PET) is a nuclear medicine imaging technique which produces a three-dimensional image or picture of functional processes in the body. The system detects pairs of gamma rays emitted indirectly by a positron-emitting radionuclide (tracer), which is introduced into the body on a biologically active molecule. Images of tracer concentration in 3-dimensional or 4-dimensional space within the body are then reconstructed by computer analysis. In modern scanners, this reconstruction is often accomplished with the aid of a CT X-ray scan performed on the patient during the same session, in the same machine (Fig. 18.19).

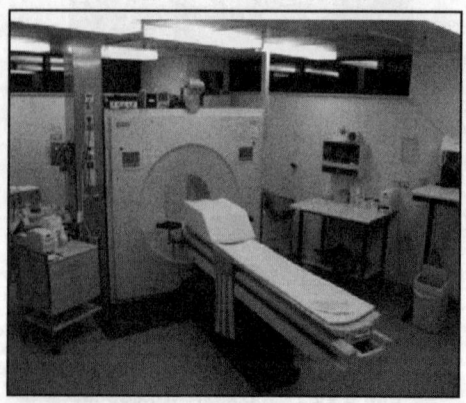

Fig. 8.19. Image of a typical positron emission tomography (PET) facility.

If the biologically active molecule chosen for PET is FDG, an analogue of glucose, the concentrations of tracer imaged then give tissue metabolic activity, in terms of regional glucose uptake. Although use of this tracer results in the most common type of PET scan, other tracer molecules are used in PET to image the tissue concentration of many other types of molecules of interest.

To conduct the scan, a short-lived radioactive tracer isotope is injected into the living subject (usually into blood circulation).

The tracer is chemically incorporated into a biologically active molecule. There is a waiting period while the active molecule becomes concentrated in tissues of interest; then the research subject or patient is placed in the imaging scanner. The molecule most commonly used for this purpose is fluorodeoxyglucose (FDG), a sugar, for which the waiting period is typically an hour. During the scan a record of tissue concentration is made as the tracer decays. As the radioisotope undergoes positron emission decay (also known as positive beta decay), it emits a positron, an antiparticle of the electron with opposite charge. After travelling up to a few millimetres the positron encounters an electron. Figure 8.20 shows schema of a PET acquisition process.

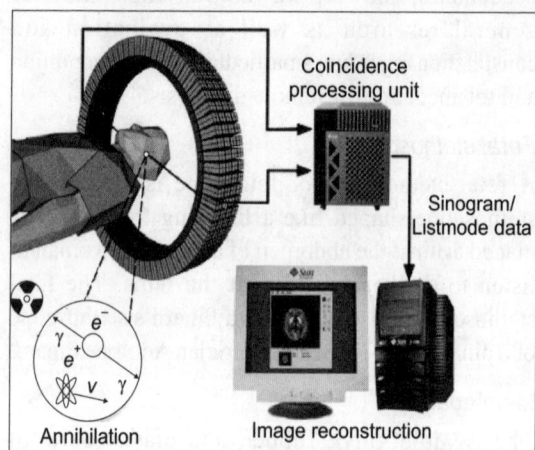

Fig. 8.20. Schema of a PET acquisition process.

The encounter annihilates them both, producing a pair of annihilation (gamma) photons moving in opposite directions. These are detected when they reach a scintillator in the scanning device, creating a burst of light which is detected by photomultiplier tubes or silicon avalanche photodiodes (Si APD). The technique depends on simultaneous or coincident detection of the pair of photons moving in approximately opposite direction (it would be exactly opposite in their centre of mass frame, but the scanner has no way to know this, and so has a built-in slight direction-error tolerance). Photons that do not arrive in temporal 'pairs' (i.e. within a timing-window of few nanoseconds) are ignored.

Localisation of the positron annihilation event

The most significant fraction of electron-positron decays result in two 511 keV gamma photons being emitted at almost 180 degrees to each other; hence it is possible to localise their source along a straight line of coincidence (also called formally the line of response or LOR). In practice the LOR has a finite width as the emitted photons are not exactly 180 degrees apart. If the resolving time of the detectors is less than 500 picoseconds rather than about 10 nanoseconds, it is possible to localise the event to a segment of a chord, whose length is determined by the detector timing resolution. As the timing resolution improves, the signal-to-noise ratio (SNR) of the image will improve, requiring fewer events to achieve the same image quality. This technology is not yet common, but it is available on some new systems.

Image reconstruction using coincidence statistics

More commonly, a technique much like the reconstruction of computed tomography (CT) and single photon emission computed tomography (SPECT) data is used, although the data set collected in PET is much poorer than CT, so reconstruction techniques are more difficult.

Using statistics collected from tens-of-thousands of coincidence events, a set of simultaneous equations for the total activity of each parcel of tissue along many LORs can be solved by a number of techniques, and thus a map of radioactivities as a function of location for parcels or bits of tissue (also called voxels), may be constructed and plotted. The resulting map shows the tissues in which the molecular probe has become concentrated, and can be interpreted by a nuclear medicine physician or radiologist in the context of the patient's diagnosis and treatment plan.

CIRCULATORY SYSTEM

The circulatory system is an organ system that passes nutrients (such as amino acids and electrolytes), gases, hormones, blood cells, etc. to and from cells in the body to help fight diseases and help stabilise body temperature and pH to maintain homeostasis. This system may be seen strictly as a blood distribution network, but some consider the circulatory system as composed of the cardiovascular system, which distributes blood, and the lymphatic system, which distributes lymph. While humans, as well as other vertebrates, have a closed cardiovascular system (meaning that the blood never leaves the network of arteries, veins and capillaries), some invertebrate groups have an open cardiovascular system. The most primitive animal phyla lack circulatory system. The lymphatic system, on the other hand, is an open system.

The main components of the human circulatory system are the heart, the blood, and the blood vessels. The circulatory system includes: the pulmonary circulation, a loop through the lungs where blood is oxygenated; and the systemic circulation, a loop through the rest of the body to provide oxygenated blood. An average adult contains five to six quarts (roughly 4.7 to 5.7 litres) of blood, which consists of plasma, red blood cells, white blood cells, and platelets. Also, the digestive system works with the circulatory system to provide the nutrients the system needs to keep the heart pumping.

Two types of fluids move through the circulatory system: blood and lymph. The blood, heart, and blood vessels form the cardiovascular system. The lymph, lymph nodes, and lymph vessels form the lymphatic system. The cardiovascular system and the lymphatic system collectively make up the circulatory system.

BLOOD FLOW

Blood flow is the flow of blood in the cardiovascular system. It can be calculated by dividing the vascular resistance into the pressure gradient.

Blood is a heterogeneous medium consisting mainly of plasma and a suspension of red blood cells. Red cells tend to coagulate when the flow shear rates are low, while increasing shear rates break these formations apart, thus reducing blood viscosity. This results in two non-Newtonian blood properties, shear thinning and yield stress. In healthy large arteries blood can be successfully approximated as a homogeneous, Newtonian fluid since the vessel size is much greater than the size of particles and shear rates are sufficiently high that particle interactions may have a negligible effect on the flow. In smaller vessels, however, non-Newtonian blood behaviour should be taken into account.

The flow in healthy vessels is generally laminar, however in diseased (e.g. atherosclerotic) arteries the flow may be transitional or turbulent.

Disturbed blood flow: Disturbed blood flow may cause ischemia and even infarction of the dependent tissue supplied by the struck vessels.

Causes include: (i) thrombosis, (ii) atherosclerosis, (iii) prolonged bedrest or immobilisation, (iv) myocardial infarction, (v) atrial fibrillation, (vi) prosthetic cardiac valves.

Disturbed blood flow is a factor in Virchow's triad for thrombosis.

Electromagnetic Blood Flowmeter

The most commonly used instrument of blood flow is of the electromagnetic type. With this type of instrument, blood flow can be measured in intact blood vessels without cannulation and under conditions which would otherwise be impossible. However, this method requires that the blood vessel be exposed so that the flow head or the measuring probe can be put across it.

The operating principle underlying all electromagnetic type flowmeters is based upon Faraday's law of electromagnetic induction which states that when a conductor is moved at right angles through a magnetic field in a direction at right angles both to the magnetic field and its length, an emf is induced in the conductor. In the flowmeter, an electromagnetic assembly provides the magnetic field placed at right angles to the blood vessel (Fig. 8.21) in which the flow is to be measured. The blood stream, which is a conductor, cuts the magnetic field and voltage is induced in the blood stream. This induced voltage is picked up by two electrodes incorporated in the magnetic assembly. The magnitude of the voltage picked up is directly proportional to the strength of the magnetic field, the diameter of the blood vessel

and the velocity of blood flow, i.e.

$$e = CHVd$$

where, e = induced voltage
H = strength of the magnetic field
V = velocity of blood flow
d = diameter of the blood vessel
C = constant of proportionality

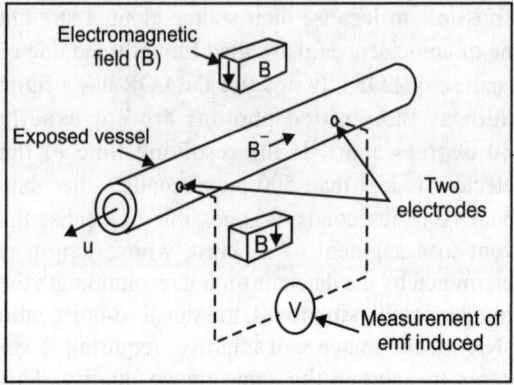

Fig. 8.21. Principle of electromagnetic flowmeter.

If the strength of the magnetic field and the diameter of the blood vessel remain unchanged, then the induced voltage will be a linear function of the blood flow velocity. Therefore,

$$e = C_1 V$$

where, C_1 is a constant and equal to CHd.

Further, the flow rate Q through a tube is given by:

$$Q = VA$$

therefore,

$$V = Q/A$$

where, A is the area of cross-section of the tube, hence

$$e = C_1 \times Q/A = C_2 \times Q$$

where, C_2 is a general constant and is given by C_1/A. This equation shows that the induced voltage is directly proportional to the flow rate through the blood vessel.

The induced voltage picked up by the electrodes is amplified and displayed/recorded on a suitable system. The system is calibrated in terms of volume flow as a function of the induced voltage. The diameter of the blood vessel is held constant by the circumference of the hole in the probe that surrounds it. The above relationship is true only if there exist conditions of axial symmetry and the blood velocity is considered independent of the velocity profile. Only then, the induced voltage is directly related to the blood volume flow.

Design of the flow transducer: In actual practice, the electromagnetic flowmeter transducer is a tube of nonmagnetic material to ensure that the magnetic flux does not bypass the flowing liquid and go into the walls of the tube. The tube is made of a conducting material and generally has an insulating lining to prevent short circuiting of the induced emf. The induced emf is picked up by point electrodes made from stainless steel or platinum. The flow head contains a slot through which the intact blood vessel can be inserted to make a snug fit. Several probes of different sizes must therefore accompany the flowmeter to match the full range of sizes of the blood vessels which have various diameters. It is naturally more difficult to construct flow heads suitable for use with very small blood vessels. However, flow heads having as small as 1 mm external diameter have been reported in literature.

The flow-induced voltage of an electromagnetic flowmeter is, within certain limitations, proportional to the velocity of the flow. This velocity is the average across the flow stream with an axis symmetric velocity profile. The average flow velocity appears to be 20 to 25 cm/s in arteries and 10 to 12 cm/s in veins. For designing the probe, velocity for the cardiovascular system is taken as 15 cm/s. For non-cannulated probes, a uniform magnetic field over the measuring area is so selected that it has a convenient shape and the smallest size. Iron cored electromagnets are used in probes having a diameter between 1 to 8.2 mm, and air cored electromagnets are use in diameters above 8.2 mm. Cannulated probes for extracorporeal use can have greater field strengths and magnet size as the constraint of small size is no longer present.

To obtain a reliable recording of the flow, a certain constriction of the vessel within the probe is necessary to maintain good contact. In order to limit the amount of constriction, a 20 per cent incremental range of sizes is chosen. To protect the probe from chemical attack, it must be encapsulated in a biologically inert material having a high electrical and chemical resistance, e.g. silicone rubber. The probes can generally be sterilised by chemical means. Probe calibration is carried out in 0.9 per cent saline during manufacture and each probe is given a calibration factor that is engraved on the connector. This factor is set on a multi-turn potentiometer to adjust the amplification to give a full scale output on the display meter.

The transducers are usually equipped with an internal ground electrode so that no external grounding is necessary. The cable from the transducer to the instrument should comprise of a teflon insulated wire completely shielded with a tinned copper braid. The entire cable is sleeved with medical grade silicone rubber tubing and impregnated with silicone rubber to minimise leakage and electrical noise. The transducers should be tested for 1000 megaohms minimum resistance between the coil and electrodes, after prolonged immersion in saline.

Common-mode rejection is influenced by the difference between the impedances of the pick-up electrodes of a transducer and is maximum only when these impedances are identical. Electrode impedances in saline generally lie between 1 kΩ and about 10 kΩ, values of 1.5–2 kΩ being typical of platinised platinum and dull gold electrodes. The common-mode impedance of the measuring circuit should be at least 100 MΩ to ensure that variations of several hundred ohms between the impedances of a pair of transducer electrodes do not significantly affect the common mode rejection.

The early models of electromagnetic blood flowmeters employed permanent magnets which were subsequently replaced by electromagnets powered at mains frequencies. However, the tremendous interference from mains voltages at the transducer electrodes resulted in baseline drifts and poor signal-to-noise ratio. Various types of waveforms at different frequencies have since been tried to overcome these difficulties. Today, we have electromagnetic flowmeters whose magnetic coils work on sine, square or trapezium current waveforms.

The probes have an open slot on one side which makes it possible to slip it over a blood vessel without cutting the vessel. The probe must fit the vessel during diastole so that the electrodes make good contact. Probes are made in 1 mm increments in the range of 1 to 24 mm to ensure that they can be used on a variety of sizes of arteries. The probes generally do not operate satisfactorily on veins because the electrodes do not make good contact when the vein collapses. Attempts have been made to miniaturise the flow head to an extent that it can be mounted on the tip of a catheter. Such devices are needed in experimental as well as in clinical cardiology for mapping the velocity conditions of the entire circulatory system.

Types of electromagnetic flowmeters

Basically all modern flowmeters consist of a generator of alternating current, a probe assembly, a series of capacitance coupled amplifiers, a demodulator, a dc amplifier and a suitable recording device. The shape of the energising current waveform for the electromagnet may be sinusoidal or square.

Sine wave flowmeters

In a sine wave flowmeter, the probe magnet is energised with a sine wave and consequently the induced voltage will also be sinusoidal in nature. The major problem encountered with the sinusoidal type of magnetic field is that the blood vessel and the fluid contained in it act as the secondary coil of a transformer when the probe magnet is excited. As a result, in addition to the induced flow voltage, there is an induced artefact voltage generally referred to as 'transformer voltage'.

The 'transformer voltage' is much larger than the signal or flow induced voltage and is 90° out of phase with it. This also causes baseline drift which necessitates high phase stability in the amplifier and demodulator circuits.

In earlier versions of sine wave flowmeters, this unwanted voltage was eliminated by injecting into the signal a voltage of equal strength, but having an opposite phase. The artefact signal is thus cancelled and only the flow induced voltage is left behind for display.

An alternative method to eliminate the transformer induced voltage in sinewave flowmeters is by using a gated amplifier. The function of this amplifier is to permit the amplification of the signals only during the portion of the cycle where flow induced voltages are maximum and the transformer induced voltages are minimum. By this method, the artefact voltage is prevented from getting amplified. This type of instrument is known as a 'gated sine wave flowmeter'.

The sine wave flowmeters require complicated electronic circuitry for the removal of transformer induced voltage from the flow induced voltage. As both the waveforms are of the same type, complete elimination of the artefact voltage becomes extremely difficult. The sine wave system, no doubt yields good signal-to-noise ratio, but imposes stringent phase stability requirements with increasing frequency.

Square wave electromagnetic flowmeters

This differs from a sine wave flowmeter in that the energising voltage given to the magnet is a square wave and therefore, the induced voltage is also a square wave. The square wave flowmeter has less stringent requirements of phase stability than the sine wave type as it can suppress the quadrature voltages relatively easily. Also, it is easier to control the magnitude and wave shape of the energising current in the case of a square wave system.

The transformer induced voltage in this case is only a spike, superimposed on the beginning of the square wave flow induced voltage. Separation of these two voltages becomes easier as the amplifier can be gated only for a very short period. In a square wave flowmeter, blanking is required only during the portion when the current in the magnet is reversing and the amplifier works during the flat portion of the square wave.

The square wave is amplitude modulated by the variation in blood flow and requires to be demodulated before it can be fed to a recorder.

Figure 8.22 shows the block diagram of a square wave electromagnetic blood flowmeter.

Transducer: The flow transducer consists of an electromagnet, which provides a magnetic field perpendicular to the direction of flow and lying within the field are a pair of pick-up electrodes whose axis is perpendicular to both the field and the flow axis. The electrodes may be in contact with either the flowing blood or the outer surface of the blood vessel carrying the flowing blood.

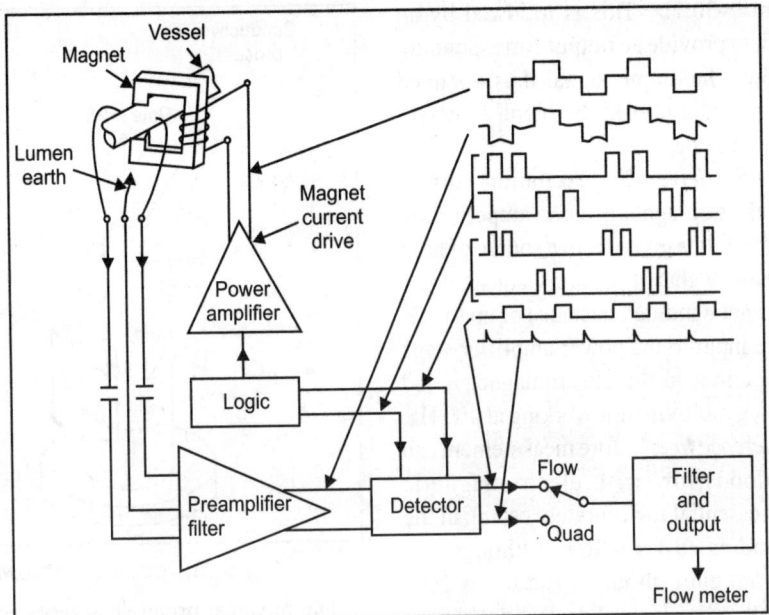

Fig. 8.22. Block diagram of a square wave electromagnetic flowmeter.

The former is called 'cannulating flowmeter' and the latter 'cuff flowmeter'.

Preamplifier: The induced voltage picked up by the electrodes is given to a low noise differential amplifier through a capacitive coupling. The preamplifier must have a very high common-mode rejection ratio and input impedance. The preamplifier used by Goodman has a CMRR of 106 dB (2,00,000:1) with a common mode input impedance of 150 MΩ. The preamplifier gain is of the order of 1000. The preamplifier also must incorporate the facility for 'probe balance' by which signals in phase with the magnet current can be selected to balance background voltages in phase with flow voltages. A calibrating signal of 30 μV amplitude can be connected to the preamplifier with an input selector switch.

Noise voltage generated in the preamplifier is an important factor in the performance of an electromagnetic flowmeter. The noise voltage is seen as a random movement of the baseline of the recorded flow. When expressed in terms of flow, it is typically 1–2 per cent of the full scale output of the chosen probe. For example, a 2.7 mm probe gives full scale deflection for 500 ml/min., so the noise is equivalent to 10 ml/min.

Gating circuit: A gating amplifier helps to remove spurious voltages generated during magnet current reversal. For the flowmeter to exhibit a satisfactory base line stability, it is essential that the spurious signals produced during the magnet current reversal and those in phase with flow voltages are made negligible. The gating action is controlled by the circuit which provides an excitation current to the electromagnet.

Bandpass amplifier: Following the gating amplifier is an active RC bandpass amplifier, which selectively passes through it the amplified square wave signal. The peak response is kept for 400 Hz. The 3 dB points are at 300 and 500 Hz. The gain of this amplifier is typically 50. The shape of the wave after this amplifier is a distorted sinusoid.

Detector: A phase sensitive detector is used to recover the signal, which is an analogue of the flow rate being measured. This type of demodulator not only offers maximum signal-to-noise ratio but also helps in the rejection of interfering voltages at frequencies well below the carrier frequency.

Low-pass filter and output stage: The demodulated signal is given to an active RC low-pass filter, which provides a uniform frequency response and a linear phase shift from 0–30 Hz. This is followed by an integrator circuit to provide an output corresponding to the mean flow. The output signal thus obtained can be put to a recorder to read the blood flow rate from the calibrated scale.

Magnet current drive: The excitation current supplied to the electromagnet is a one ampere peak square wave current. It is given from a source of high impedance to ensure that it remains constant for variations in magnet winding resistance of up to 5Ω. The square wave input to the power amplifier stage which supplies current to the electromagnet is fed from a free running multivibrator working at 400 Hz.

Zero-flow reference line: Before measurement can be made for blood flow with electromagnetic flowmeters, it is essential to accurately establish the signal corresponding to zero-flow. Although de-energising the magnet should produce a zero reference line, unfortunately this line does not always coincide with the physiological zero-flow line. This is owing to some effects at the electrode vessel interface. An alternative method could be to occlude the blood vessel in which flow is to be measured. Several arrangements have been used to act as occluders. However, there is a serious objection to their use because the necessity for occlusion of the vessel, in order to obtain a zero flow reference, introduces the possibility of producing a spasm and hence a change in the blood flow.

Electromagnetic, Ultrasonic and Coriolis Flowmeters

Modern innovations in the measurement of flow rate incorporate electronic devices that can correct for varying pressure and temperature (i.e. density) conditions, non-linearities, and for the characteristics of the fluid.

Magnetic flowmeters

The most common flow meter apart from mechanical flow meters is the magnetic flow meter, commonly referred to as a 'mag meter' or an 'electromag'. A magnetic field is applied to the metering tube, which results in a potential difference proportional to the flow velocity perpendicular to the flux lines (Fig. 8.23).

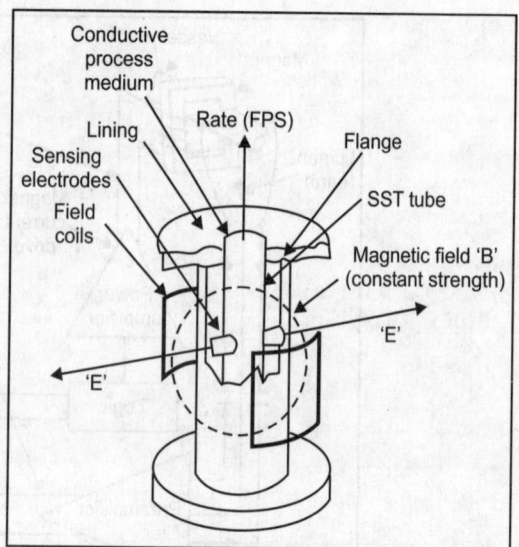

Fig. 8.23. The magnetic flowmeter.

The physical principle at work is Faraday's law of electromagnetic induction. The magnetic flow meter requires a conducting fluid, e.g. water, and an electrical insulating pipe surface, e.g. a rubber lined nonmagnetic steel tube.

Ultrasonic (Doppler, transit time) flow meters

Ultrasonic flow meters measure the difference of the transit time of ultrasonic pulses propagating in and against flow direction. This time difference is a measure for the average velocity of the fluid along the path of the ultrasonic beam. By using the absolute transit times both the averaged fluid velocity and the speed of sound can be calculated. Using the two transit times t_{up} and t_{down} and the distance between receiving and transmitting transducers L and the inclination angle α one can write the equations:

$$v = \frac{L}{2\sin(\alpha)}\frac{t_{up} - t_{down}}{t_{up}\, t_{down}} \text{ and } c = \frac{L}{2}\frac{t_{up} - t_{down}}{t_{up}\, t_{down}}$$

where, v is the average velocity of the fluid along the sound path and c is the speed of sound.

Ultrasonic flow meters are used for the measurement of natural gas flow. One can also calculate the expected speed of sound for a given sample of gas; this can be compared to the speed of sound empirically measured by an ultrasonic flow meter and for the purposes of monitoring the quality of the flow meter's measurements. A drop in quality is an indication that the meter needs servicing.

Measurement of the Doppler shift resulting in reflecting an ultrasonic beam off the flowing fluid is another recent innovation. By passing an ultrasonic beam through the tissues, bouncing it off a reflective plate, then reversing the direction of the beam and repeating the measurement, the volume of blood flow can be estimated.

The frequency of the transmitted beam is affected by the movement of blood in the vessel and by comparing the frequency of the upstream beam versus downstream the flow of blood through the vessel can be measured. The difference between the two frequencies is a measure of true volume flow. A wide-beam sensor can also be used to measure flow independent of the cross-sectional area of the blood vessel. Figure 8.24 shows schematic view of a flow sensor.

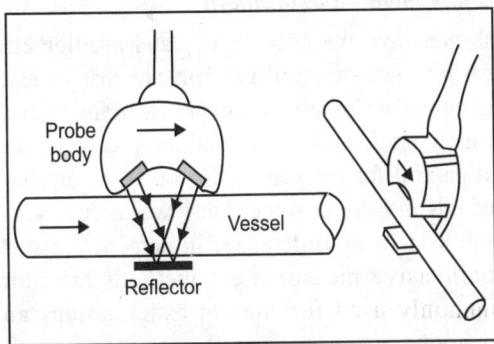

Fig. 8.24. Schematic view of a flow sensor.

For the doppler principle to work in a flowmeter it is mandatory that the flow stream contains sonically reflective materials, such as solid particles or entrained air bubbles. A related technology is acoustic doppler velocimetry.

Coriolis flow meters

Using the Coriolis effect that causes a laterally vibrating tube to distort, a direct measurement of mass flow can be obtained in a coriolis flow meter. Furthermore a direct measure of the density of the fluid is obtained. Coriolis measurement can be very accurate irrespective of the type of gas or liquid that

is measured; the same measurement tube can be used for hydrogen gas and bitumen without recalibration. Coriolis flow meters can be used for the measurement of natural gas flow.

Laser Doppler Flow Measurement

Blood flow can be measured through the use of a monochromatic laser diode. The laser probe is inserted into a tissue and turned on, where the light scatters and a small portion is reflected back to the probe. The signal is then processed to calculate flow within the tissues. There are limitations to the use of a laser doppler probe; flow within a tissue is dependent on volume illuminated, which is often assumed rather than measured and varies with the optical properties of the tissue (Fig. 8.25). In addition, variations in the type and placement of the probe within identical tissues and individuals result in variations in reading. The laser doppler has the advantage of sampling a small volume of tissue, allowing for great precision, but does not necessarily represent the flow within an entire organ. The flow meter is much more useful for relative rather than absolute measurements.

BLOOD PRESSURE

Blood pressure (BP) is a force exerted by circulating blood on the walls of blood vessels, and is one of the principal vital signs. During each heartbeat, BP varies between a maximum (systolic) and a minimum (diastolic) pressure. The mean BP, due to pumping by the heart and resistance in blood vessels, decreases as the circulating blood moves away from the heart through arteries. It has its greatest decrease in the small arteries and arterioles, and continues to decrease as the blood moves through the capillaries and back to the heart through veins. Gravity, valves in veins, and pumping from contraction of skeletal muscles, are some other influences on BP at various places in the body.

The term blood pressure usually refers to the pressure measured at a person's upper arm. It is measured on the inside of an elbow at the brachial artery, which is the upper arm's major blood vessel that carries blood away from the heart. A person's BP is usually expressed in terms of the systolic pressure and diastolic pressure, for example 115/75.

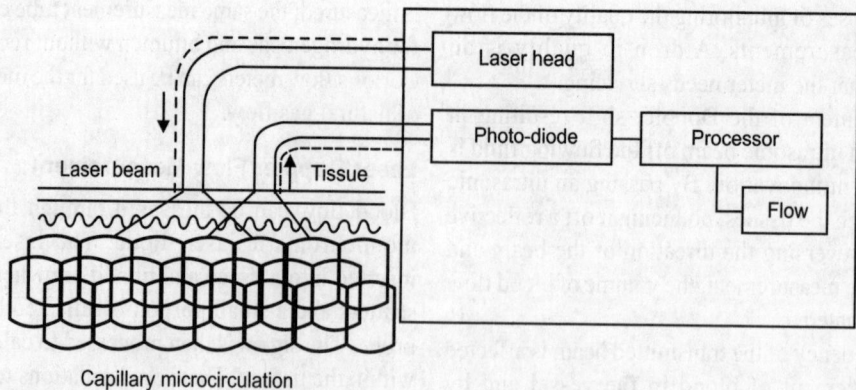

Fig. 8.25. Laser doppler flowmeter.

Measurement

Arterial pressure is most commonly measured via a sphygmomanometer, which historically used the height of a column of mercury to reflect the circulating pressure. Today BP values are still reported in millimeters of mercury (mmHg), though aneroid and electronic devices do not use mercury.

For each heartbeat, BP varies between systolic and diastolic pressures. Systolic pressure is peak pressure in the arteries, which occurs near the end of the cardiac cycle when the ventricles are contracting. Diastolic pressure is minimum pressure in the arteries, which occurs near the beginning of the cardiac cycle when the ventricles are filled with blood. An example of normal measured values for a resting, healthy adult human is 115 mmHg systolic and 75 mmHg diastolic (written as 115/75 mmHg, and spoken [in the US] as 'one-fifteen over seventy-five'). Systolic and diastolic arterial BPs are not static but undergo natural variations from one heartbeat to another and throughout the day (in a circadian rhythm). They also change in response to stress, nutritional factors, drugs, disease, exercise, and momentarily from standing up. Sometimes the variations are large. Hypertension refers to arterial pressure being abnormally high, as opposed to hypotension, when it is abnormally low. Along with body temperature, respiratory rate, and pulse rate, BP measurements are the most commonly measured physiological parameters.

Arterial pressures are usually measured noninvasively, without penetrating skin or artery. Measuring pressure invasively, by penetrating the arterial wall to take the measurement, is much less common, and usually restricted to a hospital setting.

Noninvasive measurement

The non invasive auscultatory and oscillometric measurements are simpler and quicker than invasive measurements, require less expertise in fitting, have virtually no complications, and are less unpleasant and painful for the person. However, noninvasive methods may yield somewhat lower accuracy and small systematic differences in numerical results. Noninvasive measurement methods are more commonly used for routine examinations and monitoring.

Palpation method

A minimum systolic value can be roughly estimated without any equipment by palpation, most often used in emergency situations. Historically, students have been taught that palpation of a radial pulse indicates a minimum BP of 80 mmHg, a femoral pulse indicates at least 70 mmHg, and a carotid pulse indicates a minimum of 60 mmHg. However, at least one study indicated that this method often overestimates patients' systolic BP. A more accurate value of systolic BP can be obtained with a sphygmomanometer and palpating for when a radial pulse returns. The diastolic blood pressure can not be estimated by this method. Sometimes palpation is used to get an estimate before using the auscultatory method.

Auscultatory method

The auscultatory method uses a stethoscope and a sphygmomanometer (Fig. 8.26). This comprises an inflatable (*Riva-Rocci*) cuff placed around the upper arm at roughly the same vertical height as the heart, attached to a mercury or aneroid manometer. The mercury manometer measures the height of a column of mercury, giving an absolute result without need for calibration, and consequently not subject to the errors and drift of calibration which affect other methods. The use of mercury manometers is often required in clinical trials and for the clinical measurement of hypertension in high risk patients, such as pregnant women.

A cuff of appropriate size is fitted smoothly and snugly, then inflated manually by repeatedly squeezing a rubber bulb until the artery is completely occluded. Listening with the stethoscope to the brachial artery at the elbow, the examiner slowly releases the pressure in the cuff. When blood just starts to flow in the artery, the turbulent flow creates a 'whooshing' or pounding (first Korotkoff sound). The pressure at which this sound is first heard is the systolic BP. The cuff pressure is further released until no sound can be heard (fifth Korotkoff sound), at the diastolic arterial pressure.

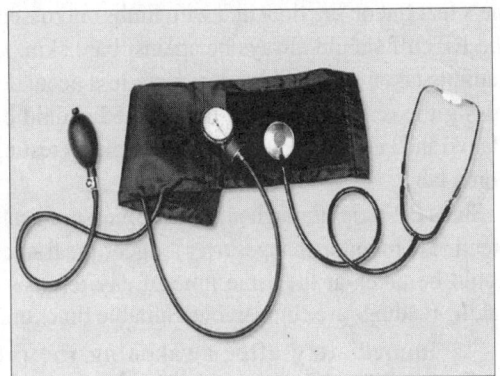

Fig. 8.26. Auscultatory method aneroid sphygmomanometer with stethoscope.

The auscultatory method has been predominant since the beginning of BP measurements but in other cases it's being replaced by other noninvasive techniques. Figure 8.27 shows mercury manometer.

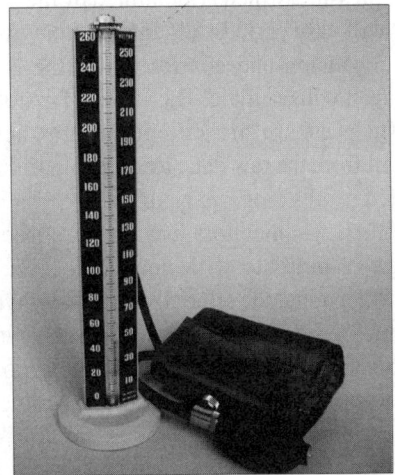

Fig. 8.27. Mercury manometer.

Oscillometric method

The oscillometric method was first demonstrated in 1876 and involves the observation of oscillations in the sphygmomanometer cuff pressure which are caused by the oscillations of blood flow, i.e. the pulse. The electronic version of this method is sometimes used in long-term measurements and general practice. It uses a sphygmomanometer cuff like the auscultatory method, but with an electronic pressure sensor (transducer) to observe cuff pressure oscillations, electronics to automatically interpret them, and automatic inflation and deflation of the cuff. The pressure sensor should be calibrated periodically to maintain accuracy.

Oscillometric measurement requires less skill than the auscultatory technique, and may be suitable for use by untrained staff and for automated patient home monitoring.

The cuff is inflated to a pressure initially in excess of the systolic arterial pressure, and then reduces to below diastolic pressure over a period of about 30 seconds. When blood flow is nil (cuff pressure exceeding systolic pressure) or unimpeded (cuff pressure below diastolic pressure), cuff pressure will be essentially constant. It is essential that the cuff size is correct: undersized cuffs may yield too high a pressure, whereas oversized cuffs yield too low a pressure. When blood flow is present, but restricted, the cuff pressure, which is monitored by the pressure sensor, will vary periodically in synchrony with the cyclic expansion and contraction of the brachial artery, i.e. it will oscillate. The values of systolic and diastolic pressure are computed, not actually measured from the raw data, using an algorithm; the computed results are displayed.

Oscillometric monitors may produce inaccurate readings in patients with heart and circulation problems, that include arterial sclerosis, arrhythmia, preeclampsia, pulsus alternans, and pulsus paradoxus.

In practice the different methods do not give identical results; an algorithm and experimentally obtained coefficients are used to adjust the oscillometric results to give readings which match the auscultatory results as well as possible. Some equipment uses computer-aided analysis of the instantaneous arterial pressure waveform to determine the systolic, mean, and diastolic points. Since many oscillometric devices have not been validated, caution must be given as most are not suitable in clinical and acute care settings.

The term NIBP, for noninvasive blood pressure, is often used to describe oscillometric monitoring equipment.

White-coat hypertension

For some patients, BP measurements taken in a doctor's office may not correctly characterise their typical BP. In up to 25 per cent of patients, the office measurement is higher than their typical BP. This type of error is called white-coat hypertension (WCH) and can result from anxiety related to an examination by a health care professional. The misdiagnosis of hypertension for these patients can result in needless and possibly harmful medication. WCH can be reduced (but not eliminated) with automated BP measurements over 15 to 20 minutes in a quiet part of the office or clinic.

Debate continues regarding the significance of this effect. Some reactive patients will also react to many other stimuli throughout their daily lives, and require treatment. In some cases a lower BP reading occurs at the doctor's office.

Home monitoring

Ambulatory blood pressure devices that take readings every half hour throughout the day and night have been used for identifying and mitigating measurement problems like white-coat hypertension. Except for periods during sleep, home monitoring could be used for these purposes instead of ambulatory blood pressure monitoring. Home monitoring may also be used to improve hypertension management and to monitor the effects of lifestyle changes and medication related to BP. Compared to ambulatory blood pressure measurements, home monitoring has been found to be an effective and lower cost alternative.

Aside from the white coat effect, BP readings outside of a clinical setting are usually slightly lower in the majority of people. The studies that looked into the risks from hypertension and the benefits of lowering BP in affected patients were based on readings in a clinical environment.

When measuring BP, an accurate reading requires that one not drink coffee, smoke cigarettes, or engage in strenuous exercise for 30 minutes before taking the reading. A full bladder may have a small effect on BP readings, so if the urge to urinate exists, one should do so before the reading. For 5 minutes before the reading, one should sit upright in a chair with one's feet flat on the floor and with limbs uncrossed. The BP cuff should always be against bare skin, as readings taken over a shirt sleeve are less accurate. During the reading, the arm that is used should be relaxed and kept at heart level, for example by resting it on a table.

Since BP varies throughout the day, measurements intended to monitor changes over longer time frames should be taken at the same time of day to ensure that the readings are comparable. Suitable times are:

1. Immediately after awakening (before washing/dressing and taking breakfast/drink), while the body is still resting.
2. Immediately after finishing work.

Automatic self-contained BP monitors are available at reasonable prices, some of which are capable of Korotkoff's measurement in addition to oscillometric methods, enabling irregular heartbeat patients to accurately measure their blood pressure at home.

Invasive measurement

Arterial blood pressure (BP) is most accurately measured invasively through an arterial line. Invasive arterial pressure measurement with intravascular cannulae involves direct measurement of arterial pressure by placing a cannula needle in an artery (usually radial, femoral, dorsalis pedis or brachial). This procedure can be done by any licensed doctor or a Respiratory Therapist.

The cannula must be connected to a sterile, fluid-filled system, which is connected to an electronic pressure transducer. The advantage of this system is that pressure is constantly monitored beat-by-beat, and a waveform (a graph of pressure against time) can be displayed. This invasive technique is regularly employed in human and veterinary intensive care medicine, anesthesiology, and for research purposes.

Cannulation for invasive vascular pressure monitoring is infrequently associated with complications such as thrombosis, infection, and bleeding.

Patients with invasive arterial monitoring require very close supervision, as there is a danger of severe bleeding if the line becomes disconnected. It is generally reserved for patients where rapid variations in arterial pressure are anticipated.

Invasive vascular pressure monitors are pressure monitoring systems designed to acquire pressure information for display and processing. There are a variety of invasive vascular pressure monitors for trauma, critical care, and operating room applications. These include single pressure, dual pressure, and multi-parameter (i.e. pressure/temperature). The monitors can be used for measurement and follow-up of arterial, central venous, pulmonary arterial, left atrial, right atrial, femoral arterial, umbilical venous, umbilical arterial, and intracranial pressures.

Intravascular Ultrasound

Intravascular ultrasound (IVUS) is a medical imaging methodology using a specially designed catheter with a miniaturised ultrasound probe attached to the distal end of the catheter. The proximal end of the catheter is attached to computerised ultrasound equipment. It allows the application of ultrasound technology to see from inside blood vessels out through the surrounding blood column, visualising the endothelium (inner wall) of blood vessels in living individuals.

The arteries of the heart (the coronary arteries) are the most frequent imaging target for IVUS. IVUS is used in the coronary arteries to determine the amount of atheromatous plaque built up at any particular point in the epicardial coronary artery. The progressive accumulation of plaque within the artery wall over decades is the setup for vulnerable plaque which, in turn, leads to heart attack and stenosis (narrowing) of the artery (known as coronary artery lesions). IVUS is of use to determine both plaque volume within the wall of the artery and/or the degree of stenosis of the artery lumen. It can be especially useful in situations in which angiographic imaging is considered unreliable; such as for the lumen of ostial lesions or where angiographic images do not visualise lumen segments adequately, such as regions with multiple overlapping arterial segments. It is also used to assess the effects of treatments of stenosis such as with hydraulic angioplasty expansion of the artery, with or without stents, and the results of medical therapy over time.

Angiography

Angiography or arteriography is a medical imaging technique used to visualise the inside, or lumen, of blood vessels and organs of the body, with particular interest in the arteries, veins and the heart chambers. This is traditionally done by injecting a radio-opaque contrast agent into the blood vessel and imaging using X-ray based techniques such as fluoroscopy. The word itself comes from the Greek words angeion, 'vessel', and graphein, 'to write or record'. The film or image of the blood vessels is called an angiograph, or more commonly, an angiogram.

Although the term angiography is strictly defined as based on projectional radiography, the term has been applied to newer vascular imaging techniques such as CT angiography and MR angiography.

Methods of visualisation

In experimental fluid dynamics, flows are visualised by three methods:

1. Surface flow visualisation: This reveals the flow streamlines in the limit as a solid surface is approached. Coloured oil applied to the surface of a wind tunnel model provides one example (the oil responds to the surface shear stress and forms a pattern).

2. Particle tracer methods: Particles, such as smoke, can be added to a flow to trace the fluid motion. We can illuminate the particles with a sheet of laser light in order to visualise a slice of a complicated fluid flow pattern. Assuming that the particles faithfully follow the streamlines of the flow, we can not only visualise the flow but also measure its velocity using a method known as particle image velocimetry.

3. Optical methods: some flows reveal their patterns by way of changes in their optical refractive index. These are visualised by optical methods known as the shadowgraph, schlieren photography, and interferometry.

Diagnostic Sonography

Medical sonography (ultrasonography) is an ultrasound-based diagnostic medical imaging technique used to visualise muscles, tendons, and many internal organs, to capture their size, structure and any pathological lesions with real time tomographic images. Ultrasound has been used by sonographers to image the human body for at least 50 years and has become one of the most widely used diagnostic tools in modern medicine. The technology is relatively inexpensive and portable, especially when compared with other modalities, such as magnetic resonance imaging (MRI) and computed tomography (CT). Ultrasound is also used to visualise fetuses during routine and emergency prenatal care.

Such diagnostic applications used during pregnancy are referred to as obstetric sonography.

As currently applied in the medical field, properly performed ultrasound poses no known risks to the patient. Sonography is generally described as a 'safe test' because it does not use mutagenic ionising radiation, which can pose hazards such as chromosome breakage and cancer development. However, ultrasonic energy has two potential physiological effects: it enhances inflammatory response; and it can heat soft tissue. Ultrasound energy produces a mechanical pressure wave through soft tissue.

This pressure wave may cause microscopic bubbles in living tissues and distortion of the cell membrane, influencing ion fluxes and intracellular activity. When ultrasound enters the body, it causes molecular friction and heats the tissues slightly. This effect is typically very minor as normal tissue perfusion dissipates most of the heat, but with high intensity, it can also cause small pockets of gas in body fluids or tissues to expand and contract/collapse in a phenomenon called cavitation; however this is not known to occur at diagnostic power levels used by modern diagnostic ultrasound units.

In 2008, the AIUM published a 130-page report titled 'American Institute of Ultrasound in Medicine Consensus Report on Potential Bioeffects of Diagnostic Ultrasound' stating that there are indeed some potential risks to administering ultrasound tests, which include 'postnatal thermal effects, fetal thermal effects, postnatal mechanical effects, fetal mechanical effects, and bioeffects considerations for ultrasound contrast agents'. The long-term effects of tissue heating and cavitation have shown decreases in the size of red blood cells in cattle when exposed to intensities higher than diagnostic levels. However, long term effects due to ultrasound exposure at diagnostic intensity is still unknown.

There are several studies that indicate the harmful side effects on animal fetuses associated with the use of sonography on pregnant mammals. A Yale study in 2006 suggested exposure to ultrasound affects fetal brain development in mice. A typical fetal scan, including evaluation for fetal malformations, typically takes 10–30 minutes. The study showed that rodent brain cells failed to migrate to their proper positions and remained scattered in incorrect parts of the brain. This misplacement of brain cells during their development is linked to disorders ranging from 'mental retardation and childhood epilepsy to developmental dyslexia, autism spectrum disorders and schizophrenia'.

However, this effect was only detectable after 30 minutes of continuous scanning. No link has yet been made between the test results on animals such as mice and the possible effects on humans. Although the possibility exists that biological effects on humans may be identified in the future, currently most doctors feel that based on available information the benefits to patients outweigh the risks.

Obstetric ultrasound can be used to identify many conditions that would be harmful to the mother and the baby.

Many health care professionals consider the risk of leaving these conditions undiagnosed to be much greater than the very small risk, if any, associated with undergoing an ultrasound scan. According to Cochrane Review, routine ultrasound in early pregnancy (less than 24 weeks) appears to enable better gestational age assessment, earlier detection of multiple pregnancies and earlier detection of clinically unsuspected fetal malformation at a time when termination of pregnancy is possible.

Sonography is used routinely in obstetric appointments during pregnancy, but the FDA discourages its use for non-medical purposes such as fetal keepsake videos and photos, even though it is the same technology used in hospitals.

Obstetric ultrasound is primarily used to:

1. Date the pregnancy (gestational age).
2. Confirm fetal viability.
3. Determine location of fetus, intrauterine vs ectopic.
4. Check the location of the placenta in relation to the cervix.
5. Check for the number of fetuses (multiple pregnancy).
6. Check for major physical abnormalities.
7. Assess fetal growth (for evidence of intrauterine growth restriction (IUGR)).
8. Check for fetal movement and heartbeat.
9. Determine the sex of the baby.

Unfortunately, results are occasionally wrong, producing a false positive (the Cochrane Collaboration is a relevant effort to improve the reliability of health care trials). False detection may result in patients being warned of birth defects when no such defect exists. Sex determination is only accurate after 12 weeks gestation. When balancing risk and reward, there are recommendations to avoid the use of routine ultrasound for low risk pregnancies. In many countries ultrasound is used routinely in the management of all pregnancies.

9

Lung, Kidney, Bone and Skin

INTRODUCTION

The chapter describes four major organs in the body: lung, kidney, bone, and skin. Each of these organs has its own properties and functions: the lungs help respiration, the kidneys help clean the blood, bone supports the body, and skin protects the body. Various bioinstrumentation methods are performed to confirm whether each of these organs is functioning properly, and also to measure some of their properties.

LUNG

The lung or pulmonary system is the essential respiration organ in all air-breathing animals, including most tetrapods, a few fish and a few snails. In mammals and the more complex life forms, the two lungs are located in the chest on either side of the heart. Their principal function is to transport oxygen from the atmosphere into the bloodstream, and to release carbon dioxide from the bloodstream into the atmosphere. This exchange of gases is accomplished in the mosaic of specialised cells that form millions of tiny, exceptionally thin-walled air sacs called alveoli (Fig.9.1).

In order to completely explain the anatomy of the lungs, it is necessary to discuss the passage of air through the mouth to the alveoli. Once air progresses through the mouth or nose, it travels through the oropharynx, nasopharynx, the larynx, the trachea, and a progressively subdividing system of bronchi and bronchioles until it finally reaches the alveoli where the gas exchange of carbon dioxide and oxygen takes place (Fig. 9.2).

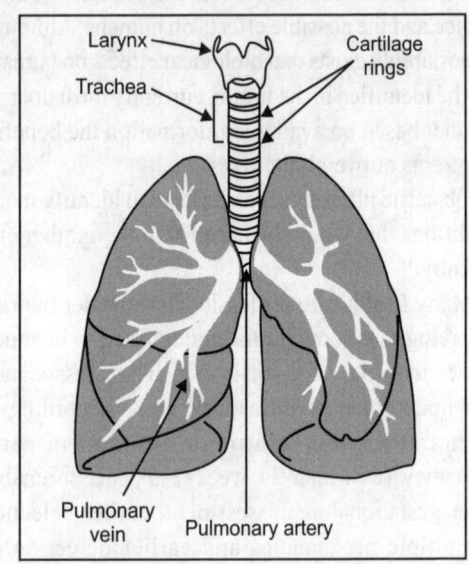

Fig. 9.1. The human lungs flank the heart and great vessels in the chest cavity.

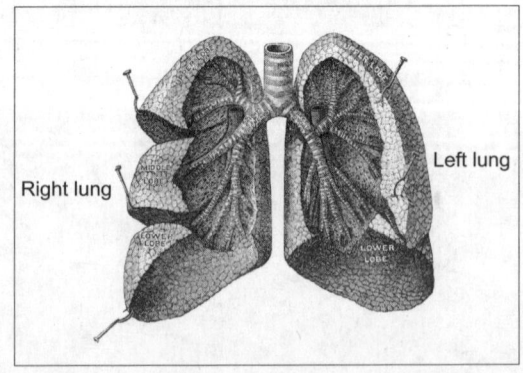

Fig. 9.2. Air enters and leaves the lungs via a conduit of cartilaginous passageways—the bronchi and bronchioles. In this image, lung tissue has been dissected away to reveal the bronchioles

The drawing and expulsion of air (ventilation) is driven by muscular action; in early tetrapods, air was driven into the lungs by the pharyngeal muscles, whereas in reptiles, birds and mammals a more complicated musculoskeletal system is used.

MEASUREMENT OF LUNG VOLUMES

The spirometer (Latin *spirare*, to breathe) is the traditional device used to measure the volume of air moved in respiration. The most popular type of spirometer consists of a hollow cylinder closed at one end, inverted and suspended in an annular space filled with water to provide an airtight seal. Figure 9.3 illustrates the method of suspending the cylinder (bell), which is free to move up and down to accommodate the volume, is usually recorded by a stylus applied to a chart that is caused to move with a constant velocity in a direction perpendicular to the movement of the recording stylus (Fig. 9.3). Below the cylinder, in the space that accommodates the volume of air, are inlet and outlet breathing tubes. At the end of one or both of these tubes is a check valve designed to maintain a unidirectional flow of gas through the spirometer. Outside the spirometer, the two breathing tubes are brought to a Y tube that is connected to a mouthpiece. With a pinchclamp placed on the nose, inspiration diminishes the volume of gas under the bell, which descends, causing the stylus to rise on the graphic record. Expiration produces the reverse effect. Thus, starting with the spirometer half-filled, quiet respiration causes the bell to rise and fall. By knowing the 'bell factor,' the volume of gas moved per centimeter excursion of the bell, the tidal volume can be measured. A maximum gas volume inhaled, which is called the inspiratory capacity. A maximum expiratory effort started from the resting expiratory level will causes the spirometer to display the expiratory reserve volume. Likewise, starting from the maximum expiratory level, a maximum inspiration will allow measurement of the vital capacity. Thus the simple spirometer can be used to measure all of the lung compartments except the residual volume.

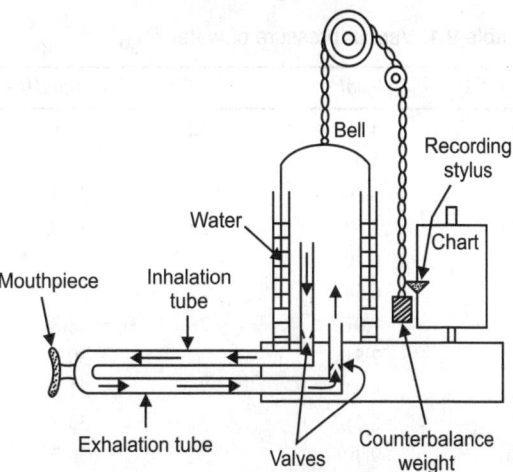

Fig. 9.3. The simple spirometer.

Standardisation of Volume

When spirometers are used to measure respiratory volumes, certain corrections must be applied. This is especially true when the volumes measured are to be compared to those in blood.

The volume of gas in the lungs exists at body temperature and atmospheric pressure and is saturated with water vapour (BTPS). Measurement of respired volumes is carried out at ambient temperature and atmospheric pressure, and the gas is saturated (ATPS). Because measurements are made in this way, it is necessary to correct the measured volumes to body temperature (37°C) and a saturated water vapour pressure of 47 mmHg. The following equation, derived directly from the gas laws, permits application of the temperature and pressure corrections:

$$\text{Volume (BTPS)} = \left(\begin{array}{c} \text{Volume collected} \\ \text{at } t°C \end{array} \right) \left[\frac{273+37}{273+t} \right]$$

$$\left[\frac{P_B - P_{H_2O}}{P_B - 47} \right]$$

where,

t = temperature of the gas in the spirometer (°C).

P_B = barometric pressure (mmHg).

P_{H_2O} = water vapour pressure (mmHg) of the gas in the spirometer at $t°C$. (See values in Table 9.1).

Table 9.1. Vapour pressure of water P_{H_2O}.

$T\,(°C)$	$P_{H_2O}\,(mmHg)$	$T\,(°C)$	$P_{H_2O}\,(mmHg)$
0	4.58	22	19.8
1	4.93	23	21.1
2	5.29	24	22.4
3	5.68	25	23.8
4	6.10	26	25.2
5	6.54	27	26.7
6	7.01	28	28.3
7	7.51	29	30.0
8	8.04	30	31.8
9	8.61	31	33.7
10	9.20	32	35.7
11	9.84	33	37.7
12	10.5	34	39.9
13	11.2	35	42.2
14	12.0	36	44.6
15	12.8	37	47.1
16	13.6	38	49.7
17	14.5	39	52.4
18	15.5	40	55.3
19	16.5	41	58.3
20	17.5	42	61.5
21	18.6	43	64.8

In practice, use of the above expression is time consuming; the temperature and pressure corrections can be obtained from published tables and nomograms.

Oxygen Uptake and Concentration

The simple water-sealed spirometer used for measuring lung volumes can be used to determine oxygen uptake if a CO_2 absorber is included inside the bell. Without such an absorber, the exhaled CO_2 will accumulate and produce hyperventilation, because CO_2 is a potent respiratory stimulant.

The CO_2 absorber incorporated into the spirometer is soda lime, a mixture of calcium hydroxide, soldium hydroxide, and silicates of sodium and calcium. The exhaled carbon dioxide combines with the soda lime and forms solid carbonates. A small amount of heat is liberated by this reaction.

Starting with a spirometer filled with oxygen (or air) and connected to a subject wearing a noseclip to prevent nasal breathing, respiration causes the bell to move up and down, indicating tidal volume, as shown in Fig. 9.4. Examination of the spirogram shows that with continued respiration the baseline of the recording rises, reflecting the disappearance of oxygen from under the bell. By measuring the slope of the baseline of the spirogram in milliliters per minute, the volume of oxygen consumed per minute can be determined.

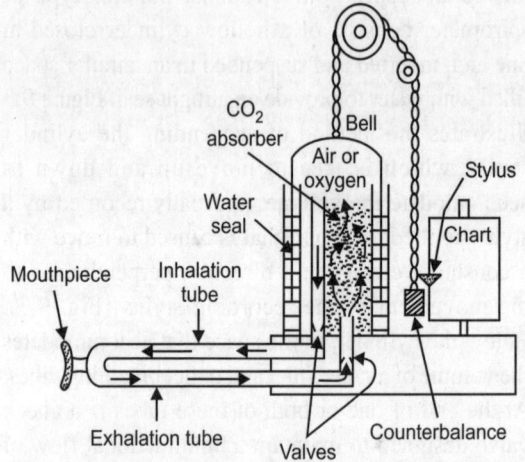

Fig. 9.4. The spirometer with carbon dioxide absorber.

Body Plethysmography

Body plethysmography is a very sensitive lung measurement used to detect lung pathology that might be missed with conventional pulmonary function tests. This method of obtaining the absolute volume of air within one's lungs may also be used in situations where several repeated trials are required or where the patient is unable to perform the multibreath tests. The technique requires moderately complex coaching and instruction for the subject. In the USA, such tests are usually performed by Certified or Registered pulmonary function technologists (CPFT or RPFT) who are credentialed by the National board for respiratory care NBRC.

More specifically, the test is done by enclosing the subject in an airtight chamber often referred to as a body box; a pneumotachometer is used to measure airflow while a mouth pressure transducer with a shutter measures the alveolar pressure. The most common measurements made using body plethysmographs are thoracic gas volume (VTG) and airway resistance (R_{AW}). This test is used mainly in the Pulmonary Function Testing laboratories.

Using body plethysmography, doctors can examine the lungs' resistance to airflow, distinguish between restrictive and obstructive lung diseases, determine the response to bronchodilators, and determine bronchial hyperreactivity in response to methacholine (Fig. 9.5).

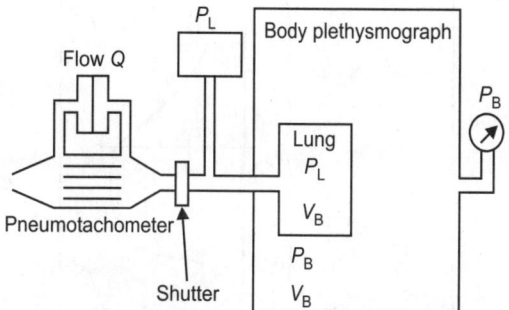

Fig. 9.5. The total body plethysmograph measures lung volume with the shutter closed and the airway resistance via a pneumotachometer with the shutter open.

Flow and pressure plethysmographs

There are two types of plethysmographs: flow and pressure. In flow plethysmography, airway resistance is measured by two maneuvers. The patient first pants while the mouth shutter is open to allow flow changes to be measured. Then, the mouth shutter closes at the patient's end expiratory or FRC level and the patient continues panting while maintaining an open glottis. This provides a measure of the driving pressure used to move air into the lungs.

Pressure plethysmographs are usually measured at the end-expiratory level and are then equal to FRC. The patient sits in the box, which has the pressure transducer in the wall of the device, and breathes through a mouthpiece connected to a device that contains an electronic shutter and a differential pressure pneumotachometer. The mouth pressure and box pressure changes that are measured during tidal breathing and panting maneuvers which are performed during the test by the patient at the end of expiration are sent to a microprocessor unit that calculates thoracic gas volume.

Impedance Phlebography

Impedance phlebography, or impedance plethysmography (IPG), is a non-invasive medical test that measures small changes in electrical resistance of the chest, calf or other regions of the body. These measurements reflect blood volume changes, and can indirectly indicate the presence or absence of venous thrombosis. This procedure provides an alternative to venography, which is invasive and requires a great deal of skill to execute adequately and interpret accurately. A model for two electrode impedance plethysmography is given in Fig. 9.6.

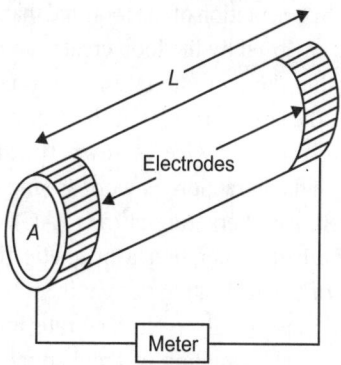

Fig. 9.6. A model for two electrode impedance plethysmography for cylindrical vessels.

For the chest, the technique was developed by NASA to measure the split second impedance changes within the chest, as the heart beats, to calculate both cardiac output and lung water content. This technique has progressed clinically (often now called BioZ, i.e. biologic impedance, as promoted by the leading manufacturer in the US) and allows low cost, non-invasive estimations of cardiac output and total peripheral resistance, using only 4 skin electrodes, oscillometric blood pressure measurement and lung water volumes with minimal removal of clothing in physician offices having the needed equipment.

For leg veins, the test measures blood volume in the lower leg due to temporary venous obstruction. This is accomplished by inflating a pneumatic cuff around the thigh to sufficient pressure to cut off venous flow but not arterial flow, causing the venous blood pressure to rise until it equals the pressure under the cuff. When the cuff is released there is a rapid venous runoff and a prompt return to the resting blood volume. Venous thrombosis will alter the normal response to temporary venous obstruction in a highly characteristic way, causing a delay in emptying of the venous system after the release of the tourniquet. The increase in blood volume after cuff inflation is also usually diminished.

Respiratory Inductance Plethysmography (RIP)

RIP relies on the principle that a current applied through a loop of wire generates a magnetic field normal to the orientation of the loop and that a change in the area enclosed by the loop creates an opposing current within the loop directly proportional to the change in the area. An elastic belt into which a zigzagging (coiled) wire is sewn (to allow for expansion and contraction) is worn around the chest or abdomen. An alternating current (AC) is passed through the belt, generating a magnetic field. The frequency of the alternating current is set to be more than twice the typical respiratory rate in order to achieve adequate sampling of the respiratory effort waveform. The act of breathing changes the cross-sectional area of the patient's body, and thus changes the shape of the magnetic field generated by the belt, 'inducing' an opposing current that can be measured, most easily as a change in the frequency of the applied current. With RIP, no electrical current passes through the body (a weak magnetic field is present that does not affect the patient or any surrounding equipment). The signal produced is linear and is a fairly accurate representation of the change in cross-sectional area. In addition, RIP does not rely on belt tension, thus is not affected by belt trapping.

Technical considerations

RIP equipment consists of the following:
1. Effort belt, consisting of an elastic material with a zigzagging (coiled) wire sewn into the belt.
2. Connecting wire sets.
3. Driver module consisting of a frequency generator, signal processor and analog/digital converter.

Applications of respiratory inductance plethysmography (RIP)

RIP can be in tandem with nasal/oral airflow to produce a flow-volume hysteresis loop. This technique can be employed to assess inspiratory and expiratory flow limitation as a function of body position, sleep stage, etc (Fig. 9.7).

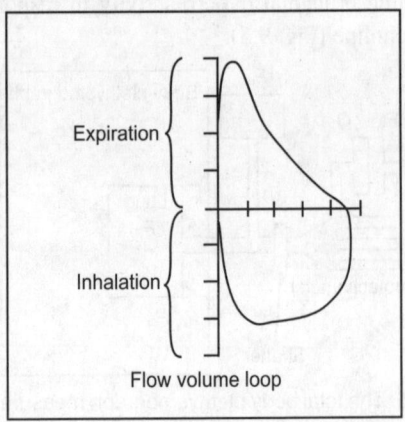

Fig. 9.7. RIP showing expiration, inhalation and flow volume loop.

The chest and abdominal signals can be represented independently, or they can be mathematically summed. Mathematical summing of the signals is particularly useful as a screen for paradoxical breathing. Because there are differences in the amplitudes of chest and abdominal output signals, these values are typically normalised prior to summation (Fig. 9.8).

The summing channel can also be thought of as an indicator of the phase relationship of the chest and abdominal belts. The more out of phase the signals are becoming (moving toward paradox), the smaller the sum channel will be. When expansion and contraction of chest and abdomen are completely out of phase, the sum channel will be flat. However, due to the method in which the sum channel is created, a completely flat sum signal is rare due to the delay in the summing and normalisation of the channels in the summing process. The sum signal does provide a very useful function by presenting a definite decrease in the signal amplitude during events which include paradoxical breathing signals.

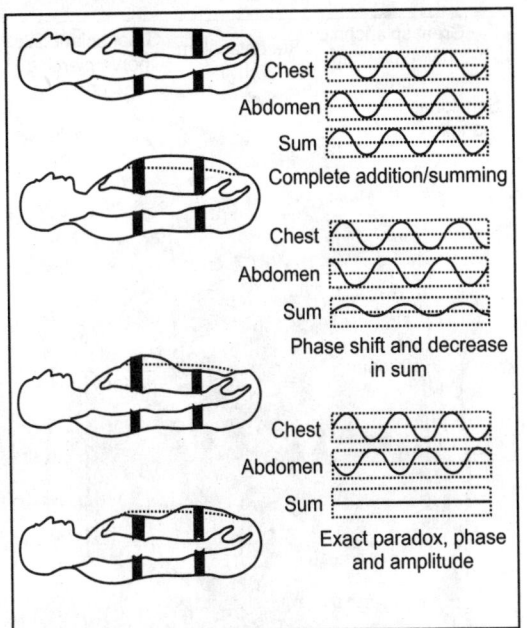

Fig. 9.8. RIP showing chest and abdominal signals.

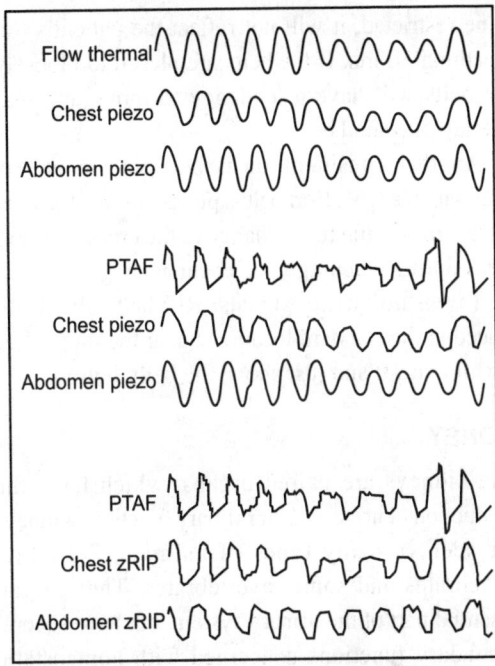

Fig. 9.9. Shows how the RIP belts can parallel the output of a pressure transducer used for flow.

Recording RIP effort signals

When recording through an AC channel the following settings would be used:

Low frequency filter	0.1 Hz or lower (0.05–0.01 Hz)
(High pass filter)	0.1 Hz or lower (0.05–0.01 Hz)
(Time constant)	1.0 Sec or longer (3–5 Sec)

Using a low frequency setting of 0.05 to 0.01 Hz can allow visualisation of possible flattening in the thorax belt which sometimes occurs along with a flattening of the observed signal from a pressure transducer.

High frequency filter	35 Hz
(Low pass filter)	35 Hz

An average resting respiratory rate is 12 breaths per minute. This is equal to approximately 0.2 Hz a relatively low setting of the high frequency Filter (low pass filter) should not influence this signal.

Sampling rate	10 Hz or higher

Figure 9.9 shows how the RIP belts can parallel the output of a pressure transducer used for flow.

Comparing RIP to piezo crystal effort belts

The sensing element, a zigzagging wire, on a RIP effort belt runs the entire length of the belt. When placed on the patient the sensing element covers their entire circumference. As such, all changes in breathing are detected regardless of the position the patient is in. The sensing element, a piezo crystal, on a piezo effort belt is located only on a very small section of the belt's length. As such, there are situations, for example when a patient is lying on top of the piezo crystal, where the effort signal can be dampened, not detected, producing erroneous readings or unexplained changes in polarity that look like paradoxical effect.

Poor Signals

RIP technology has been shown to be very accurate in determining the effort of breathing. However, there are conditions that can decrease the accuracy of the device. If the belts are placed too tight causing the actual cross sectional change of the chest or abdomen to be restricted, it will not reflect the patient's true breathing efforts. If the belts are placed too loosely, the belts will have a tendency to move and may overlap one another.

Another consideration is belt placement. For example, if a RIP effort belt is placed around the hips, there will be little to no change in the cross sectional areas during diaphragmatic excursions.

To ensure quality signals, RIP belts should be placed at the standard locations: near the nipple line (or mid-chest) and just above the belly button.

KIDNEY

The kidneys are paired organs, which have the production of urine as their primary function. Kidneys are seen in many types of animals, including vertebrates and some invertebrates. They are an essential part of the urinary system, but have several secondary functions concerned with homeostatic functions. These include the regulation of electrolytes, acid-base balance, and blood pressure. In producing urine, the kidneys excrete wastes such as urea and ammonium; the kidneys also are responsible for the reabsorption of glucose and amino acids. Finally, the kidneys are important in the production of hormones including calcitriol, renin and erythropoietin (Fig. 9.10).

Located behind the abdominal cavity in the retroperitoneum, the kidneys receive blood from the paired renal arteries, and drain into the paired renal veins. Each kidney excretes urine into a ureter, itself a paired structure that empties into the urinary bladder (Fig. 9.11).

Renal physiology is the study of kidney function, while nephrology is the medical specialty concerned with diseases of the nephron, which is the functional unit of the kidney. Diseases of the kidney are diverse, but individuals with kidney disease frequently display characteristic clinical features. Common clinical presentations include the nephritic and nephrotic syndromes, acute kidney failure, chronic kidney disease, urinary tract infection, nephrolithiasis, and urinary tract obstruction.

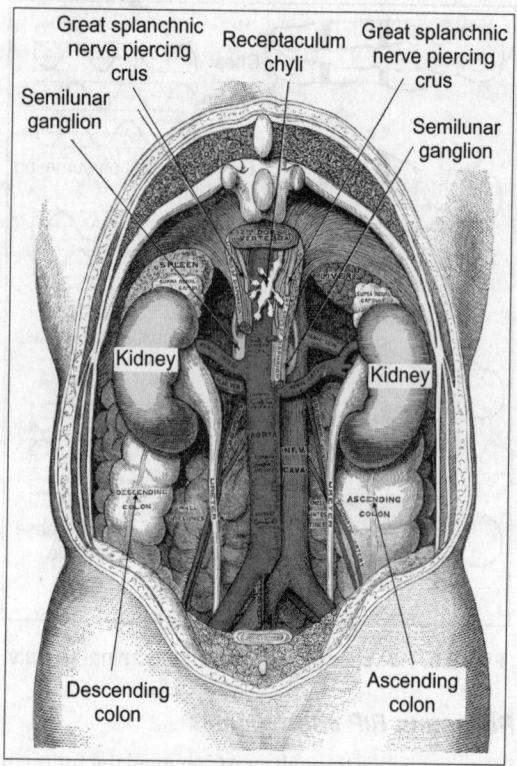

Fig. 9.10. Human kidneys viewed from behind with spine removed.

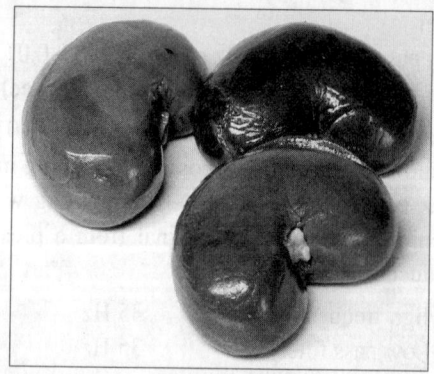

Fig. 9.11. Lamb kidneys.

Kidney Clearance

Creatine

Creatine is naturally produced in the human body from amino acids primarily in the kidney and liver.

It is transported in the blood for use by muscles. Approximately 95 per cent of the human body's total creatine is located in skeletal muscle. The rest is located in the brain or heart.

Creatine is not an essential nutrient as it is manufactured in the human body from L-arginine, glycine, and L-methionine.

In humans and animals, approximately half of stored creatine originates from food (mainly from fresh meat). Since vegetables do not contain creatine, vegetarians show lower levels of muscle creatine. With the help of creatine supplementation vegetarians can compensate for this loss.

Kidney Imaging

Retrograde pyelogram

Retrograde Pyelogram is a urologic procedure where the physician injects contrast into the ureter in order to visualise the ureter and kidney. The flow of contrast (up from the bladder to the kidney) is opposite the usual flow of urine, hence the *retrograde* name.

Reasons for performing a retrograde pyelogram include identification of filling defects (e.g. stones or tumors), as an adjunct during the placement of ureteral stents or ureteroscopy, or to delineate renal anatomy in preparation for surgery. Retrograde pyelography is generally done when an intravenous excretory study (IVP or contrast CT scan) cannot be done because of renal disease or allergy to intravenous contrast.

Relative contraindications include the presence of infected urine, pregnancy and contrast allergy.

The procedure requires cystoscopy and the placement of a small tube into the lower part of the ureter to inject contrast and opacify the ureter and renal pelvis. Fluoroscopy, or dynamic X-rays, is typically used for visualisation. The procedure is usually done under general or regional anesthesia.

Intravenous pyelogram

An intravenous pyelogram (also known as IVP, pyelography, intravenous urogram or IVU) is a radiological procedure used to visualise abnormalities of the urinary system, including the kidneys, ureters, and bladder.

An injection of X-ray contrast media is given to a patient via a needle or cannula into the vein, typically in the arm. The contrast is excreted or removed from the bloodstream via the kidneys, and the contrast media becomes visible on X-rays almost immediately after injection. X-rays are taken at specific time intervals to capture the contrast as it travels through the different parts of the urinary system. This gives a comprehensive view of the patient's anatomy and some information on the functioning of the renal system.

Immediately after the contrast is administered, it appears on an X-ray as a 'renal blush'. This is the contrast being filtered through the cortex. At an interval of 5 minutes, the renal blush is still evident (to a lesser extent) but the calices and renal pelvis are now visible. At 15 minutes the contrast begins to empty into the ureters and travel to the bladder which has now begun to fill. To visualise the bladder correctly, a post micturition X-ray is taken, so that the bulk of the contrast (which can mask a pathology) is emptied. An IVP can be performed in either emergency or routine circumstances.

Emergency IVP

This procedure is carried out on patients who present to an Emergency department, usually with severe renal colic and a positive hematuria test. In this circumstance the attending physician requires to know whether a patient has a kidney stone and if it is causing any obstruction in the urinary system.

Patients with a positive find for kidney stones but with no obstruction are usually discharged with a follow-up appointment with a urologist.

Patients with a kidney stone and obstruction are usually required to stay in hospital for monitoring or further treatment. An emergency IVP is carried out roughly as follows:

1. Plain KUB or Abdominal X-ray.
2. An injection of contrast media, typically 50 ml.
3. Delayed Abdominal X-ray, taken at roughly 15 minutes post injection.

If no obstruction is evident on this film a post-micturition film is taken and the patient is sent back to the emergency department. If an obstruction is visible, a post-micturition film is still taken, but is followed up with a series of radiographs taken at a 'double time' interval. For example, at 30 minutes post-injection, 1 hour, 2 hours, 4 hours, and so forth, until the obstruction is seen to resolve. This time delay can give important information to the urologist on where and how severe the obstruction is.

Routine IVP

This procedure is most common for patients who have unexplained microscopic or macroscopic hematuria. It is used to ascertain the presence of a tumour or similar anatomy-altering disorders. The sequence of images are roughly as follows:

1. Plain or control KUB image.
2. Immediate X-ray of just the renal area.
3. 5 minute X-ray of just the renal area.

Note: At this point, compression may or may not be applied (this is contraindicated in cases of obstruction).

1. If compression is applied: a 10 minutes post-injection X-ray of the renal area is taken, followed by a KUB on release of the compression.
2. If compression is not given: a standard KUB is taken to show the ureters emptying. This may sometimes be done with the patient lying in a prone position.
3. A post-micturition X-ray is taken afterwards. This is usually a coned bladder view.

Image assessment

The kidneys are assessed and compared for: Regular appearance, smooth outlines, size, position, equal filtration and flow.

The ureters are assessed and compared for: Size, a smooth regular and symmetrical appearance. A 'standing column' is suggestive of a partial obstruction.

The bladder is assessed for: Regular smooth appearance and complete voiding.

An IVP can and should be used in conjunction with the following tests: (i) ultrasound, and (ii) cstoscopy.

DIALYSIS

In medicine, dialysis is primarily used to provide an artificial replacement for lost kidney function (renal replacement therapy) due to renal failure. Dialysis may be used for very sick patients who have suddenly but temporarily, lost their kidney function (acute renal failure) or for quite stable patients who have permanently lost their kidney function (stage 5 chronic kidney disease). For patients with stage 5, or end-stage kidney disease (ESKD), the decline in kidney function occurred over a period of months to years until a level was reached at which treatment was needed for survival. Unlike acute renal failure (ARF) (acute kidney injury (AKI)), chronic kidney failure cannot be cured or reversed and long-term treatments are needed to replace the lost functions of the kidney. The treatment for ESKD that most naturally replaces lost kidney function is a kidney transplant. However, some patients are not good candidates for a transplant due to medical or other reasons, some cannot receive a transplant because of the short supply of donor kidneys, and others simply decide that a transplant is not the best option for them. As a result, most patients with ESKD must rely on dialysis to replace the water and waste removal functions of the healthy kidneys.

The kidneys have important roles in maintaining health. When healthy, the kidneys maintain the body's internal equilibrium of water and minerals (sodium, potassium, chloride, calcium, phosphorus, magnesium, sulphate). Those acidic metabolism end products that the body cannot get rid of via respiration are also excreted through the kidneys. The kidneys also function as a part of the endocrine system producing erythropoietin and 1,25-dihydroxy-cholecalciferol (calcitriol). Erythropoietin is involved in the production of red blood cells and calcitriol plays a role in bone formation. Dialysis is an imperfect treatment to replace kidney function because it does not correct the endocrine functions of the kidney. Dialysis treatments replace some of these functions through diffusion (waste removal) and ultrafiltration (fluid removal).

Principle

Dialysis works on the principles of the diffusion of solutes and ultrafiltration of fluid across a semipermeable membrane. Diffusion describes a property of substances in water. Substances in water tend to move from an area where they are in a high concentration to an area of low concentration. Blood flows by one side of a semi-permeable membrane, and a dialysate, or special dialysis fluid, flows by the opposite side. A semipermeable membrane is a thin layer of material that contains various sized holes, or pores. Smaller solutes and fluid pass through the membrane, but the membrane blocks the passage of larger substances (for example, red blood cells, large proteins).

The two main types of dialysis, Haemodialysis (HD) and Peritoneal dialysis (PD), remove wastes and excess water from the blood in different ways. Haemodialysis removes wastes and water by circulating blood outside the body through an external filter, called a dialyser, that contains a semipermeable membrane. The blood flows in one direction and the dialysate flows in the opposite. The counter-current flow of the blood and dialysate maximises the concentration gradient of solutes between the blood and dialysate, which helps to remove more urea and creatinine from the blood. The concentrations of solutes (for example potassium, phosphorus, and urea) are undesirably high in the blood, but low or absent in the dialysis solution and constant replacement of the dialysate ensures that the concentration of undesired solutes is kept low on this side of the membrane. The dialysis solution has levels of minerals like potassium and calcium that are similar to their natural concentration in healthy blood. For another solute, bicarbonate, dialysis solution level is set at a slightly higher level than in normal blood, to encourage diffusion of bicarbonate into the blood, to act as a pH buffer to neutralise the metabolic acidosis that is often present in these patients. The levels of the components of dialysate are typically prescribed by a nephrologist according to the needs of the individual patient. In peritoneal dialysis, wastes and water are removed from the blood inside the body using the peritoneal membrane as a natural semipermeable membrane. Wastes and excess water move from the blood, across the peritoneal membrane, and into a special dialysis solution, called dialysate, in the abdominal cavity which has a composition similar to the fluid portion of blood.

Types of Dialysis

There are two primary types of dialysis, haemodialysis and peritoneal dialysis, and a third investigational type, intestinal dialysis.

Haemodialysis

In haemodialysis, the patient's blood is pumped through the blood compartment of a dialyser, exposing it to a partially permeable membrane. The dialyser is composed of thousands of tiny synthetic hollow fibres. The fibre wall acts as the semipermeable membrane. Blood flows through the fibres, dialysis solution flows around the outside the fibres, and water and wastes move between these two solutions. The cleansed blood is then returned via the circuit back to the body. Ultrafiltration occurs by increasing the hydrostatic pressure across the dialyser membrane. This usually is done by applying a negative pressure to the dialysate compartment of the dialyser. This pressure gradient causes water and dissolved solutes to move from blood to dialysate, and allows the removal of several litres of excess fluid during a typical 3 to 5 hours treatment. In the US, haemodialysis treatments are typically given in a dialysis center three times per week. Studies have demonstrated the clinical benefits of dialysing 5 to 7 times a week, for 6 to 8 hours. These frequent long treatments are often done at home, while sleeping but home dialysis is a flexible modality and schedules can be changed day to day, week to week. In general, studies have shown that both increased treatment length and frequency are clinically beneficial (Fig. 9.12).

The amount of fluid removed from the blood each hour is calculated using the formula:

$$mL/h = TMP \times KUF \qquad ... (9.1)$$

where TMP is the transmembrane pressure (mmHg) and KUF is the Coefficient of ultrafiltration of the dialyser ((mL/h)mmHg). Transmembrane pressure is the arithmetic difference between the pressure on the blood side of the dialyser (usually positive) and the dialysate pressure (usually negative). The negative pressure is calculated using the formula:

$$NP = TMP - \frac{AP + VP}{2} \qquad ... (9.2)$$

where NP is the negative pressure, AP is the arterial pressure, and VP is the venous pressure. The transmembrane pressure can be calculated using the formula:

$$TMP = \frac{\text{Total fluid to be removed} \div \text{hours on dialysis}}{\text{KUF of a dialyser}}$$

$$... (9.3)$$

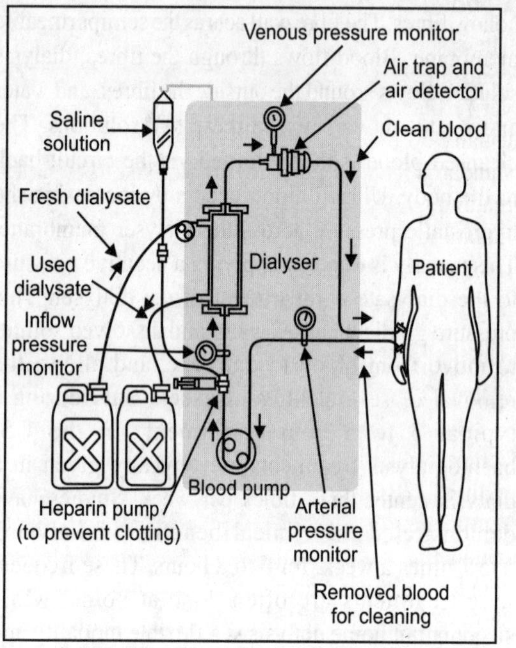

Venous pressure monitor

Air trap and air detector

Saline solution

Clean blood

Fresh dialysate

Used dialysate

Dialyser

Patient

Inflow pressure monitor

Heparin pump (to prevent clotting)

Blood pump

Arterial pressure monitor

Removed blood for cleaning

Fig. 9.12. Haemodialysis schematic.

Dialysate temperature control and measurement

The dialysis is normally done at the body temperature. The temperature of the dialysate is, therefore, monitored and controlled before it is supplied to the dialyser. In case the dialysate gets over-heated, the system should stop the flow to the dialyser and pass it to the bypass. Dialysis at temperatures lower than the body temperature is less efficient and requires rewarming of the blood before its return to the patient's body. Temperatures in excess of 40°C tend

to damage components of the blood. A temperature control system is used to raise the temperature of the dialysate to the required temperature which can be varied from 36° to 42°C. A secondary safety cut-out ensures that the heaters are switched off if the temperature exceeds 43°C.

Two types of circuits can be used for effecting control of temperature: (i) A bi-metallic thermostat which would connect or disconnect supply to the heater coil depending upon the temperature of the dialysate, and (ii) A completely electronic single-term proportional controller which makes use of a thermistor for sensing the temperature and a triac for control of power to the heater. A typical circuit for such a system is shown in Fig. 9.13. Normally, the uni-junction transistor is 'off' until the capacitor C charges to a point of breakdown voltage. When this occurs, the transistor conducts and the capacitor is discharged through the pulse transformer T. The triac thus gets a triggering pulse and switches on the heaters. The triac switches off at the end of each half-cycle and remains so until triggered once again. Since a triac conducts in both directions, it can be switched on during each half-cycle.

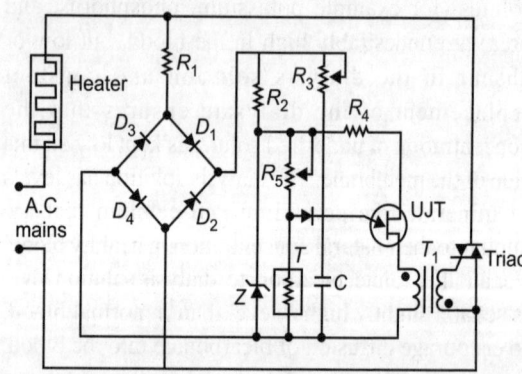

Fig. 9.13. Simplified circuit diagram for controlling dialysate temperature.

The thermistor has a negative temperature coefficient. With an increase in temperature from the set value, its resistance decreases, thereby reducing the rate of charge of C. Therefore, the frequency of charge and discharge (oscillations) reduces and less power is delivered to the heaters which results in a reduction in temperature. With this method, it is possible to control the temperature with an accuracy of 0.2°C. The temperature can also be controlled by varying resistance R_2 and therefore, any temperature can be set with the help of this control.

A thermistor connected in one arm of a Wheatstone bridge may be used as a sensor of temperature of the dialysate in the header tank. The output of the bridge can be amplified in a differential amplifier and displayed on' a panel metre. The amplified signal would also operate alarm circuits in case the temperature of dialysate crosses the preset limits.

Some machines have facilities for automatic sterilisation. Sterilisation is carried out by passing water at 85° to 90°C, through the total hydraulic system. In these machines, sequence interlocks ensure that a dialysis cannot be started without sterilisation and that minimum requirements, for adequate sterilisation are achieved before the dialysis phase can be selected.

In the modern microprocessor-based haemo-dialysis machines, the temperature monitor and control circuitry generate a signal that the CPU utilises to generate display of the fluid temperature and to control the heaters. A dual element heater assembly, which has a 150 W and a 300 W element, is used to bring the fluid up to and to maintain the operating temperature. When the fluid temperature rises to within 2.5°C of the preset temperature (between 35°C to 39°C), the 300 W heater is turned off and the 150 W heater is used to maintain the set temperature (Fig. 9.14).

As a secondary fault monitor, the system incorporates a mercury type temperature switch which is normally open when the dialysate temperature is below 40°C (±0.5°C) and closed when the dialysate temperature exceeds 40°C (±0.5°C). In case the fluid temperature exceeds 40°C, the microprocessor removes the heater elements. In addition to the thermistor probe and temperature switch, the enabling of the heaters is dependent upon the flow rate. The microprocessor reads the flow pulses and determines if there is adequate flow within the system. If the flow is inadequate, the heater elements are disconnected.

The flow is measured using a flow-thrugh transducer which produces a precise number of pulses

per unit of flow (26,000/litre or 108 pulses/second at 250 ml/min). This is achieved by monitoring the rotation of a disk which contains light reflective white spots. Light pulses from the rotating disk are transmitted by internal fibre optics. The sensor assembly includes a light source and a photo-transistor to provide the optical coupling with the sensor. The pulses generated by the flow transducer are amplified, filtered and counted to determine the flow rate. These pulses are also used to control the flow rate in the hydraulic circuit. This circuit supplies a computer-generated variable drive signal to the dialysate pump and flow rate feedback signal to the CPU.

Conductivity measurement

The conductivity of the dialysate being produced is continuously monitored by a conducting cell, to verify the accuracy of proportioning. The result is usually displayed as a percentage deviation from the standard. In practice, a fluctuation about the mean reading will occur and conductivity will normally be maintained with 1 per cent. If an alarm occurs due to the conductivity not remaining within limits, an alarm is given. The effluent pump motor will be switched off automatically which effectively prevents further circulation of dialysate through the dialyser, and dialysate production will be by-passed to the drain.

The composition of the dialysate is checked by comparing the electrical conductivity of the dialysate with a standard sample of the dialysate. Proper temperature compensation is essential as the conductivity of the dialysate changes by about 2 per cent for every 1°C change in temperature. Figure 9.15 shows a block diagram of the conductivity measuring system. It comprises a 1.5 kHz oscillator which drives a bridge circuit, one arm of which contains a conductivity cell. The conductivity cell is of the flow type and is mounted directly downstream of the header tank. In order to provide a fast response to changes of solution temperature which would otherwise considerably affect the conductivity measurements, a temperature compensation thermistor is placed in another arm of the bridge. The output from the bridge, after amplification, is capacitively coupled to a phase-sensitive detector where its phase is compared with the phase of the 1.5 kHz oscillator output. The magnitude and phase

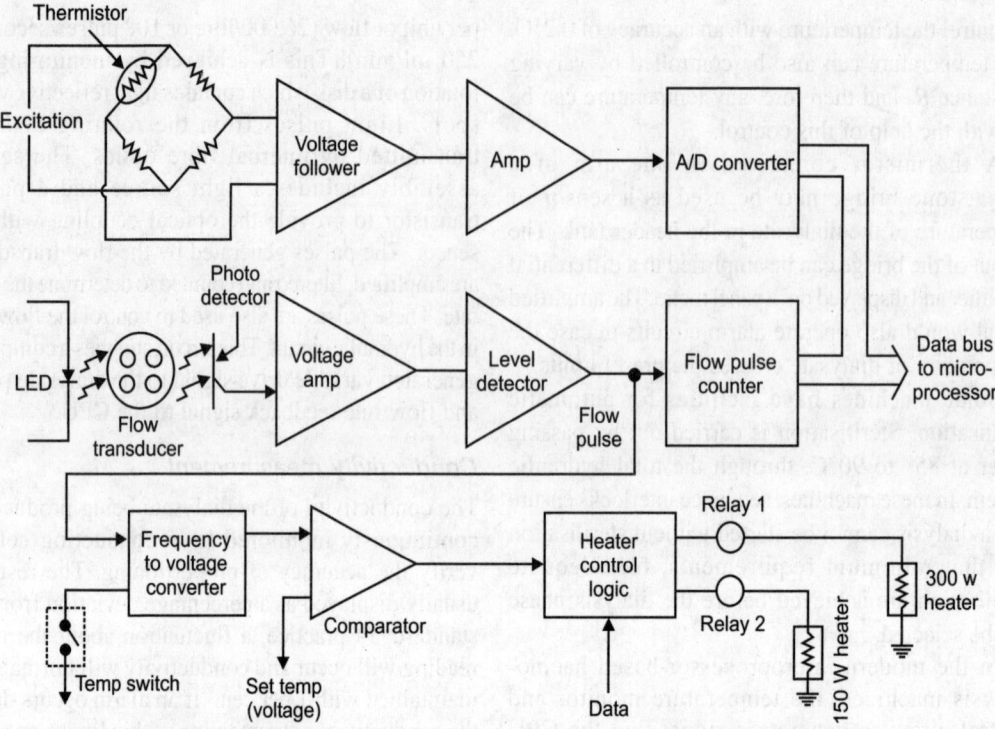

Fig. 9.14. Temperature monitor and control circuit using multiple heaters.

of the output from the phase-sensitive detector determine the direction and amount of deviation from the pre-set value.

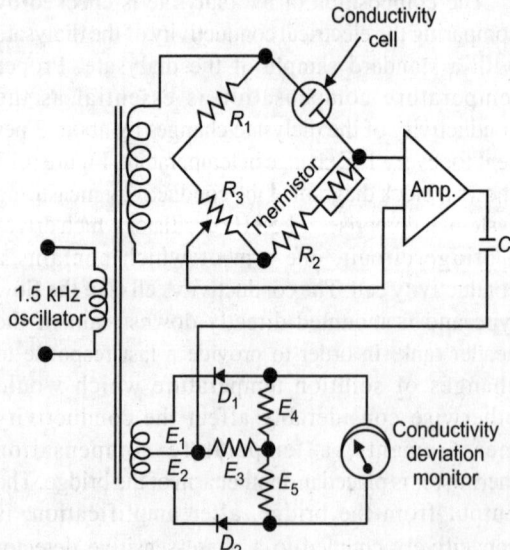

Fig. 9.15. Simplified circuit diagram for monitoring conductivity of dialysate.

An alternative arrangement for conductivity measurement is to make use of a conductivity flow cell consisting of two probes. Each probe consists of four ring — electrodes. Two of the electrodes provide a fixed current through the solution, while the other two electrodes sense the differential voltage generated due to the solution conductance. The current source consists of two parts: a constant amplitude oscillator (10 kHz) and a voltage-to-current converter. The constant amplitude oscillator (A) on probe 1, and oscillator on probe 2, have a positive feedback to ensure oscillation and a negative feedback to set the frequency and the output amplitude. The voltage-to-current converters provide an output of approximately 1.0 mA. The output of the current source is transformer-coupled to the two current electrodes to minimise leakage current through the solution.

The two sensing electrodes are AC-coupled to a differential-amplifier, U1on probe-1 and U2 on probe-2. The output is then AC-coupled into an AC to DC converter whose output is given to the A/D converter, after making offset and gain adjustments.

The output of the A/D converter is given to the system microprocessor.

In practice, the mEq/1 of sodium, calcium, chloride, potassium, magnesium and acetate are added to obtain the total ionic content of the dialysate in mEq/1. For example: for total ionic content of 270 mEq/l, the conductivity is 12.9 milli-ohms and for 304 mEq/l, it is 13.8 milli-ohms.

Dialysis must never commence unless it is known that the conductivity circuit calibration and concentrate in use are both correct for the intended dialysis. Therefore, it is recommended that once per month a sample of the dialysate from the machine's dialysate outlet connector be analysed in a laboratory to check conductivity monitor calibration.

Dialysate pressure control and measurement

Negative pressure upon the dialysate is created by the effluent pump. The effluent pump is a fixed flow, motor-driven gear pump. A small plastic housing encloses stainless steel gears driven by an electric motor. Pressures between zero and maximum are available by adjustment of a needle valve mounted on the machine panel. A relief valve (preset to suit the type of dialyser) limits the maximum negative pressure available, thus minimising the risk of a burst in the dialyser membrane which may be caused by high transient pressures. Pressure adjustments should not produce any significant change in the flow rate. The pressure is measured by a strain gauge transducer connected immediately downstream of the dialysate return side. Pressures within the range 0 to –400 mmHg are generally made available and any value can be adjusted in this range.

The pressure indicated on the gauge will be the dialysate pressure on one side of the dialyser membrane. On the other side of the membrane will be the venous pressure. The effective pressure across the membrane, which is so important in consideration of filtration and weight control, will be the algebraic sum of the dialysate pressure and venous pressure. If the pressure goes beyond the alarm limits, the effluent pump is switched off automatically and dialysate production by-passed to drain by way of the header tank overflow and the waste funnel.

Venous pressure measurement

Venous pressure is normally measured at the bubble trap. A length of tubing connects the trap to a small plastic housing to which a strain gauge transducer is attached. The sensor diaphragm is fragile and should not be roughly handled. The elevation above the floor of the point of connection to the blood line produces a small change in the pressure reading. For maximum accuracy, the sensor connection should be maintained in the same, altitude during dialysis, preferably with the luer connector downwards to prevent blood, reaching the diaphragm in the event of a leak. If the venous pressure passes beyond one of the alarm limits, power to the blood pump will be isolated and the blood pump, if in use, will cease to operate.

Blood leak detector

In a dialysis machine, a thin membrane separates the patient's blood from the dialysate. Normally, the pressure on the blood side of the membrane is maintained at a much higher level than the pressure on the dialysate side. This is necessary to minimise the time required for the dialysis procedure. Besides this, in order to reduce the total time required for dialysis, the membrane area is made as large as possible. Therefore, these two conditions of a high pressure differential across a large fragile membrane may result in a leak in the membrane. In fact, even a relatively small tear in the membrane can result in major blood loss in a very short time, with the consequent immediate threat to the patient.

Blood-to-dialysate leaks usually occur at the beginning of dialysis and can be detected by examination of the effluent from the dialyser. However, it is not rare to have instances wherein blood leaks have been found to start several hours after setting up dialysis. The detection of blood leaking through imperfection in the membrane into the dialysate is best achieved by monitoring the effluent from the dialyser for changes in transmission of light resulting from the presence of haemoglobin. If there is any blood leak across the dialyser membrane, it can be detected by using a photo-electric transducer.

The dialysis membrane leak detector basically examines the light absorption of the dialysate at

560 nm, the absorption wavelength for haemoglobin. This spectral tuning of the system makes it sensitive and stable, and reduces false alarm situations. An LED is available which has a peak spectral emission at 560 nm with a spectral line half width of 27 nm.

Figure 9.16 shows a block diagram of the blood leak detector. In order to minimise drift over a period of several hours required for the dialysis, a chopped light system with AC amplifiers is employed. Chopping is achieved by driving the LED with a square wave of current. The light is detected with a cadmium sulphide (CdS) photo-conductive cell. This has peak response at 565 nm. After amplification of the AC response signal, an absolute value circuit provides a signal whose peak value is proportional to the received 560 nm light. The peak value is compared to a reference voltage which is preset. When the peak value falls below the selected threshold, visual and audible alarms are activated.

Blood leak detectors are liable to give false alarms when used over a long period of several weeks. This is the result of a gradual build-up of contaminants on the lenses of the LED and CdS cell. This needs gradual change in the setting of the threshold. Careful cleaning of the transducer can, however, restore the original threshold. This does not materially affect system performance since in almost all machines, the threshold is set at the beginning of each dialysis procedure.

Blood leak level, for normal operation, is set at 25 mg of haemoglobin per litre of dialysate. The maximum setting detects blood leaks at the rate of 65 mg/I of dialysate. If a blood leak is detected, the effluent pump is switched off automatically and dialysate production by-passed to drain by way of header tank overflow. The blood pump is de-energised and, if in use, ceases to operate.

Ultra-filtrate monitor

The ultra-filtrate monitor circuit is used to monitor the amount of fluid removed from the patient and in conjunction with the negative pressure, to control the rate at which it is removed. This circuit generates a signal that the CPU utilises to generate display of the total UF(ultra-filtrate). The CPU also uses this signal to calculate the TMP required to maintain the UF rate required by the operator.

$$\text{UF Rate (L/hr)} = \frac{\text{Total fluid removal required (liers)}}{\text{Treatment time (hours)}}$$

This is done by measuring the amount of fluid removed during a measured time period by the amount of fluid removed. This calculation helps determine the coefficient (K) of the dialyser.

Dialyser K = Total UF (6 min period)/TMP (Avg.)

The CPU then divides the required UF Rate by the dialyser K factor to determine how much IMP is needed to achieve this UF rate.

Required TMP = Required UF Rate (L/hr)/ dialyser K

The CPU will then subtract the measured blood pressure from the TMP calculated to determine how much negative pressure is required to achieve the calculated TMP.

Blood pressure = Venous blood pressure + Arterial blood pressure /2

Negative pressure required = TMP–Blood pressure

If the calculated negative pressure is less than 30 mmHg or greater than 350 mmHg, the CPU will generate an alarm signal.

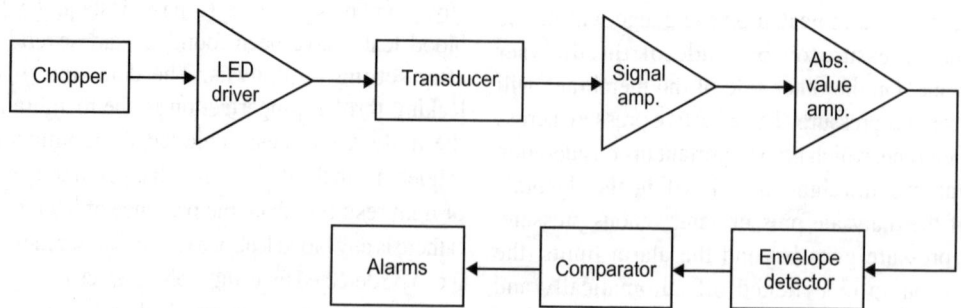

Fig. 9.16. Block diagram of blood leak detector using LED as a light source.

Figure 9.17 is a block diagram of the ultra-filtrate monitor. The load cell and associated electronics are used to monitor the weight changes of the fluid in the reservoir during the haemodialysis treatment. The load cell utilises a strain gauge that produces a differential resistance proportional to the applied force. An excitation of 10V DC is supplied to the strain gauge bridge from a reference source. The differential output from the strain gauge bridge is typically 13.3 m V for a 10 kg load. The differential input is first connected to the instrumentation amplifier which gives a gain of 100 and produces a single-ended output. The following amplifier stage includes provisions for offset and gain adjustments. The weight is represented at this stage by a DC voltage. It is changed to a proportional frequency by a voltage-to-frequency converter. The pulses corresponding to the weight are then counted and given to the microprocessor.

Peritoneal dialysis

In peritoneal dialysis, a sterile solution containing minerals and glucose is run through a tube into the peritoneal cavity, the abdominal body cavity around the intestine, where the peritoneal membrane acts as a semipermeable membrane.The peritoneal membrane or peritoneum is a layer of tissue containing blood vessels that lines and surrounds the peritoneal, or abdominal, cavity and the internal abdominal organs (stomach, spleen, liver, and intestines). The dialysate is left there for a period of time to absorb waste products, and then it is drained out through the tube and discarded (Fig. 9.18). This cycle or 'exchange' is normally repeated 4–5 times during the day, (sometimes more often overnight with an automated system). Ultrafiltration occurs via osmosis; the dialysis solution used contains a high concentration of glucose, and the resulting osmotic pressure causes fluid to move from the blood into

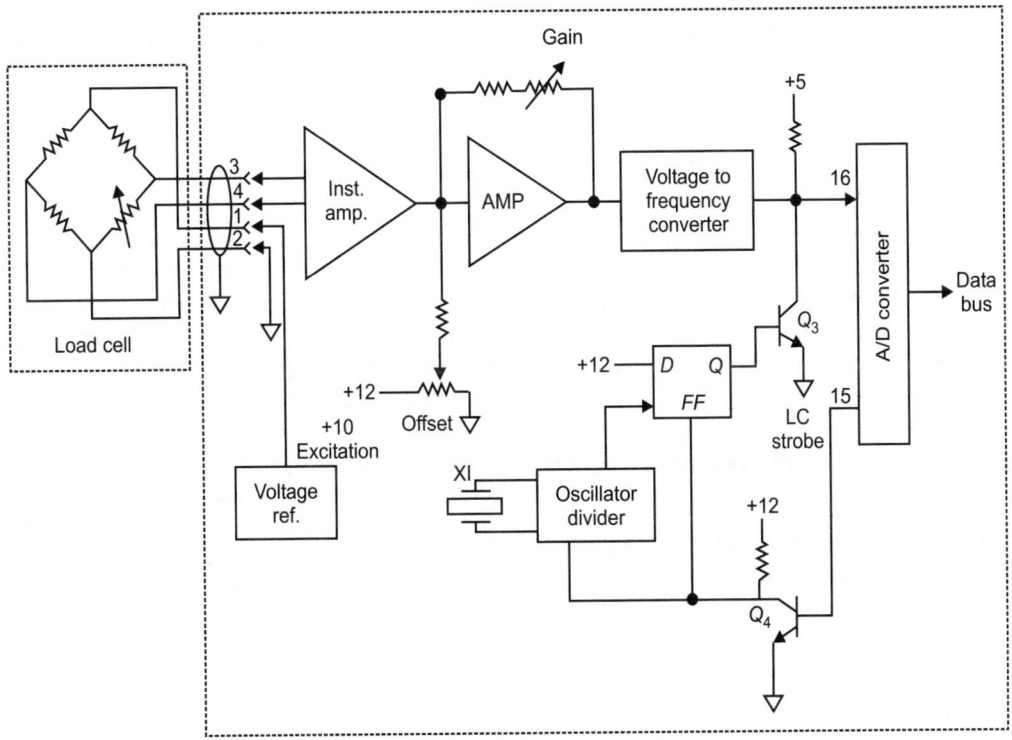

Fig. 9.17. Block diagram of ultrafiltration monitor.

the dialysate. As a result, more fluid is drained than was instilled. Peritoneal dialysis is less efficient than haemodialysis, but because it is carried out for a longer period of time the net effect in terms of removal of waste products and of salt and water are similar to haemodialysis. Peritoneal dialysis is carried out at home by the patient. Although support is helpful, it is not essential. It does free patients from the routine of having to go to a dialysis clinic on a fixed schedule multiple times per week, and it can be done while travelling with a minimum of specialised equipment.

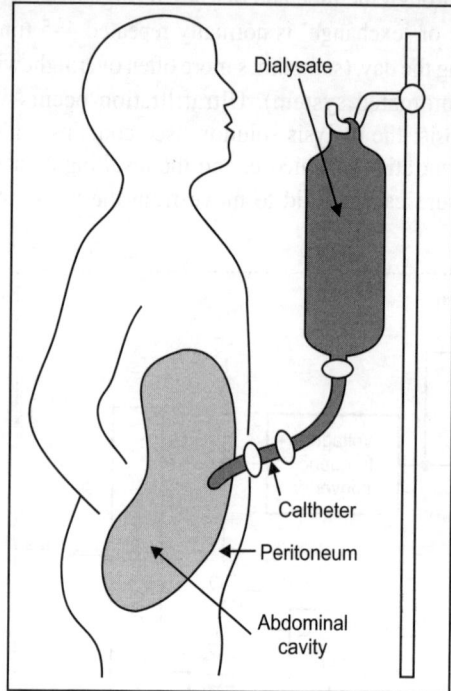

Fig. 9.18. Schematic diagram of peritoneal dialysis.

The key measurement in the peritoneal dialysis process is the weight of the fluids. It is not practical to attempt to measure the change in concentration of the dialysate. Therefore, the amount of fluid pumped into the peritoneal cavity and the amount of fluid removed are measured as the means of monitoring the amount of water and waste diffused from the body fluids. The circuit in Fig. 9.19 shows a possible means of measuring the fluid weight.

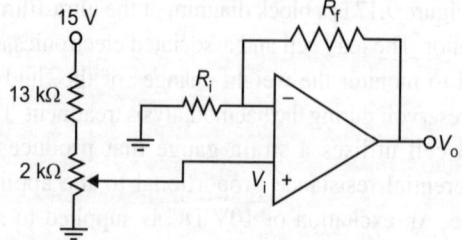

Fig. 9.19. Dialysate weight measuring circuit.

The weight of the fluid determines the position of the wiper on a potentiometer. The fluid may be suspended from a spring-loaded mechanism that varies the wiper position. In this case, the value of the variable 2 kΩ resistor is dependent upon the weight of the fluid and has been installed in a voltage divider powered by the 15 V power supply to the op amp. A change in the resistance varies the input voltage, v_i, to the noninverting op amp circuit. The input voltage is amplified by $(R_f + R_i)/R_i$. The amplification is limited by the 12 V saturation of the op amp. Acceptable resistance values for R_i and R_f are 1 kΩ, and 5 kΩ respectively. The maximum value of v_i is 2 V, which results in a 12 V output voltage can be sent to an analog-to-digital converter and then to CPU for data storage and processing.

The greater the osmotic pressure difference across the membrane, the more diffusion occurs. As the pressure decreases, less diffusion occurs. The concentration of body fluid waste is exponentially removed. It is important to understand that it is this relationship that is used to determine the frequency with which the dialysate should be refreshed. If peritoneal dialysis can accurately be simplified, a relationship can be developed to determine the rate at which the body fluid wastes or solutes diffuse across the membrane.

The concentration of the solutes are defined as:

$$C = \frac{N}{V} \qquad \dots (9.4)$$

where C is the concentration of solute (molecules/m³), N is the number of particles in the solute, and V is the volume of the solute.

The solute flow rate through a membrane, J_s, due to diffusion is defined as:

$$J_s = \omega RT(C_b - C_d)$$

$$J_s = \omega RT \left(\frac{N_b}{V_b} - \frac{N_d}{V_d} \right) \qquad \dots (9.5)$$

where R is the gas constant ($J/(\text{mol K})$), T is the absolute temperature, 310 K , and ω is the solute permeability of the peritoneal membrane (1×10^{-5} moles/(N $\cdot$ s)). The designations of b and d stand for the body fluid and dialysate, respectively.

Through some algebra and knowing J_s, the surface area of the peritoneum and the initial concentrations, the concentration in the body determined as a function of time is:

$$C(t) = C_0 \left[\frac{V_d}{V_b + V_d} e^{-\alpha t} + \frac{V_b}{V_b + V_d} \right] \quad \dots (9.6)$$

This relationship can be plotted to determine at what point the dialysate should be refreshed. Normally, 30 min cycles are done. After 30 min, the body fluid concentration is approximately $0.9524C_0$ using the values given above. The concentration after n cycles is simply computed as:

$$C(t) = (0.9524)^n C_0$$

and may be used to estimate the reduction in body fluid solute concentration following the dialysis. As mentioned previously, the rate of dialysis is monitored by weighing the dialysate and spent dialysate.

Haemofiltration

Hemofiltration is a similar treatment to hemodialysis, but it makes use of a different principle. The blood is pumped through a dialyser or 'hemofilter' as in dialysis, but no dialysate is used. A pressure gradient is applied; as a result, water moves across the very permeable membrane rapidly, 'dragging' along with it many dissolved substances, importantly ones with large molecular weights, which are cleared less well by hemodialysis. Salts and water lost from the blood during this process are replaced with a 'substitution fluid' that is infused into the extracorporeal circuit during the treatment. Hemodiafiltration is a term used to describe several methods of combining hemodialysis and hemofiltration in one process.

Intestinal dialysis

In intestinal dialysis, the diet is supplemented with soluble fibres such as acacia fibre, which is digested

by bacteria in the colon. This bacterial growth increases the amount of nitrogen that is eliminated in fecal waste (Fig. 9.20).

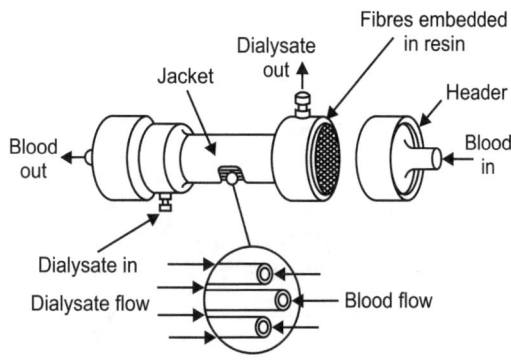

Fig. 9.20. Constructional details of hollow-fibre dialyser.

Parallel Flow Dialysers

The parallel flow dialyser has a low internal resistance which allows adequate blood flow through the dialyser with the patient's arterial blood pressure, eliminating the need for a blood pump. The dialysing surface area of a parallel flow dialyser is about 1 sq m. At a blood flow rate of 200 ml/min and a dialysate flow of 500 ml/min, the urea and creatinine clearance is about 80 and 64 ml/min. The rigid supports used in parallel flow dialysers permit negative pressure to be created on the dialysate side of the membrane for ultra-filtration. The water is ultra-filtered at a rate of 9.2 ml/min with a negative pressure of 130 mmHg. This rate is 1.8 ml/min without negative pressure. The dialysate flows continuously at 500 ml/min in a direction counter current to the blood, permitting exchange to take place throughout the dialyser.

The KIIL dialyser has earlier been the most commonly used form of parallel flow dialyser. It consists of (Fig. 9.21) three polypropylene boards with dialysing membranes laid between them. The boards are held firmly with a frame on the top and bottom and are fastened by a series of bolts on the side. A rubber gasket runs along the periphery of the boards inner surface to prevent blood and dialysate leakage. The dialysate enters through a stainless steel port and is distributed to grooves running across the end of the board both above and below the membrane of each layer. After flowing down longitudinal grooves in the boards, it is collected and flowed out at the opposite end of the board. The outside measurements of a KIIL dialyser are $125 \times 40 \times 16.5$ cm.

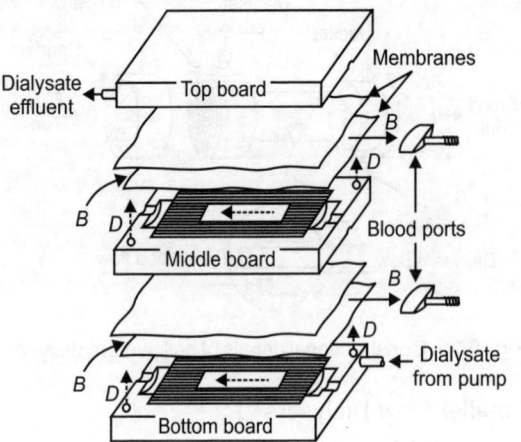

Fig. 9.21. Constructional details of KIIL dialyser showing plates separated out.

The KIIL dialyser is not disposable. It needs to be cleaned and re-built after each dialysis operation. With this type of dialyser, a single-pass body temperature dialysate passes through the dialyser once before going to the drain to obtain higher operational efficiency and to minimise bacterial infection.

Several modifications have been introduced in the basic KIIL system. The parallel grooves have been replaced by pyramidal grooves which allow multiple point support for the membranes. This arrangement provides greater clearance of urea and creatinine under the same flow conditions because of increased surface area.

Coil Haemodialyser

A coil hemodialyser comprises a tubular membrane placed between flexible support wrapped around a rigid cylindrical core. The coil is immersed in a dialysing bath. The tubular membrane can be of cellophane or cuprophane. The average wall thickness of cellophane membrane is 20–30 μm and that of cuprophane in the range of 18–75 μm. The coil membrane supports are woven screens or unwoven lattice. Usually, the 'twin-coil' is made with three layers of woven, polyvinyl chloride-coated fibre glass

screen separated by four narrow strips of the same material, which are sewn into place with cotton thread. Coil dialysers are available with several design variations, which include the type of membrane, the membrane support, the number of blood channels (1,2 or 4), the width of the blood channels (38–100 mm) and surface area (0.7–1.9 m^2). Coil dialysers can be pre-fabricated because of their simple design. They are characterised by high dialysate flow rates and high resistance to blood.

Performance Analysis of Dialysers

The dialyser performance can be compared in terms of their clearance of urea and creating priming volume, residual blood volume, ultra-filtration rate, convenience of handling and cost, etc.

Clearance

The overall performance of the dialyser is expressed as the clearance, analogous to that of a natural kidney. It represents that part of the total blood flow rate through the dialyser which is completely cleared of solute. Uremic patients carry a number of toxic solutes in their blood, which are generated daily. Despite the uncertainty as to which solutes and how much should be removed, the performance of a dialyser is generally assessed for a spectrum of molecular weight solutes. The molecular weight of urea is 60, of creatinine, 113, Vitamin B_{12}, 1355 and of insulin, 5200.

The clearance of urea and creatinine is measured at clinically useful blood flow rates and standard dialysis fluid addition or flow rate. It is calculated as:

$$\text{Clearance} = \frac{\text{Blood flow rate}}{A + B \times \text{blood flow rate}}$$

(where A and B are constants) with 95 per cent confidence limits of the mean by least square approximation. The blood flow rate is measured by bubble transit time over a two-metre track using the mean of three measurements. Urea and creatinine concentrations are measured in the plasma from 1 ml sample of heparinised blood. Usually, the blood flow is maintained between 75–300 ml/min and dialysis fluid flow rate at 500 ml/min.

The performance of hemodialysers is usually compared by employing the dialysance curve which is a graph of dialysance versus the blood flow rate.

$$\text{Dialysance } D = \frac{Q_b(C_{bi} - C_{bo})}{C_{bi} - C_{di}} \quad \text{... (9.7)}$$

where,

Q_b = Blood flow rate.

C_{bi} = Blood solute concentration at the dialyser inlet.

C_{bo} = Blood solute concentration at the dialyser outlet.

C_{di} = Dialysate solute concentration at the inlet.

Figure 9.22 and (Eq. 9.7) show that dialysance rises rapidly at low blood flow rates and tends to stabilise at high flow rates. Therefore, for comparing the performance of the dialyser, it is important to specify the blood flow at which the measurements are made. The equation also shows that more waste is likely to be removed early in the treatment when the blood dialysate gradient is high.

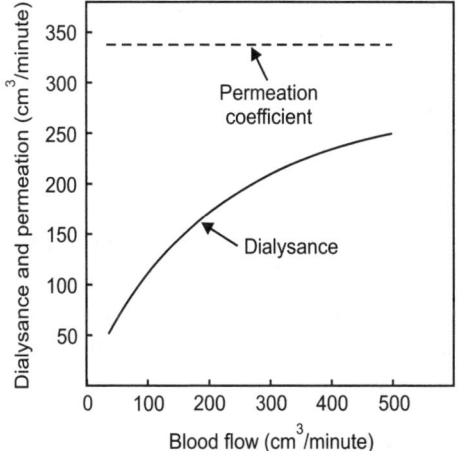

Fig. 9.22. Dialysance vs blood flow.

The dialysance is also used to calculate the clearance, by the following relationship:

$$\text{Clearance} = \frac{\text{Dialysance}}{1 + \dfrac{\text{Dialysance}}{\text{dialysis fluid addition rate}}}$$

It may be noted that the clearance may vary with time despite quasi-steady state conditions. If the dialysate is recirculated, its solute concentration increases, which effectively reduces the concentration driving force. For a given blood flow rate, the clearance is greater for the smaller molecular sized constituents.

This is due to less membrane resistances and higher liquid diffusion coefficients for smaller-molecular weight solutes. On the other hand, the contribution of the membrane resistance to the overall value becomes greater with the increase in solute molecular weight. Bobb and others suggested 'square meter hour' concept for increased removal of middle molecules by either increasing dialysis time or increasing membrane area.

They illustrated that inadequate removal of solutes of 300–2000 daltons (middle molecules) might be associated with the neurological dysfunction in chronic uraemic patients. Keeping in view this study, attempts have been made to design dialysers with large surface area (2.5 m^2) and development of more permeable membranes. Another method of comparing the performance capacity of dialysers is given by:

$$\text{Performance capacity} = K_s A = \frac{A}{R_s} \text{c... (9.8)}$$

where,

A = surface area.

K_s = permeability coefficient.

R_s = mass transfer resistance, i.e. reciprocal of permeability.

Mass transfer resistance is composed of resistance due to a blood film layer, resistance of the membrane itself and the dialysate film resistance layer. (Eq. 9.8) is independent of blood flow rate and can be considered as a measure of dialyser performance.

Ultra-filtration rate

The fluid removal during dialysis (ultra-filtration) takes place due to hydrostatic and osmotic transmembrane pressure gradients. The rate of fluid removal due to hydrostatic pressure effects depends upon the specifications of the dialyser in terms of mass-transfer coefficient and surface area. It, however, has a linear function of the transmembrane pressure (TMP) gradient. It is given by:

Mean transmembrane pressure

$$= \frac{1}{2}[PB_i + PB_o] - \frac{1}{2}[PD_i + PD_o]$$

where PB_i and PB_o are the blood inlet and outlet pressures and PD_i and PD_o are the dialysate inlet and outlet pressures respectively.

The pressure losses generated by blood and dialysate flows in their respective flow paths should be small. This ensures that the local transmembrane pressure (ΔPm) will not vary excessively from the mean pressure. High values of ΔPm can result in deformation of the membrane and its possible rupture.

In actual clinical practice, only one blood pressure and one dialysate pressure are normally measured. Therefore, in order to obtain reasonable control over ultra-filtration, the pressure loss in the blood and dialysate compartments should be known as a function of the respective flow rates. The pressure drop (difference between blood inlet and outlet pressures, ΔPb) across a dialyser is directly proportional to the length of the passage and the viscosity of the fluid and inversely proportional to the number of blood passage and some function of their cross-sectional area. Blood passage width may change with changing blood compartment pressures. Therefore, the relationship of pressure drop to blood flow is not linear at increased flows which are accompanied by increased pressures that can cause a widening of the blood passage and a decrease in $\Delta P_b/Q_b$. The viscosity of the blood is not constant as the blood is an anomalous fluid. Its viscosity tends to increase with haematocrit and decrease in small passage. The area of cross-section is important as with small areas, an inordinately high pressure is required to yield a given flow or flow is reduced to very low levels for a given pressure source.

Residual blood volume

Residual blood volume can be measured after an 800 ml saline wash in. The fluid remaining in the dialyser and lines is circulated through a 0.1 litre bottle of 0.04 per cent ammonia solution for 10 mm.

The residual blood volume is calculated from the formula.

Residual blood volume =

$$\frac{U\,(1000 + \text{volume of dialyser and lines in ml})}{200S}$$

where,

U = the haemoglobin concentration of the re-circulated fluid.

S = the haemoglobin concentration of a sample of arterial blood taken at the end of dialysis and diluted 1:200 with 0.04 per cent ammonia.

Residual volumes of 1.8 to 6.3 ml are quoted in the literature depending upon the dialyser type and washback volume.

Priming volume

The volume of blood within the dialyser is known as priming volume. It is desirable that this should be minimal. Priming volume of present day dialysers range from 75 to 200 ml, depending on the membrane area geometry and operating conditions. Requirement of low priming volume permits the use of patients own blood to prime the circuit without serious hypovolemic effects. This is particularly significant in the case of long-term dialysis therapy.

Extra-corporeal blood volumes become important in those dialysers which require priming. Priming is usually accompanied at relatively low pressures. Recent innovations have considerably reduced the extra-corporeal volume and a saline prime is frequently used.

Pyrogenicity

Pyrogen reactions are rare with all disposable dialysers. However, they are known to exist with KIIL dialysers but at rates well lower than 1 per cent.

Leakage rate

Blood-to-dialysis-fluid leak with the KIIL dialyser is found to be 3 per cent, but it varies with the dialyser, the batch of membrane and the skill of the operator. The leak rate from all cuprophan coils is, however, high.

Starting indications

The decision to initiate dialysis or haemofiltration in patients with renal failure depends on several factors. These can be divided into acute or chronic indications.

Indications for dialysis in the patient with acute kidney injury are:

1. Metabolic acidosis in situations where correction with sodium bicarbonate is impractical or may result in fluid overload.
2. Electrolyte abnormality, such as severe hyperkalemia, especially when combined with AKI.
3. Intoxication, that is, acute poisoning with a dialysable drug, such as lithium, or aspirin.
4. Fluid overload not expected to respond to treatment with diuretics.
5. Complications of uremia, such as pericarditis, encephalopathy, or gastrointestinal bleeding.

Chronic indications for dialysis:

1. Symptomatic renal failure
2. Low glomerular filtration rate (GFR) (RRT often recommended to commence at a GFR of less than 10–15 mls/min/1.73m^2). In diabetics dialysis is started earlier.
3. Difficulty in medically controlling fluid overload, serum potassium, and/or serum phosphorus when the GFR is very low.

KIDNEY FUNCTION

Body Water

In medicine, body water is all of the water content of the human body. A significant fraction of the human body is water.

'The total amount of water in a man of average weight (70 kilograms) is approximately 40 litres, averaging 57 per cent of his total body weight. In a newborn infant, this may be as high as 75 per cent of the body weight, but it progressively decreases from birth to old age, most of the decrease occurring during the first 10 years of life. Also, obesity decreases the percentage of water in the body, sometimes to as low as 45 per cent'. These figures are statistical averages, so are illustrative, and like all biostatistics, will vary with things like type of population, age and number of people sampled, and methodology. So there is not, and cannot be, a figure that is exactly the same for all people, for this or any other physiological measure.

Regarding specific tissues: Lean muscle tissue contains about 75 per cent water by weight. Blood contains almost 70 per cent water, body fat contains 10 per cent water and bone has 22 per cent water. Skin also contains much water. The human body is about 60 per cent water in adult males and 55 per cent in adult females.

In diseased states where body water is affected, the compartment or compartments that have changed can give clues to the nature of the problem. Body water is regulated by hormones, including anti-diuretic hormone (ADH), aldosterone and atrial natriuretic peptide.

There are many methods to determine body water. One way to get a simple estimate is by calculation.

Per *Netter's Atlas of Human Physiology*, body water is broken down into the following *compartments:*

1. Intracellular fluid (2/3 of body water). Per Guyton, in a body containing 40 litres of fluid, about 25 litres is intracellular, which amounts to 62.5 per cent (5/8), close enough to the 2/3 rule of thumb. Jackson's texts states 70 per cent of body fluid is intracellular.
2. Extracellular fluid (1/3 of body water). Per Guyton's illustration, for a 40 litre body, about 15 litres is extracellular, which amounts to 37.5 per cent again, this is close to the 1/3 rule of thumb cited here.
   (a) Plasma (1/5 of extracellular fluid). Per Guyton's illustration, of the 15 litres of extracellular fluid, plasma volume averages 3 litres. This amounts to 20 per cent, the same as per Netter's Atlas.
   (b) Interstitial fluid (4/5 of extracellular fluid).
   (c) Transcellular fluid (a.k.a. 'third space,' normally ignored in calculations).

The simplest calculation is the 60–40–20 rule.

1. Total body water = 60 per cent of body weight.
2. Intracellular fluid = 40 per cent of body weight.
3. Extracellular fluid = 20 per cent of body weight.

This is consistent with the above relations between total body water and the compartmental fluids.

These proportions are not preserved in fluid interventions, however. For example, pure water added to total body water will distribute throughout the above compartments, but isotonic saline will remain in the extracellular compartment.

Measurement of body water

Dilution and equilibration

Total body water can be determined using flowing afterglow mass spectrometry FA-MS measurement of deuterium abundance in breath samples from individuals. A known dose of deuterated water (Heavy water, D_2O) is ingested and allowed to equilibrate within the body water. The FA-MS instrument then measures the deuterium-to-hydrogen (D:H) ratio in the exhaled breath water vapour. The total body water is then accurately measured from the increase in breath deuterium content in relation to the volume of D_2O ingested.

Different substances can be used to measure different fluid compartments:

1. Total body water: Tritiated water or heavy water.
2. extracellular fluid: Inulin.
3. blood plasma: Evans blue.

Intracellular fluid may then be estimated by subtracting extracellular fluid from total body water.

Bioelectrical impedance analysis

Another method of determining total body water percentage (TBW%) is via Bioelectrical Impedance Analysis (BIA). In the traditional BIA method, a person lies on a cot and spot electrodes are placed on the hands and bare feet. Electrolyte gel is applied first, and then a current of 50 kHz is introduced. BIA has emerged as a promising technique because of its simplicity, low cost, high reproducibility and noninvasiveness. BIA prediction equations can be either generalised or population-specific, allowing this method to be potentially very accurate. Selecting the appropriate equation is important to determining the quality of the results.

For clinical purposes, scientists are developing a multi-frequency BIA method that may further improve the method's ability to predict a person's hydration level. New segmental BIA equipment that uses more electrodes may lead to more precise measurements of specific parts of the body.

Fluid loss

Volume contraction is a decrease in body fluid volume, with or without a concomitant loss of osmolytes. The loss of the body water component of body fluid is specifically termed dehydration.

Na^+ loss approximately correlates with fluid loss from extracellular fluid (ECF), since Na^+ has a much higher concentration in ECF than intracellular fluid (ICF). In contrast, K^+ has a much higher concentration in ICF than ECF, and therefore its loss rather correlates with fluid loss from ICF, since K^+ loss from ECF causes the K^+ in ICF to diffuse out of the cells, dragging water with it by osmosis.

BONE AND JOINTS

Bones are rigid organs that form part of the endoskeleton of vertebrates. They function to move, support, and protect the various organs of the body, produce red and white blood cells and store minerals. Bone tissue is a type of dense connective tissue. Because bones come in a variety of shapes and have a complex internal and external structure they are lightweight, yet strong and hard, in addition to fulfilling their many other functions. One of the types of tissue that makes up bone is the mineralised osseous tissue, also called bone tissue, that gives it rigidity and a honeycomb-like three-dimensional internal structure. Other types of tissue found in bones include marrow, endosteum and periosteum, nerves, blood vessels and cartilage. There are 206 bones in the adult human body and 270 in an infant.

Functions of Bone

Mechanical

1. Protection—Bones can serve to protect internal organs, such as the skull protecting the brain or the ribs protecting the heart and lungs.

2. Shape—Bones provide a frame to keep the body supported.

3. Movement—Bones, skeletal muscles, tendons, ligaments and joints function together to generate and transfer forces so that individual body parts or the whole body can be manipulated in three-dimensional space. The interaction between bone and muscle is studied in biomechanics.

4. Sound transduction—Bones are important in the mechanical aspect of overshadowed hearing.

Synthetic

Blood production—The marrow, located within the medullary cavity of long bones and interstices of cancellous bone, produces blood cells in a process called haematopoiesis.

Metabolic

1. Mineral storage—Bones act as reserves of minerals important for the body, most notably calcium and phosphorus.

2. Growth factor storage—Mineralised bone matrix stores important growth factors such as insulin-like growth factors, transforming growth factor, bone morphogenetic proteins and others.

3. Fat Storage—The yellow bone marrow acts as a storage reserve of fatty acids.

4. Acid-base balance—Bone buffers the blood against excessive pH changes by absorbing or releasing alkaline salts.

5. Detoxification—Bone tissues can also store heavy metals and other foreign elements, removing them from the blood and reducing their effects on other tissues. These can later be gradually released for excretion.

6. Endocrine organ—Bone controls phosphate metabolism by releasing fibroblast growth factor - 23 (FGF-23), which acts on kidneys to reduce phosphate reabsorption.

Bone Density

Bone density (or bone mineral density) is a medical term referring to the amount of matter per square centimeter of bones. Note that this is not a true 'density', which would be measured in mass per cubic area. It is measured by a procedure called densitometry, often performed in the radiology or nuclear medicine departments of hospitals or clinics. The measurement is painless and non-invasive and involves minimal radiation exposure. Measurements are most commonly made over the lumbar spine and over the upper part of the hip. The forearm is scanned if either the hip or the lumbar spine can't be. Average density is around 1500 kg m^{-3} (Fig.9.23) .

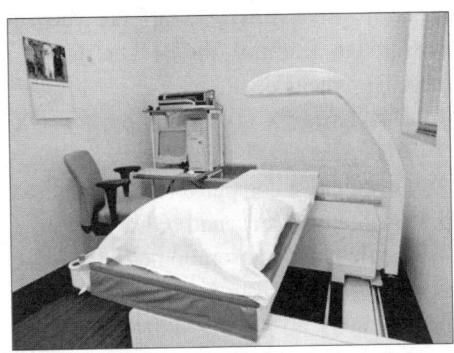

Fig. 9.23. A scanner used to measure bone density with dual energy X-ray absorptiometry.

Results are often reported in three terms:

1. Measured density in g cm^{-3}.

2. z-score, the number of standard deviations above or below the mean for the patient's age, sex and ethnicity.

3. t-score, the number of standard deviations above or below the mean for a healthy 30 year old adult of the same sex and ethnicity as the patient.

Limitations

The technique has several limitations:

1. Measurement can be affected by the size of the patient, the thickness of tissue overlying the bone, and other factors extraneous to the bones.

2. Bone density is a proxy measurement for bone strength, which is the resistance to fracture and the truly significant characteristic. Although the two are usually related, there

are some circumstances in which bone density is a poorer indicator of bone strength.

3. Reference standards for some populations (e.g. children) are unavailable for many of the methods used.

4. Crushed vertebrae can result in falsely high bone density so must be excluded from analysis.

Types of tests

While there are many different types of BMD tests, all are non-invasive. Most tests differ in which bones are measured to determine the BMD result.

These tests include:

1. Dual energy X-ray absorptiometry (DXA or DEXA).
2. Quantitative computed tomography (QCT).
3. Qualitative ultrasound (QUS).
4. Single photon absorptiometry (SPA).
5. Dual photon absorptiometry (DPA).
6. Digital X-ray radiogrammetry (DXR).
7. Single energy X-ray absorptiometry (SEXA).

DEXA is currently the most widely used, but ultrasound has been described as a more cost-effective approach to measure bone density.

The test works by measuring a specific bone or bones, usually the spine, hip, and wrist. The density of these bones is then compared with an average index based on age, sex, and size. The resulting comparison is used to determine risk for fractures and the stage of osteoporosis in an individual.

Average bone mineral density = BMC/W[g/cm²]:

1. BMC = bone mineral content = g/cm.
2. W   = width at the scanned line.

Photon absorptiometry test is most commonly used. Dual-energy bone densitometry can be performed with two types of scanners. The traditional dual-photon absorptiometry (DPA) machines use an isotope source, whereas the newly introduced dual-energy radiography (DER) devices use an incorporated X-ray tube (Fig. 9.24).

The short-term precision error *in vivo* was 1.2 per cent for femoral neck measurements with DER. Long-term precision error *in vitro* was reduced from

1.30 per cent (DPA) to 0.44 per cent (DER). The scanning time for both spine and hip measurements was reduced from 20–40 minutes to 6–7 minutes. Intraosseous fat sensitivity remained the same, at a level of 12 mg/cm² apparent decrease of bone mineral density (BMD) per 10 per cent fat by volume change, and for both devices there was no shift in BMD when phantom thickness was increased by 1.5 inches. The correlation of DPA and DER was high: r = 0.98 for the spine and r = 0.95 for the femoral neck. Correlation of DPA versus quantitative computed tomography (CT) (r = 0.83) and DER versus quantitative CT (r = .085) was good. The advent of DER represents a significant advance for the field of bone densitometry.

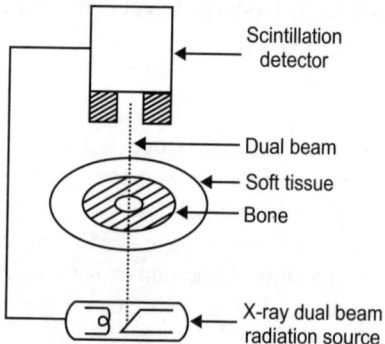

Fig. 9.24. In a dual photon absorptiometer, an X-ray source is filtered to emit at two discrete energies.

Stress–Strain Curve

During testing of a material sample, the stress–strain curve is a graphical representation of the relationship between stress, derived from measuring the load applied on the sample, and strain, derived from measuring the deformation of the sample, i.e. elongation, compression, or distortion. The nature of the curve varies from material to material. The following diagrams illustrate the stress–strain behaviour of typical materials in terms of the engineering stress and engineering strain where the stress and strain are calculated based on the original dimensions of the sample and not the instantaneous values (Fig. 9.25).

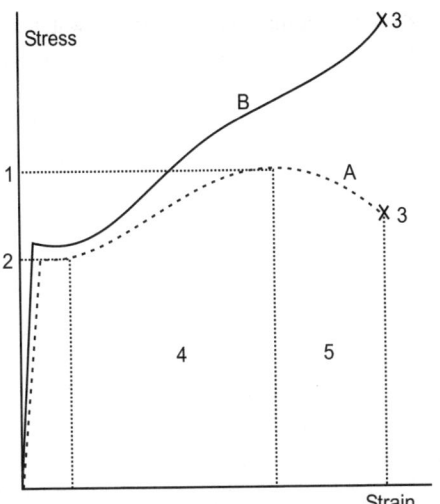

Fig. 9.25. A stress–strain curve typical of structural steel 1. Ultimate strength 2. Yield strength 3. Rupture 4. Strain hardening region 5. Necking region. A: Apparent stress (F/A_0) B: Actual stress (F/A).

Linear Variable Differential Transformer (LVDT)

The linear variable differential transformer (LVDT) is a type of electrical transformer used for measuring linear displacement. The transformer has three solenoidal coils placed end-to-end around a tube. The centre coil is the primary, and the two outer coils are the secondaries. A cylindrical ferromagnetic core, attached to the object whose position is to be measured, slides along the axis of the tube.

An alternating current is driven through the primary, causing a voltage to be induced in each secondary proportional to its mutual inductance with the primary. The frequency is usually in the range 1 to 10 kHz.

As the core moves, these mutual inductances change, causing the voltages induced in the secondaries to change. The coils are connected in reverse series, so that the output voltage is the difference (hence 'differential') between the two secondary voltages. When the core is in its central position, equidistant between the two secondaries, equal but opposite voltages are induced in these two coils, so the output voltage is zero.

When the core is displaced in one direction, the voltage in one coil increases as the other decreases,

causing the output voltage to increase from zero to a maximum. This voltage is in phase with the primary voltage. When the core moves in the other direction, the output voltage also increases from zero to a maximum, but its phase is opposite to that of the primary. The magnitude of the output voltage is proportional to the distance moved by the core (up to its limit of travel), which is why the device is described as 'linear'. The phase of the voltage indicates the direction of the displacement.

Because the sliding core does not touch the inside of the tube, it can move without friction, making the LVDT a highly reliable device. The absence of any sliding or rotating contacts allows the LVDT to be completely sealed against the environment (Fig. 9.26).

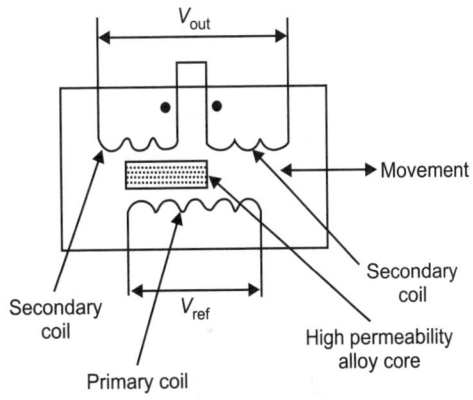

Fig. 9.26. LVDT transformer.

The AC excitation is typically 5 V at 3 kHz. The coupling between these two coils is changed by the motion of the high permeability magnetic alloy between them. When the alloy is symmetrically placed, the two secondary voltages are equal and the output signal is zero. When the alloy moves up, a greater voltage is transformed to the top secondary coil and the output voltage is linearly proportional to the displacement. The LVDT is useful in determining the strain on tendons and ligaments.

The most commonly used technique for measurement of stress and strain on bone specimens is the Uniaxial tension test using the LVDT. Figure 9.27 shows the set up for this test. It consists of one fixed and one moving head with attachments to grip the test specimen. A specimen is placed and firmly fixed in the equipment, a tensile force of known magnitude is applied through the moving head, and the corresponding elongation is measured.

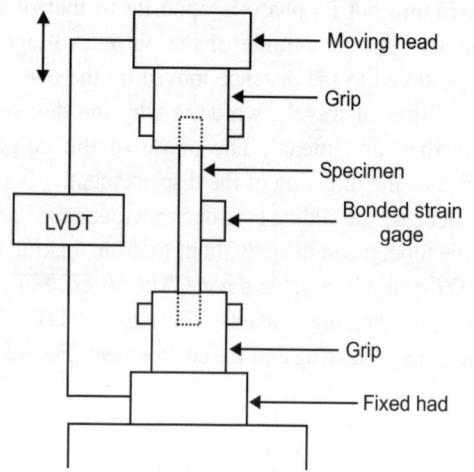

Fig. 9.27. The uniaxial tension test measures force versus elongation.

Soft Tissue Strain Measurement

The measurement of strain in soft tissues has proven to be a difficult task. Thus many different techniques have been proposed, optical and otherwise. None of the techniques, however, has been widely accepted. It is therefore worth examining why it is so difficult to measure strains on soft tissues before reviewing the optically based techniques which have been developed.

The soft tissues of the body are in many architectural forms. These tissues are composites, typically being made up of a combination of collagen and elastin fibres arranged in some way in a matrix of other substances including hydrophilic glycosaminoglycan molecules. Tissues with a large proportion of hydrophilic components can have high water contents. For example, the soft tissues of the musculoskeletal system-articular cartilage, ligaments and tendons-have water contents in the range 65–80 per cent. The tissues are prestressed with the swelling of the hydrophilic molecules being restrained by the collagen fibre arrangement. Mechanically, soft tissues are anisotropic with mechanical properties which

depend on time, temperature and tissue water content. As a result, mechanical tests on soft tissues are usually performed with the specimen immersed in a physiological solution at constant temperature. But recent work suggests that even this might not keep water contents at *in vivo* levels.

A direct method of measuring ligament strain is by mounting a strain gage load cell within cadaveric knees. A noncontact method for measuring ligament strain is the video dimension analyser (VDA) Reference lines are drawn on the specimen using stain, and the test is videotaped. The VDA system tracks the reference lines, yielding strain versus time. Tendon and ligament tissues contain low-modulus elastin, which bears the majority of the load for strains up to about 0.07. At higher strains, collagen fibres, which possess a zigzag crimp, take an increasing portion of the load, resulting in an upward curvature of the stress–strain curve.

Proteoglycans are important components of the extracellular matrix of articular cartilage and other soft tissues. Viscosity of proteoglycans extracted from cartilage can be measured using a cone-on-plate viscometer described. The angle of the cone α is 0.04 and the diameter of the plate $2a$ is 50 mm. The shear rate $\gamma = \omega/\alpha$, where ω is the rotational speed of the plate (rad/s). Apparent viscosity $\eta_{app} = 3T(2\omega a3\gamma)$, where T = torque. Another viscometer is the Ostwald capillary viscometer, which calculates the coefficient of viscosity η from the pressure gradient dp/dL, the volume rate of flow Q, and the tube radius R using the equation $\eta = (\pi R^4/(8Q))(dp/dL)$. Another viscometer is the Couette coaxial viscometer, in which an outer rotating cylinder transmits torque through the test fluid to an inner coaxial cylinder.

Joint Friction

A Synovial joint is the most common and most movable type of joint in the body of a mammal. As with most other joints, synovial joints achieve movement at the point of contact of the articulating bones. Structural and functional differences distinguish synovial joints from cartilaginous joints (synchondroses and symphyses) and fibrous joints (sutures, gomphoses, and syndesmoses). The main structural differences between synovial and fibrous joints is the existence of capsules surrounding the articulating surfaces of a synovial joint and the presence of lubricating synovial fluid within that capsule (synovial cavity).

Diarthrodial (synovial) joints have a large motion between opposing bones. To diagnose disease and design artificial joints, we desire to measure friction between them. The resistance to motion between two bodies in contact is given by frictional force $F = \mu W$, where μ is the coefficient of friction and W is the applied load. Surface friction comes either from adhesion of one surface to another due to roughness on the two surfaces, or from the viscosity of the sheared lubricant film between the two surfaces. Lubrication of bone joints is an important factor in determining coefficient of friction. Rheumatoid arthritis results in overproduction of synovial fluid in the joint and commonly causes swollen joints. The synovial fluid is the lubricating fluid that is used by the joints. The lubricating properties of the fluid depend on its viscosity; thin oil is less viscous and a better lubricant than thick oil. The viscosity of synovial fluid decreases under the large shear stresses found in the joint.

The coefficient of friction is measured in the laboratory using arthrotripsometers (pendulum devices). Here (in Fig. 9.28), a normal hip joint from a fresh cadaver is mounted upside down with heavy weights pressing the head of femur into the socket. The weight on the joint is varied to study the effect of different loads. The whole unit acts like a pendulum with the joint serving as the pivot. From the rate of decrease of the amplitude with time, the coefficient of friction is calculated. It can be concluded that fat in the cartilage helps to reduce the coefficient of friction. When synovial fluid is removed, the coefficient of friction is increased considerably. Figure 9.28 shows an arrangement for measuring the coefficient of friction.

We wish to measure wear in joints of artificial materials such as ultra-high-molecular-weight polyethylene (UHMWPE). For polymeric materials, the volume $V = kPX$ produced by wear during sliding against metallic or ceramic countersurfaces is proportional to the applied load P and the total sliding distance X. k is a wear factor indicative of the wear resistance of a material.

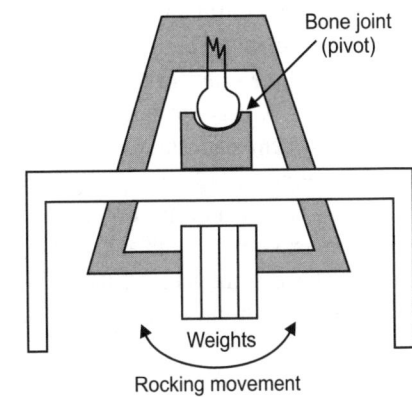

Fig. 9.28. Decay of oscillation amplitude in the pendulum device permits calculation of the coefficient of friction of a joint.

Bone Position

Bone position is important for calculating the loading forces that act on it. The most complicated bones in the body, on which these forces are calculated, are in the spinal cord. Calculating forces for other bones, such as the femur, is relatively easy. These loading forces are static and dynamic in nature.

A goniometer is an electric potentiometer that can be attached to a joint to measure its angle of rotation.

Human joint and gross body motions can be measured by simple protractor type goniometers, electrogoniometers, exoskeletal linkage devices, interrupted light or normal and high speed photography, television-computer, X-ray or cineradiographic techniques, sonic digitisers, photo-optical technique, and accelerometers.

Bone Strain-Related Potentials

Bending a slab of cortical or whole living or dead bone yields piezoelectric potentials of about 10 mV, which we can measure using electrodes. If the strain is maintained, the potentials rapidly decay to a very low value, called the offset potential. Some workers hypothesise that these potentials have a role in directing growth, healing, and remodelling.

SKIN

The skin is a soft outer covering of an animal, in particular a vertebrate. Other animal coverings such the arthropod exoskeleton or the seashell have different developmental origin, structure and chemical composition. The adjective cutaneous literally means 'of the skin' (from Latin *cutis*, skin). In mammals, the skin is the largest organ of the integumentary system made up of multiple layers of ectodermal tissue, and guards the underlying muscles, bones, ligaments and internal organs. Skin of a different nature exists in amphibians, reptiles, birds. All mammals have some hair on their skin, even marine mammals which appear to be hairless. Because it interfaces with the environment, skin plays a key role in protecting (the body) against pathogens and excessive water loss. Its other functions are insulation, temperature regulation, sensation, and the protection of vitamin B folates. Severely damaged skin will try to heal by forming scar tissue. This is often discoloured and depigmented (Fig. 9.29).

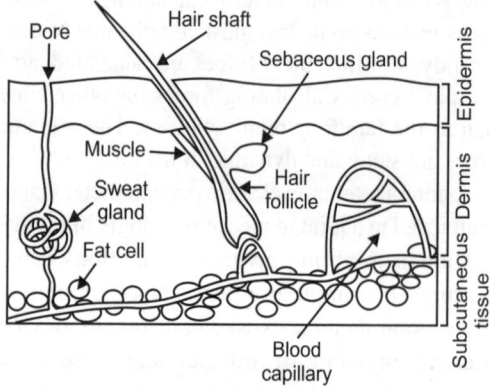

Fig. 9.29. Layers of mammal skin: epidermis, dermis, and subcutis, showing a hair follicle, sweat gland and sebaceous gland.

Hair with sufficient density is called fur. The fur mainly serves to augment the insulation the skin provides, but can also serve as a secondary sexual characteristic or as camouflage. On some animals, the skin is very hard and thick, and can be processed to create leather. Reptiles and fish have hard protective scales on their skin for protection, and birds have hard feathers, all made of tough β-keratins.

Amphibian skin is not a strong barrier to passage of chemicals and is often subject to osmosis. A frog sitting in an anesthetic solution could quickly go to sleep (Fig. 9.30).

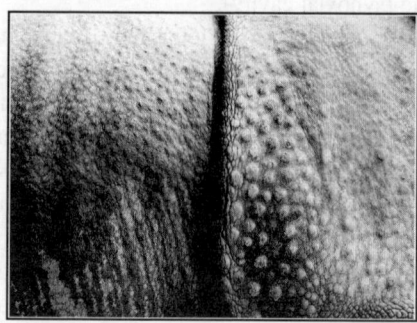

Fig. 9.30. A close up picture of a rhinoceros skin.

Transepidermal Water Loss

Transepidermal water loss (TWL) or (TEWL) is a term associated with dermatology and connected sciences.

It is defined as the measurement of the quantity of water that passes from inside a body (animal or plant) through the epidermal layer (skin) to the surrounding atmosphere via diffusion and evaporation processes.

Transepidermal water loss in mammals is also known as 'insensible water loss' as it is a process over which organisms have little physiological control.

Measurements of TWL may be useful for identifying skin damage caused by certain chemicals, physical insult (such as 'tape stripping') or pathological conditions such as eczema, as rates of TWL increase in proportion to the level of damage. However, TWL is also affected by environmental factors such as humidity, temperature, the time of year (season variation) and the moisture content of the skin (hydration level). Therefore, care must be taken when interpreting the meaning of TWL rates.

There is at present some confusion over the correct acronym for transepidermal water loss, with some references using TWL others using TEWL. It is thought that TEWL is often used to avoid confusion with the term 'total water loss' commonly used in some disciplines.

Measurement of the transepidermal water loss (TEWL, expressed in grams per squaremeter and per hour) is used for studying the water barrier function of the human skin. The more perfect the skin protective coat, the higher the water content and the lower the TEWL (Fig. 9.31).

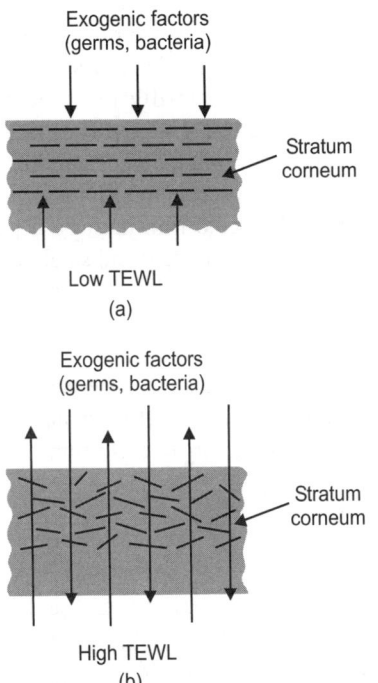

Fig. 9.31. Schematic illustration of the barrier function of the stratum corneum. (a) healthy skin , (b) disturbed skin.

The outer part of the skin is the stratum corneum which forms a barrier against diffusion of water and is also an effective barrier for microbes and chemical substances. The stratum corneum contains much water and is flexible in the healthy state, but it becomes hard and brittle when dehydrated. Disorders such as atopic dermatitis arise when this barrier function does not work properly.

Several techniques have been developed to measure the skin properties that are influenced by the water content. One possibility is the measurement of the transepidermal water loss of the skin.

TEWL measurements allow to discover disturbances in the skin protective function in an early stage, even before they are visible. Normal skin allows water loss only in small amounts. In the case of atopic skin the water loss is much higher. The determination of the TEWL is an important support to investigate the skin irritation that occurs by various physical and chemical influences. Typical fields of application are allergic tests, occupational medicine, observation of the newborn, supervision the healing process of skin damages and burns or testing the effectiveness and biocompatibility of cosmetic products. Different methods for TEWL measurement from local skin sites have been described: Closed chamber methods and open chamber methods.

Operating Principles

In this section we report on two novel TEWL instruments based on the closed chamber method. The microsensor is placed in a housing which forms a closed measuring chamber after touching the skin. The water vapour emitted from the skin fills the small measuring chamber and causes an increasing relative humidity inside the chamber. The growing rate of the humidity is a measure for the TEWL value of the skin. Some recovery time is necessary after each measurement. The sensor chip must have enough time to try up and to reach its initial condition before starting a new measurement.

The first instrument (later on called instrument A, Fig. 9.32) is based on a ceramic chip carrying an interdigital electrode structure which is covered by a hygroscopic an organic salt film.

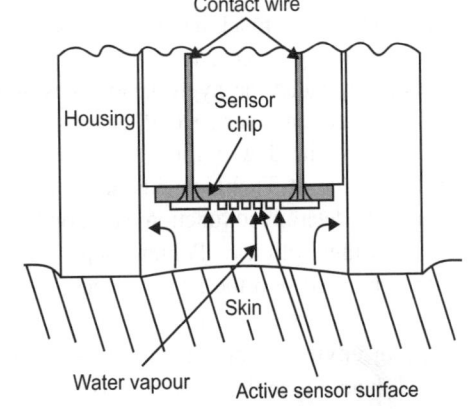

Fig. 9.32. Schematic cross section of the measuring head of the instrument A (conductivity method).

The main sensing effect used in this instrument is the conductance change of the hygroscopic film represented by the real part of the admittance. The measuring frequency is 500 kHz. The admittance Y is measured by using a Precision LCR Meter. Furthermore, it is necessary to measure the relative humidity RH of the ambient air. After a time interval t_m (30 s) starting at the moment of touching the skin the change of admittance (Y_s at the starting time, Ym after the measuring interval t_m) is recorded. The TEWL value is calculated from t_m, ($Y_m - Y_s$) and RH by using an experimentally determined function.

The second instrument described here (later on called instrument B, Fig. 9.33) is based on a silicon chip, which is mounted on a Peltier couple. The sensing effect of this instrument is the change of the dew point temperature by the emission of water from the skin.

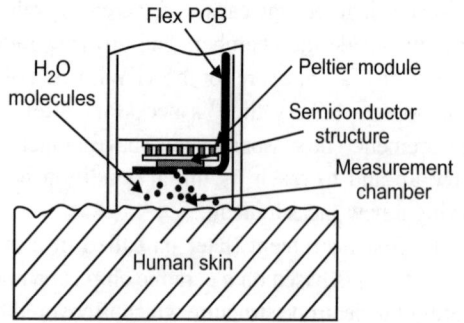

Fig. 9.33. Schematic cross section of the measuring head of the instrument B (dew point method).

At the moment of touching the skin the actual dew point recording process is started. Depending on the humidity value the hygrometer takes about 5 readings (detections) per second. After the time interval t_m (5 s) the dew point temperature T_s is recorded. A value of TEWL is calculated with an experimentally determined function based on T_s and t_m. The algorithm optimises Peltier couple current and energy injected into the heater to achieve fast detections and to follow humidity changes in the surrounding environment. The hygrometer can measure air humidity in the range from 0 to 30°C of dew point temperatures with resolution 0.1°C and accuracy 0.4°C (with detections of every 0.2 – 0.3 s).

Technology

In the case of instrument A a ceramic chip with the dimensions of 5 mm × 5 mm × 0.6 mm is used. The chip is mounted in a distance of about 1.4 mm away from the skin surface. The lead-in wires are guided through funnel-shaped holes to the rear substrate surface (Fig. 9.32). They are bonded to the contact pads of the chip by using an isotropically conductive adhesive. The width of the electrodes is about 55 μm, the gap between interdigital electrodes is approximately 15 μm (Fig. 9.34). The electrodes are made of a double layer of molybdenum (0.2 μm) and gold (8 μm). The molybdenum film is deposited by RF-sputtering. The gold film must be deposited in such a way that it completely and safely covers the underlying molybdenum electrode including side walls. Therefore, the gold film is produced by electroplating. It has an important protective function against chemical degradation. The active moisture sensing area is 1.75 mm × 3.15 mm and is covered with a hygroscopic an organic salt film.

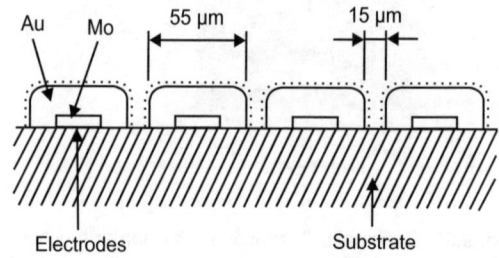

Fig. 9.34. Schematic cross sectional view of the electrode system of the instrument A (conductivity method). Sensing area covered by an an organic salt film.

In the case of instrument B the hygrometer is based on a silicon semiconductor structure, which contains a dew point interdigital impedance detector (on level II), and thermistor and heater (on level I). The chip face is positioned in a distance of 8 mm away from the skin surface. On the silicon substrate (385 μm thick) the following layers were formed and patterned: thermal silicon dioxide (0.3 μm), gold (0.25 μm as thermoresistor and heater), silicon dioxide (0.6 μm) and gold (0.15 μm) as impedance detector. The impedance detector electrodes pitch was set to 6 μm (Fig. 9.35). The sensitive detector area opened in the flexible PCB is approximately 2 mm ×

2 mm. Finally a flip-chip technology was used for electrical structure input/output bonding into flexible PCB ribbon.

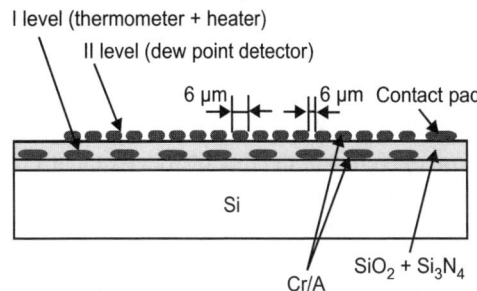

Fig. 9.35. Schematic cross sectional view of the electrode system of the instrument B (dew point method).

Calibration

The experimental methods used for the calibration of the instruments A and B are practically the same and differ only in marginal details. To generate a certain TEWL value we have used a small and light vessel containing some water and covered by a semipermeable diaphragm. The water evaporation rate (ER) can be calculated from the formula:

$$ER = \frac{\Delta m}{A \cdot \Delta t} \qquad \text{... (9.9)}$$

with the mass loss Δm in grams, the time interval Δt in hours and the area of the diaphragm A in squaremeter. To determine the water loss the vessel is arranged on a precision balance. First a stable value of ER is generated by using a proper diaphragm. Then the TEWL sensor to be tested is placed on top of the diaphragm whereby the sensor head touches the diaphragm forming a closed measuring chamber (Fig. 9.36). The evaporation rate defined by corresponds to the TEWL in case of a measurement on the human skin. Hence the evaporation rate of the calibration configuration is also called TEWL. It is supposed that the evaporation rate is uniformly distributed over the surface of the diaphragm. Different TEWL values can be adjusted either by applying a different number of membrane layers or different types of membrane materials (methods used at WUT). Different TEWL values can also be achieved during a long term drying process of the vessel (method used at VUT).

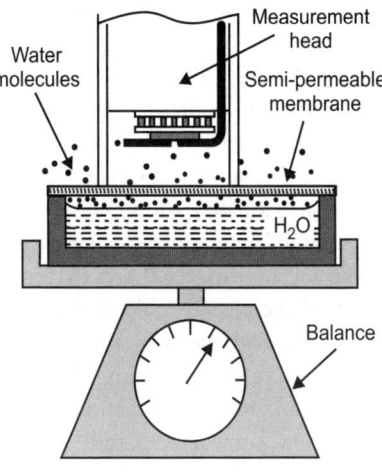

Fig. 9.36. Schematic illustration of a TEWL generator used for the calibration of the instruments.

The instrument A (developed at VUT) has been calibrated at different values of relative humidity of the ambient air in the range from 31 per cent to 64 per cent. We have investigated five persons in the age between 19 and 65 years. The measurements were carried out in the crook of the left arm. The test persons have been asked to rest at least 30 minutes before starting the measurement in order to avoid errors caused by perspiration. One characteristic result is shown in Fig. 9.37. The persons (all male) are ordered in their age: person 1:19 y, person 2:27 y, person 3:27 y, person 4:32 y, person 5:65 y.

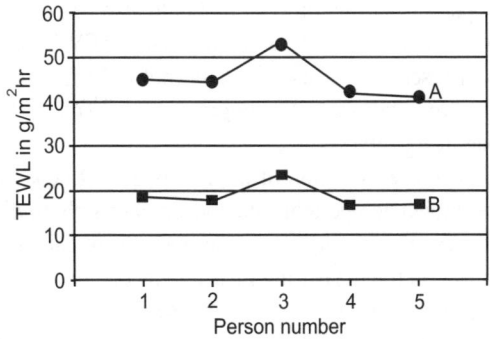

Fig. 9.37. Comparison of measurement results. The upper curve refers to instrument A (conductivity method), the lower curve belongs to instrument B (dew point method).

Discussion

The results presented in Fig. 9.37 show that both instruments indicate the individual differences in the TEWL value of the investigated persons. It can be clearly seen that the TEWL of subject 3 differs significantly from the other subjects. Furthermore, we find that the old person 5 has a lower TEWL compared with the young person 1. This is in good agreement with results found in the literature. However, the absolute values of the two curves A and B shown in Fig.9.37 are different. One explanation of the considerable shift is based on a biological effect. With the instrument B the skin sees a rather cold surface during the period of measurement because of the action of the Peltier couple. The dew point temperature is significantly below room temperature. Therefore, the emission of water from the skin will be lower, resulting in a lower TEWL. Another contribution to the shift is the difference in the measuring times (30 s for the instrument A and 5 s for the instrument B) and the non-linearity of the relationship between the air humidity inside the closed chamber and the measuring time.

Measured humidity curves show a part with increasing slope at the begin of the measuring interval followed by a part with decreasing slope which approaches a saturation value. Furthermore, the rate of water evaporation from the skin is not constant during the measuring time. Therefore, further research is necessary to find a way how to define a proper measuring interval. It should also be possible to create new ideas how to calculate a TEWL value from a series of sensor signals (not only from two humidity values at the begin and the end of the measuring interval).

A further question of interest is the influence of the ambient temperature and the ambient air humidity on measuring results. Both quantities do not only have impact on the measuring instruments but also on the measuring subjects itself. TEWL measurements should be carried out in a special room with standard conditions (stable temperature and stable relative humidity). It is also known that the TEWL value depends not only on the type of skin, but also on the emotional condition of a person and of other parameters, like the day time and the season of measurements (differences in summer and winter). Therefore, the medical interpretation of a measured TEWL value is difficult.

Flow hygrometry

In flow hygrometry, the flux of water vapour out of a fixed area of skin is determined by measuring the increase in water vapour concentration in the flowing gas stream. The increase in humidity is read at a sensor output once steady-state conditions have been reached. TWL can be calculated using the formula:

$$TWL = \frac{K \times V \times R}{A} \qquad ... (9.10)$$

where K is the instrument constant, V is the increase in the sensor output, R is the gas flow rate and A the skin area isolated by the measuring chamber. TWL is usually measured in $mg/(cm^2 \cdot h)$. Numerous possible sources of error in the flow hygrometry system include uncertainty in the gas flow rate, uncertainty in the actual area of skin exposed to flowing gas, absorption of water vapour in tubing connecting the skin chamber with the sensor, and leaks in the seal of the chamber to the skin site. These errors can be minimised by careful design of the system.

In this method, transfer of water vapour to the sensor is by convection which normally requires gas tanks or pumps, valves, and tubing, in addition to the sensor and the skin chamber. Figure 9.38 shows a flow hygrometer.

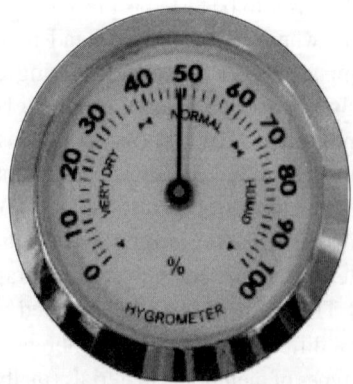

Fig. 9.38. Flow hygrometer.

Closed cup method

In the close cup method, the humidity sensor is sealed into one end of a cylinder of known length. The cylinder is placed on the skin, trapping a volume of unstirred air between the skin and the deterctor as shown in Fig. 9.39. Within a few seconds, the sensor voltage begins to rise steadily followed by a gradual decrease in rate of change.

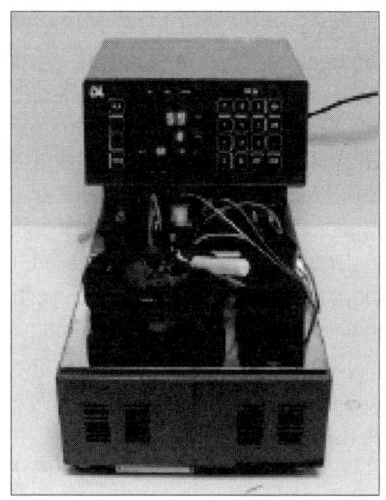

Fig. 9.39. Closed cup hygrometer.

The application of diffusion principles to the water vapour in the volume of trapped air predicts this behaviour and shows that the TWL is directly proportional to the slope of the transient linear portion of the detector output curve. The TWL is found from:

$$\text{TWL} = K \times l \times \frac{dv}{dt} \qquad ... (9.11)$$

where K is an instrument calibration constant, l is the distance between the detector and the skin surface, v is the detector voltage, and t is the time. The closed chamber method does not permit recordings of continuous TWL because when the air inside the chamber is saturated, skin evaporation ceases.

Open cup method

Figure 9.40(a) shows the open cup hygrometer. The sensor is mounted in the wall of the cylindrical chamber with the top end of the chamber open and the bottom end placed against the skin. As in the closed cup method, the cylindrical chamber defines a volume of undisturbed air in which the transfer of water vapour is controlled by diffusion in air. A few minutes after applying the chamber to the skin, the sensor reaches a new equilibrium in which the rate of flow of vapour out of the open end of the cylinder is equal to the rate of flow of vapour out of the skin, the TWL. In this condition the rate of flow can be calculated, according to the principles of diffusion, from the product of diffusion coefficient of water vapour in the air and the concentration gradient. For the configuration shown in Fig. 9.40(a) the sensor is mounted at a distance l from the end of the cylinder where the humidity is determines by the room condition. Thus the increase in sensor response divided by the length determines the humidity gradient. The equation for TWL measurement with the open cup method is then

$$\text{WL} = \frac{(V - V_0) \times K \times D}{l} \qquad ... (9.12)$$

where V and V_0 are equilibrium and initial sensor voltages, respectively, K is an instrument constant, D is the diffusion coefficient of water in air, and l is the distance between the sensor and the end of the cylindrical chamber open to the room air. Air movement and humidity are the greatest drawbacks of this method. This method is currently used in commercially available devices.

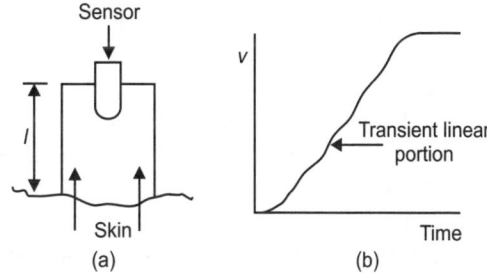

Fig. 9.40. The open cup hygrometer: (a) configuration of measurement cylinder, (b) typical sensor output curve.

In the flow hygrometry method, the investigator has the option of selecting the water content of the sweep gas within the limits of the humidity sensor. For indirect methods, unless measurements are made in humidity-controlled room, the variable ambient condition can have a profound effect on the resulting measurements.

Colour

Among the physical skin parameters, colour is important in clinical dermatology. The experienced dermatologist uses colour information in several ways. First, he frequently bases his first-view diagnosis or elaboration of differential diagnosis to a considerable amount on specific colours of the skin lesions themselves. Second, the colour differences often allow the clinician to judge the distribution of lesions on the human body, even without close inspection and palpation. Finally, the intensity of colour may provide useful information about the severity of a pathological process, and changes in colour to normal tell the dermatogist if the treatment works.

Ultraviolet radiation in the sun's rays or from a discharge lamp will cause skin tanning (pigmentation), which is a photochemical response involving the release of the skin pigment melanin. In the basal skin layer are located the melanocytes that contain melanin. On exposure to ultraviolet radiation the melanocytes take up tyrosine from the circulation to synthesise melanin. The preexisting melanin in the skin also darkens; both contribute to skin drakening. It should be recognised that skin pigmentation is also affected by hormones. Melanocytes are not uniformly distributed over the skin surface, being about three times as dense on the face as on the thigh. Thus the response to the same amount of ultraviolet radiation will be different on different parts of the body.

Melanin strongly absorbs ultraviolet radiation and provides protection for the deeper skin layers. About 80 per cent of the radiation is absorbed in the first 0.2 mm of the skin, i.e. the epidermis is the major site of absorption. In regions where the skin is thick, such as the palms of the hands and soles of the feet, very little of the radiation reaches the melanocytes. Consequently, these sites pigment very little. It is important to note that pigmentation is a delayed process, requiring about 0.5 day for the pigment to be released from the melanocytes. Suntan protection preparations act as filters that absorb the ultraviolet radiation so that less reaches the melanocytes.

In using ultraviolet radiation to induce pigmentation, it is essential that the eyes be protected. Exposure can cause conjunctivitis and temporary or permanent blindness. Ordinary glass is virtually opaque to ultraviolet radiation, and eyeglasses afford protection. However, they should fit snugly.

Dermaspectrometer and erythema meter

The instruments used to measure the variations in skin colour are the Dermaspectrometer and the Erythema meter. Their working principle can be explained as follows: Inflammatory skin erythema is the result of an increased presence of erythrocytes in skin structures. In inflammation, cutaneous vessels are dilated, and blood flow is increased. Because oxyhaemoglobin has absorption in the spectral range from 520 to 580 nm, it absorbs green light, while red light is reflected to the absorber. Changes in skin redness affect the absorption of green light, but affect red light less. An erythema index of the skin can therefore be based on the ratio between the reflection of red and green light.

Erythema index =

$$\log_{10} \frac{(\text{Intensity of reflected red light})}{(\text{Intensity of reflected green light})} \quad \dots (9.13)$$

Similarly, melanin pigmentation of the skin leads to an increased absorption both in the green and red parts of the spectrum. A melanin index may be defined as follows:

Melanin index = $\log_{10}$
(intensity of reflected red light) ... (9.14)

The Dermaspectrometer emits green and red light (568 and 655 nm) from an LED source. The Erythema meter emits green and red light (546 and 671 nm) from a tungsten lamp. Figure 9.41 shows that the light reflected from the skin is detected with a photosensor. A microprocessor calculates the erythema and melanin index, with is then displayed.

The skin erythema meter is a fibre optic, dual-wavelength reflectance metre that measures the reflectance of the skin on two wavelengths, one the blood/haemoglobin absorption band (555 nm) and another a reference (660 nm). The instrument consists of a fibre optic sensor head, a microprocessor-based control and analysis unit, and a plotter, and it presents the relation between the measured reflectance results in terms of a reflectance index [R(555 nm): R(660 nm)]. The measurement cycle, including printing, takes 5s. Stability tests on the erythema meter (constant distance, reference object) showed the standard deviation of the reflectance index to be +/–0.1 per cent, whereas that in repeatability tests was less than +/–0.5 per cent for skin and less than +/– 0.2 per cent for paper with hand-held positioning and repetition. The dynamic change in the reflectance index was about 30 per cent with strong irritation. Results of various irritation test series on human skin are also presented. Finally, the performance and applicability of the skin erythema meter with respect to allergy test procedures, irritancy testing, and measurement of UV-induced erythema are discussed.

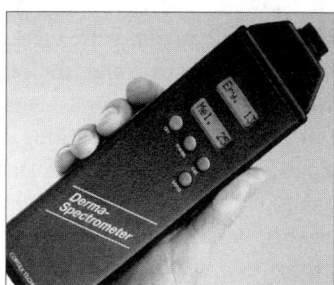

Fig. 9.41. Dermaspectrometer.

Chromameter

Applications

1. Measure tristimulus values, chromaticity, colour difference, correlated colour temperature, and illuminance of light sources.

2. R & D and colour inspection of light in a variety of industries such as lamp manufacturers, building and interior design.

3. Set-up projectors for presentation purposes.

4. Adjust colour of CRTs, flat panel, and other display devices.

5. Evaluate and control colour of light boxes and light booths

Chromameter measures chromaticity, tristimulus values, colour difference, correlated colour temperature and the illuminance of light sources. Also used for colour inspection and illuminance measurement of light sources.

The chromameter uses one main body for single and multi-point measurements. You can add up to 30 receptor heads to one body. Applications include: colour adjustment of CRTs, flat panel and other display devices projector set-ups R & D and colour inspection of light sources (Fig. 9.42).

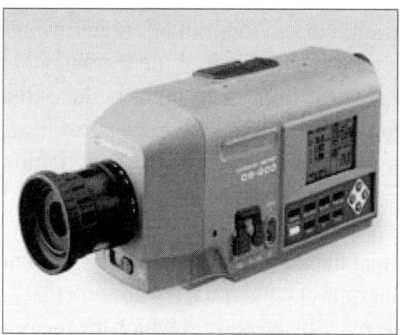

Fig. 9.42. Chromameter.

To use the Receptor head off of the body, you will need one adapter for the body and one adapter for each head. To connect, use any standard Cat 5 LAN cable. Recommended length is not to exceed 100M.

10

Body Temperature, Heat, Fat and Movement

INTRODUCTION

This chapter deals with measurements of physical parameters from the total body, such as temperature, heat, fat, and movement. These four parameters are somewhat related because they all deal with energy. Heat is the thermal energy content of a body. It is defined as the vibratory motion of its component particles. Body heat is the result of a balance between heat production and heat loss, which occurs through conduction, convection, radiation and evaporation. Temperature is a measure of the tendency of a body to transfer heat from or to other bodies. Balancing heat production within the body against heat loss to the surroundings determines the body temperature. Body fat is energy related in that it is part of the heat storage process.

Normal human body temperature, also known as normothermia or euthermia, is a concept that depends upon the place in the body at which the measurement is made, and the time of day and level of activity of the body. Although the value 37.0°C (98.6°F) is the commonly accepted average core body temperature, the value of 36.8°±0.7°C, or 98.2°±1.3°F is an average oral (under the tongue) measurement. Rectal measurements, or measurements taken directly inside the body cavity, are typically slightly higher. In Russia and former Soviet countries, the commonly quoted value is 36.6°C (97.9°F), based on an armpit reading. The core body temperature of an individual tends to have the lowest value in the second half of the sleep cycle; the lowest point, called the nadir, is one of the primary markers for circadian rhythms.

Temperature control (thermoregulation) is part of a homeostatic mechanism that keeps the organism at optimum operating temperature, as it affects the rate of chemical reactions. In humans the average oral temperature is 36.8°C (98.2°F), though it varies among individuals, as well as cycling regularly through the day, as controlled by one's circadian rhythms with the lowest temperature occurring about two hours before one normally wakes up (Fig. 10.1).

Body temperature normally fluctuates over the day, with the lowest levels around 4 am and the highest in the late afternoon, between 4 and 6 pm (assuming the person sleeps at night and stays awake during the day). Therefore, an oral temperature of 37.2°C (99.0°F) would, strictly speaking, be normal in the afternoon but not in the morning. An individual's body temperature typically changes by about 0.5 °C (0.9 °F) between its highest and lowest points each day (Fig. 10.2).

Temperature is increased after eating, and psychological factors also influence body temperature.

Many outside factors affect the measured temperature as well. 'Normal' values are generally given for an otherwise healthy, non-fasting adult, dressed comfortably, indoors, in a room that is kept at a normal room temperature (22.7° to 24.4°C or 73° to 76°F), during the morning, but not shortly after arising from sleep. Furthermore, for oral temperatures, the subject must not have eaten, drunk, or smoked anything in at least the previous fifteen to twenty minutes, as the temperature of the food, drink, or smoke can dramatically affect the reading.

Children develop higher temperatures with activities like playing, but this is not fever because their set-point is normal. Elderly patients may have a decreased ability to generate body heat during a

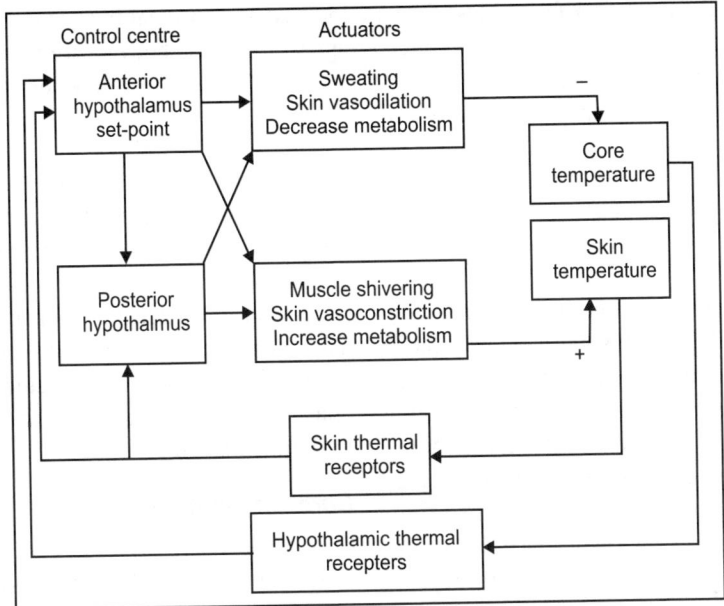

Fig. 10.1. The human temperature regulation system can increase or decrease body temperature.

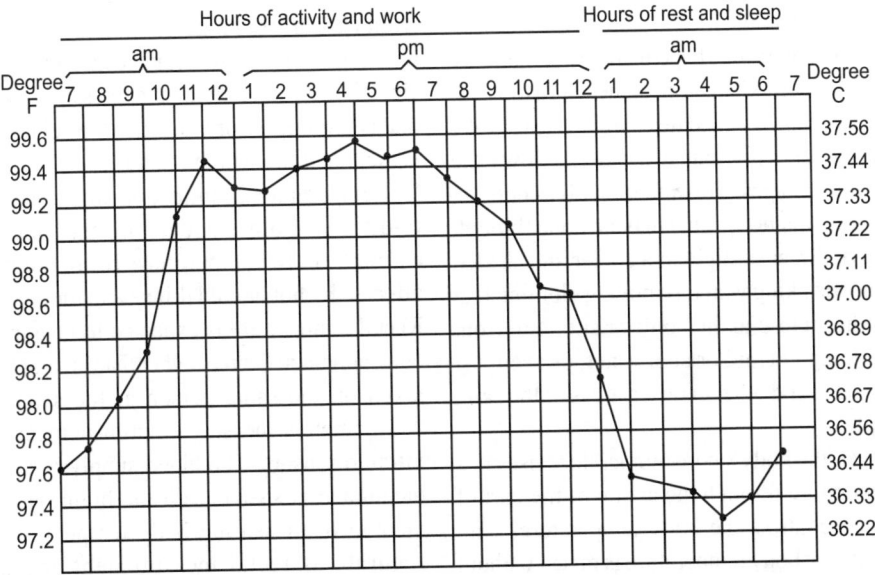

Fig. 10.2. Diurnal variation in body temperature, ranging from about 37.5°C from 10 am to 6 pm, and falling to about 36.4°C from 2 am to 6 am.

fever, so even a low-grade fever can have serious underlying causes in geriatrics.

Normal body temperature may differ as much as 1.0°F between individuals or from day to day.

Specific Temperature Concepts

Fever

A temperature setpoint is the level at which the body attempts to maintain its temperature. When the setpoint is raised, the result is a fever. Most fevers are caused by infectious disease and can be lowered, if desired, with antipyretic medications.

An organism at optimum temperature is considered *a febrile* or *apyrexic*, meaning 'without fever'. If temperature is raised, but the setpoint is not raised, then the result is hyperthermia.

Hyperthermia

Hyperthermia is an acute condition which occurs when the body produces or absorbs more heat than it can dissipate. It is usually caused by prolonged exposure to high temperatures. The heat-regulating mechanisms of the body eventually become overwhelmed and unable to deal effectively with the heat, causing the body temperature to climb uncontrollably. Hyperthermia at or above about 40°C (104°F) is a life-threatening medical emergency and requires immediate treatment. Common symptoms include headache, confusion, and fatigue. If sweating has resulted in dehydration, then the affected person may have dry, red skin.

In a medical setting, mild hyperthermia is commonly referred to as heat exhaustion or heat prostration; severe hyperthermia is called heat stroke. Heat stroke may come on suddenly, but it usually follows the untreated milder stages. Treatment involves cooling and rehydrating the body. This may be done through moving out of direct sunlight to a cooler and shaded environment, drinking water, removing clothing that might keep heat close to the body, or sitting in front of a fan. Bathing in tepid or cool water, or even just washing the face and other exposed areas of the skin, can be helpful.

With fever, the body's core temperature rises to a higher temperature through the action of the part of the brain that controls the body temperature; with hyperthermia, the body temperature is raised without the consent of the heat control centres.

Hypothermia

In hypothermia, the body temperature drops below that required for normal metabolism and bodily functions. In humans, this is usually due to excessive exposure to cold air or water, but it can be deliberately induced as a medical treatment. Symptoms usually appear when the body's core temperature drops by 1°–2°C (1.8°–3.6°F) below normal temperature.

Basal body temperature

Basal body temperature is the lowest temperature attained by the body during rest (usually during sleep). It is generally measured immediately after awakening and before any physical activity has been undertaken, although the temperature measured at that time is somewhat higher than the true basal body temperature. In women, temperature differs at various points in the menstrual cycle, and this can be used for family planning.

Core temperature

Core temperature, also called core body temperature, is the operating temperature of an organism, specifically in deep structures of the body such as the liver, in comparison to temperatures of peripheral tissues. Core temperature is normally maintained within a narrow range so that essential enzymatic reactions can occur. Significant core temperature elevation (hyperthermia) or depression (hypothermia) that is prolonged for more than a brief period of time is incompatible with human life.

Temperature examination in the rectum is the traditional gold standard measurement used to estimate core temperature (oral temperature is affected by hot or cold drinks and mouth-breathing). Rectal temperature is expected to be approximately one Fahrenheit degree higher than an oral temperature taken on the same person at the same time. Ear thermometers measure eardrum temperature using infrared sensors. The blood supply to the tympanic membrane is shared with the brain. However, this method of measuring body temperature is not as accurate as rectal measurement and has a low sensitivity for fevers, missing three or four out of every ten fevers in children. Ear temperature measurement may be acceptable for observing trends in body temperature but is less useful in consistently identifying fevers.

Until recently, direct measurement of core body temperature required invasive insertion of a probe —

a procedure that is not clinically possible—so a variety of indirect methods have commonly been used. While the rectal or vaginal temperature is generally considered to give the most accurate assessment of core body temperature, particularly in hypothermia, its recording is disliked by patients and medical staff alike. In the early 2000s, ingestible thermistors in capsule form were produced, allowing the temperature inside the digestive tract to be transmitted to an external receiver; one study found that these were comparable in accuracy to rectal temperature measurement.

METHODS OF MEASUREMENT

Taking a patient's temperature is an initial part of a full clinical examination (Fig. 10.3).

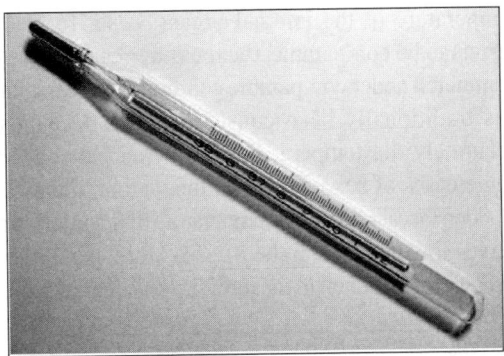

Fig. 10.3. A medical/clinical thermometer showing the temperature of 38.7°C.

The temperature reading depends on which part of the body is being measured. Measurements are commonly taken in the mouth, the ear, the anus, or the armpit. In females, the vagina can also be used. The median daytime temperature among healthy adults are as follows:

1. Temperature in the anus (rectum/rectal), vagina, or in the ear (otic) is about 37.6°C (98.6°F).
2. Temperature in the mouth (oral) is about 36.8°C (98.2°F).
3. Temperature under the arm (axillary) is about 36.4°C (97.6°F).

Normal human body temperature varies slightly from person to person and by the time of day.

Consequently, each type of measurement has a range of normal temperatures. The range for normal human body temperatures, taken orally, is 36.8±0.7°C (98.2±1.3 °F). This means that any oral temperature between 36.1 and 37.5 °C (96.9 and 99.5 °F) is likely to be normal.

Problems of Various Measurements

It is claimed that changes in core body temperature are reflected sooner and more accurately in the ear than at other sites.

Influencing factors on other areas where temperatures are taken:

1. Oral temperatures are influenced by drinking, eating and breathing.
2. Rectal temperatures lag behind changes in core body temperature and there is a risk of cross-contamination.
3. Skin temperatures, measured under the arm or at the forehead, are not always reliable indicators of core body temperature, especially during those critical times when core body temperature is increasing or decreasing. This is because the skin is a tool the body uses to control core body temperature. For example, when fever is increasing people are likely to react by shivering and drawing in heat from the increased core body temperature. Skin temperatures are further influenced by factors such as fever-lowering medication, clothing and external temperature.

MEASUREMENT DEVICES

There is a risk of injury from cracking the original glass thermometers if too much force is applied by the teeth to hold them in place and the alcohol or mercury contents are poisonous. This is avoided by the use of electronic thermometers which are made from solid plastic and use a metal (thermocouple) sensor.

A plastic thermometer strip placed on the forehead gives an approximate local reading, which depends to a great extent on ambient air temperature and local circulation effects. Using a thermometer to record the temperature under the armpit is less affected by surrounding air temperature, but is still prone to diverge from true core temperature if there are alterations in blood circulation.

Since the year 2000, small ear thermometers have become available and it is thought that the eardrum closely mirrors core temperature values. These work by detecting the infrared heat emission from the tympanic membrane and a measurement is quickly taken within one second making them popular for use with children. While the electronic display of the temperature value is easier to read than interpreting the graduation marks on a thermometer, there are some concerns for the accuracy of ear thermometers in home use.

THERMOREGULATION

Thermoregulation is the ability of an organism to keep its body temperature within certain boundaries, even when the surrounding temperature is very different. This process is one aspect of homeostasis: a dynamic state of stability between an animal's internal environment and its external environment (the study of such processes in zoology has been called ecophysiology or physiological ecology).

If the body is unable to maintain a normal temperature and it increases significantly above normal, a condition known as hyperthermia occurs. The opposite condition, when body temperature decreases below normal levels, is known as hypothermia (Fig. 10.4).

Whereas an organism that thermoregulates is one that keeps its core body temperature within certain limits, a thermoconformer is subject to changes in body temperature according to changes in the temperature outside of its body. It was not until the introduction of thermometers that any exact data on the temperature of animals could be obtained. It was then found that local differences were present, since heat production and heat loss vary considerably in different parts of the body, although the circulation of the blood tends to bring about a mean temperature of the internal parts. Hence it is important to identify the parts of the body that most closely reflect the temperature of the internal organs. Also, for such results to be comparable, the measurements must be conducted under comparable conditions. The rectum has traditionally been considered to reflect most accurately the temperature of internal parts, or in some cases of sex or species, the vagina, uterus or bladder. Occasionally the temperature of the urine as it leaves the urethra may be of use. More usually the temperature is taken in the mouth, axilla, ear or groin.

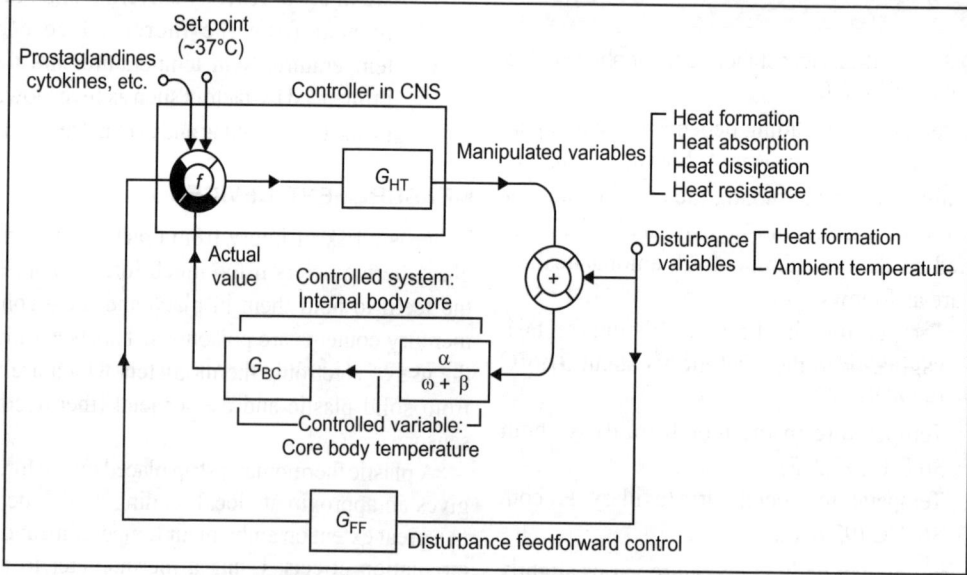

Fig. 10.4. Human thermoregulation (simplified).

Thermoregulation in Humans

As in other mammals, thermoregulation is an important aspect of human homeostasis. Most body heat is generated in the deep organs, especially the liver, brain, and heart, and in contraction of skeletal muscles. Humans have been able to adapt to a great diversity of climates, including hot humid and hot arid. High temperatures pose serious stresses for the human body, placing it in great danger of injury or even death.

For humans, adaptation to varying climatic conditions includes both physiological mechanisms as a by-product of evolution, and the conscious development of cultural adaptations.

There are four avenues of heat loss: convection, conduction, radiation, and evaporation. If skin temperature is greater than that of the surroundings, the body can lose heat by radiation and conduction. But if the temperature of the surroundings is greater than that of the skin, the body actually gains heat by radiation and conduction. In such conditions, the only means by which the body can rid itself of heat is by evaporation. So when the surrounding temperature is higher than the skin temperature, anything that prevents adequate evaporation will cause the internal body temperature to rise. During sports activities, evaporation becomes the main avenue of heat loss. Humidity affects thermoregulation by limiting sweat evaporation and thus heat loss.

The skin assists in homeostasis (keeping different aspects of the body constant, e.g. temperature). It does this by reacting differently to hot and cold conditions so that the inner body temperature remains more or less constant. Vasodilation and sweating are the primary modes by which humans attempt to lose excess body heat. The brain creates much heat through the countless reactions which occur. Even the process of thought creates heat. The head has a complex system of blood vessels, which keeps the brain from overheating by bringing blood to the thin skin on the head, allowing heat to escape. The effectiveness of these methods is influenced by the character of the climate and the degree to which the individual is acclimatised.

In hot conditions

Sweat glands under the skin secrete sweat (a fluid containing mostly water with some dissolved ions) which travels up the sweat duct, through the sweat pore and onto the surface of the skin. This causes heat loss via evaporative cooling; however, a lot of essential water is lost.

The hairs on the skin lie flat, preventing heat from being trapped by the layer of still air between the hairs. This is caused by tiny muscles under the surface of the skin called erector pili muscles relaxing so that their attached hair follicles are not erect.

These flat hairs increase the flow of air next to the skin increasing heat loss by convection. When environmental temperature is above core body temperature, sweating is the only physiological way for humans to lose heat.

Arterioles vasodilation occurs, this is the process of relaxation of smooth muscle in arteriole walls allowing increased blood flow through the artery. This redirects blood into the superficial capillaries in the skin increasing heat loss by convection and conduction.

Note: Most animals can not sweat efficiently. Cats and dogs only have sweat glands on the pads of their feet. Horses and humans are two of the few animals capable of sweating. Many animals pant rather than sweat, this is because the lungs have a large surface area and are highly vascularised. Air is inhaled, cooling the surface of the lungs and is then exhaled losing heat and some water vapour.

Liquid Crystal Thermometer

A liquid crystal thermometer or plastic strip thermometer is a type of thermometer that contains heat-sensitive (thermochromic) liquid crystals in a plastic strip that change colour to indicate different temperatures. Liquid crystals possess the mechanical properties of a liquid, but have the optical properties of a single crystal. Temperature changes can affect the colour of a liquid crystal, which makes them useful for temperature measurement. The resolution of liquid crystal sensors is in the 0.1°C range. Disposable liquid crystal thermometers have been developed for home and medical use. For example if the thermometer is black and it is put onto someones forehead it will change colour depending how much temperature the person has (Fig. 10.5).

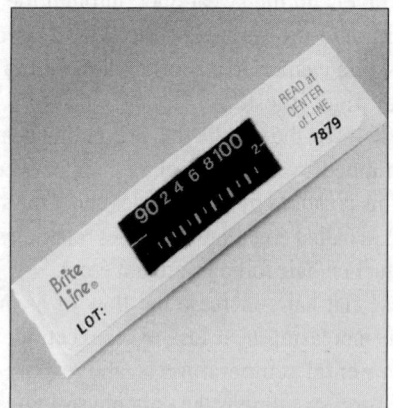

Fig. 10.5. Liquid crystal thermometer.

There are two stages in the liquid crystals, (i) the hot nematic stage is the closest to the liquid phase where the molecules are freely moving around and only partly ordered, and (ii) the cold smectic stage is closest to the solid phase where the molecules align themselves into tightly wound chiral matrixes.

Liquid crystal thermometers portray temperatures as colours and can be used to follow temperature changes caused by heat flow. They can be used to observe that heat flows by conduction, convection, and radiation.

In medical applications, liquid crystal thermometers may be used to read body temperature by placing against the forehead. These are safer than a mercury-in-glass thermometer, and may be advantageous in some patients, but do not always give an exact result, especially the smaller ones.

Liquid crystal thermometers are also commonly used in aquariums in homebrewing, and in mood rings.

Mercury-in-Glass Thermometer

A mercury-in-glass thermometer, invented by German physicist Daniel Gabriel Fahrenheit, is a thermometer consisting of mercury in a glass tube. Calibrated marks on the tube allow the temperature to be read by the length of the mercury within the tube, which varies according to the heat given to it. To increase the sensitivity, there is usually a bulb of mercury at the end of the thermometer which contains most of the mercury; expansion and contraction of this volume of mercury is then amplified in the much narrower bore of the tube. The space above the mercury may be filled with nitrogen or it may be less than atmospheric pressure, which is normally known as a vacuum (Fig. 10.6).

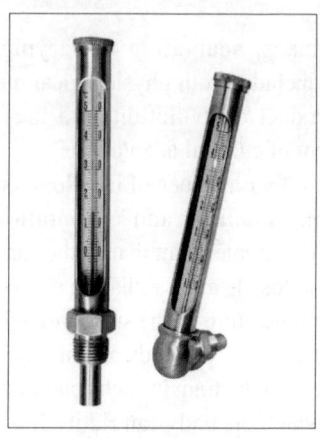

Fig. 10.6. Mercury-in-glass thermometer.

When Celsius decided to use his own temperature scale, he originally defined his scale 'upside-down', i.e. he chose to set the boiling point of pure water at $0°C$ ($212°F$) and the freezing point at $100°C$ ($32°F$). One year later Frenchman Jean Pierre Cristin proposed to invert the scale with the freezing point at $0°C$ ($32°F$) and the boiling point at $100°C$ ($212°F$). He named it Centigrade. Finally, Celsius proposed a method of calibrating a thermometer:

1. Place the cylinder of the thermometer in melting pure water and mark the point where the fluid in the thermometer stabilises. This point is the freeze/thaw point of water.

2. In the same manner mark the point where the fluid stabilises when the thermometer is placed in boiling water vapour.

3. Divide the length between the two marks into 100 equal pieces.

These points are adequate for approximate calibration but both vary with atmospheric pressure.

Nowadays, the triple point of water is used instead (the triple point occurs at 273.16 kelvins (K), 0.01°C).

Maximum thermometer

A special kind of mercury thermometer, called a maximum thermometer, works by having a constriction in the neck close to the bulb. As the temperature rises the mercury is pushed up through the constriction by the force of expansion. When the temperature falls the column of mercury breaks at the constriction and cannot return to the bulb thus remaining stationary in the tube. The observer can then read the maximum temperature over the set period of time. To reset the thermometer it must be swung sharply. This is similar to the design of a medical thermometer. Mercury will solidify (freeze) at –38.83°C (–37.89°F) and so may only be used at higher temperatures.

Mercury, unlike water, does not expand upon solidification and will not break the glass tube, making it difficult to notice when frozen. If the thermometer contains nitrogen the gas may flow down into the column and be trapped there when the temperature rises. If this happens the thermometer will be unusable until returned to the factory for reconditioning.

To avoid this some weather services require that all mercury thermometers be brought indoors when the temperature falls to –37°C (–34.6°F).

In areas where the maximum temperature is not expected to rise above –38.83°C (–37.89°F) a thermometer containing a mercury-thallium alloy may be used. This has a solidification (freezing) point of –61.1°C (–78°F).

Phase out

Today, many mercury thermometers are still widely used in meteorology, however in other usage they are becoming increasingly rare, as many countries have banned them outright from medical use. Some manufacturers use galinstan, a liquid alloy of gallium, indium, and tin, as a replacement for mercury.

The typical 'fever thermometer' contains between 0.5 to 3 g (0.3 to 1.7 dr) of elemental mercury. Swallowing this amount of mercury would, it is said, pose little danger but the inhaling of the vapour could lead to health problems.

Infrared Thermometer

Infrared thermometers measure temperature using blackbody radiation (generally infrared) emitted from objects. They are sometimes called laser thermometers if a laser is used to help aim the thermometer, or noncontact thermometers to describe the device's ability to measure temperature from a distance. By knowing the amount of infrared energy emitted by the object and its emissivity, the object's temperature can be determined (Fig. 10.7).

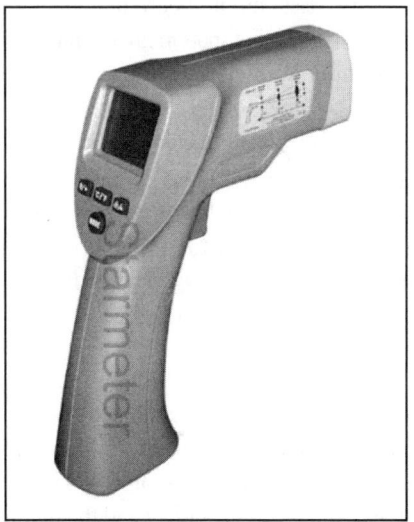

Fig. 10.7. Infrared thermometer.

The most basic design consists of a lens to focus the infrared energy on to a detector, which converts the energy to an electrical signal that can be displayed in units of temperature after being compensated for ambient temperature variation. This configuration facilitates temperature measurement from a distance without contact with the object to be measured. As such, the infrared thermometer is useful for measuring temperature under circumstances where thermocouples or other probe type sensors cannot be used or do not produce accurate data for a variety of reasons. Some typical circumstances are where the object to be measured is moving; where the object is surrounded by an electromagnetic field, as in induction heating; where the object is contained in a vacuum or other controlled atmosphere; or in applications where a fast response is required.

Infrared thermometers can be used to serve a wide variety of temperature monitoring functions. A few examples provided to this article include:

1. Detecting clouds for remote telescope operation
2. Checking mechanical equipment or electrical circuit breaker boxes or outlets for hot spots
3. Checking heater or oven temperature, for calibration and control purposes
4. Detecting hot spots/performing diagnostics in electrical circuit board manufacturing
5. Checking for hot spots in fire fighting situations
6. Monitoring materials in process of heating and cooling, for research and development or manufacturing quality control situations.

There are many varieties of infrared temperature sensing devices available today, including configurations designed for flexible and portable hand-held use, as well many designed for mounting in a fixed position to serve a dedicated purpose for long periods.

Specifications of portable hand-held sensors available to the home user will include ratings of temperature accuracy (usually ±2°C/±4°F) and other parameters. The distance-to-spot ratio (D:S) is the ratio of the distance to the object and the diameter of the temperature measurement area. For instance if the D:S ratio is 12:1, measurement of an object 12 inches away will average the temperature over a 1-inch diameter area. The sensor may have an adjustable emissivity setting, which can be set to measure the temperature of reflective (shiny) and non-reflective surfaces. A nonadjustable thermometer can be used to measure the temperature of a shiny surface by applying a non-shiny paint or tape to the surface.

The most usual infrared thermometers are the:

1. Spot infrared thermometer or infrared pyrometer, which measures the temperature at a spot on a surface (actually a relatively small area determined by the D:S ratio).

Related equipment, although not strictly thermometers, are:

1. Infrared line scanning systems scan a larger area, typically by using what is essentially a spot thermometer pointed at a rotating mirror. These devices are widely used in manu facturing involving conveyors or 'web' processes, such as large sheets of glass or metal exiting an oven, fabric and paper, or continuous piles of material along a conveyor belt.
2. Infrared cameras are essentially infrared thermometers which measure the temperature at many points over a relatively large area to generate a two-dimensional image, called a thermogram, with each pixel representing a temperature. This technology is more processor- and software-intensive than spot or scanning thermometers, and is used for monitoring large areas. Typical applications include perimeter monitoring used by military or security personnel, inspection/process quality monitoring of manufacturing processes, and equipment or enclosed space hot or cold spot monitoring for safety and efficiency maintenance purposes. A photographic camera using infrared film and suitable lens, etc. is also called an infrared camera.

CALORIMETRY

Calorimetry is the science of measuring the heat of chemical reactions or physical changes. Calorimetry involves the use of a calorimeter. The word calorimetry is derived from the Latin word calor, meaning heat. Scottish physician and scientist Joseph Black, who was the first to recognise the distinction between heat and temperature, is said to be the founder of calorimetry.

Calorimeters are special containers used to measure the exchange of heat when substances are mixed. The name comes from the old unit of energy, the calorie (Fig. 10.8).

Calorimeters are designed so that virtually all of the heat is transferred from one substance to another inside the container—with no heat loss to the surroundings. The insulated lid, ring, and dead air space are central to preventing heat loss to the surroundings.

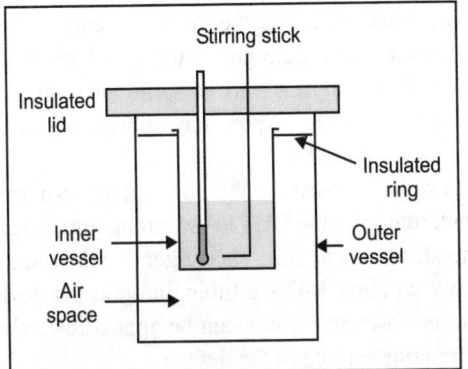

Fig. 10.8. Calorimeter containers used to measure the exchange of heat when substances are mixed.

Indirect calorimetry calculates heat that living organisms produce from their production of carbon dioxide and nitrogen waste (frequently ammonia in aquatic organisms, or urea in terrestrial ones), OR from their consumption of oxygen. Lavoisier noted in 1780 that heat production can be predicted from oxygen consumption this way, using multiple regression. The Dynamic Energy Budget theory explains why this procedure is correct. Of course, heat generated by living organisms may also be measured by direct calorimetry, in which the entire organism is placed inside the calorimeter for the measurement.

The specific heat formula is as follows:

$$q = mc\Delta T$$

where,

q is energy, or heat,

m is mass,

c is specific heat,

ΔT is change in temperature.

Constant-Volume Calorimetry (Bomb Calorimetry)

Constant-volume calorimetry is calorimetry performed at a constant volume. This involves the use of a constant-volume calorimeter.

No work is performed in constant-volume calorimetry, so the heat measured equals the change in internal energy of the system. The equation for constant-volume calorimetry is (the heat capacity at constant volume is assumed to be constant):

$$q = Cv\Delta T = \Delta U$$

where,

ΔU is change in internal energy,

ΔT is change in temperature and

C_V is the heat capacity at constant volume.

Since in constant-volume calorimetry the pressure is not kept constant, the heat measured does not represent the enthalpy change.

Differential scanning calorimetry

A widely used modern instrument is the Differential scanning calorimeter, a device which allows thermal data to be obtained on small amounts of material. It involves heating the sample at a controlled rate and recording the heat flow either into or from the specimen.

Synchronous Direct Gradient Layer and Indirect Room Calorimetry

A dual direct/indirect room-sized calorimeter is used at the Beltsville Human Nutrition Research Centre to measure heat emission and energy expenditure in humans. Because the response times of a gradient layer direct calorimeter and an indirect calorimeter are not equivalent, the respective rate of heat emission and energy expenditure cannot be directly compared. A system of equations has been developed and tested that can correct the respective outputs of the direct gradient layer calorimeter and indirect calorimeter for delays due to the response times of the measurement systems. Performance tests using alcohol combustion to simulate a human subject indicate accurate measurements of heat production from indirect (99.9+/–0.4 per cent), indirect corrected for response time (99.9+/–0.5 per cent), direct (99.9+/–0.8 per cent), and direct corrected for response time (99.9+/–0.8 per cent) calorimetry systems. Results from 24-hr measurements in 10 subjects indicate that corrected heat emission is equivalent to (99.8+/–2.0 per cent) corrected energy expenditure. However, heat emission measured during sleep was significantly greater (14 per cent) than energy expenditure, suggesting a change in the energy stored as heat in the body. This difference was reversed during the day. These results illustrate how the simultaneous measurement of heat emission and energy expenditure provides insights into heat regulation.

Water-Flow Calorimeter

This unique system permits on-site calorimetric evaluation of a wide variety of devices ranging in power from a few watts to hundreds of watts. The calorimetry is based upon the fact that 1 calorie of heat (4.186 joules) is required to raise 1 gram of water at 1°C. By circulating water at a known flow rate through a heat exchanger wrapped around the device under test (DUT) and measuring the temperature rise that occurs in the water, the heat being dissipated by the DUT can be determined (Fig. 10.9).

A constant delivery pump (FMI) circulates water around a loop that contains a Peltier heater/cooler, an inlet temperature probe, the heat exchanger, an outlet temperature probe, and an open reservoir. The Peltier heater/cooler, under control of the system computer, provides constant temperature water. The probes, DUT, and heat exchanger are well insulated to reduce heat losses to negligible levels.

Electrical power to the DUT is monitored and reported to the system computer by a Clarke-Hess 2330 power analyser. This versatile instrument can accurately measure the power in arbitrary waveforms from DC to 400 kHz.

In order to measure the heat energy it must be transferred from the DUT to the circulating water. In general, a custom heat exchanger is fabricated by simply winding 1/4″ Cu tubing around the device. In some cases the tubing can be applied directly to the exterior surface of the device.

Indirect Calorimetry

There are various methods of measuring and estimating caloric burn rate energy expenditure. Estimating energy expenditure is usually done using equations such as the Harris-Benedict equation. Other estimation techniques may make use of directly

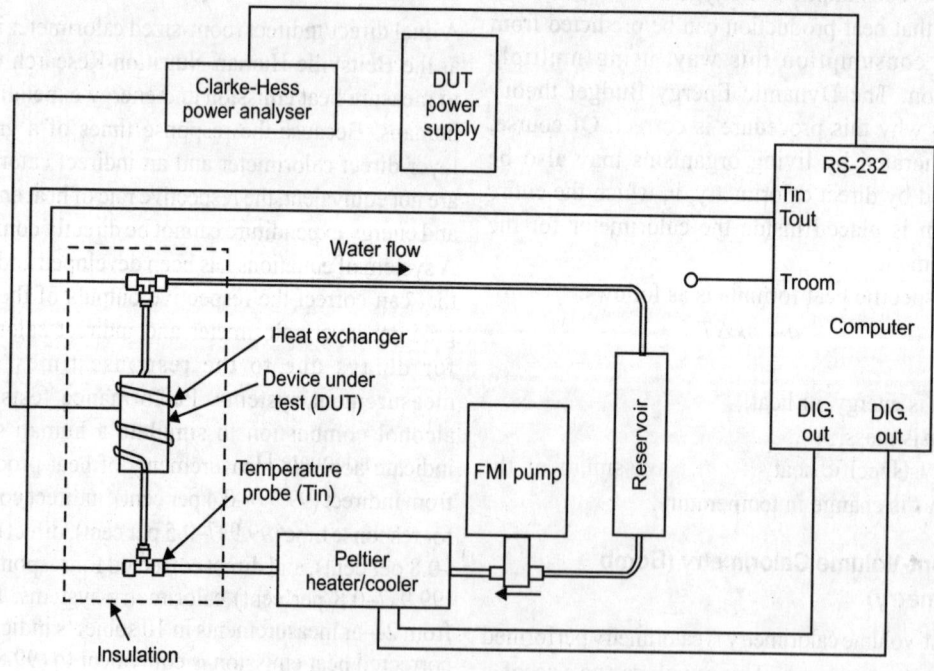

Fig. 10.9. Water-flow calorimeter.

measured per cent body fat, heart rate, etc. The only methods of directly measuring energy expenditure are doubly labelled water (DLW) and indirect calorimetry (IC). The doubly labelled water technique is primarily a laboratory-based research method in which energy expenditure is calculated from carbon dioxide production measured over a multiple day period.

Indirect calorimetry is the only accurate and clinically feasible method of measuring energy expenditure.

It is called 'indirect' because the caloric burn rate is calculated from a measurement of oxygen uptake. Direct calorimetry implies a measurement of heat released by the body, which is technically difficult and clinically impractical.

Indirect calorimetry relies on the fact that burning 1 calorie (Kilocalorie) requires 208.06 millilitres of oxygen. Because of this very direct relationship between caloric burn and oxygen consumed, measurements of oxygen uptake (V_{O_2}) and caloric burn rate are virtually interchangeable. Oxygen uptake requires a precise measurement of the volume of expired air and of the concentration of oxygen in the expired air.

Metabolic Measurement Using Indirect Calorimetry during Mechanical Ventilation

Procedure

Metabolic measurements using indirect calorimetry for determination of oxygen consumption (V_{O_2}), carbon dioxide production (V_{CO_2}), respiratory quotient (RQ), and resting energy expenditure (REE) as an aid to patient nutritional assessment and management; assessment of weaning success and outcome; assessment of the relationship between O_2 delivery (D_{O_2}) and V_{O_2}; and assessment of the contribution of metabolism to ventilation. The guideline addresses metabolic measurement during mechanical ventilation.

Description/Definition

Metabolic measurements use an indirect calorimeter to measure V_{O_2} and V_{CO_2} via expired gas analysis.

The measurements of V_{O_2} and V_{CO_2} are used to calculate RQ (V_{CO_2}/V_{O_2}) and REE using the Weir equation:

$$REE = [V_{O_2} (3.941) + V_{CO_2} (1.11)] \ 1440 \ min./day$$

The measurement of REE in mechanically ventilated neonatal, pediatric, and adult patients has been shown to be more accurate than published formulas used to predict REE, to reduce the incidence of overfeeding and underfeeding, and to decrease costs associated with total parenteral nutrition (TPN). Measurement of REE and RQ has been shown to be helpful in designing nutritional regimens to reduce V_{CO_2} in patients with chronic obstructive pulmonary disease (COPD) and patients requiring mechanical ventilation. Despite this evidence, studies demonstrating improved outcome, decreased time spent on the ventilator, or shorter intensive care unit (ICU)/hospital stay are lacking. The objectives of metabolic measurements by indirect calorimetry are:

1. To accurately determine the REE of mechanically ventilated patients to guide appropriate nutritional support.
2. To accurately determine RQ to allow nutritional regimens to be tailored to patient needs.
3. To accurately determine REE and RQ to monitor the adequacy and appropriateness of current nutritional support.
4. To allow determination of substrate utilisation when urinary nitrogen values are concomitantly measured.
5. To determine the O_2 cost of breathing as a guide to the selection of ventilator mode, settings, and weaning strategies.
6. To monitor the V_{CO_2} as a guide to targeting adequate D_{CO_2}.
7. To assess the contribution of metabolism to ventilation.

Setting

Mechanically ventilated patients:
1. In the hospital.
2. In the extended care facility.

Indications

Metabolic measurements may be indicated:

1. In patients with known nutritional deficits or derangements. Multiple nutritional risk and stress factors that may considerably skew prediction by Harris-Benedict equation include:
   (a) Neurologic trauma.
   (b) Paralysis.
   (c) COPD.
   (d) Acute pancreatitis.
   (e) Cancer with residual tumour burden.
   (f) Multiple trauma.
   (g) Amputations.
   (h) Patients in whom height and weight cannot be accurately obtained.
   (i) Patients who fail to respond adequately to estimated nutritional needs.
   (j) Patients who require long-term acute care.
   (k) Severe sepsis.
   (l) Extremely obese patients.
   (m) Severely hypermetabolic or hypometabolic patients.

2. When patients fail attempts at liberation from mechanical ventilation to measure the O_2 cost of breathing and the components of ventilation.

3. When the need exists to assess the V_{O_2} in order to evaluate the haemodynamic support of mechanically ventilated patients

4. To measure cardiac output by the Fick method.

5. To determine the cause(s) of increased ventilatory requirements.

Limitations of procedure

Limitations of the procedure include:

1. Accurate assessment of REE and RQ may not be possible because of patient condition or certain bedside procedures or activities.

2. Inaccurate measurement of REE and RQ may be caused by leaks of gas from the patient/ventilator system preventing collection of expired gases including:

(a) Leaks in the ventilator circuit.
(b) Leaks around tracheal tube cuffs or uncuffed tubes.
(c) Leaks through chest tubes or bronchopleural fistula.

3. Inaccurate measurement of REE and RQ occurs during peritoneal and haemodialysis due to removal across the membrane of CO_2 that is not measured by the indirect calorimeter.

4. Inaccurate measurement of REE and RQ during open circuit measurement may be caused by:
   (a) Instability of delivered oxygen concentration (F_{IO_2}) within a breath or breath to breath due to changes in source gas pressure and ventilator blender/mixing characteristics
   (b) $F_{IO_2} > 0.60$.
   (c) Inability to separate inspired and expired gases due to bias flow from flow-triggering systems, IMV systems, or specific ventilator characteristics.
   (d) The presence of anaesthetic gases or gases other than O_2, CO_2, and nitrogen in the ventilation system.
   (e) The presence of water vapour resulting in sensor malfunction.
   (f) Inappropriate calibration.
   (g) Connection of the indirect calorimeter to certain ventilators, with adverse effect on triggering mechanism, increased expiratory resistance, pressure measurement, or maintenance of the ventilator.
   (h) Total circuit flow exceeding internal gas flow of indirect calorimeter that incorporates the dilutional principle.
   (i) Internal leaks within the calorimeter.
   (j) Inadequate length of measurement.

5. Inaccurate measurement of REE and RQ during closed circuit measurement may be caused by:
   (a) Short duration of the measurement period (a function of CO_2 absorber life

and V_{CO_2}) that may not allow REE state to be achieved.

(b) Changes in functional residual capacity (FRC) resulting in changes in spirometer volume unassociated with V_{O_2}.

(c) Leaks drawing gas into the system during spontaneous breathing measurements that adds volume to the system and cause erroneously low V_{O_2} readings.

(d) Increased compressible volume in the circuit that prevents adequate tidal volume delivery resulting in alveolar hypoventilation and changes in V_{CO_2}/V_{O_2}.

(e) Increased compressible volume and resistance that results in difficulty triggering the ventilator and increased work of breathing.

Assessment of need

Metabolic measurements should be performed only on the order of a physician after review of indications and objectives.

Assessment of test quality and outcome

Test quality can be evaluated by determining whether:

1. RQ is consistent with the patient's nutritional intake.
2. RQ rests in the normal physiologic range (0.67 to 1.3).
3. Variability of the measurements for V_{O_2} and V_{CO_2} should be <5 per cent for a 5-minute data collection.
4. The measurement is of sufficient length to account for variability in V_{O_2} and V_{CO_2} if the above conditions (<5 per cent for a 5-minute data collection) are not met.

Outcome may be assessed by comparing the measurement results with the patient's condition and nutritional intake. Outcome may be assessed by observation of the patient prior to and during the measurement to determine if the patient is at steady state.

Resources

Indirect calorimeter, open- or closed-circuit design:

1. The calibration gas mixture should be relevant to the concentration of gas to be measured clinically.
2. The indirect calorimeter should be calibrated on the day of measurement and more often if errors in measurement are suspected.
3. When the measurement results are suspect and/or when repeated calibration attempts are marked by instability, the indirect calorimeter may be tested via an independent test method (burning ethanol or other substance with a known RQ or adding known flows of C_{O_2} and nitrogen to simulate V_{O_2} and V_{CO_2}). As a simple test, ventilation of a leak-free system should yield V_{O_2} and V_{CO_2} values of near 0. Routinely scheduled measurement of normal control subjects (volunteers) may be useful.

A method of stabilising V_{IO_2} during open-circuit measurements should be available and may include:

1. An air-oxygen blender connected between the gas source and the ventilator inlets for high pressure gas.
2. An inspiratory mixing chamber between the ventilator main flow circuit and the humidifier.
3. Ventilator changes, which may include mode, inspiratory flow rate, positive end-expiratory pressure (PEEP), or tidal volume to improve patient-ventilator synchrony.

An isolation valve, double-piloted exhalation valve, or other device to separate inspiratory and expiratory flow should be incorporated when using continuous flow in the ventilator circuit.

Personnel: Due to the level of technical and patient assessment skills required, metabolic measurements using indirect calorimeters should be performed by individuals trained in and with the demonstrated and documented ability to:

1. Calibrate, operate, and maintain an indirect calorimeter.

2. Operate a mechanical ventilator, including knowledge of the air-oxygen blending system, the spontaneous breathing mechanisms, and the alarm and monitoring functions.

3. Recognise metabolic measurement values within the normal physiologic range and evaluate the results in light of the patient's current nutritional and clinical status.

4. Assess patient haemodynamic and ventilatory status and make recommendations on appropriate corrective/therapeutic maneuvers to improve or reverse the patient's clinical course. A relevant credential (e.g. RRT, CRT, RN, or RPFT) is desirable.

A hood canopy system in combination with airway sampling may be employed to capture gas that leaks around an uncuffed endotracheal tube.

If a stable F_{IO_2} cannot be achieved, V_{CO_2} may be used to estimate REE by assuming an RQ of 0.83 and the largest expected error is an:

1. Underestimation of 25 per cent for RQ of 1.2.
2. Overestimation of 19 per cent for RQ of 0.67.

A simultaneous measure of P_{aCO_2} and V_{CO_2} will allow calculation of pulmonary dead space and components of ventilation using the Bohr equation:

$$V_E = V_{CO_2} \times 0.863\, P_{aCO_2} \times (1 - VD/VT)$$

Monitoring

The following should be evaluated during the performance of a metabolic measurement to ascertain the validity of the results:

1. Clinical observation of the resting state.
2. Patient comfort and movement during testing.
3. Values in concert with the clinical situation.
4. Equipment function.
5. Results within the specifications listed in 'Assessment of test quality and outcome' above.
6. F_{IO_2} stability.

Measurement data should include a statement of test quality and list the current nutritional support, ventilator settings, F_{IO_2} stability, and vital signs.

Frequency

Metabolic measurements should be repeated according to the clinical status of the patient and indications for performing the test. The literature suggests that more frequent measurement may be necessary in patients with a rapidly changing clinical course as recognised by:

1. Haemodynamic instability.
2. Spiking fevers.

Patients in the immediate postoperative period and those being weaned from mechanical ventilation may also need more frequent measurement.

Infection control

Metabolic measurements using indirect calorimetry are relatively safe procedures, but a remote possibility of cross-contamination exists either via patient-patient or patient-caregiver interface. The following guidelines should be followed when a metabolic measurement is performed.

1. Standard precautions should be exercised whenever there is potential for contamination with blood or other body fluids.
2. Appropriate use of barriers and hand washing is recommended.
3. Tubing used to direct expiratory gas from the ventilator to the indirect calorimeter should be disposed of or cleaned between patients.
4. Connections used in the inspiratory limb of the circuit proximal to the humidifier should be wiped clean between patients; equipment distal to the humidifier should be disposed of or subjected to high-level disinfection between patients.
5. Bacteria filters may be used to protect equipment in both the inspired and expired lines, but caution should be used that moisture does not increase filter resistance resulting in poor gas sampling flow or increased resistance to exhalation.

Scuba Set

A scuba set is an independent breathing set that provides a scuba diver with the breathing gas necessary to breathe underwater during scuba diving. It is much used for sport diving and some sorts of work diving. The word SCUBA was originally an acronym for Self-Contained Underwater Breathing Apparatus.

These initials originated in 1939 in the United States Navy to refer to their military diver's rebreather sets. As with radar, the acronym has become so familiar that it is often not capitalised and is treated as an ordinary noun; for example, it has been taken into the Welsh language as 'sgwba'.

Figure 10.10 shows a diving cylinder with its various components.

Types of scuba sets

Modern scuba sets are of two types:
1. Open-circuit (In Europe, it is often called an 'aqualung'. Here the diver breathes in from the equipment and all the exhaled gas goes to waste in the surrounding water. This type of equipment is relatively simple, making it cheaper and more reliable. The two-hose design originally used was the one designed by Cousteau and Gagnan. The single-hose design generally used today was invented in Australia by Ted Eldred.
2. Closed-circuit/semi-closed circuit (also referred to as a rebreather). Here the diver breathes in from the set, and breathes back into the set, where the exhaled gas is processed to make it fit to breathe again. These existed before the open-circuit sets and are still used, but less so than open-circuit sets.

Both types of scuba provide a means of supplying air or other breathing gas, nearly always from a high pressure diving cylinder, and a harness to strap it to the diver's body. Most open-circuit scuba and some rebreathers have a demand regulator to control the supply of breathing gas. Some 'semi-closed' rebreathers only have a constant-flow regulator, or occasionally a set of constant-flow regulators of various outputs.

Some divers use the word 'scuba' to mean open-circuit sets only.

Open circuit scuba sets

The duration of open-circuit dives is shorter than a rebreather dive, in proportion to the weight and bulk of the set. Open-circuit can be less economic than a rebreather when used with expensive gas mixes such as heliox and trimix. Most divers breathe normal air i.e. 21 per cent oxygen and 79 per cent nitrogen. The cylinder is nearly always worn on the back. 'Twin sets' with two backpack cylinders were much more common in the 1960s than now; although twin cylinders (doubles) are commonly used by technical divers for increased dive duration and redundancy. At one time a firm called Submarine Products sold a

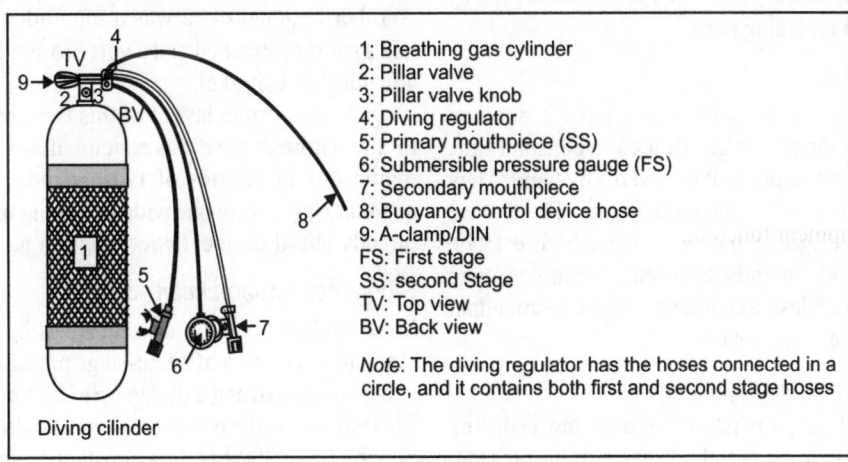

1: Breathing gas cylinder
2: Pillar valve
3: Pillar valve knob
4: Diving regulator
5: Primary mouthpiece (SS)
6: Submersible pressure gauge (FS)
7: Secondary mouthpiece
8: Buoyancy control device hose
9: A-clamp/DIN
FS: First stage
SS: second Stage
TV: Top view
BV: Back view

Note: The diving regulator has the hoses connected in a circle, and it contains both first and second stage hoses

Diving cilinder

Fig. 10.10. A diving cylinder with its various components.

sport air scuba with three backpack cylinders. Cave divers sometimes have cylinders slung at their sides instead, allowing them to swim through narrower spaces.

Until Enriched Air Nitrox was widely accepted in the late 1990s, almost all sport scuba used simple compressed air. This allowed the scuba industry in the US to avoid regulation by the US Food and Drug Administration (FDA), which defines non-air gas mixtures intended to prevent or treat diseases as 'drugs'. Exotic gas mixtures presently used in scuba are intended to prevent decompression illness in diving, but officially, the FDA appears to continue to believe that scuba divers all use compressed air.

At partial pressures over about 2.1 atmospheres, oxygen becomes toxic. Open-circuit scuba sets may supply various breathing gases, but rarely pure oxygen, except during decompression stops in technical diving.

Some divers use Enriched Air Nitrox, which has a higher percentage of oxygen, usually 32 or 36 per cent (EAN32 and EAN36, respectively). This lets them stay underwater longer, because less nitrogen is absorbed into the body's tissues. The drawback to the higher oxygen content is that the maximum diving depth is decreased in order to avoid oxygen toxicity. The common nitrox blending method by partial pressure requires that the cylinder is in 'oxygen service', which is a cylinder that has had any non-oxygen-compatible grease or rubber removed, by cleaning and replacing parts.

Constant flow

Constant flow scuba sets do not have a demand regulator; the breathing gas flows at a constant rate, unless the diver switches it on and off by hand. They run out of air quicker than aqualungs. There were attempts at designing and using these before 1939, for diving and for industrial use. Examples were 'Ohgushi's Peerless Respirator', and Commandant le Prieur's breathing sets.

With a demand regulator

This type of set consists of one or more diving cylinders containing breathing gas at high pressure (typically 200–300 Bar) connected to a diving regulator. The regulator supplies the diver with as much of the gas as needed, at a pressure suitable for breathing at the depth of the diver.

Colloquially this type of breathing set is sometimes (depending on the country of the English speaker) often called an aqualung. The word Aqua-Lung, which first appeared in the Cousteau-Gagnan patent, is a trademark, currently owned by US divers.

Twin-hose open-circuit scuba

This is the first type of diving demand valve to come into general use, and the one that can be seen in classic 1960s television scuba adventures, such as Sea Hunt. They often had two cylinders.

In this type of set, the two (or occasionally one or three) stages of the regulator are in a large circular valve assembly mounted on top of the cylinder pack. This type has two wide bellows-like breathing tubes like those on many modern rebreathers, one for intake and one for exhalation. The return tube was not for rebreathing, but because the air exhaust needed to be as near as possible to the regulator's second stage diaphragm, to avoid pressure differences, which would cause a free-flow of gas, or extra resistance to breathing, according to the diver's orientation in the water—head-up, head-down, level. In modern single-hose sets this problem is avoided by moving the second-stage regulator to the diver's mouthpiece. The twin-hose sets came with a mouthpiece as standard, but a full-face diving mask was an option. Another optional extra was a mouthpiece that also had a snorkel attached and a valve to switch between aqualung and snorkel.

Note the correct layout of this type, in the image to the right. There have been many incorrect depictions in comics of two-cylinder twin-hose aqualungs, showing one wide breathing tube coming directly out of each cylinder top with no regulator.

Single-hose open-circuit scuba

Most modern open-circuit scuba sets have a diving regulator consisting of a first-stage pressure-reducing valve fastened over the diving cylinder's output valve. This valve cuts the pressure from the cylinder, which may be up to 300 bar, to a constant lower pressure, often about 10 bar above the ambient pressure, which is used in the 'low pressure' part of the system. A relatively thin low-pressure hose links this with the second-stage regulator, or 'demand valve', which is located in the mouthpiece. Exhalation occurs out of a one-way diaphragm in the chamber of the demand valve, directly into the water quite close to the diver's mouth. This configuration type is called 'single hose'. The first make of this sort of scuba was the Porpoise, which was made in Melbourne, Australia by Ted Eldred. Some early single hose scuba sets used full-face masks instead of a mouthpiece, such as those made by Desco and Scott Aviation (who continue to make breathing units of this configuration for use by firefighters).

The first Porpoise scuba set design was a rebreather, but when a demonstration resulted in a diver passing out, Eldred began to develop the single-hose open-circuit scuba system. Its regulator's first stage and second stage had to be separated to avoid the Cousteau-Gagnan patent, which protected the double-hose scuba. In the process, Eldred also improved performance.

Safety second regulator on an octopus, and integrated into the BC

Most modern scuba sets have a spare second-stage demand valve on a separate hose, a configuration called an octopus, because it often has two or more hoses for other purposes coming out of the primary regulator on the cylinder top. This separate second-stage regulator and hose, or alternate air source, safe secondary or safe-second for short, is typically yellow in colour, signalling that it is an emergency or backup device. It is often worn secured into a clip on the buoyancy compensator (BC) or a special friction plug on a diver's chest, easily available to be grabbed by, or offered to, a second diver short of air. In so doing, this second mouthpiece eliminates the need for two divers who need to share a cylinder to 'buddy-breathe', by trading off the same mouthpiece. Diving instructors still continue to teach buddy-breathing as a now obsolete but still useful technique to know; then they show the new method that has superseded it, since availability of two secondary regulators per diver is now assumed in all modern scuba sets.

The original octopus idea was conceived by cave-diving pioneer Sheck Exley as a way for single-file-swimming cave divers to share air in a narrow tunnel, but has now become the standard in recreational diving. Modern "octopus" type primary-stage regulators also typically feature high-pressure ports for use by dive-computer pressure sensors, and additional ports for additional low-pressure hoses for inflation of dry suits and BC devices.

Increasingly, in the 21st century, the second 'safety' second-stage regulator/mouthpiece has been combined with the inflator and exhaust assembly of the integrated weight BC device. This combination eliminates the need for a separate low pressure hose for the BC (though the low pressure hose for the combined use must be larger than dedicated BC inflation hoses, because demand on it will be higher if it is used for breathing). In this configuration, the safety spare regulator is now integral to the BC, rather than deriving as a separate hose/regulator from the octopus.

No matter which configuration of safety secondary regulator is used, many diving schools now suggest that a diver routinely offer another diver in trouble their 'primary' mouthpiece, i.e. the one in their mouth, before going to their own safe-secondary regulator. The idea behind this technique is that the primary mouthpiece is certain to be working, and the diver not in trouble has much more time to sort things out with his/her own equipment after temporarily losing ability to breathe (in a great many instances, panicked out-of-air divers have grabbed the primary regulators out of the mouths of other divers, so changing breathing regulators suddenly in an out-of-air emergency becomes necessary for the rescue diver, in any case). With integrated regulator/BC designs, the safe-secondary regulator is at the end of an even shorter hose (the BC mouthpiece/exhaust) than is the case with the traditional octopus safe-secondary, so deliberate use of the primary regulator and hose to help another diver becomes even more natural, and almost necessary, with the BC-integrated-regulator configuration.

Doubly-labelled water

Doubly-labelled water is water in which both the hydrogen and the oxygen has been partly or completely replaced for tracing purposes (i.e. labelled) with an uncommon isotope of these elements.

In theory, radioactive forms of hydrogen and oxygen could be used for such labelling, and this was the case in many early applications of the method. In practice, for both practical and safety reasons, almost all recent applications of the 'doubly-labelled water' method use water labelled with the heavy, non-radioactive forms of the elements deuterium and oxygen-18 (O-18 or ^{18}O).

In particular, use of the doubly-labelled water method (or DLW method) generates a particular type of measurement of metabolic rate, in which average metabolic rate of an organism is measured over a period of time. This is done by administering a dose of doubly-labelled water, and then measuring the elimination rates of deuterium and O-18 in the subject, over time, through the regular sampling of heavy isotope concentrations in the body water (by sampling saliva, urine, or blood). The minimum number of samples required is two — an initial sample after the isotopes have reached equilibrium in the body, and a second sample some time later the period between these samples depends on size of the animal involved. In small animals the period may be as short as 24 hours, and in larger animals like adult humans, the period may be as long as 14 days. In animals this average daily metabolic rate measured by the DLW method is often also called the Field metabolic rate or FMR. The method was invented in the 1950s by Nathan Lifson and colleagues at the University of Minnesota, however its use was restricted to small animals until the 1980s because of the high costs of the oxygen-18 isotope. Advances in mass spectrometry over the 1970s and early 1980s reduced the amount of isotope needed to be used and this made it feasible to apply the method to humans. The first application to humans was made in 1982, by Dale Schoeller, over 25 years after the method was initially discovered.

Mechanism of the test

The technique measures a subject's carbon dioxide production over the interval between first and last body water samples. The key concept which allows this, is that oxygen in body water (including the marker dose of O-18) equilibriates with the body's bicarbonate and dissolved carbon dioxide pool (through the action of the enzyme carbonic anhydrase), and is therefore lost from the body, in carbon dioxide. This was discovered by Lifson in 1949. Additionally the oxygen in water is lost through body water loss (urine and evaporative water losses). However, since deuterium (as a second label and marker for body water) is only lost in water, the deuterium change in body water over time can be used to mathematically compensate for the loss of tracer O-18 by the water-loss route. This leaves only the remaining net loss of O-18 in carbon dioxide, and thus an estimate for total carbon dioxide production. Once this is known, the total metabolic rate may be estimated from simplifying assumptions, regarding the ratio of oxygen used in metabolism (and therefore heat generated), to carbon dioxide eliminated.

Practical isotope administration

Doubly-labelled water may be administered by injection, or orally (the usual route in humans). Since the isotopes will be diluted in body water, there is no need to administer them in a state of high isotopic purity, no need to employ water in which all or even most atoms are heavy atoms, or even to begin with water which is doubly-labelled. In practice, doses of doubly-labelled water for metabolic work are prepared by simply mixing a dose of deuterium oxide (heavy water) (90 to 99 per cent) with a second dose of $H_2^{18}O$, which is water which has been separately enriched with O-18 (though usually not to a high level, since this is expensive and unnecessary for this use), but otherwise contains normal hydrogen. The mixed water sample then contains both types of heavy atoms, in a far higher degree than normal water, and is now doubly-labelled. The free interchange of hydrogens between water molecules (via normal ionisation) in liquid water ensures that the pools of oxygen and hydrogen in any sample of water will be separately equilibriated in a short time with any added heavy isotope(s).

Applications

The doubly-labelled water method is particularly useful for measuring average metabolic rate (Field metabolic rate) over relatively long periods of time (a few days or weeks), in subjects for which other types of direct or indirect calorimetric measurements of metabolic rate would be difficult or impossible. For example, the technique can measure the metabolism of animals in the wild state, with the technical problems being related mainly to how to administer the dose of isotope, and collect several samples of body water at later times to check for differential isotope elimination.

Most animal studies involve capturing the subject animals and injecting them, then holding them for a variable period before the first blood sample has been collected.

This period depends on the size of the animal involved and varies between 30 minutes for very small animals to 6 hours for much larger animals. In both animals and humans, the test is made more accurate if a single determination of respiratory quotient has been made for the organism eating the standard diet at the time of measurement, since this value changes relatively little (and more slowly) compared with the much larger metabolic rate changes related to thermoregulation and activity.

Because the heavy hydrogen and oxygen isotopes used in the standard doubly-labelled water measurement are non-radioactive, and also nontoxic in the doses used, the doubly-labelled water measurement of mean metabolic rate has been used extensively in human volunteers, and even in infants and pregnant women. The technique has been used on over 200 species of wild animals (mostly birds, mammals and some reptiles).

Body Fat Percentage

A person's body fat percentage is the total weight of the person's fat divided by the person's weight and consists of essential body fat and storage body fat. Essential body fat is necessary to maintain life and reproductive functions. The percentage for women is greater than that for men, due to the demands of childbearing and other hormonal functions. Essential fat is 3–5 per cent in men, and 8–12 per cent in women. Storage body fat consists of fat accumulation in adipose tissue, part of which protects internal organs in the chest and abdomen. The minimum recommended total body fat percentage exceeds the essential fat percentage value reported above. A number of online tools are available for calculating estimated body fat percentage.

Some regard the body fat percentage as the better measure of an individual's fitness level, as it is the only body measurement which directly calculates the particular individual's body composition without regard to the individual's height or weight.

The widely-used body mass index (BMI), on the other hand, simply makes blanket assumptions as to what every individual of a certain height should ideally weigh, regardless of the body composition which makes up that weight. The BMI gives particularly inaccurate information with regard to individuals with above-average lean muscle mass, classifying such individuals as 'overweight' or 'obese' despite the fact that their body fat percentage would indicate they are in excellent physical condition. Different cultures value different body compositions differently at different times, and some are related to better health or improved athletic performance. Levels of body fat are epidemiologically dependent on gender and age.

Measurement techniques

A living person's exact body fat percentage generally cannot be determined, but there are several techniques which can be used to estimate it accurately.

Near-infrared interactance

A beam of infrared light is transmitted into the biceps. The light is reflected from the underlying muscle and absorbed by the fat. The method is safe, noninvasive, rapid and easy to use.

Dual energy X-ray absorptiometry

Dual energy X-ray absorptiometry, or DXA (formerly DEXA), is a newer method for estimating body fat percentage, and is commonly cited as the current gold standard for body composition testing.

Two different types of X-ray scans the body, one that detects all tissues and another that doesn't detect fat. A computer can subtract the second picture from the first one, giving only fat detection. The mass of this can be estimated by the grade of exposure.

Expansions

There are several more complicated procedures that more accurately determine body fat percentage. Some, referred to as multicompartment models, can include DXA measurement of bone, plus independent measures of body water (using the dilution principle with isotopically labelled water) and body volume (either by water displacement or air plethysmography).

Various other components may be independently measured, such as total body potassium.

In vivo neutron activation can quantify all the elements of the body and use mathematical relations among the measured elements in the different components of the body (fat, water, protein, etc.) to develop simultaneous equations to estimate total body composition, including body fat.

Body average density measurement

Prior to the adoption of DXA, the most accurate method of estimating body fat percentage was to measure that person's average density (total mass divided by total volume) and apply a formula to convert that to body fat percentage.

Since fat tissue has a lower density than muscles and bones, it is possible to estimate the fat content. This estimate is distorted by the fact that muscles and bones have different densities: for a person with a more-than-average amount of bone mass, the estimate will be too low. However, this method gives highly reproducible results for individual persons (± 1 per cent), unlike the methods discussed below, which can have an uncertainty up to ± 10 per cent. The body fat percentage is commonly calculated from one of two formulas:

1. Brozek formula: $BF = (4.57/\rho - 4.142) \times 100$.
2. Siri formula is: $BF = (4.95/\rho - 4.50) \times 100$.

Bioelectrical impedance analysis

The Bioelectrical impedance analysis (BIA) method is a more affordable but less accurate way to estimate body fat percentage. The general principle behind BIA: two conductors are attached to a person's body and a small electrical current is sent through the body. The resistance between the conductors will provide a measure of body fat, since the resistance to electricity varies between adipose, muscular and skeletal tissue. Fat-free mass (muscles) is a good conductor as it contains a large amount of water (approximately 73 per cent) and electrolytes, while fat is anhydrous and a poor conductor of electrical current. Factors that affect the accuracy and precision of this method include instrumentation, subject factors, technician skill, and the prediction equation formulated to estimate the Fat Free Mass. Criticism of this methodology is based on where the conductors are placed on the body; typically they are placed on the feet, with the current sent up one leg, across the abdomen and down the other leg. As technician error is minor, factors such as eating, drinking and exercising must be controlled since hydration level is an important source of error in determining the flow of the electrical current to estimate body fat. As men and women store fat differently around the abdomen and thigh region, the results can be less accurate as a measure of total body fat percentage. Another variable that can affect the amount of body fat this test measures is the amount of liquid an individual has consumed before the test. As electricity travels more easily through water, a person who has consumed a large amount of water before the test will measure as a lower body fat percentage. Less water will increase the percentage of body fat. Also reducing the reliability of this method is the variation between models of the BIA devices: for instance when comparing outputs from a Tanita scale to an Omron Body Logic hand-held device the Tanita scale overestimated the percentage body fat in college-aged men by 40 per cent and in college aged women by 55 per cent. Bioelectrical impedance analysis is available in a laboratory, or for home use in the form of body fat scales and hand held body fat analysers.

Anthropometric methods

There exist various anthropometric methods for estimating body fat. The term anthropometric refers to measurements made of various parameters of the human body, such as circumferences of various body parts or thicknesses of skinfolds. Most of these methods are based on a statistical model. Some measurements are selected, and are applied to a population sample. For each individual in the sample, the method's measurements are recorded, and that individual's body density is also recorded, being determined by, for instance, underwater weighing, in combination with a multi-compartment body density model. From this data, a formula relating the body measurements to density is developed.

Because most anthropomorphic formulas such as the Durnin-Womersley skinfold method, the Jackson-Pollock skinfold method, and the US Navy circumference method, actually estimate body density, not body fat percentage, the body fat percentage is obtained by applying a second formula, such as the Siri or Brozek described in the above section on density. Consequently, the body fat percentage calculated from skin folds or other anthropometric methods carries the cumulative error from the application of two separate statistical models.

These methods are therefore inferior to a direct measurement of body density and the application of just one formula to estimate body fat percentage. One way to regard these methods is that they trade accuracy for convenience, since it is much more convenient to take a few body measurements than to submerge individuals in water tanks.

The chief problem with all statistically derived formulas is that in order to be widely applicable, they must be based on a broad sample of individuals. Yet, that breadth makes them inherently inaccurate. The ideal statistical estimation method for an individual is based on a sample of similar individuals. For instance, a skinfold based body density formula developed from a sample of male collegiate rowers is likely to be much more accurate for estimating the body density of a male collegiate rower than a method developed using a sample of the general population, because the sample is narrowed down by age, sex, physical fitness level, type of sport, and lifestyle factors. On the other hand, such a formula is unsuitable for general use.

Skinfold methods

The skinfold estimation methods are based on a skinfold test, whereby a pinch of skin is precisely measured by calipers at several standardised points on the body to determine the subcutaneous fat layer thickness. These measurements are converted to an estimated body fat percentage by an equation. Some formulas require as few as three measurements, others as many as seven. The accuracy of these estimates is more dependent on a person's unique body fat distribution than on the number of sites measured. As well, it is of utmost importance to test in a precise location with a fixed pressure. Although it may not give an accurate reading of real body fat percentage, it is a reliable measure of body composition change over a period of time, provided the test is carried out by the same person with the same technique.

Skinfold-based body fat estimation is sensitive to the type of caliper used, and technique. This method also only measures one type of fat: subcutaneous adipose tissue (fat under the skin). Two individuals might have nearly identical measurements at all of the skin fold sites, yet differ greatly in their body fat levels due to differences in other body fat deposits such as visceral adipose tissue: fat in the abdominal cavity. Some models partially address this problem by including age as a variable in the statistics and the resulting formula. Older individuals are found to have a lower body density for the same skinfold measurements, which is assumed to signify a higher body fat percentage. However, older, highly athletic individuals might not fit this assumption, causing the formulas to underestimate their body density.

Height and circumference methods

There also exist formulas for estimating body fat percentage from an individual's weight and girth measurements. For example, the US Navy Circumference method compares abdomen or waist and hips measurements to neck measurement and height and other sites claim to estimate one's body fat percentage by a conversion from the body mass index. In the US Navy the method is known as the 'rope and choke'.

The US Marine Corps and US Army also rely on the Height and Circumference method. For males, they measure the neck and waist just above the navel. Females are measured around the hips, waist, and neck. These measurements are compared to a height/weight chart with age factored in as well. This method is used because it is a cheap and convenient way to implement a body fat test throughout the entire Department of Defense.

Due to different body compositions, those with larger necks may artificially generate lower body fat percentage calculations than those with smaller necks.

From BMI

Body fat can be estimated from your Body mass index or BMI. There are a number of alternative formulae that relate body fat to BMI. The body mass index is calculated from an individual's weight divided by the square of the height.

Densitometry

Densitometry is the quantitative measurement of optical density in light-sensitive materials, such as photographic paper or film, due to exposure to light. Optical density is a result of the darkness of a developed picture and can be expressed absolutely as the number of dark spots (i.e. silver nitrate grains in developed films) in a given area, but usually it is a relative value, expressed in a scale.

Since density is usually measured by the decrease in the amount of light which shines through a transparent film, it is also called absorptiometry, the measure of light absorption through the medium. The corresponding measuring device is called a densitometer (absorptiometer). The logarithm of the reciprocal of the transmittance is called the absorbance or density. Figure 10.11 shows the principle of spot light densitometry.

DMax and DMin refer to the maximum and minimum density that can be recorded on the material. The difference between the two is the density range. The density range is related to the exposure range (dynamic range), which is the range of light intensity that is represented by the recording, via the Hurter–Driffield curve. The dynamic range can be measured in 'stops', which is the binary logarithm of the ratio of highest and lowest distinguishable exposures.

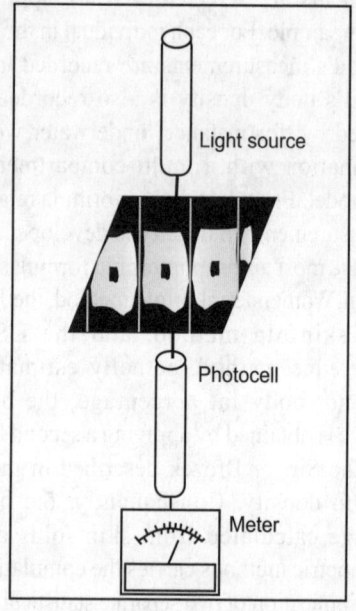

Fig. 10.11. Principle of spot light densitometry.

According to the principle of operation of the densitometer, one can have:

1. Spot densitometry: the value of light absorption is measured at a single spot.
2. Line densitometry: the values of successive spots along a dimension are expressed as a graph.
3. Bidimensional densitometry: the values of light absorption are expressed as a 2D synthetic image, usually using false-colour shading.

Dual energy X-ray absorptiometry is used in medicine to evaluate calcium bone density, which is altered in several diseases such as osteopenia and osteoporosis. Special devices have been developed and are in current use for clinical diagnosis, called bone densitometers.

Underwater weighing (hydrostatic weight)

Underwater weighing, or hydrostatic weighting is a method of determining body composition or the various components that make up a person's total body density using Archimedes' principle of displacement. Underwater weighing has been considered the gold standard for body composition assessment, however new, more sophisticated methods may make underwater weighing obsolete in the near future.

Underwater weighing is based upon the assertion that the density of fat mass and fat-free mass are constant, lean tissue such as bone and muscle are more dense than water, and fat tissue is less dense than water. Therefore, a person with more body fat will weigh less underwater and be more buoyant. Someone with more muscle will weigh more underwater.

To perform underwater weighing, a person is first weighted on land. Next the individual will get into a large tank of water. While sitting on a special scale, he is lowered underwater and asked to expel all the air from his lings and remain motionless while the underwater weight is measured. This procedure is repeated three times and averaged.

A special calculation is then used to determine lean weight and fat weight and determine a person's percentage of body fat.

Dual energy X-ray absorptiometry

Dual energy X-ray absorptiometry (DXA, previously DEXA) is a means of measuring bone mineral density (BMD). Two X-ray beams with differing energy levels are aimed at the patient's bones. When soft tissue absorption is subtracted out, the BMD can be determined from the absorption of each beam by bone. Dual energy X-ray absorptiometry is the most widely used and most thoroughly studied bone density measurement technology (Fig. 10.12).

DXA scans are primarily used to evaluate bone mineral density. DXA scans can also be used to measure total body composition and fat content. However, it has been suggested that while very accurately measuring minerals, DXA does not reliably measure fat content since this was not DXA's original purpose. It is suggested that for total body composition, DXA be used in conjunction with another method (underwater weighing, etc.).

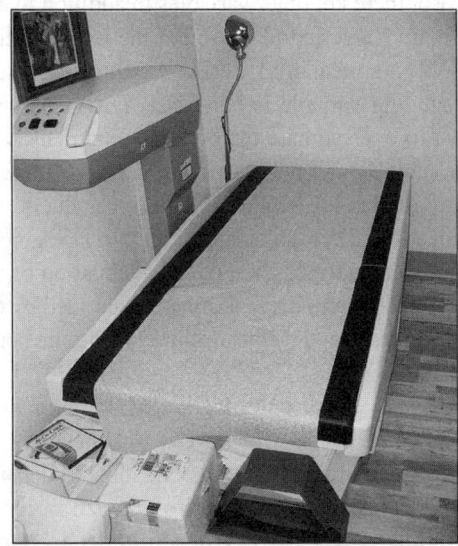

Fig. 10.12. A scanner used to measure bone density with dual energy X-ray absorptiometry.

Women at risk of osteoporosis, especially if over the age of 50 years should get a DXA scan. 'At risk' includes many different clinical risk factors including: prior fragility fracture, use of glucocorticoids, heavy smoking, excess alcohol intake, rheumatoid arthritis, history of parental hip fracture, chronic renal and liver disease, chronic respiratory disease, long-term use of phenobarbitone or phenytoin, celiac disease, inflammatory bowel disease and other risks. The same clinical risk factors in men over 50 years should prompt getting a DXA scan too.

Scoring

A T-score equal to or less than −2.5 is indicative of osteoporosis. This test is very reliable.

Special considerations are involved in the use of DXA to assess bone mass in children. Specifically, comparing the bone mineral density of children to the reference data of adults (to calculate a T-score) will underestimate the BMD of children, because children have less bone mass than fully developed adults. This would lead to an over diagnosis of osteopenia for children. To avoid an overestimation of bone mineral deficits, BMD scores are commonly compared to reference data for the same gender and age (by calculating a Z-score).

Also, there are other variables in addition to age which are suggested to confound the interpretation of BMD as measured by DXA. One important confounding variable is bone size. DXA has been shown to overestimate the bone mineral density of taller subjects and underestimate the bone mineral density of smaller subjects. This error is due to the way in which DXA calculates BMD. In DXA, bone mineral content (measured as the attenuation of the X-ray by the bones being scanned) is divided by the area (also measured by the machine) of the site being scanned.

Because DXA calculates BMD using area (aBMD: areal Bone Mineral Density), it is not an accurate measurement of true bone mineral density, which is mass divided by a volume. In order to distinguish DXA BMD from volumetric bone-mineral density, researchers sometimes refer to DXA BMD as an areal bone mineral density (aBMD). The confounding effect of differences in bone size is due to the missing depth value in the calculation of bone mineral density. Despite DXA technology's problems with estimating volume, it is still a fairly accurate measure of bone mineral content. Methods to correct for this shortcoming include the calculation of a volume which is approximated from the projected area measure by DXA. DXA BMD results adjusted in this manner, are referred to as the bone mineral apparent density (BMAD) and are a ratio of the bone mineral content versus a cuboidal estimation of the volume of bone.

Like aBMD, BMAD results do not accurately represent true bone mineral density, since they use approximations of the bone's volume. BMAD is used primarily for research purposes and is not yet used in clinical settings.

Other imaging technologies such as computed quantitative computer tomography (QCT) are capable of measuring the bone's volume, and are therefore not susceptible to the confounding effect of bone-size in the way that DXA results are susceptible.

DXA uses X-rays to assess bone mineral density. However, the radiation dose is approximately 1/10th that of a standard chest X-ray.

The quality of DXA operators varies widely. DXA is not regulated like other radiation based imaging techniques because of its low dosage. Each state has a different policy as to what certifications are needed to operate a DXA machine. Because BMD testing with DXA is very susceptible to operator error, it is important to find out what qualifies the technician to operate the machine.

It is important for patients to get repeat BMD measurements done on the same machine each time, or at least a machine from the same manufacturer. Error between machines, or trying to convert measurements from one manufacturer's standard to another can introduce errors large enough to wipe out the sensitivity of the measurements.

DXA results need to be adjusted if the patient is taking strontium supplements.

Current clinical practice in paediatrics

DXA is, by far, the most widely used technique for bone measurements since it is considered to be cheap, accessible, easy to use, and able to provide an accurate estimation of bone mineral density in adults.

The official position of the ISCD (International Society for Clinical Densitometry) is that a patient may be tested for BMD if; he suffers from a condition which could precipitate bone loss or is going to be prescribed pharmaceuticals known to cause bone loss or he is being treated and needs to be monitored. The ISCD states that there is no clearly understood correlation between BMD and the risk of a child suffering a fracture; the diagnosis of osteoporosis in children cannot be made using the basis of a densitometry criteria. T-scores are prohibited with children and should not even appear on DXA reports, and thus, the WHO classification of osteoporosis and osteopenia in adults cannot be applied to children but Z-scores can be used to assist diagnosis.

Some clinics may routinely carry out DXA scans on paediatric patients with conditions such as nutritional rickets, lupus and Turner Syndrome. DXA has been demonstrated to measure skeletal maturity and body fat composition and has been used to evaluate the effects of pharmaceutical therapy. It may also aid paediatricians in diagnosing and monitoring treatment of disorders of bone mass acquisition in childhood. However it seems that DXA is still in its early days in paediatrics and there are widely acknowledged limitations and disadvantages with DXA. A view exists that DXA scans for diagnostic purposes should not even be performed outside specialist centres and if a scan is done outside one of these centres, it should not be interpreted without consultation with an expert in the field. Furthermore, most of the pharmaceuticals that are given to adults with low bone mass can be given to children only in strictly monitored clinical trials.

Whole-body calcium measured by DXA has been validated in adults using *in vivo* neutron activation of total body calcium but this is not suitable for paediatric subjects and studies have been carried out on paediatric-sized animals.

Indirect Measurement of Body Fat

Indirect measurement techniques of body fat such as anthropometry and BIA require empirically derived regression equations to estimate body fat or total body water (TBW). These techniques are suitable for population studies where individual distinction is less critical. They often need to be validated by reference methods such as densitometry and the isotope dilution method. Anthropometry is a rapid and inexpensive way to evaluate nutritional status for a population in a field study, but it requires a skilled technician and anthropometrist to achieve accurate measurement. Single or multiple frequency BIA also provides a rapid and simple method to allow the investigator to predict TBW and extracellular water (ECW). In general, both techniques are less likely to be useful for prediction of change in body composition.

Anthropometry

Anthropometry, in physical anthropology, refers to the measurement of the human individual for the purposes of understanding human physical variation.

Today, anthropometry plays an important role in industrial design, clothing design, ergonomics and architecture where statistical data about the distribution of body dimensions in the population are used to optimise products. Changes in life styles, nutrition and ethnic composition of populations lead to changes in the distribution of body dimensions (e.g. the obesity epidemic), and require regular updating of anthropometric data collections.

Modern anthropometry and biometrics

Anthropometric studies are today conducted for numerous different purposes. Academic anthropologists investigate the evolutionary significance of differences in body proportion between populations whose ancestors lived in different environmental settings. Human populations exhibit similar climatic variation patterns to other large-bodied mammals, following Bergmann's rule, which states that individuals in cold climates will tend to be larger than ones in warm climates, and Allen's rule, which states that individuals in cold climates will tend to have shorter, stubbier limbs than those in warm climates.

Today people are performing anthropometry with three-dimensional scanners. The subject has a three-dimensional scan taken of their body, and the anthropometrist extracts measurements from the scan rather than directly from the individual. This is beneficial for the anthropometrist in that they can use this scan to extract any measurement at any time and the individual does not have to wait for each measurement to be taken separately.

Goniometers and Accelerometers

Goniometer

A goniometer is an instrument that either measures angle or allows an object to be rotated to a precise angular position. The term goniometry is derived from two Greek words, gonia, meaning angle and metron, meaning measure (Fig. 10.13).

There are many types of goniometers, each specialised for its particular application.

Audio: An audio goniometer is used to see the amount of stereo in a signal.

Communications: Goniometers are used for direction finding in signals intelligence applications for military and civil purposes, e.g. interception of satellite and naval communications as performed on the French warship Dupuy de Lôme uses multiple goniometers.

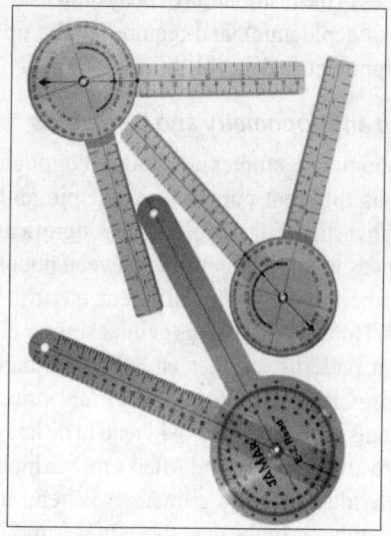

Fig. 10.13. Goniometer.

Crystallography: In crystallography, goniometers are used for measuring angles between crystal faces. They are also used in X-ray diffraction to rotate the samples (Fig. 10.14).

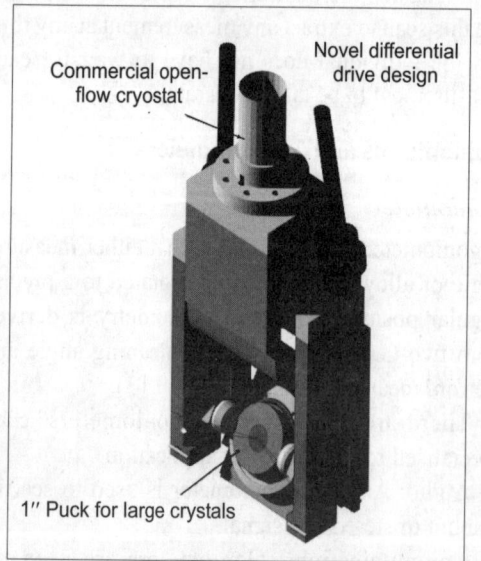

Fig. 10.14. A goniometer for crystallography.

Light measurement: Goniophotometers measure the spatial distribution of light visible to the human eye at a specific angular position.

Physical therapy: In occupational therapy and physical therapy, a goniometer is an instrument which measures an axis and range of motion. If a patient or client is suffering from decreased range of motion in a joint (e.g. a knee or elbow), the therapist can use a goniometer to assess what the range of motion is prior to intervention, and then make sure the intervention is working by using the goniometer in subsequent interventions.

Surface science: In surface science, an instrument generally called a contact angle goniometer is used to measure the static contact angle, advancing and receding contact angles, and surface tension.

Accelerometer

An accelerometer is a device that measures proper acceleration; the acceleration it experiences relative to freefall. Single- and multi-axis models are available to detect magnitude and direction of the acceleration as a vector quantity, and can be used to sense orientation, vibration and shock. Micro-machined accelerometers are increasingly present in portable electronic devices and video game controllers, to detect the orientation of the device or provide for game input.

Most accelerometers are designed for motion sensitivity in one major axis. Normally, the accelerometer will transduce shock and vibration that is input normal to the accelerometers mounting base (Fig. 10.15).

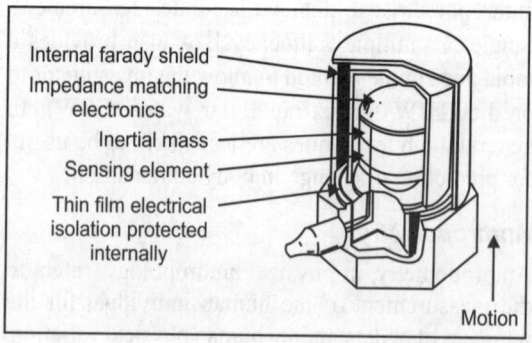

Fig. 10.15. Accelerometers are designed for motion sensitivity in one major axis.

An accelerometer measures proper acceleration which is the acceleration it experiences relative to freefall, and is the acceleration that is felt by people and objects. Put another way, at any point in spacetime the equivalence principle guarantees the existence of a local inertial frame, and an accelerometer measures the acceleration relative to that frame.

As a consequence an accelerometer at rest relative to the Earth's surface will indicate approximately 1 g upwards, because any point on the earth's surface is accelerating upwards relative to a local inertial frame. To obtain the acceleration due to motion with respect to the earth, this 'gravity offset' should be subtracted.

The reason for the appearance of a gravitational offset is Einstein's equivalence principle, which states that the effects of gravity on an object are indistinguishable from acceleration of the reference frame. When held fixed in a gravitational field by, for example, applying a ground reaction force or an equivalent upward thrust, the reference frame for an accelerometer (its own casing) accelerates upwards with respect to a free-falling reference frame.

The effect of this reference frame acceleration is indistinguishable from any other acceleration experienced by the instrument.

An accelerometer will read zero during free fall. This includes use in a spaceship orbiting earth, but not a (non-free) fall with air resistance where drag forces reduce the acceleration until terminal velocity is reached, at which point the device would once again indicate 1 g acceleration upwards.

Acceleration is quantified in the SI unit metres per second per second (m/s^2), in the cgs unit gal (Gal), or popularly in terms of g-force (g).

For the practical purpose of finding the acceleration of objects with respect to the earth, such as for use in an inertial navigation system, a knowledge of local gravity is required. This can be obtained either by calibrating the device at rest, or from a known model of gravity at the approximate current position.

Accelerometers are used to measure the depth of CPR chest compressions.

Optoelectronics

Optoelectronics is the study and application of electronic devices that source, detect and control light, usually considered a sub-field of photonics. In this context, light often includes invisible forms of radiation such as gamma rays, X-rays, ultraviolet and infrared, in addition to visible light.

Optoelectronic devices are electrical-to-optical or optical-to-electrical transducers, or instruments that use such devices in their operation. Electro-optics is often erroneously used as a synonym, but is in fact a wider branch of physics that deals with all interactions between light and electric fields, whether or not they form part of an electronic device.

Optoelectronics is based on the quantum mechanical effects of light on semiconducting materials, sometimes in the presence of electric fields.

1. Photoelectric or photovoltaic effect, used in:
   (a) Photodiodes (including solar cells).
   (b) Phototransistors.
   (c) Photomultipliers.
   (d) Integrated optical circuit (IOC) elements.

2. Photoconductivity, used in:
   (a) Photoresistors.
   (b) Photoconductive camera tubes.
   (c) Charge-coupled imaging devices.

3. Stimulated emission, used in:
   (a) Injection laser diodes.
   (b) Quantum cascade lasers.

4. Lossev effect, or radiative recombination, used in:
   (a) Light-emitting diodes or LED.

5. Photoemissivity, used in:
   (a) Photoemissive camera tube.

Important applications of optoelectronics include:
1. Optocoupler.
2. Optical fibre communications.

11

Chemical Transducers

INTRODUCTION

Chemical transducers play an important role in medicine and physiology in the assessment of metabolism. In general, there are two types: (i) those that measure chemical composition of the blood, tissue, and organ fluids, and (ii) those that measure the composition of the respiratory gases. The most commonly encountered transducers are those used for measuring the blood gases (in solution). Such transducers measure the partial pressure of oxygen (pO_2) and carbon dioxide (pCO_2) and the concentration of hydrogen ions (pH). Complementing these transducers are those for the respiratory gases O_2, CO_2, and N_2. The latter is a diluent the measurement of which permits determining the only lung volume not measurable with a spirometer-the residual volume (RV), which is the quantity of air remaining in the lungs after a maximal expiration.

Although some chemical transducers employ a colour change to identify a chemical species (for example, the oximeter), many are electrochemical cells in which the quantity to be measured causes a change in cell potential or a change in current flow through the cell. All such cells contain electrodes, sometimes of unusual design. Often one electrode constitutes the sensor, and the other (reference) electrode plays no active part. It is well to recall that such reference electrodes have a potential with respect to their environmental solutions.

BLOOD GASES

Accurate assessment of blood gases is fundamental to supportive care in critical care medicine.

Traditionally, blood gases have been measured by invasive sampling, either through an indwelling arterial catheter or by arterial puncture, and analysed in the laboratory by blood gas analysers. This presents significant drawbacks, mainly because of the prolonged delay between sample acquisition and the availability of the laboratory results. In neonatal applications, for example, frequent blood sampling can cause significant blood loss, especially for very small infants, unless microblood samples are used for analysis. Furthermore, blood gas values are available only intermittently and therefore indicate the status of the patient only at the time the blood sample was drawn. The inevitable delay and lack of continuous information can lead to potential diagnostic errors, particularly in critically ill patients, in whom rapid and often life-threatening cardiopulmonary changes can occur during short periods of time. Continuous monitoring of blood gases, on the other hand, offers a major advantage since instantaneous changes in blood gas levels can be recognised and adequately corrected before irreversible tissue damage occurs. Furthermore, it provides trending information to assist in assessing the therapeutic response and predicting prognosis.

Recent advances in biosensors and medical instrumentation have made continuous blood gas monitoring a widely accepted diagnostic practice. There are three major groups of patients in whom blood gas monitoring is especially essential: patients suffering from acute respiratory or cardiovascular failure, premature neonates, and patients undergoing cardiac surgery. The most important clinical applications of blood gas monitoring include

(i) assessment of acid-base disorders, (ii) detection and management of hyperoxia, hypoxia, and hypercapnia, and (iii) detection of right-to-left shunts and dead space ventilation.

In this chapter we present the basic methods that have been developed for continuous blood gas monitoring. It is intended not to provide an exhaustive coverage of the topic, but rather to give the reader a fundamental knowledge of this emerging new field. In this chapter we review the principles of invasive and noninvasive monitoring of mixed venous oxygen saturation (SvO_2), arterial oxygen saturation (SaO_2), oxygen tension (pO_2), pH, and carbon dioxide tension (pCO_2) utilising electrochemistry, spectrophotometry, gas chromatography, and mass spectrometry techniques.

BLOOD GAS TRANSPORT

O_2 Transport

Oxygen is transported by the blood from the lungs to the tissues in two distinct states. Under normal physiological conditions, approximately 2 per cent of the total amount of O_2 carried by the blood is dissolved in the plasma. The remaining 98 per cent is carried inside the red blood cells in a loose reversible combination with haemoglobin (Hb), as oxyhaemoglobin (HbO_2). The amount of O_2 in the blood depends on its pO_2. The amount of dissolved O_2 is linearly proportional to the blood pO_2. The amount of O_2 chemically combined with Hb, on the other hand, is related to the pO_2 nonlinearly and is described by the sigmoidshaped oxyhaemoglobin dissociation curve (ODC). Accordingly, as the pO_2 increases, there is a progressive but nonlinear increase in the blood oxygen saturation (i.e. the ratio between the O_2 content to the maximum O_2 carrying capacity expressed as a percentage). This nonlinear relationship ensures efficient transport of O_2 to the tissues by the blood. Using this curve, and assuming a healthy patient, an approximate oxygen saturation value can be calculated from the pO_2 measured in the laboratory by *in vitro* blood gas analysis, or vice versa. However, large errors may result in unhealthy patients or under abnormal physiological conditions.

This is due mainly to variations in the blood pH, body temperature, the elevated level of 2,3-diphospho-glycerate (DPG), pCO_2, and type of functional Hb (e.g. adult HbA or fetal HbF). These factors play an important role in controlling the affinity with which Hb binds and releases O_2, and thus can cause a shift in the ODC. Therefore, to avoid errors inherent in this relationship, it is preferred to measure oxygen saturation directly rather than to measure pO_2 and then estimate oxygen saturation from the ODC if the factors causing the shift in the curve are not taken into account. Normally, arterial blood has a pO_2 of about 100 mm Hg (13.3 kPa), which corresponds to an oxygen saturation of approximately 98 per cent. The pO_2 of venous blood is normally about 40 mm Hg (5.3 kPa), which corresponds to an oxygen saturation of approximately 75 per cent.

CO_2 Transport

CO_2 is carried by the blood both in a dissolved state and in combination with Hb and plasma proteins as carbamino compounds. The dissolved CO_2 in the blood reacts with water to form carbonic acid, which is subsequently dissociated into hydrogen and bicarbonate ions. The reversible combination of CO_2 with water accounts for approximately 70 per cent of the total CO_2 transported by the blood under normal resting conditions. The remaining CO_2 is transported in the dissolved state (approximately 7 per cent) and in a loose reversible combination with Hb as carbaminohaemoglobin (approximately 23 per cent). The total amount of CO_2 carried by the blood is a function of the blood pCO_2. It is important to note that this relationship is a function of the blood pO_2, since binding of O_2 with Hb tends to displace CO_2 from the blood. The normal pCO_2 of arterial blood is about 40 mm Hg (5.3 kPa), whereas that of venous blood is about 45 mm Hg (6 kPa).

ELECTROCHEMISTRY OF pO_2 AND pCO_2 MEASUREMENT

pO_2 Measurement

Measurement of pO_2 is based on the principle of polarography as shown schematically in Fig. 11.1. Accordingly, O_2 molecules dissolved in an electrolyte (e.g. KCl) are reduced at the surface of a noble metal cathode (e.g. platinum or gold). A constant polarising voltage of approximately –600 mV is applied between the cathode and an adjacent reference Ag/AgCl anode. This polarising voltage is required to minimise the interference of other gases that can also be reduced and to assure rapid oxygen reduction at the cathode. The electrochemical reduction at the cathode can be described by the following chemical reaction:

$$O_2 + 2H_2O + 4e^- \longrightarrow 4OH^-$$

According to this reaction, an O_2 molecule takes four electrons from the cathode, then reacts with two water molecules, generating four hydroxyl ions. The hydroxyl ions created in this reaction are buffered by the electrolyte. At the Ag/AgI reference anode, the chemical reaction is:

$$Ag \longleftrightarrow Ag^+ + e^-$$

$$Ag^+ + Cl^- \longleftrightarrow AgCl$$

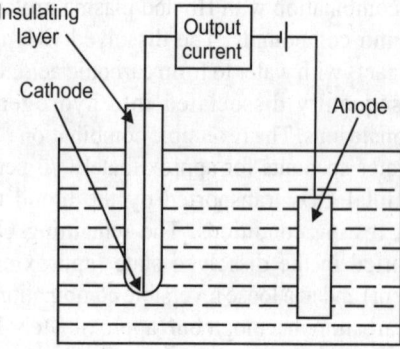

Fig. 11.1. Principle of polarographic pO_2 measurement.

Silver from the electrode is first oxidised to silver ions and electrons are liberated to the anode. The silver ions immediately combine with chloride ions to form silver chloride which precipitates on the electrode surface. Consequently, there is a continuous flow of electrons (current) between the cathode and the anode, the rate of which is linearly proportional to the supply of O_2 to the cathode. Since all O_2 molecules reaching the cathode will react with it, the pO_2 at the cathode surface is zero. In practice, the current generated is linearly proportional to the pO_2 in the electrolyte. Thus, by measuring the change in current between the cathode and the anode, one can determine the amount of oxygen dissolved in the electrolyte. For medical applications, bare electrodes are seldom used. Instead, the sensor is separated from the blood by a semipermeable membrane that permits either O_2, CO_2, or hydrogen ions to diffuse slowly into the polarographic electrode. This significantly decreases the instability of the electrode due to flow-dependent effects.

pCO₂ Measurement

The pCO_2 electrode operates according to the Stow-Severinghaus principle, in which a CO_2 change is sensed by a pH electrode. The principle of pCO_2 measurement is illustrated schematically in Fig. 11.2. In practice, the CO_2 molecules diffuse into a bicarbonate solution through a semipermeable membrane. Subsequently, hydrogen and bicarbonate ions are formed according to the following chemical reaction:

$$CO_2 + H_2O \longleftrightarrow H_2CO_3 \longleftrightarrow H^+ + HCO_3^-$$

As a result of this chemical reaction, a potential is generated between the glass pH and the reference electrode (e.g. Ag/AgCl). This potential can be calibrated knowing the CO_2 concentration in the solution. By means of the Henderson-Haselbach relationship, it can be shown that the measured pH is proportional to the negative logarithm of the pCO_2.

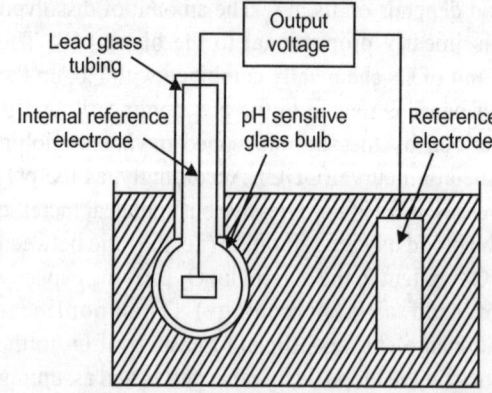

Fig. 11.2. Principle of electrochemical pCO_2 measurment.

PRINCIPLE OF OPTICAL OXIMETRY

The basis of oxygen saturation measurement relies on the difference in optical absorption spectra of Hb and HbO_2, as illustrated in Fig. 11.3. Consequently, various optical methods for measuring oxygen saturation have been developed based on measuring the light transmission through, or reflection from, blood at two wavelengths: λ_1, where a large difference in light absorption between Hb and HbO_2 exist (e.g. 660 nm), and λ_2, an isobestic wavelength, where the absorption of light is independent of blood oxygenation (e.g. 805 nm). The absorption of light by a Hb solution (i.e. hemolysed blood) can be accurately determined using Beer-Lambert's law, which can be written as:

$$P_t = P_0 \times 10^{-\alpha cd} \qquad \dots (11.1)$$

where P_t is the transmitted light power, P_0 the incident light power, α the specific absorption coefficient of the sample, c the concentration of the sample, and d the lightpath distance.

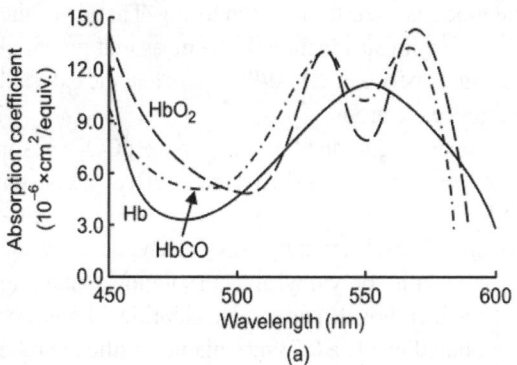

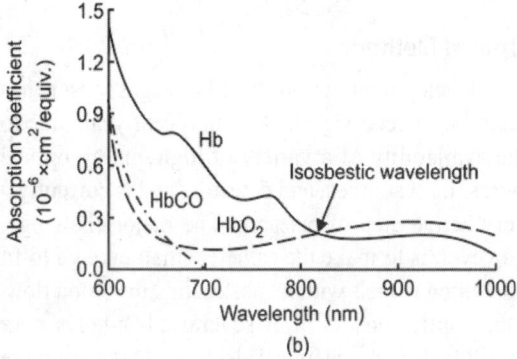

Fig. 11.3. Optical absorption spectra of Hb, HbO_2, and HbCO.

Assuming that a haemolysed blood solution consists of a two-component mixture (e.g. Hb and HbO_2) and that light absorption by a homogeneous mixture of these two components is additive, the following relationship can be derived:

$$\text{Oxygen saturation} = A - B \frac{OD(\lambda_1)}{OD(\lambda_2)} \qquad \dots (11.2)$$

where A and B are functions of the specific absorption coefficients of Hb and HbO_2, and OD is the optical density [i.e. $\log_{10}(P_0/P_t)$] of the sample. It is important to keep in mind that this relationship is derived based on the assumption that hemolysed blood obeys Beer Lambert's law, which requires a monochroamtic light source and collimated light transmission through the sample. Furthermore, the solution cannot contain any particles that cause light scattering.

INVASIVE INTRAVASCULAR BLOOD GAS MONITORING

Efforts have been ongoing over the last decade to develop blood gas sensors which can be sufficiently miniaturised to enable intravascular placement. Several approaches have been developed utilising electrochemical sensors, optical sensors, and indwelling sampling catheters connected to an external gas chromatograph or mass spectrometer.

Electrochemical Methods

pO₂ sensors

Direct intravascular monitoring of pO_2 can be performed by a miniaturised bipolar polarographic sensor placed at the tip of a catheter. Figure 11.4 illustrates a pO_2 sensor that consists of thin silver cathode and anode wires embedded in a 0.65-mm-diameter polyethylene tubing that acts as a gas-permeable membrane. The Teflon insulation of the cathode wire is removed from the wire end over a length of 5 mm. The oxygen molecules diffuse through the walls of the polyethylene tube into an electrolyte gel and then reduced in an electrochemical reaction. The advantage of this particular catheter-tip configuration is that the measurement is performed on the sides of the probe and not at its tip, which has been shown to be particularly sensitive to fibrin deposits.

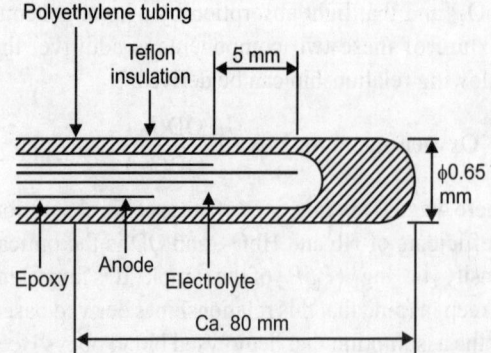

Fig. 11.4. Cross-section of an intravascular pO_2 catheter sensor.

The sensor described above can be introduced into a femoral, brachial, or radial artery through a 4F (1.33-mm-diameter) plastic catheter. The tip of the sensor is then pushed forward so that it protrudes approximately 5 to 10 cm beyond the tip of the catheter. A special adapter can be used to monitor blood pressure and withdraw blood samples. The sensor is calibrated *in situ* by withdrawing and analysing the pO_2 of a blood sample using a standard blood gas analyser and adjusting the instrument reading accordingly.

A different type of polarographic sensor was described by Kimmich using solid-state fabrication techniques. The advantages of semiconductor integrated-circuit technologies were utilised because they allow one to design different miniature cathode and anode structures with good reproducibility and reasonable low cost. This particular pO_2 sensor was constructed in the shape of two rectangular spirals. The gold cathode and silver anode were deposited on a silicone substrate by vapour deposition. A porous cross-linked polymer matrix was used between the cathode and anode. A rubber membrane was utilised as a carrier for the electrolyte. The chip was then incorporated into a 4F (1.33-mm-diameter) catheter for intravascular measurements.

Neuman described a multicathode polarographic oxygen sensor which can be fabricated using either thick- or thin-film metallisation techniques. This approach can be used to deposit defined structures of gold and silver films on an alumina substrate. In this particular sensor, a silicone dioxide film was used to delineate the exposed surface of the multiple gold cathode sites and the silver anode.

pCO₂ sensors

A catheter-tip sensor for simultaneous monitoring of blood pCO_2 and pH has been developed by Coon. This sensor consists of a palladium oxide (PdO) hydrogenion-sensitive electrode and an Ag/AgCl reference electrode. The electrodes are surrounded by a thin layer of bicarbonate solution and enclosed with a silicone polycarbonate pH sensitive copolymer membrane. The entire catheter size is approximately 0.6 mm in diameter.

Blood pCO_2 is measured according to the Severinghous-Stow technique with the PdO electrode being used to detect changes in the pH of the bicarbonate solution. An additional reference electrode outside the sensor but in direct contact with the blood is used for pH monitoring. The pH of the blood is a linear function of the measured potential generated between the Pd/PdO wire and the external reference electrode.

Kohama described a catheter-tip pCO_2 sensor based on a pH-ion-selective field-effect transistor (ISFET) technique. The sensor consists of a pH-sensitive ISFET and a Ag/AgCl reference electrode covered with a polyvinyl alcohol solution containing sodium bicarbonate and sodium chloride. The sensor is mounted inside a 0.73 mm-diameter silicone tube sealed with silicone resin.

Optical Methods

The development of fibre optic blood gas sensors has taken on special significance in recent years due to the availability of a variety of high-quality optical fibres, light sources, and detectors and is currently a very active area of research. The major challenge, however, is to make the catheter small enough to fit into blood vessels without obstructing the blood flow. Fibre optic sensors offer several advantages over traditional electrochemical electrodes. Some of these advantages include: immunity to electrical and electromagnetic interference, low drift (which is essential for long-term monitoring), and small size. The major challenges in developing a fibre optic blood gas sensor for medical application have been in the immobilisation of the reagents used on the fibre tip, and making these sensors both biocompatible and sterilisable. Intravascular optical blood gas sensors fall into two categories: those that sense changes in the optical absorption of the blood directly (i.e. SvO_2 sensors) and those that use a reagent that changes its optical properties in response to changes in the analyte and the optical measurement is performed indirectly (i.e. pO_2, pH, and pCO_2 sensors).

The basic construction of a fibre optic blood gas sensing system is shown schematically in Fig. 11.5. Light from a suitable source (LED, laser diode, or a combination of incandescent light and an interference optical filter) travels along an optical fibre by total internal reflection at the interface between a core and a cladding material having different refractive indices to a sensor at its tip. There the light interacts with the sample either directly or indirectly through a specific reagent. The collected light then returns to a photodetector along either the same or a separate optical fibre, where it is processed.

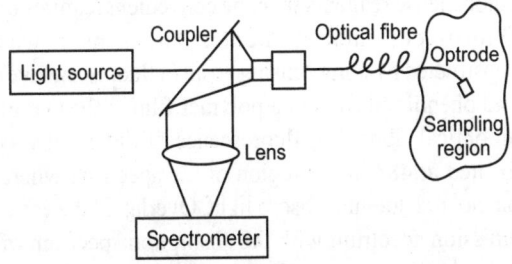

Fig. 11.5. Principle of fibre optic blood gas sensing.

Indirect fibre optic blood gas sensors use an immobilised reagent indicator that reacts with a specific analyte. An optical signal is produced in response to changes in the analyte concentration. The chemical reaction between the blood and the reagent can be reversible (the reagent used is not consumed) or irreversible (the reagent is eventually consumed). The measurement is performed by illuminating the sample with light at a known wavelength and intensity. Multiple wavelengths can also be used to measure several analytes simultaneously if the specific optical reaction results in sufficiently distinct absorption spectra.

Depending on the specific reaction monitored, either the attenuation of the incident light intensity due to absorption, reflection outside the fibre, or reflection along the surface of an uncladded fibre (attenuated total reflection or evanescent wave absorption) or the optical fluorescence produced (both emission and quenching) can be utilised to monitor the unknown sample concentration. Fluorescence-based sensors have many inherent advantages over the other optical sensing techniques. This advantage results from the fact that absorption measurements produce very small light attenuation that must be measured against a strong background light intensity. In fluorescence, on the other hand, the dye emits light at a wavelength different from that at which the excitation energy is absorbed. This too results in a small amount of light detected, but the measurement is made against a dark background that produces a much more sensitive and selective signal. Furthermore, a single fibre optic can be used to carry the excitation energy to the sample and return the fluorescence signal to the detector for analysis.

pO_2 sensors

Oxygen quenching of luminescence occurs due to the transfer of energy from an excited molecule to molecular oxygen. The greater the collision frequency of oxygen molecules with excited molecules, the fewer excited molecules remain for optical detection. Therefore, the luminescence intensity decreases with increasing pO_2. Utilising this concept, Lubbers and Opitz developed a fluorescence pO_2 sensor based on the O_2 quenching of pyrene butyric acid. A similar approach was devised by Peterson using the dye perylene dibutyrate. The dye was absorbed on polystyrene and contained in a porous polypropylene envelope. The pO_2 of the blood is measured by illuminating the dye with blue light and detecting the yellow-green fluorescence intensity emitted. The ratio of the returned yellowgreen to blue light intensity is processed according to the Stem-Volmer relationship, providing a readout proportional to pO_2 according to

$$\frac{I_0}{I} = 1 + K(pO_2) \qquad \text{... (11.3)}$$

where I is the relative fluorescence intensity, I_0 the intensity without O_2 quenching, an K a calibration constant.

pH sensors

Since most pCO_2 measurements involve the measurement of pH, a brief discussion of relevant intravascular pH sensors is provided below. The first fibre optic blood pH sensor was developed by Peterson. The basic design of this sensor is shown in Fig. 11.6. The sensing is performed in a miniature spectrophotometric cell made from an ionpermeable cellulose hollow fibre attached to the tip of two optical fibres. The special cell contains a pH-sensitive dye (phenol red) which is covalently bound to polyacrylamide microspheres.

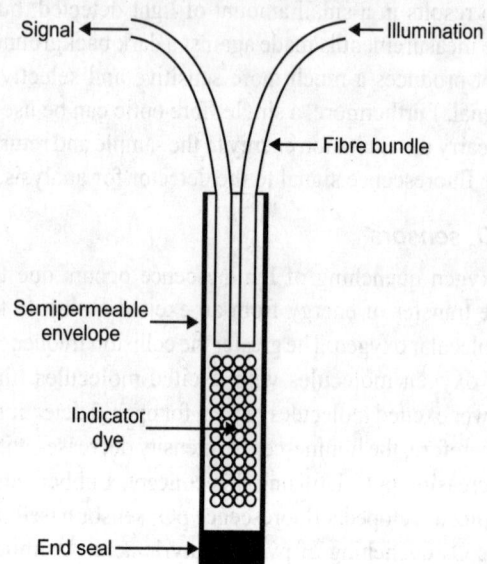

Fig. 11.6. Fibre optic pH sensor.

The dye is reversible and has two tautometric forms, each with a different light absorption spectra. The relative proportions of the base form (absorbing green light) and the acid form (absorbing blue light) vary with pH. Green (560 nm) and red (600 nm) light is passed into the cell from one optical fibre. The green light is partially absorbed by the dye, while the red light that is not absorbed acts as a reference beam. A separate optical fibre collects the emitted light and passes it to a photodetector for processing.

The ratio r of the green to red light intensities detected by the photodetector is related to the sample pH according to the equation

$$r = k \times 10^{-c/(10^{-d}+1)} \qquad \ldots (11.4)$$

where k is a constant of the system, c the optical density at 560 nm when the dye is in its base form, and d the difference between the pH and pK of the dye. The sensor has been shown to be sensitive to pH in the range between 7.0 and 7.4 units with a precision of approximately ±0.01 pH units.

Saari described a pH sensor using an immobilised fluoresceinamine dye bound covalently to cellulose. The pH is measured by exciting the dye at 480 nm and detecting the fluorescence emission produced at 520 nm. Jordon developed a different type of fibre optic pH sensor based on the work of Hirschfeld. This approach is based on an absorption-emission technique in which a colorimetric reagent turns a fluorescent indicator dye on and off by radiationless resonance energy transfer (quantum tunneling). This technique combines the general availability of colorimetric reagents with the convenient features of fluorescent measurements. The sensor was constructed by immobilising eosin (a fluorescent dye) and phenol red dyes in a polymer film at the end of an optical fibre. The fluorescence of the eosin was excited at 488 nm, a region of the spectrum where phenol red does not absorb light. Overlap of the eosin emission spectrum with the absorption spectrum of phenol red produces efficient energy transfer from the eosin, which is used as a donor molecule, to the phenol red, which is used as the acceptor molecule, resulting in a decrease of the eosin emission. As the pH is decreased, the phenol red absorbance shifts to shorter wavelengths, resulting in less efficient energy transfer and an increased eosin emission.

Recently, Gehrich developed a fibre optic pH sensor using a hydroxypyrene trisulphonic acid dye bonded covalently to a cellulose matrix which is attached to the fibre tip. Blood pH is calculated from the ratio of fluorescence intensity emitted at 520 nm measured with 460 nm excitation to that measured with 410 nm excitation light. This sensor is incorporated in one fibre optic catheter together with other proprietary pO_2 and pCO_2 sensitive dyes to measure simultaneously all three blood gas parameters. A similar optical fluorescence technique has been used also to develop an extracorporeal sensor for blood gases. This particular sensor was designed to monitor pO_2, pH, and pCO_2 simultaneously in arterial and venous blood during open heart surgery. The sensor consists of proprietary fluorescence dyes and membranes for gases and hydrogen ions mounted inside a special disposable flowthrough cell which is attached to the extracorporeal circuit of a heart-lung machine.

pCO₂ sensors

A fibre optic pCO_2 sensor has been developed by Vurek based on an extension of Peterson's work. The sensor is comprised of two optical fibres and a gas-permeable silicone rubber tube filled with a pH indicator dye (phenol red), an isotonic solution of $KHCO_3$, and KCl. Ambient pCO_2 controls the pH of the solution, which influences the optical transmission of the phenol red dye. Lubbers and Opitz devised a pCO_2 sensor utilising β-methylumbelliferone as a pH indicator dye. The basic sensing mechanism is this dye, which detects changes in hydrogen ion concentration in a bicarbonate containing solution that in turn varies as a function of the pCO_2 in the solution.

SvO₂ sensors

The development of inexpensive plastic fibre optics, solid-state LEDs, and photodetectors has enabled direct *in vivo* monitoring of blood SvO_2. The measurement is performed by placing a flexible fibre catheter in the bloodstream and monitoring the relative change in backscattered light intensity from the flowing red blood cells with variations in SvO_2. The optical fibres are incorporated into a disposable balloon-tipped bilumen catheter similar to a Swan-Ganz thermodilution catheter which is used for cardiac output measurement. The flow-directed catheter is typically inserted through the right heart into the pulmonary artery for monitoring mixed venous SvO_2. Central venous SvO_2 monitoring is useful for detecting congenital heart defects that allow oxygenated blood to shunt into the venous side of the heart.

Figure 11.7 illustrates the principle of this measurement. The fibre optic catheter is connected to an optical module which contains the LEDs and photodetector. The incident light is transmitted to the blood through a source fibre.

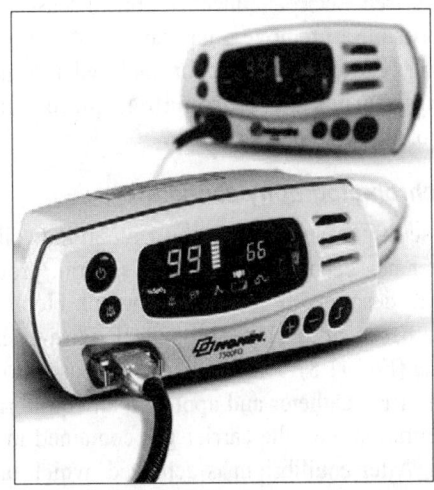

Fig. 11.7. Fibre optic SO_2 sensor and oximeter.

The backscattered light from the blood is collected by a second optical fibre located adjacent to the tip of the source fibre. Since SvO_2 measurement is affected by blood flow and haematocrit, two wavelengths and the possibility of entering blood haematocrit by the user or three wavelengths are typically used to compensate for these effects. Further corrections for haematocrit variations can be achieved if two unequally spaced detecting fibres are incorporated in the catheter. The light intensities emanating from the catheter tip are usually normalised by placing a standard reflecting surface over the catheter tip before the catheter is inserted into the blood. An empirically derived equation relating SvO_2 to the infrared (IR)/red (R) reflectance ratio such as:

$$SvO_2 = K_1 - K_2 \frac{IR}{R} \qquad \dots (11.5)$$

where K_1 and K_2 are constants depending on the catheter configuration and the optical properties of the blood, is typically used for processing the signals by the oximeter.

Gas Chromatography and Mass Spectrometry Methods

In addition to indwelling catheters where the measurement is performed intravascularly using a miniaturised electrochemical or optical sensor, it is also possible to remove a gas sample of the blood utilising a carrier gas or a vacuum and feed the sample to an external gas chromatograph or mass spectrometer for analysis.

Gas chromatography sensors

The use of gas chromatography with an indwelling catheter has been investigated by several, groups. Massaro described a gas chromatograph blood gas sensor based on a closed-tipped 2F intra-arterial catheter (Fig. 11.8). The blood gases diffuse into the lumen of the catheter and approach an equilibrium concentration with the carrier gas contained in the lumen. After equilibrium is achieved, which takes approximately 4 min, a bolus of the gas content in the lumen is delivered to the gas chromatograph for separation and analysis. Helium gas is delivered from the analyser through the outer annular supply line in the catheter. The helium gas containing the equilibrated blood gases is drawn back into the analyser through the central return line. Silicone rubber tubing which is highly permeable to the dissolved gases facilitates their rapid diffusion into the catheter lumen. Carlon and Hall tested an indwelling arterial catheter for blood gases connected to a Sentorr gas analyser. The blood gases are aspirated into the gas analyser through a heparin-coated helium-filled probe that was inserted into a peripheral artery through an 18-gauge catheter. Common problems with all of these sensors are inadequate reliability and safety.

Mass spectrometry sensors

The continuous analysis of gases in blood with a mass spectrometer has been adapted for use with indwelling catheters. Brantigan described the characteristics of different indwelling catheters for blood gas measurements using mass spectrometers.

The catheters consist of a semipermeable polymer membrane mounted over a mandril of narrowgauge flexible stainless steel tubing. In operation, the distal tip is placed in the blood and the proximal end is attached through 6 ft of connecting tubing to a vacuum inlet of the spectrometer. A pressure gradient is established which continuously draws a minute amount of gas across the membrane at a sampling rate of about 2×10^{-6} mL/s. The gases entering the mass spectrometer are analysed according to their molecular weights.

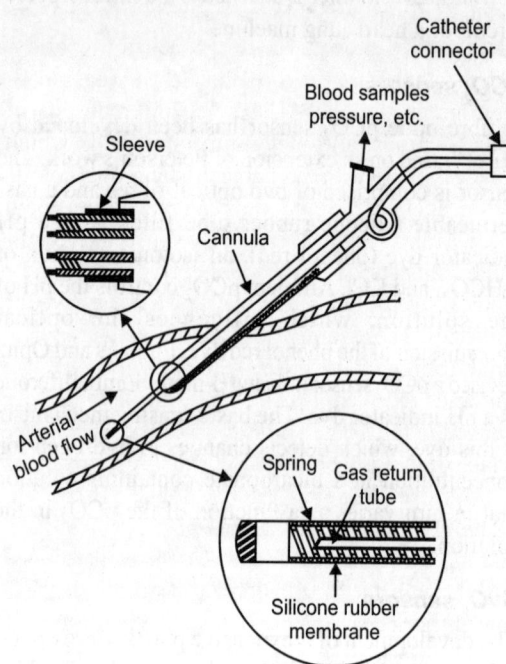

Fig. 11.8. Gas chromatograph blood gas catheter.

NONINVASIVE BLOOD GAS MONITORING

Intravascular monitoring is not without limitations. Probe failure due to thrombotic deposition on the sensing element can be a serious problem and can provide a source of emboli and infection. Noninvasive monitoring (i.e. where there is no direct contact between the blood or other tissue fluids and the sensor) has, therefore, been the subject of extensive research and immense development for many years.

Gas Diffusion Through the Skin

To understand the basics of O_2 and CO_2 diffusion through the skin, and some of the factors that affect noninvasive blood gas monitoring, it is important first to understand the physiology and anatomy of the human skin. The skin consists of three principal layers: the stratum corneum, epidermis, and dermis. The thickness of the human skin varies with age, sex, and region of the body. The outermost layer of the skin; the stratum corneum, is a nonliving layer composed mainly of dehydrated cells. Thus this dead layer does not consume any O_2 or produce CO_2. The thickness of the stratum corneum varies from 0.1 to 0.2 mm, depending on the part of the body. Underneath the stratum corneum is the living, blood-free, epidermis layer. The epidermis consists of proteins, lipids, and melaninforming cells which provide the skin with its characteristic brown colour. The thickness of the epidermis can range from about 0.05 to 1 mm. The third layer of the skin is the dermis, which consists of dense connective tissue, hair follicles, sweat glands, fat cells, and a dense layer of capillaries. These capillaries are arranged in vertical loops approximately 0.2 to 0.4 mm long. The capillaries receive blood from arterioles, which are arranged in the form of a flat network parallel to the surface of the skin below the dermis. Arteriovenous anastomoses innervated by nerve fibres are commonly found in the dermis of the palms, face, and ears. These shunting blood vessels regulate blood flow through the skin. Blood flow through these channels can increase nearly 30 fold in response to heat.

Gas diffusion through the skin occurs due to a partial pressure between the blood in the dermis and the outermost surface of the skin. Diffusion of O_2 and CO_2 through the skin is normally very low. For example, it has been shown that under normal physiological conditions, the pO_2 measured on the surface of the skin is less than 2.5 mm Hg (0.33 kPa). However, when the skin is heated to approximately 43°C, it becomes much more permeable to gases.

Electrochemical Methods

Transcutaneous pO_2 sensors

In 1951, Baumberger and Goodfriend reported that they had been able to determine arterial pO_2 successfully through the intact human skin. By immersing a finger in a phosphate buffer solution heated to 45°C, they found that the pO_2 of the buffer approached that of the alveolar air. Soon thereafter, the physiologic observations of Evans and Naylor and the development by Clark of the membrane-covered polarographic pO_2 electrode led to the development by Lubbers, Huch and Eberhard in the early 1970, of a skin sensor for transcutaneous pO_2 measurements.

The transcutaneous pO_2 electrode is operated in the 'plateau' region of the polarogram, which is dependent on the rate of O_2 diffusion to the cathode and is independent of the applied polarisation voltage. The process takes place behind a membrane that is permeable to O_2, but separates the electrode from its surroundings. The thickness and composition of the membrane determines the rate of O_2 diffusion. For example, thicker membranes prolong the response time by significantly increasing the diffusion time. The most commonly used membrane materials in polarographic pO_2 electrodes include Teflon, polypropylene, and polyethylene. Since the O_2-dependent current flow exhibits a linear relationship, only two known gas mixtures are required for calibrating a pO_2 electrode. Two *in vitro* calibration techniques can be employed: (i) using two precision gas mixtures (e.g. nitrogen and oxygen), and (ii) using a 'zero solution' (e.g. sodium sulphite) and ambient air. Once calibrated, sufficient stability is usually maintained. Typically, the drift of a transcutaneous pO_2 electrode is on the order of ±2 mm Hg/h (±0.3 kPa/h).

Figure 11.9 illustrates a cross section of a typical Clark-type transcutaneous pO_2 sensor. This sensor consists of three glass-sealed Pt cathodes that are separately connected via current amplifiers to a surrounded Ag/AgCl cylindrical anode ring. A buffered KCl electrolyte, which has a low water content to reduce drying of the sensor, is used. The two electrodes are covered with a thin layer of the electrolytic solution that is maintained in place by a membrane. This allows a slow diffusion of O_2 from the skin into the sensor.

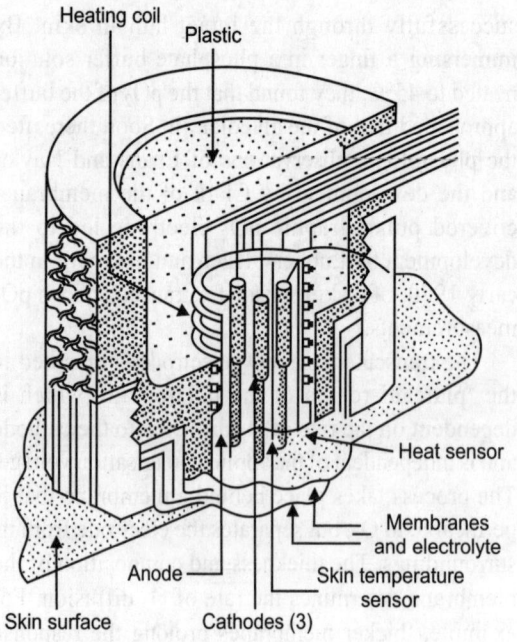

Heating coil
Plastic
Heat sensor
Membranes and electrolyte
Anode
Skin temperature sensor
Cathodes (3)
Skin surface

Fig. 11.9. Cross-section diagram of a transcutaneous pO_2 sensor.

The diffusion of O_2 through the skin is normally very low. Under normal physiological conditions, the pO_2 measured at the surface of the skin using a nonheated transcutaneous pO_2 electrode is nearly zero, regardless of the underlying blood pO_2. To facilitate O_2 diffusion through the skin, abrasion of the skin and drug-induced hyperemia through the application of nicotinic acid cream were used initially. However, since direct skin heating gives a more prolonged and consistent effect, a heating element is now used in all commercial transcutaneous pO_2 sensors. Generally, temperatures between 43°C in premature infants and 44°C in term infants yield adequate vasodilation of the cutaneous blood vessels with minimal skin damage. Heating the skin speeds up O_2 diffusion through the stratum corneum. In addition, it causes vasodilation of the dermal capillaries, which increases blood flow to the region of skin in contact with the sensor. With increased blood flow, more O_2 is available to the tissues surrounding the capillaries in the skin, and consequently, the pO_2 of the blood in these capillary loops more closely approximates that of the arterial blood. Thus measurement by the transcutaneous

sensor approaches more closely the pO_2 of the arterial blood. Heating the blood also shifts the ODC to the right. Therefore, binding of Hb with O_2 is reduced and the release of O_2 to the cells 'is increased. Note also that simultaneously, heat also increases local tissue O_2 consumption. Fortunately, however, these two factors tend to cancel each other.

Typical transcutaneous pO_2 sensors have a round, snap-on plastic ring for mounting purposes. Attachment of the sensor to the skin is achieved using a double-sided, self-adhesive transparent tape. It is essential to ensure a gastight seal around the electrode; otherwise, ambient air will diffuse into the electrode. This will result in erroneous high pO_2 readings. Approximately 10 to 15 min is normally required after mounting of the electrode before adequate skin vasodilation is achieved. Monitoring duration depends on the sensitivity of the skin to possible bums, as well as electrode drift. Usually, 4 to 6 hr of continuous monitoring is possible before changing skin sites is recommended.

Some commercially available transcutaneous pO_2 monitors measure and display the power required to heat the skin and maintain a constant sensor temperature. This power can be used to indicate 'relative local tissue perfusion.' For example, a decrease in the power level is indicative of a decrease in skin circulation, and vice versa. However, accurate determination of skin blood flow is not possible using this approach mainly because the heater power is susceptible to a great extend to surrounding ambient air and body temperature fluctuations.

During the past decade, transcutaneous pO_2 monitoring has found numerous applications in both clinical medicine and physiological research. A wealth of information on the application of transcutaneous pO_2 is available in several excellent monographs. To date, the principal application has been in intensive' care of newborns. This is due primarily to the relatively thin layer of the epidermis at birth and the frequent need to measure O_2 in infants suffering from respiratory distress. The main rationale for monitorig pO_2 in sick infants relates to the need for administering supplemental O_2 while preventing dangerous high arterial pO_2 that, in preterm infants, can lead to retinal and pulmonary tissue damage. Low pO_2, on the other hand, may cause death.

Under appropriate physiological conditions, good correlation between transcutaneous and arterial pO_2 is normally obtained when the patient is not in shock or in hypothermia. During shock, it has been observed in dogs and humans that transcutaneous pO_2 correlates well with cardiac output and therefore may be used to tissue.

In hemodynamically unstable patients, transcutaneous pO_2 does not usually equal arterial pO_2. Even with proper sensor heating, 'any significant decrease in skin perfusion that alters the flow of blood beneath the sensor, and thus the diffusion of O_2 through the skin, will lead to low pO_2 readings that may be as high as 50 per cent of the true arterial pO_2. For example, in severe hypothermia, acidemia, anemia, or shock, skin perfusion may be compromised, and thus transcutaneous pO_2 readings will no longer correlate with central arterial pO_2.

In adults, transcutaneous pO_2 is usually 20 to 40 per cent lower than arterial pO_2 even at a sensor temperature of 45°C. This is attributed to the greater skin thickness, which requires intolerably high sensor temperatures to compensate for the greater effect of metabolism. Although transcutaneous pO_2 monitoring is not widely used in the care of adult patients, studies have shown that it can be useful for evaluating the adequacy of cutaneous circulation in patients with peripheral vascular disease, during shock and cardiopulmonary resuscitation, and during exercise.

Transcutaneous pCO_2 sensors

Continuous pCO_2 monitoring can be advantageous in monitoring lung dysfunction and preventing respiratory alkalosis and acidosis. For example, early respiratory failure is often recognised from an abnormal rise in arterial pCO_2. Furthermore, when artificial ventilation is required, pCO_2 monitoring makes it easier to adjust the parameters of the respirator to suit the specific physiological needs of the patient.

A typical transcutaneous pCO_2 sensor, which is similar in many respects to a transcutaneous pO_2 sensor, is illustrated in Fig. 11.10. This sensor consists

of a glass pH electrode with a concentric Ag/AgCl reference electrode that also serves as a temperature-controlled heater. A small amount of buffer electrolyte (e.g. HCO_3) is placed on the surface of the electrodes and a thin CO_2 permeable membrane (e.g. Teflon) is stretched over the electrode to separate the sensor from its surroundings.

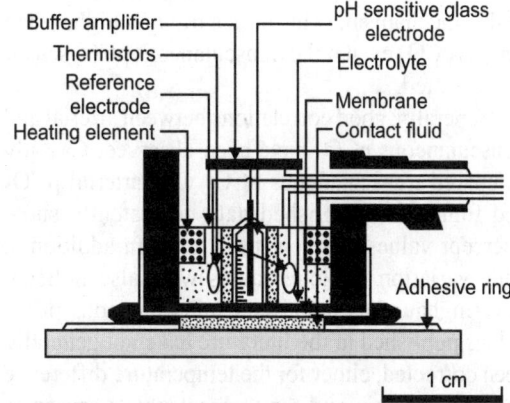

Fig. 11.10. Cross-section diagram of a transcutaneous pCO_2 sensor.

Since a pCO_2 sensor has a high temperature coefficient, it must be calibrated at a temperature at which it will be operated. The effects of heating a transcutaneous pCO_2 sensor must therefore be considered when interpreting the measurements. Heating the sensor results in an increase in (i) pCO_2, since the solubility of CO_2 gas decreases, (ii) local tissue metabolism, and (iii) the rate of CO_2 diffusion through the stratum corneum layer. Therefore, transcutaneous pCO_2 values are higher than the corresponding arterial pCO_2. Despite this difference, the correlation between transcutaneous pCO_2 and arterial pCO_2 is usually satisfactory. Because the electrical signal obtained from a transcutaneous pCO_2 sensor is proportional to the logarithm of the CO_2 concentration, there is no 'zero-point' calibration as in a transcutaneous pO_2 sensor. Therefore, one needs two different precisely analysed gas mixtures for calibration. Usually, gas mixtures containing 5 and 10 per cent CO_2 are used for calibrating a transcutaneous pCO_2 sensor.

Since CO_2 produced by epidermal cells diffuses to the dermal capillaries, transcutaneous pCO_2 values are higher than the corresponding blood pCO_2. The countercurrent blood gas exchange mechanism in the dermal capillaries causes CO_2 diffusion between the parallel arterial and venous sides of the capillary bed. The rising arterial side picks up CO_2 from the existing venous side. Therefore, venous pCO_2 is lower than arterial blood and a maximum pCO_2 gradient is established at the tips of the capillary loops. Because of this mechanism, skin surface pCO_2 is higher than venous pCO_2 even if the transcutaneous pCO_2 sensor is not heated.

Generally, good correlations between arterial and transcutaneous pCO_2 have been observed. Cassady compared transcutaneous pCO_2 with arterial pCO_2 and found that published data consistently show intercept values different from zero. In addition, a wide variation in slope values were also noticed. Severinghaus has noted that transcutaneous pCO_2 values published in the literature have not generally been corrected, either for the temperature difference between the skin and the transcutaneous sensor or for skin metabolism. When these corrections are made, transcutaneous and arterial pCO_2 values are in satisfactory agreement.

Tremper studied the relationship between transcutaneous pCO_2, arterial pCO_2, and cardiac output in dogs during hypercarbia and shock. By haemorrhaging dogs, it was observed that arterial pCO_2 remained unchanged throughout the experiment. On the other hand, transcutaneous pCO_2 increased when cardiac output decreased below 50 per cent of the control. As blood volume was replaced, transcutaneous pCO_2 returned to its original baseline. These findings demonstrated that in hypovolemic shock, transcutaneous pCO_2 can be used as a good indicator of tissue CO_2 levels.

Generally, it is accepted that transcutaneous pCO_2 is a valuable trend monitor in neonates and adults who are not in shock. Since arterial pCO_2 varies inversely with alveolar ventilation, transcutaneous pCO_2 can provide immediate information concerning the effectiveness of spontaneous or mechanical ventilation. Tremper observed that in adult patients transcutaneous pCO_2 values accurately follow the trend in arterial pCO_2 when blood flow is normal. During severe low-flow shock conditions, when the cardiac index falls below 1.5 L/min per square metre,

transcutaneous pCO_2 rises relative to arterial pCO_2 and the transcutaneous readings become primarily flow dependent.

Optical Methods

pCO$_2$ sensors

Besides electrochemical techniques, CO_2 diffusion through the skin has been measured using an infrared absorption technique. An example of such an application uses the Hewlett-Packard model 47210A capnometer and a special sensor. This specially designed miniature sensor, which is normally used with the capnometer for airway measurement of pCO_2, has been adapted for transcutaneous pCO_2 monitoring. The sensor consists of a light source, a filter wheel, and a detector mounted inside a small sealed chamber. The absorption of light emitted from the infrared source is a function of the pCO_2 inside the sealed chamber. The chamber is applied to a flat part of the skin, which must be previously prepared by removing the top dry layer of the skin with repeated applications of a specially designed adhesive tape. To enhance CO_2 diffusion through the skin, the sensor is heated and maintained at a constant temperature of 39°C. This relatively low skin temperature minimises the risk of skin burns and facilities prolonged monitoring without the need for frequent site changes. Although satisfactory correlation between arterial and transcutaneously measured pCO_2 has been demonstrated, this technique has had only limited clinical success mainly because of the inconvenience associated with preparing the skin prior to each measurement.

SaO$_2$ sensors

Ear oximetry: The first application of Beer-Lambert's law to noninvasive arterial SaO_2 measurement was suggested by Wood and Geraci in 1949. Since the ear tissue is an imperfect optical cuvette and thus the light transmitted undergoes partial reflection and multiple scattering by both tissue and blood, initial attempts to measure arterial SaO_2 noninvasively required the subtraction of the light attenuated by the bloodless tissue from the total amount of light transmitted through the ear. This was accomplished by compressing the ear using a transparent pressure capsule that is initially inflated to a pressure that exceeds the arterial blood pressure (e.g. 200 mm Hg), thus rendering the ear pinna almost bloodless. After the light transmission through the bloodless ear is measured and a baseline is established, the pressure in the capsule is released and a second measurement is taken. Arterial SaO_2 was then determined from the difference in these two measurements. Although this approach was the first significant step toward an accurate noninvasive measurement of arterial SaO_2, it was not very successful, due mainly to problems associated with the calibration of the ear probe, inadequate accuracy and reproducibility, and inconvenience.

The first widely used commercial ear oximeter was developed by Hewlett-Packard in 1970. A photograph of the Hewlett-Packard model 47201A ear oximeter sensor is shown in Fig. 11.11, and the principle of its operation is shown in Fig. 11.12. A highintensity tungsten lamp generates a broad spectrum of light. Eight narrow-band interference filters are mounted on a rotating wheel that intercepts the light path sequentially and provide a source of wavelength selection. These filtered light beam pulses enters a fibre optic cable that carries it to the ear. A second fibre optic cable carries the light pulses transmitted through the ear back to the instrument for detection and analysis. To measure arterial SaO_2, the ear probe is attached to the pinna of the ear after the ear has been rubbed briskly for about 20 s to increase local blood flow. A temperature-controlled heater within the probe maintains a temperature of 41°C, causing an increase in local blood flow an proper blood 'arterialisation' after the ear probe has been properly positioned on the ear.

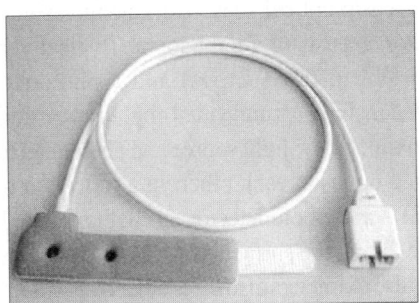

Fig. 11.11. Hewlett-packard model 47201A ear oximeter sensor.

The Hewlett-Packard ear oximeter measures SaO_2 by comparing the intensity of the light passing through the ear at eight selective wavelengths between 650 and 1050 nm. It is assumed that the ear pinna acts as an optical cuvette and consists of a mixture of different light absorbers. The oximeter determines the light transmissions T_n of the ear by comparing the transmitted light intensity at each wavelength to the corresponding value stored during a brief standardisation procedure before the ear probe is applied to the ear. The computation circuits derive SaO_2 according to Beer-Lambert's model of the ear using the equation:

$$\% \ SaO_2 = \frac{A_0 + \sum_{n=1}^{8} A_n \log T_n}{B_0 + \sum_{n=1}^{8} B_n \log T_n} \times 100 \qquad ... \ (11.6)$$

where A_n and B_n are constants that were determined empirically on a diverse range of subjects breathing varying O_2 concentrations. The Hewlett-Packard ear oximeter measures arterial SaO_2 continuously, accurately, and without involving the subject in any calibration or standardisation procedures. The accuracy of the measurement is better than 2.6 per cent saturation regardless of skin colour and ear thickness. The response time of the oximeter can be selected by the operator and is changeable between 1.5 and 4.7s. Bilirubin concentration greater than 10 mg per cent will cause erroneously low readings. Furthermore, cardiogreen dye in concentrations used during cardiac output determination will cause transiently high SaO_2 readings.

The major disadvantage of the Hewlett-Packard ear oximeter is the weight of the fibre optic cable (approximately 100 g) and the size of the ear probe (approximately 10 × 10 cm). This is a particular disadvantage in applications where monitoring of neonates and premature infants is desired. The Hewlett-Packard ear oximeter is no longer being manufactured.

Pulse oximetry

A different optical approach to measure arterial SaO_2 noninvasively has been suggested by Yoshiya. The method is based on the assumption that the change

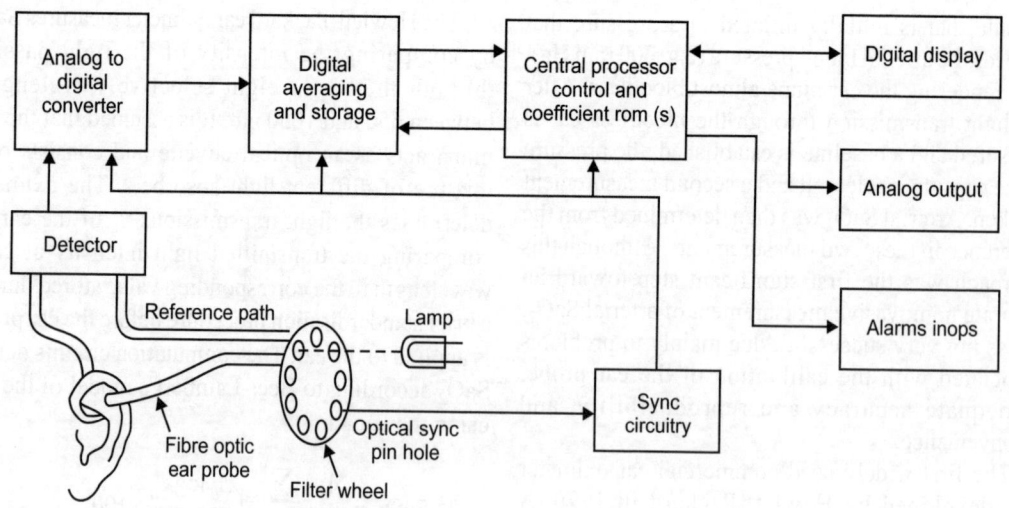

Fig. 11.12. Simplified diagram of the Hewlett-Packard model 47201A ear oximeter.

in light transmitted through tissue during the inflow phase of the cardiac cycle (i.e. systole) is caused solely by the arterial blood. This is illustrated as a photoplethysmogram in Fig. 11.13. It is assumed that there is no pulse from the surrounding tissue and that the pulse of venous blood is normally insignificant. Consequently, arterial SaO_2 can be derived by analysing only the changes in optical density caused by the pulsating arterial bed at a red wavelength (e. g. 660 nm) and a second (isobestic) infrared wavelength (e.g. 805 nm). Typically, a normalisation process is performed by which the pulsatile (ac) component of the red and infrared photopletysmograms is divided by the corresponding nonpulsatile (dc) components, comprised of the light absorbed by tissue, nonpulsatile arterial blood, venous blood, and capillary blood. This process results in a normalised red/infrared ratio R, which is independent of the incident light intensity. Precalibration of a pulse oximeter by the manufacturer is typically performed empirically by correlating the measured ratio R from a group of healthy volunteers with actual arterial SaO_2 values obtained from a standard *in vitro* oximeter. The advantage of this photoplethysmographic approach is that only two wavelengths are required to determine arterial SaO_2. This greatly simplifies the configuration of the optical sensor. Furthermore,

blood 'arterialisation' is not necessary, thus eliminating the need for continuous skin heating.

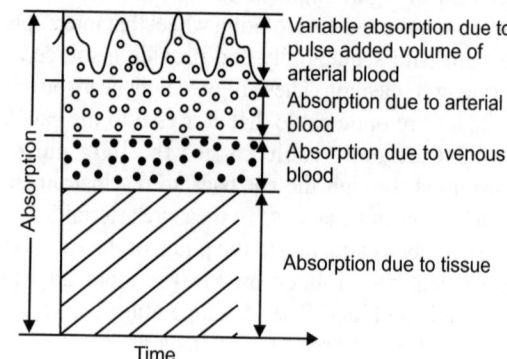

Fig. 11.13. Variations in light attenuation by tissue illustrating the rhythmic effect of arterial pulsation.

The basic optical sensor of a noninvasive pulse oximeter consists of a light source (typically, a pair of red and infrared LEDs) and a photodetector mounted inside a springloaded clip. In a transmission pulse oximeter the light source and photodetector are mounted opposite each other. In a reflection mode, the LEDs and photodetector are both mounted side by side facing the surface of the skin. Besides SaO_2, most pulse oximeters also offer other display features, including pulse rate and analog or bar graphs indicating pulse waveform or pulse amplitude.

Several locations on the body, such as the earlobes, fingertips, and toes, are suitable for monitoring arterial SaO_2 with transmission pulse oximeters. The most popular site is the fingertip, since it is convenient to use and a good photoplethysmographic signal can be obtained. A pulse oximeter and finger sensor depicting the way it is attached to a finger are illustrated in Fig. 11.14. A slightly different configuration (Fig. 11.15) is also available for attaching a transmission sensor to the earlobe and foot. Other locations on the skin that are not accessible to conventional transillumination techniques (e.g. the limbs, torso, or head) can be monitored using a reflection SaO_2 sensor (Fig. 11.16). The sensor, which has been devised by Mendelson can be attached to the surface of the skin using a transparent, self-adhesive, double-sided tape.

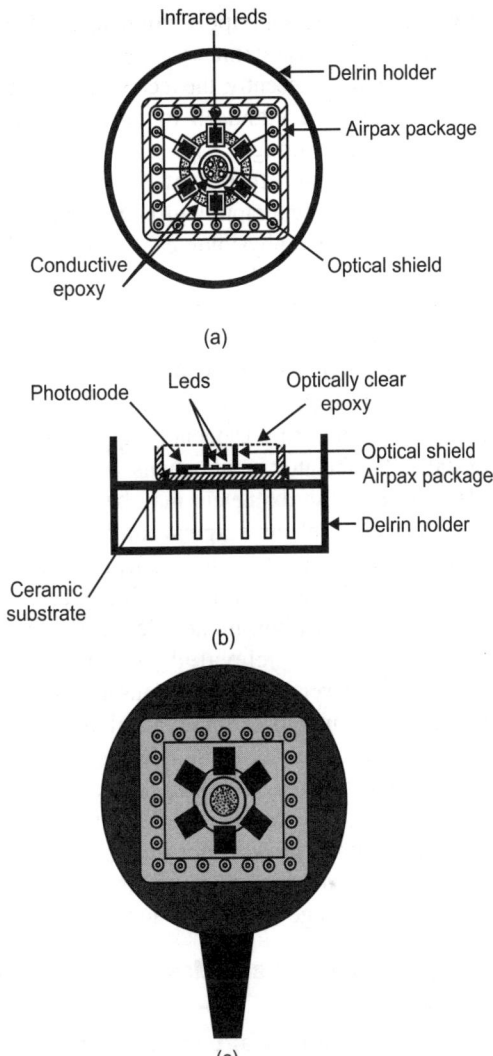

(a)

(b)

(c)

Fig. 11.16. Noninvasive reflection SaO_2 sensor.

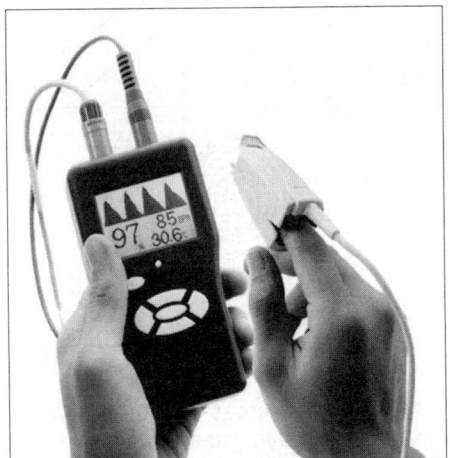

Fig. 11.14. Finger probe assemblies of the nellcor model N-100 pulse oximeter.

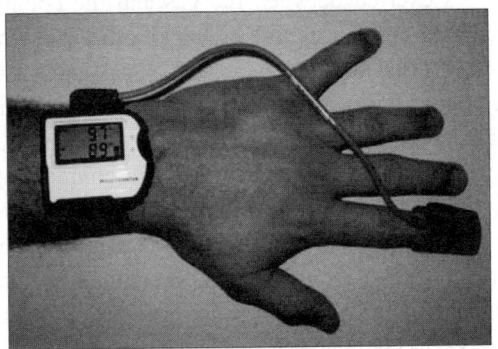

Fig. 11.15. Finger probe of datascope pulse oximeter.

Since pulse oximeters rely on adequate arterial pulsation, significant reduction in peripheral vascular pulsation, such as in hypotension, vasoconstriction, or hypothermia, can produce a signal too small to be processed reliably by the oximeter. Furthermore, motion artifacts can cause erroneous readings. Practically, these artifacts are reduced by digital processing of the analog signals and averaging the SaO_2 values over several seconds before they are displayed. Nevertheless, despite these limitations, the fact that no calibration, stabilisation time, or site preparation is required and the availability of a small, lightweight, and easy-to-apply noninvasive SaO_2 sensor has made pulse oximetry a very useful and popular technique. Recently, the technique has been recommended as a standard of care for basic intraoperative monitoring.

Noninvasive monitoring of SaO_2 by pulse oximetry is becoming a rapidly growing practice in clinical medicine and physiological research. Pulse oximetry is widely used in various applications, including surgery, ICU, hypoxemia screening, exercise monitoring, controlling oxygen administration, sleep studies, and pulmonary function tests. The availability of small, lightweight optical sensors makes SaO_2 monitoring especially applicable for neonatal and ambulatory applications.

The use of pulse oximeters may be limited by interference from electrosurgical units and high-intensity light sources such as surgical lamps. Furthermore, being a two-wavelength device, high concentrations of carbon monoxide, as in smoke inhalation victims, elevated bilirubin and methemoglobin levels, and intravenous dyes such as methylene blue, indigo carmine, and indocyanine green can cause inaccurate readings. Considering the many possible sources of errors, the accuracy of noninvasive pulse oximeters is sufficient for many clinical applications. Most manufacturers claim that their instruments are accurate to within ±2 per cent (SD) in the SaO_2 range between 70 and 100 per cent.

Gas Chromatography and Mass Spectrometry Methods

In addition to the optical and electrochemical techniques described above, other innovative methods for transcutaneous monitoring of blood gases, such as mass spectrometry and gas chromatography, have been investigated. These techniques consist of a small, lightweight, and inexpensive skin sensor that is connected to a remote gas analyser. Transcutaneously diffused gases are then collected in a heated chamber from which they are fed by a gas-impermeable line to a remote analyser where several gases can be analysed simultaneously.

Gas chromatography sensors

The gas chromatograph, like the mass spectrometer, is an instrument capable of separating and analysing

most of the gases of clinical interest using very small samples. Figure 11.17 illustrates a typical transcutaneous gas chromatograph sensor. The sensor consists of a metal body with a fine spiral groove machined across the centre of the front face. The back contains a heating coil and a thermistor. The carrier gas (e.g. He or N_2) enters the spiral groove and travels around it before it exits via the centre. A small amount of sampled gas is injected into the carrier gas stream, which passes through a chromatograph column packed with small polymer beads.

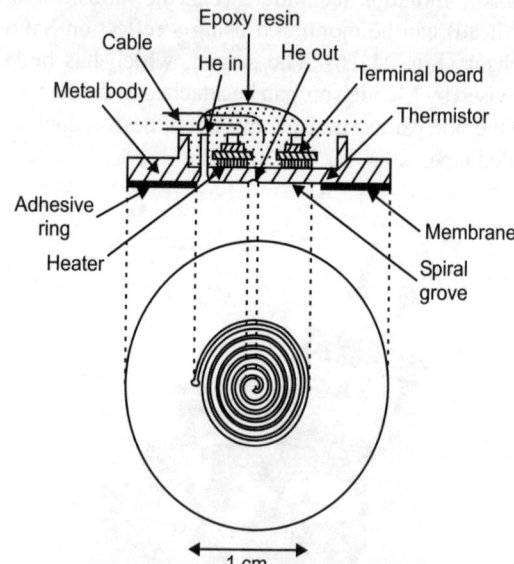

Fig. 11.17. Typical cross-section diagram of a transcutaneous gas chromatograph sensor.

The various components of the sampled gas are separated according to the difference in the molecular forces exerted between the gas and the column material. Thus gases with higher affinities will tend to stay inside the column longer than will gases with relatively lower affinities. A thermal conductivity detector produces a series of short pulses corresponding to the different gas components present in the sample. These pulses are then integrated to provide the unknown amount of sampled gas. The primary disadvantage of transcutaneous gas chromatography is that it is not possible to monitor gases on a continuous basis. This disadvantage may be outweighed by the fact that the system is less expensive and more portable compared to a mass spectrometer.

Mass spectrometry sensors

Transcutaneous mass spectrometry sensors have been utilised in limited clinical studies to demonstrate the feasibility of monitoring O_2, CO_2, N_2, and N_2O_2 gases simultaneously. A schematic diagram of a typical transcutaneous mass spectrometer sensor is shown in Fig. 11.18. This sensor consists of a small stainless-steel chamber with a porous metallic substrate across its open face. Gases collected in this chamber pass by a vacuum pump along a gas-impermeable tube into the ion source of the mass spectrometer. The back of the sensor contains a heating coil and a thermistor for controlling the temperature of the sensor. A membrane is placed across the substrate and sealed to the skin with a doublesided, self-adhesive ring.

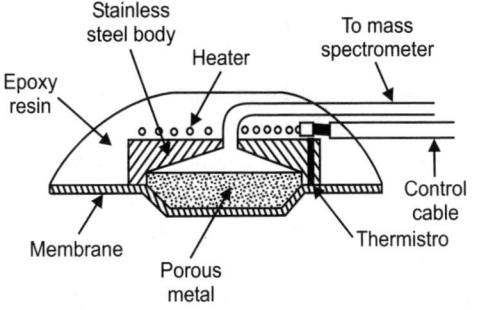

Fig. 11.18. Typical cross-section diagram of a transcutaneous mass spectrometer sensor.

The major drawbacks of transcutaneous mass spectrometry and gas chromatography includes the possibility of gas leaks and the relatively slow response time. The amount of gas that can usually be removed from the skin without disturbing the tissue gas profile is limited to approximately 10^{-7} mL/cm^2 per second. Since very low gas concentrations are obtained, there is a stringent requirement on the inlet gas connections, which must be properly sealed to avoid any leaks that can invalidate the measurements. As a consequence, the signal levels available are very small. The total response time of a mass spectrometer is a function of the time required for the gas molecules to travel from the transcutaneous sensor to the analyser. Typically, this response time is on the order of 20s.

Cerebral Oxygenation Monitoring

Cytochrome aa_3 (cytochrome c oxidase) is the terminal enzyme of the mitochrondrial respiratory chain and catalyses approximately 90 per cent of all O_2 utilisation in the body. This enzyme is of particular importance in monitoring oxidative metabolism because it donates electrons directly to O_2. Therefore, the redox state of cytochrome aa_3 is believed to be an indicator of intracellular O_2 sufficiency. In the oxidised state this enzyme exhibits a distinctive absorption band in the 820 to 870 nm region of the spectra. This band disappears upon reduction when O_2 delivery is compromised. Since Hb and HbO_2 also absorb in this spectral region, multiple wavelengths and the application of appropriate algorithms are required to eliminate the interference of Hb and HbO_2.

Jobsis described an optical method for noninvasive monitoring of cerebral O_2 delivery and utilisation. The technique involves monitoring the steady-state changes of the oxidation-reduction level of cytochrome aa_3 *in vivo* together with changes in local blood volume and hemoglobin oxygenation. Three GaAlAs laser diodes with peak emission wavelengths between 760 and 904 nm were used as light sources. The light is guided to the subject's forehead by a glass fibre optic cable. The light backscattered from the brain which is characteristic of changes in the optical absorption by cytochrome aa_3 and Hb, is collected by a second fibre optic cable located approximately 5 cm lateral from the incident entry beam. The concept has been proven to be a feasible monitoring technique in animals and humans.

Choroidal Eye Oximetry

A special eye oximeter for noninvasive measurement of choroidal blood oxygen saturation in the back of the eye has been developed by Laing and Delore. The measurement is made by shining a multiwavelength light beam into the eye and measuring the amount of light that is backscattered from the ocular fundus using a special fundus camera. Blood oxygen saturation is computed using conventional spectrophotometric oximetry techniques. Since the choroidal blood is characteristic of the blood supply to the brain, this approach has been suggested as a noninvasive diagnostic tool to monitor relative changes in oxygen saturation in the arterial blood supplying the brain.

Palpebral Conjunctiva Monitoring

A palpebral conjunctival (i.e. inner eyelid) sensor, for measuring the pO_2 in a vascular bed perfused by the ophthalmic artery has been developed by Kwan and Fatt and Markle and Fink. This eyelid sensor takes advantage of the unique function of the capillary bed in the palpebral conjunctiva, which is perfused by the internal carotid artery that supplies O_2 to the avascular cornea during sleep. The conjunctival oxygen sensor is essentially a miniaturised unheated version of a Clark-type pO_2 electrode mounted in an oval ophthalmic conformer ring as shown in Fig. 11.19.

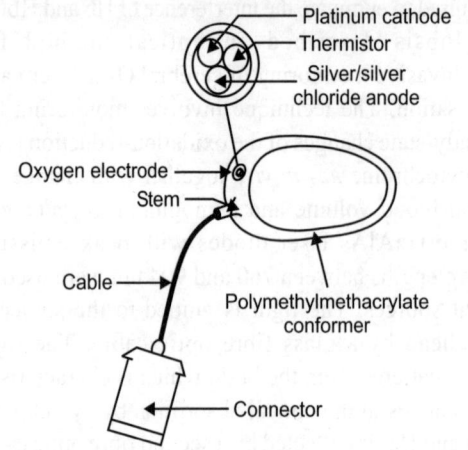

Fig. 11.19. Diagram of the palpebral conjective (eyelid) pO_2 sensor.

The conformer ring, which is made of a plastic biocompatible material (e.g. polymethyl methacrylate), is contoured to the shape of the sclera so that normal vision is not obstructed and free eye movement can be maintained.

The device is designed to fit beneath the eyelid and is positioned such that the pO_2 sensor abuts the inner surface of the superior eyelid. This maintains a close contact with the inner eyelid tissue. Wires emanating from the temporal side of the sensor are connected to the monitoring console. The primary limited applications of this pO_2 sensor to date have been in emergency and critical care medicine.

The conformer ring of the conjunctival sensor has been modified by several researchers to demonstrate the feasibility of using the inner eyelid as a potential site for monitoring blood pH, and SaO_2 in addition to pO_2. Markle and Fink have incorporated a fibre optic pH sensor which has been developed by Peterson into the conformer ring and demonstrated that tissue pH can be measured in normal adult volunteers. Wong have encapsulated a pH-ISFET and a miniature Ag/AgCl reference electrode into the conformer ring and showed that the sensor can be used to follow variations in blood pH in dogs. Mendelson has incorporated a miniature optical reflectance SaO_2 sensor and demonstrated that the palpebral conjunctiva is also a feasible location for monitoring arterial blood SaO_2 in rabbits.

12

Physiological Transducers

INTRODUCTION

Transducers are devices which convert one form of energy into another. Because of the familiar advantages of electric and electronic methods of measurement, it is the usual practice to convert all non-electric phenomenon associated with the physiological events into electric quantities. Numerous methods have since been developed for this purpose and basic principles of physics have extensively been employed. Variation in electric circuit parameters like resistance, capacitance and inductance in accordance with the events to be measured, is the simplest of such methods. Peizo-electric and photoelectric transducers are also very common. Chemical events are detected by measurement of current flow through the electrolyte or by potential changes developed across the membrane electrodes. A number of factors decide the choice of a particular transducer to the used for the study of a specific phenomenon. These factors include:

1. The magnitude of quantity to be measured.
2. The order of accuracy required.
3. The static or dynamic character of the process to be studied.
4. The site of application on the process to be studied.
5. Economic considerations.

PIEZOELECTRIC SENSOR

A piezoelectric sensor is a device that uses the piezoelectric effect to measure pressure, acceleration, strain or force by converting them to an electrical signal (Fig. 12.1).

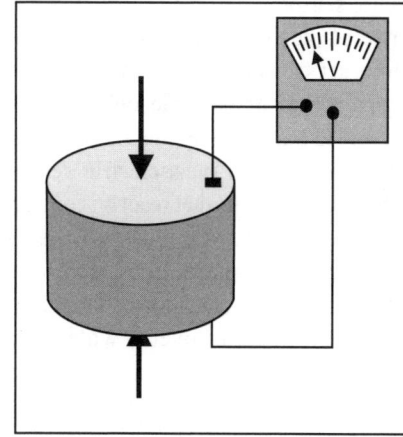

Fig. 12.1. A piezoelectric disk generates a voltage when deformed.

Piezoelectric sensors have proven to be versatile tools for the measurement of various processes. They are used for quality assurance, process control and for research and development in many different industries (Fig. 12.2).

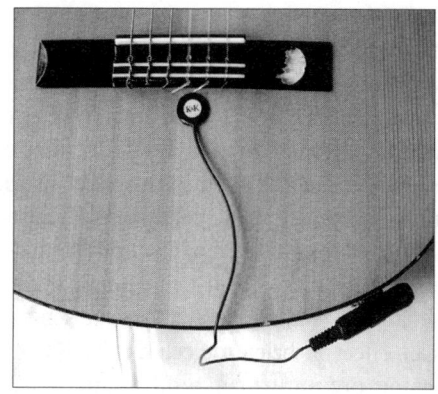

Fig. 12.2. Piezoelectric disk used as a guitar pickup.

It has been successfully used in various applications as for example in medical, aerospace, nuclear instrumentation and in mobiles' touch key pad as pressure sensor.

In the automotive industry piezoelectric elements are used as the standard devices for engine indicating in developing internal combustion engines. The combustion processes are measured with piezoelectric sensors. The sensors are either directly mounted into additional holes into the cylinder head or the spark/glow plug is equipped with a built in miniature piezoelectric sensor.

The rise of piezoelectric technology is directly related to a set of inherent advantages. The high modulus of elasticity of many piezoelectric materials is comparable to that of many metals and goes up to 105 N/m². Even though piezoelectric sensors are electromechanical systems that react on compression, the sensing elements show almost zero deflection. This is the reason why piezoelectric sensors are so rugged, have an extremely high natural frequency and an excellent linearity over a wide amplitude range. Additionally, piezoelectric technology is insensitive to electromagnetic fields and radiation, enabling measurements under harsh conditions. Some materials used (especially gallium phosphate or tourmaline) have an extreme stability over temperature enabling sensors to have a working range of up to 1000°C. Tourmaline shows pyroelectricity in addition to the piezoelectric effect; this is the ability to generate an electrical signal when the temperature of the crystal changes. This effect is also common to piezoceramic materials.

One disadvantage of piezoelectric sensors is that they cannot be used for true static measurements. A static force will result in a fixed amount of charges on the piezoelectric material. While working with conventional readout electronics, imperfect insulating materials, and reduction in internal sensor resistance will result in a constant loss of electrons, and yield a decreasing signal. Elevated temperatures cause an additional drop in internal resistance and sensitivity. The main effect on the piezoelectric effect is that with increasing pressure loads and temperature the sensitivity is reduced due to twin-formation. While quartz sensors need to be cooled during measurements at temperatures above 300°C special types of crystals like GaPo4 gallium phosphate do not show any twin formation up to the melting point of the material itself.

Anyhow, it would be a misconception that piezoelectric sensors can only be used for very fast processes or at ambient conditions. In fact, there are numerous applications that show quasi-static measurements while there are other applications that go to temperatures far beyond 500°C.

Piezoelectric sensors are also seen in nature. Dry bone is piezoelectric, and is thought by some to act as a biological force sensor.

Principle of Operation

Depending on how a piezoelectric material is cut, three main modes of operation can be distinguished: transverse, longitudinal, and shear.

Transverse effect

A force is applied along a neutral axis (y) and the charges are generated along the (x) direction, perpendicular to the line of force. The amount of charge depends on the geometrical dimensions of the respective piezoelectric element. When dimensions a, b, c apply,

$$C_x = d_{xy}F_y b/a,$$

where a is the dimension in line with the neutral axis, b is in line with the charge generating axis and d is the corresponding piezoelectric coefficient.

Longitudinal effect

The amount of charge produced is strictly proportional to the applied force and is independent of size and shape of the piezoelectric element. Using several elements that are mechanically in series and electrically in parallel is the only way to increase the charge output. The resulting charge is:

$$C_x = d_{xx}F_x n,$$

where d_{xx} is the piezoelectric coefficient for a charge in x-direction released by forces applied along x-direction (in pC/N). F_x is the applied Force in x-direction [N] and n corresponds to the number of stacked elements.

Shear effect

Again, the charges produced are strictly proportional to the applied forces and are independent of the element's size and shape. For n elements mechanically in series and electrically in parallel the charge is:

$$C_x = 2d_{xx}F_x n.$$

In contrast to the longitudinal and shear effects, the transverse effect opens the possibility to fine-tune sensitivity on the force applied and the element dimension.

Electrical Properties

Allpiezoelectric transducer has very high DC output impedance and can be modelled as a proportional voltage source and filter network. The voltage V at the source is directly proportional to the applied force, pressure, or strain. The output signal is then related to this mechanical force as if it had passed through the equivalent circuit (Fig. 12.3).

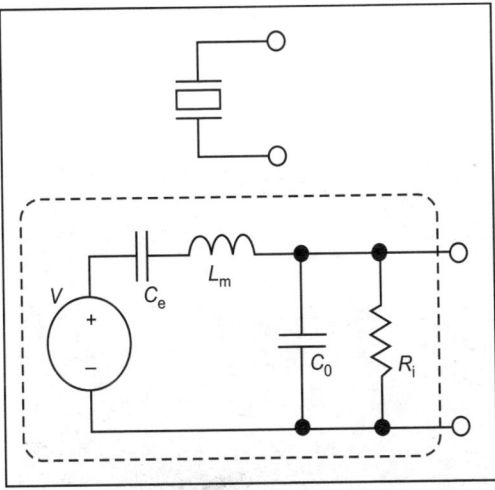

Fig. 12.3. Schematic symbol and electronic model of a piezoelectric sensor.

A detailed model includes the effects of the sensor's mechanical construction and other non-idealities. The inductance L_m is due to the seismic mass and inertia of the sensor itself. C_e is inversely proportional to the mechanical elasticity of the sensor. C_0 represents the static capacitance of the transducer, resulting from an inertial mass of infinite size. R_i is the insulation leakage resistance of the transducer

element. If the sensor is connected to a load resistance, this also acts in parallel with the insulation resistance, both increasing the high-pass cutoff frequency (Fig. 12.4).

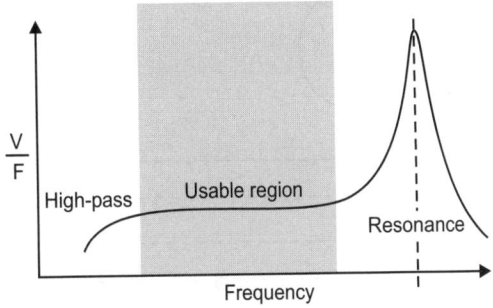

Fig. 12.4. Frequency response of a piezoelectric sensor; output voltage vs applied force.

For use as a sensor, the flat region of the frequency response plot is typically used, between the high-pass cutoff and the resonant peak. The load and leakage resistance need to be large enough that low frequencies of interest are not lost. A simplified equivalent circuit model can be used in this region, in which C_s represents the capacitance of the sensor surface itself, determined by the standard formula for capacitance of parallel plates. It can also be modelled as a charge source in parallel with the source capacitance, with the charge directly proportional to the applied force, as above (Fig. 12.5).

Based on piezoelectric technology various physical quantities can be measured; the most common are pressure and acceleration. For pressure sensors, a thin membrane and a massive base is used, ensuring that an applied pressure specifically loads the elements in one direction. For accelerometers, a seismic mass is attached to the crystal elements. When the accelerometer experiences a motion, the invariant seismic mass loads the elements according to Newton's second law of motion $F = ma$.

The main difference in the working principle between these two cases is the way forces are applied to the sensing elements. In a pressure sensor a thin membrane is used to transfer the force to the elements, while in accelerometers the forces are applied by an attached seismic mass.

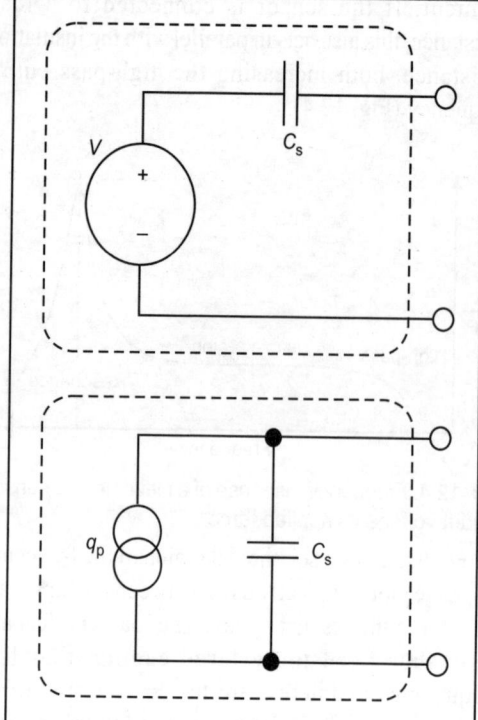

Fig. 12.5. In the flat region, the sensor can be modelled as a voltage source in series with the sensor's capacitance or a charge source in parallel with the capacitance.

Sensors often tend to be sensitive to more than one physical quantity. Pressure sensors show false signal when they are exposed to vibrations. Sophisticated pressure sensors therefore use acceleration compensation elements in addition to the pressure sensing elements. By carefully matching those elements, the acceleration signal (released from the compensation element) is subtracted from the combined signal of pressure and acceleration to derive the true pressure information. Vibration sensors can also be used to harvest otherwise wasted energy from mechanical vibrations. This is accomplished by using piezoelectric materials to convert mechanical strain into usable electrical energy.

Sensing Materials

Two main groups of materials are used for piezoelectric sensors: piezoelectric ceramics and single crystal materials. The ceramic materials (such as PZT ceramic) have a piezoelectric constant/sensitivity that is roughly two orders of magnitude higher than those of single crystal materials and can be produced by inexpensive sintering processes. The piezoeffect in piezoceramics is 'trained', so unfortunately their high sensitivity degrades over time. The degradation is highly correlated with temperature. The less sensitive crystal materials (gallium phosphate, quartz, tourmaline) have a much higher—when carefully handled, almost infinite—long term stability.

ACCELEROMETER

An accelerometer is a device that measures proper acceleration, the acceleration experienced relative to freefall. Single- and multi-axis models are available to detect magnitude and direction of the acceleration as a vector quantity, and can be used to sense orientation, vibration and shock. Micromachined accelerometers are increasingly present in portable electronic devices and video game controllers, to detect the orientation of the device or provide for game input (Fig. 12.6).

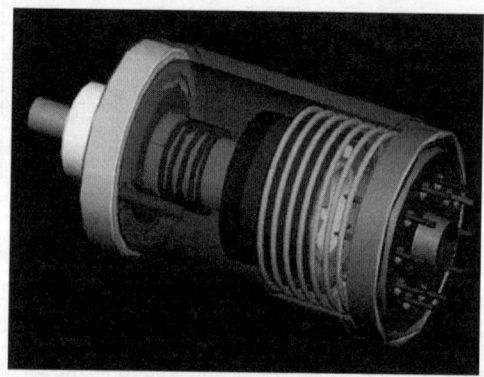

Fig. 12.6. Accelerometer.

Physical Principles

An accelerometer measures proper acceleration which is the acceleration it experiences relative to freefall, and is the acceleration that is felt by people and objects. Put another way, at any point in spacetime the equivalence principle guarantees the existence of a local inertial frame, and an accelerometer measures the acceleration relative to that frame.

As a consequence an accelerometer at rest relative to the earth's surface will indicate approximately 1 g upwards, because any point on the earth's surface is accelerating upwards relative to a local inertial frame. To obtain the acceleration due to motion with respect to the earth, this 'gravity offset' should be subtracted.

The reason for the appearance of a gravitational offset is Einstein's equivalence principle, which states that the effects of gravity on an object are indistinguishable from acceleration of the reference frame. When held fixed in a gravitational field by, for example, applying a ground reaction force or an equivalent upward thrust, the reference frame for an accelerometer (its own casing) accelerates upwards with respect to a free-falling reference frame. The effect of this reference frame acceleration is indistinguishable from any other acceleration experienced by the instrument.

An accelerometer will read *zero* during free fall. This includes use in a spaceship orbiting earth, but not a (non-free) fall with air resistance where drag forces reduce the acceleration until terminal velocity is reached, at which point the device would once again indicate 1 g acceleration upwards.

Acceleration is quantified in the SI unit metres per second per second (m/s^2), in the cgs unit gal (Gal), or popularly in terms of g-force (g).

For the practical purpose of finding the acceleration of objects with respect to the earth, such as for use in an inertial navigation system, a knowledge of local gravity is required. This can be obtained either by calibrating the device at rest, or from a known model of gravity at the approximate current position.

Conceptually, an accelerometer behaves as a damped mass on a spring. When the accelerometer experiences an acceleration, the mass is displaced to the point that the spring is able to accelerate the mass at the same rate as the casing. The displacement is then measured to give the acceleration.

Modern accelerometers are often small micro electro-mechanical systems (MEMS), and are indeed the simplest MEMS devices possible, consisting of

little more than a cantilever beam with a proof mass (also known as seismic mass). Damping results from the residual gas sealed in the device. As long as the Q-factor is not too low, damping does not result in a lower sensitivity.

Micromechanical accelerometers are available in a wide variety of measuring ranges, reaching up to thousands of *g*'s. The designer must make a compromise between sensitivity and the maximum acceleration that can be measured.

DOPPLER EFFECT

The Doppler effect (or Doppler shift), named after Austrian physicist Christian Doppler who proposed it in 1842, is the change in frequency of a wave for an observer moving relative to the source of the wave. It is commonly heard when a vehicle sounding a siren or horn approaches, passes, and recedes from an observer. The received frequency is higher (compared to the emitted frequency) during the approach, it is identical at the instant of passing by, and it is lower during the recession (Fig. 12.7).

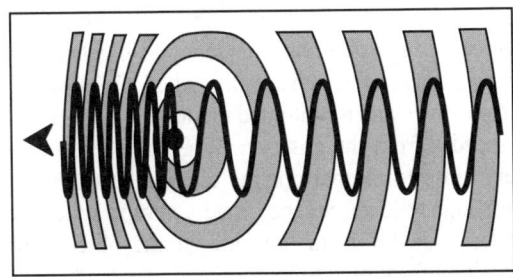

Fig. 12.7. Change of wavelength caused by motion of the source.

For waves that propagate in a medium, such as sound waves, the velocity of the observer and of the source are relative to the medium in which the waves are transmitted. The total Doppler effect may therefore result from motion of the source, motion of the observer, or motion of the medium. Each of these effects is analysed separately. For waves which do not require a medium, such as light or gravity in general relativity, only the relative difference in velocity between the observer and the source needs to be considered.

In classical physics (waves in a medium), where the source and the receiver velocities are not supersonic, the relationship between observed frequency f and emitted frequency f_0 is given by:

$$f = \left(\frac{v + v_r}{v + v_s} \right) f_0$$

where,

v is the velocity of waves in the medium.

v_r is the velocity of the receiver relative to the medium.

v_s is the velocity of the source relative to the medium.

Both velocities v_s and v_r are computed so that the observed frequency is increased when either the source is moving towards the observer or the observer is moving towards the source. The frequency is decreased if either is moving a way from the other.

The above formula assumes that the source is either directly approaching or receding from the observer. If the source approaches the observer at an angle (but still with a constant velocity), the observed frequency that is first heard is higher than the object's emitted frequency. Thereafter, there is a monotonic decrease in the observed frequency as it gets closer to the observer, through equality when it is closest to the observer, and a continued monotonic decrease as it recedes from the observer. When the observer is very close to the path of the object, the transition from high to low frequency is very abrupt. When the observer is far from the path of the object, the transition from high to low frequency is gradual.

In the limit where the speed of the wave is much greater than the relative speed of the source and observer (this is often the case with electromagnetic waves, e.g. light), the relationship between observed frequency f and emitted frequency f_0 is given by:

Observed frequency   Change in frequency

$$f = \left(1 - \frac{v_{s,r}}{C} \right) f_0 \qquad \Delta f = -\frac{v_{s,r}}{C} f_0 = \frac{v_{s,r}}{\lambda_0}$$

where,

$v_{s,r} = v_s - v_r$ is the velocity of the source relative to the receiver: it is positive when the source and the receiver are moving away.

$C =$ is the speed of wave (e.g. 3×10^8 m/s for electromagnetic waves travelling in a vacuum).

$\lambda_0 =$ is the wavelength of the transmitted wave in the reference frame of the source.

These two equations are only accurate to a first order approximation. However, they work reasonably well when the speed between the source and receiver is slow relative to the speed of the waves involved and the distance between the source and receiver is large relative to the wavelength of the waves. If either of these two approximations are violated, the formulae are no longer accurate.

Analysis

The frequency of the sounds that the source *emits* does not actually change. To understand what happens, consider the following analogy. Someone throws one ball every second in a man's direction. Assume that balls travel with constant velocity. If the thrower is stationary, the man will receive one ball every second. However, if the thrower is moving towards the man, he will receive balls more frequently because the balls will be less spaced out. The inverse is true if the thrower is moving away from the man. So it is actually the *wavelength* which is affected; as a consequence, the received frequency is also affected. It may also be said that the velocity of the wave remains constant whereas wavelength changes; hence frequency also changes.

If the source moving away from the observer is emitting waves through a medium with an actual frequency f_0, then an observer stationary relative to the medium detects waves with a frequency f given by:

$$f = \left(\frac{v}{v + v_s} \right) f_0$$

where v_s is positive if the source is moving away from the observer, and negative if the source is moving towards the observer.

A similar analysis for a moving *observer* and a stationary source yields the observed frequency (the receiver's velocity being represented as v_r):

$$f = \left(\frac{v + v_r}{v} \right) f_0$$

where the similar convention applies: v_r is positive if the observer is moving towards the source, and negative if the observer is moving away from the source.

These can be generalised into a single equation with both the source and receiver moving.

$$f = \left(\frac{v + v_r}{v + v_s} \right) f_0$$

With a relatively slow moving source, $v_{s,r}$ is small in comparison to υ and the equation approximates to

$$f = \left(1 - \frac{v_{s,r}}{v} \right) f_0$$

where, $v_{s,r} = v_s - v_r$.

However the limitations mentioned above still apply. When the more complicated exact equation is derived without using any approximations (just assuming that source, receiver, and wave or signal are moving linearly relatively to each other) several interesting and perhaps surprising results are found. For example, as Lord Rayleigh noted in his classic book on sound, by properly moving it would be possible to hear a symphony being played backwards. This is the so-called 'time reversal effect' of the Doppler effect. Other interesting conclusions are that the Doppler effect is time-dependent in general (thus we need to know not only the source and receivers' velocities, but also their positions at a given time), and in some circumstances it is possible to receive two signals or waves from a source, or no signal at all. In addition there are more possibilities than just the receiver approaching the signal and the receiver receding from the signal.

All these additional complications are derived for the classical, i.e. non-relativistic, Doppler effect, but hold for the relativistic Doppler effect as well.

ULTRASOUND

Ultrasound is cyclic sound pressure with a frequency greater than the upper limit of human hearing. Although this limit varies from person to person, it is approximately 20 kilohertz (20,000 hertz) in healthy, young adults and thus, 20 kHz serves as a

useful lower limit in describing ultrasound. The production of ultrasound is used in many different fields, typically to penetrate a medium and measure the reflection signature or supply focused energy. The reflection signature can reveal details about the inner structure of the medium, a property also used by animals such as bats for hunting. The most well known application of ultrasound is its use in sonography to produce pictures of fetuses in the human womb. There are a vast number of other applications as well (Fig. 12.8).

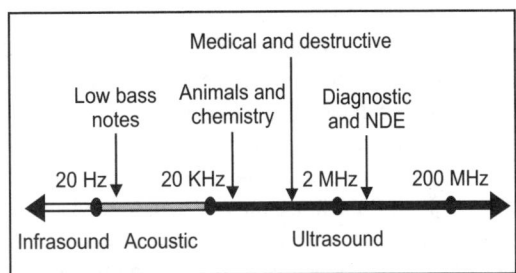

Fig. 12.8. Approximate frequency ranges corresponding to ultrasound, with rough guide of some applications.

Ability to Hear Ultrasound

The upper frequency limit in humans (approximately 20 kHz) is due to limitations of the middle ear, which acts as a low-pass filter. Ultrasonic hearing can occur if ultrasound is fed directly into the skull bone and reaches the cochlea without passing through the middle ear. Carefully-designed scientific studies have been performed supporting what the authors call the hypersonic effect—that even without consciously hearing it, high-frequency sound can have a measurable effect on the mind.

It is a fact in psychoacoustics that children can hear some high-pitched sounds that older adults cannot hear, because in humans the upper limit pitch of hearing tends to become lower with age. A cell phone company has used this to create ring signals supposedly only able to be heard by younger humans; but many older people claim to be able to hear it, which is likely given the considerable variation of age-related deterioration in the upper hearing threshold.

Some animals — such as dogs, cats, dolphins, bats, and mice — have an upper frequency limit that is greater than that of the human ear and thus can hear ultrasound, which is how a dog whistle works.

Diagnostic Sonography

Medical sonography (ultrasonography) is an ultrasound-based diagnostic medical imaging technique used to visualise muscles, tendons, and many internal organs, to capture their size, structure and any pathological lesions with real time tomographic images. Ultrasound has been used by sonographers to image the human body for at least 50 years and has become one of the most widely used diagnostic tools in modern medicine. The technology is relatively inexpensive and portable, especially when compared with other techniques, such as magnetic resonance imaging (MRI) and computed tomography (CT). Ultrasound is also used to visualise fetuses during routine and emergency prenatal care. Such diagnostic applications used during pregnancy are referred to as obstetric sonography.

As currently applied in the medical field, properly performed ultrasound poses no known risks to the patient. Sonography is generally described as a 'safe test' because it does not use mutagenic ionising radiation, which can pose hazards such as chromosome breakage and cancer development. However, ultrasonic energy has two potential physiological effects: it enhances inflammatory response; and it can heat soft tissue. Ultrasound energy produces a mechanical pressure wave through soft tissue. This pressure wave may cause microscopic bubbles in living tissues and distortion of the cell membrane, influencing ion fluxes and intracellular activity. When ultrasound enters the body, it causes molecular friction and heats the tissues slightly. This effect is typically very minor as normal tissue perfusion dissipates most of the heat, but with high intensity, it can also cause small pockets of gas in body fluids or tissues to expand and contract/collapse in a phenomenon called cavitation; however this is not known to occur at diagnostic power levels used by modern diagnostic ultrasound units.

Obstetric ultrasound is primarily used to:

1. Date the pregnancy (gestational age).
2. Confirm fetal viability.
3. Determine location of fetus, intrauterine vs ectopic.
4. Check the location of the placenta in relation to the cervix.
5. Check for the number of fetuses (multiple pregnancy).
6. Check for major physical abnormalities.
7. Assess fetal growth (for evidence of intrauterine growth restriction (IUGR)).
8. Check for fetal movement and heartbeat.
9. Determine the sex of the baby.

According to the European committee of medical ultrasound safety (ECMUS) 'Ultrasonic examinations should only be performed by competent personnel who are trained and updated in safety matters. Ultrasound produces heating, pressure changes and mechanical disturbances in tissue. Diagnostic levels of ultrasound can produce temperature rises that are hazardous to sensitive organs and the embryo/fetus. Biological effects of non-thermal origin have been reported in animals but, to date, no such effects have been demonstrated in humans, except when a microbubble contrast agent is present.' Nonetheless, care should be taken to use low power settings and avoid pulsed wave scanning of the fetal brain unless specifically indicated in high risk pregnancies.

It should be noted that obstetrics is not the only use of ultrasound. Soft tissue imaging of many other parts of the body is conducted with ultrasound. Other scans routinely conducted are cardiac, renal, liver and gallbladder (hepatic). Other common applications include musculo-skeletal imaging of muscles, ligaments and tendons, ophthalmic ultrasound (eye) scans and superficial structures such as testicle, thyroid, salivary glands and lymph nodes. Because of the real time nature of ultrasound, it is often used to guide interventional procedures such as fine needle aspiration FNA or biopsy of masses for cytology or histology testing in the breast, thyroid, liver, kidney, lymph nodes, muscles and joints.

Ultrasound scanners have different Doppler-techniques to visualise arteries and veins. The most common is colour doppler or power doppler, but also other techniques like b-flow are used to show bloodflow in an organ. By using pulsed wave doppler or continuous wave doppler bloodflow velocities can be calculated.

Biomedical Ultrasonic Applications

Ultrasound also has therapeutic applications, which can be highly beneficial when used with dosage precautions:

1. According to RadiologyInfo, ultrasounds are useful in the detection of pelvic abnormalities and can involve techniques known as abdominal (transabdominal) ultrasound, vaginal (transvaginal or endovaginal) ultrasound in women, and also rectal (transrectal) ultrasound in men.

2. Focused high-energy ultrasound pulses can be used to break calculi such as kidney stones and gallstones into fragments small enough to be passed from the body without undue difficulty, a process known as lithotripsy.

3. Treating benign and malignant tumors and other disorders via a process known as high intensity focused ultrasound (HIFU), also called focused ultrasound surgery (FUS). In this procedure, a generally lower frequencies than medical diagnostic ultrasound is used (250–2000 kHz), but significantly higher time-averaged intensities. The treatment is often guided by magnetic resonance imaging (MRI)—this is called Magnetic resonance-guided focused ultrasound (MRgFUS). Delivering chemotherapy to brain cancer cells and various drugs to other tissues is called acoustic targeted drug delivery (ATDD). These procedures generally use high frequency ultrasound (1–10 MHz) and a range of intensities (0–20 watts/cm^2). The acoustic energy is focused on the tissue of interest to agitate its matrix and make it more permeable for therapeutic drugs.

4. Therapeutic ultrasound, a technique that uses more powerful ultrasound sources to generate cellular effects in soft tissue has fallen out of favour as research has shown a lack of efficacy and a lack of scientific basis for proposed biophysical effects. Ultrasound has been used in cancer treatment.

5. Cleaning teeth in dental hygiene.

6. Focused ultrasound sources may be used for cataract treatment by phacoemulsification.

7. Additional physiological effects of low-intensity ultrasound have recently been discovered, e.g. the ability to stimulate bone-growth and its potential to disrupt the blood-brain barrier for drug delivery.

8. Ultrasound is essential to the procedures of ultrasound-guided sclerotherapy and endovenous laser treatment for the non-surgical treatment of varicose veins.

9. Ultrasound-assisted lipectomy is lipectomy assisted by ultrasound. Liposuction can also be assisted by ultrasound.

10. Doppler ultrasound is being tested for use in aiding tissue plasminogen activator treatment in stroke sufferers in the procedure called ultrasound-enhanced systemic thrombolysis.

11. Low intensity pulsed ultrasound is used for therapeutic tooth and bone regeneration.

12. Ultrasound can also be used for elastography. This can be useful in medical diagnoses, as elasticity can discern healthy from unhealthy tissue for specific organs/growths. In some cases unhealthy tissue may have a lower system Q, meaning that the system acts more like a large heavy spring as compared to higher values of system Q (healthy tissue) that respond to higher forcing frequencies. Ultrasonic elastography is different from conventional ultrasound, as a transceiver (pair) and a transmitter are used instead of only a transceiver. One transducer acts as both the transmitter and receiver to image the region of interest over time. The extra transmitter is a very low frequency trans-mitter, and perturbs the system so the unhealthy tissue oscillates at a low frequency and the healthy tissue does not. The transreciver, which operates at a high frequency (typically MHz) then measures the displacement of the unhealthy tissue (oscillating at a much lower frequency). The movement of the slowly oscillating tissue is

used to determine the elasticity of the material, which can then be used to distinguish healthy tissue from the unhealthy tissue.

13. Ultrasound has been shown to act synergistically with antibiotics in bacterial cell killing.

14. Ultrasound has been postulated to allow thicker eukaryotic cell tissue cultures by promoting nutrient penetration.

15. Ultrasound in the low MHz range in the form of standing waves is an emerging tool for contactless separation, concentration and manipulation of microparticles and biological cells, a method referred to as acoustophoresis. The basis is the acoustic radiation force, a non-linear effect which causes particles to be attracted to either the nodes or anti-nodes of the standing wave depending on the acoustic contrast factor, which is a function of the sound velocities and densities of the particle and of the medium in which the particle is immersed.

Some sorts of ultrasound can disintegrate biological cells including bacteria. This has uses in biological science and in killing bacteria in sewage. High power ultrasound at frequency of around 20 kHz produces cavitation that facilitates particle disintegration.

Ultrasonic Range Finding

A common use of ultrasound is in range finding; this use is also called SONAR, (sound navigation and ranging). This works similarly to RADAR (radio detection and ranging): An ultrasonic pulse is generated in a particular direction. If there is an object in the path of this pulse, part or all of the pulse will be reflected back to the transmitter as an echo and can be detected through the receiver path. By measuring the difference in time between the pulse being transmitted and the echo being received, it is possible to determine how far away the object is (Fig. 12.9).

The measured travel time of SONAR pulses in water is strongly dependent on the temperature and the salinity of the water. Ultrasonic ranging is also applied for measurement in air and for short distances.

Such method is capable for easily and rapidly measuring the layout of rooms.

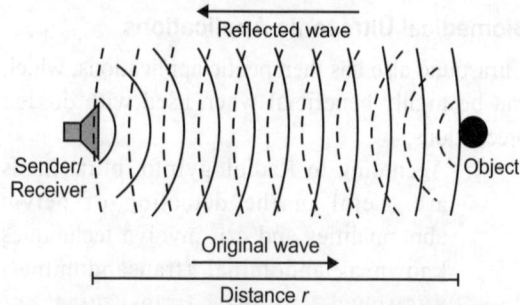

Fig. 12.9. Principle of an active sonar.

Although range finding underwater is performed at both sub-audible and audible frequencies for great distances (1 to several kilometers), ultrasonic range finding is used when distances are shorter and the accuracy of the distance measurement is desired to be finer. Ultrasonic measurements may be limited through barrier layers with large salinity, temperature or vortex differentials. Ranging in water varies from about hundreds to thousands of meters, but can be performed with centimeters to meters accuracy.

Because of their high amplitude to wavelength ratio, ultrasonic waves commonly display nonlinear propagation.

Occupational exposure to ultrasound in excess of 120 dB may lead to hearing loss. Exposure in excess of 155 dB may produce heating effects that are harmful to the human body, and it has been calculated that exposures above 180 dB may lead to death.

OPHTHALMOLOGY

Ophthalmology is a branch of medicine which deals with the diseases and surgery of the visual pathways, including the eye, hairs, and areas surrounding the eye, such as the lacrimal system and eyelids. The term ophthalmologist is an eye specialist for medical and surgical problems. Since ophthalmologists perform operations on eyes, they are considered to be both a surgical and medical specialty (Fig. 12.10).

The word ophthalmology comes from the Greek roots ophthalmos meaning eye and logos meaning word, thought or discourse; ophthalmology literally means 'the science of eyes'. 'Opthomology' is a common mis-hearing or mis-remembering of the term. As a discipline, it applies to animal eyes also, since the differences from human practice are surprisingly minor and are related mainly to differences in anatomy or prevalence, not differences in disease processes. However, veterinary medicine is regulated separately in many countries and states/provinces resulting in few ophthalmologists treating both humans and animals.

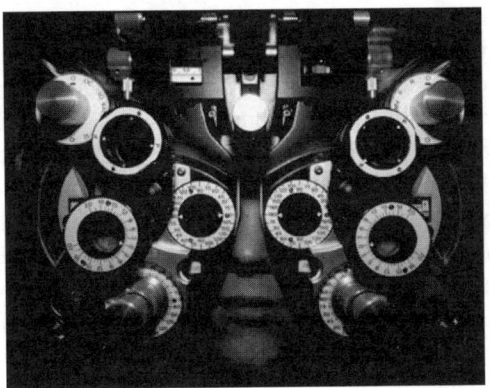

Fig. 12.10. A phoropter in use.

ECHOCARDIOGRAPHY

An echocardiogram, often referred to in the medical community as a cardiac ECHO or simply an ECHO, is a sonogram of the heart (it is not abbreviated as ECG, which in medicine usually refers to an electrocardiogram). Also known as a cardiac ultrasound, it uses standard ultrasound techniques to image two-dimensional slices of the heart. The latest ultrasound systems now employ 3D real-time imaging.

In addition to creating two-dimensional pictures of the cardiovascular system, an echocardiogram can also produce accurate assessment of the velocity of blood and cardiac tissue at any arbitrary point using pulsed or continuous wave Doppler ultrasound. This allows assessment of cardiac valve areas and function, any abnormal communications between the left and right side of the heart, any leaking of blood through the valves (valvular regurgitation), and calculation of the cardiac output as well as the ejection fraction.

Echocardiography was an early medical application of ultrasound. Echocardiography was also the first application of intravenous contrast-enhanced ultrasound. This technique injects gas-filled microbubbles into the venous system to improve tissue and blood delineation. Contrast is also currently being evaluated for its effectiveness in evaluating myocardial perfusion. It can also be used with Doppler ultrasound to improve flow-related measurements.

Echocardiography is either performed by cardiac sonographers or doctors trained in cardiology.

Echocardiography is used to diagnose cardiovascular diseases. In fact, it is one of the most widely used diagnostic tests for heart disease. It can provide a wealth of helpful information, including the size and shape of the heart, its pumping capacity and the location and extent of any damage to its tissues. It is especially useful for assessing diseases of the heart valves. It not only allows doctors to evaluate the heart valves, but it can detect abnormalities in the pattern of blood flow, such as the backward flow of blood through partly closed heart valves, known as regurgitation. By assessing the motion of the heart wall, echocardiography can help detect the presence and assess the severity of coronary artery disease, as well as help determine whether any chest pain is related to heart disease. Echocardiography can also help detect hypertrophic cardiomyopathy. The biggest advantage to echocardiography is that it is noninvasive (doesn't involve breaking the skin or entering body cavities) and has no known risks or side effects.

Transthoracic Echocardiogram

A standard echocardiogram is also known as a transthoracic echocardiogram (TTE), or cardiac ultrasound. In this case, the echocardiography transducer (or probe) is placed on the chest wall (or thorax) of the subject, and images are taken through the chest wall. This is a non-invasive, highly accurate and quick assessment of the overall health of the heart.

Transoesophageal Echocardiogram

This is an alternative way to perform an echocardiogram. A specialised probe containing an ultrasound transducer at its tip is passed into the patient's oesophagus. This allows image and Doppler evaluation which can be recorded. This is known as a transoesophageal echocardiogram, or TOE (TEE in the United States).

3-Dimensional Echocardiography

3-D echocardiography is now possible, using an ultrasound probe with an array of transducers and an appropriate processing system. This enables detailed anatomical assessment of cardiac pathology, particularly valvular defects, and cardiomyopathies. The ability to slice the virtual heart in infinite planes in an anatomically appropriate manner and to reconstruct 3-dimensional images of anatomic structures make 3-D echocardiography unique for the understanding of the congenitally malformed heart.

INTRAVASCULAR ULTRASOUND

Intravascular ultrasound (IVUS) is a medical imaging methodology using a specially designed catheter with a miniaturised ultrasound probe attached to the distal end of the catheter. The proximal end of the catheter is attached to computerised ultrasound equipment. It allows the application of ultrasound technology to see from inside blood vessels out through the surrounding blood column, visualising the endothelium (inner wall) of blood vessels in living individuals.

The arteries of the heart (the coronary arteries) are the most frequent imaging target for IVUS. IVUS is used in the coronary arteries to determine the amount of atheromatous plaque built up at any particular point in the epicardial coronary artery. The progressive accumulation of plaque within the artery wall over decades is the setup for vulnerable plaque which, in turn, leads to heart attack and stenosis (narrowing) of the artery (known as coronary artery lesions). IVUS is of use to determine both plaque volume within the wall of the artery and/or the degree of stenosis of the artery lumen.

It can be especially useful in situations in which angiographic imaging is considered unreliable; such as for the lumen of ostial lesions or where angiographic images do not visualise lumen segments

adequately, such as regions with multiple overlapping arterial segments. It is also used to assess the effects of treatments of stenosis such as with hydraulic angioplasty expansion of the artery, with or without stents, and the results of medical therapy over time.

Advantages Over Angiography

Arguably the most valuable use of IVUS is to visualise plaque, which cannot be seen by angiography. It has been increasingly used in research to better understand the behaviour of the atherosclerosis process in living people. Based on the angiographic view and long popular medical beliefs, it had long been assumed that areas of high grade stenosis (narrowing) of the lumen (opening) within the coronary arteries, visible by angiography, were the likely points at which most myocardial infarctions (heart attacks) would occur. Research using IVUS has helped to reveal the fallacy (in most instances) of this belief.

IVUS enables accurately visualising not only the lumen of the coronary arteries but also the atheroma (membrane/cholesterol loaded white blood cells) 'hidden' within the wall. IVUS has thus enabled advances in clinical research providing a more thorough perspective and better understanding.

Disadvantages Versus Angiography

The primary disadvantages of IVUS being used routinely in a cardiac catheterisation laboratory are its expense, the increase in the time of the procedure, and the fact that it is considered an interventional procedure, and should only be performed by angiographers that are trained in interventional cardiology techniques. In addition, there may be additional risk imposed by the use of the IVUS catheter.

Additionally, IVUS adds significant additional examination time and some increased risk to the patient beyond performing a standard diagnostic angiographic examination. This increase is significantly less when IVUS is part of a percutaneous coronary intervention, since much of the setup is the same for the intervention as for the IVUS imaging. IVUS continues to improve and some manufacturers have proposed building IVUS technology into angioplasty and stent balloon catheters, a potential major advance, but limited by complexity, cost and increased bulk of the catheters.

Method

To visualise an artery or vein, angiographic techniques are used and the physician positions the tip of a guidewire, usually 0.36 mm (0.014″) diameter with a very soft and pliable tip and about 200 cm long. The physician steers the guidewire from outside the body, through angiography catheters and into the blood vessel branch to be imaged.

The ultrasound catheter tip is slid in over the guidewire and positioned, using angiography techniques so that the tip is at the farthest away position to be imaged. The sound waves are emitted from the catheter tip, are usually in the 10–20 MHz range, and the catheter also receives and conducts the return echo information out to the external computerised ultrasound equipment which constructs and displays a real time ultrasound image of a thin section of the blood vessel currently surrounding the catheter tip, usually displayed at 30 frames/second image.

The guide wire is kept stationary and the ultrasound catheter tip is slid backwards, usually under motorised control at a pullback speed of 0.5 mm/s. (The motorised pullback tends to be smoother than hand movement by the physician.)

The (i) blood vessel wall inner lining, (ii) atheromatous disease within the wall, and (iii) connective tissues covering the outer surface of the blood vessel are echogenic, i.e. they return echoes making them visible on the ultrasound display.

By contrast, the blood itself and the healthy muscular tissue portion of the blood vessel wall is relatively echolucent, just black circular spaces, in the images.

Heavy calcium deposits in the blood vessel wall both heavily reflect sound, i.e. are very echogenic, but are also distinguishable by shadowing. Heavy calcification blocks sound transmission beyond and so, in the echo images, are seen as both very bright areas but with black shadows behind (from the vantage point of the catheter tip emitting the ultrasound waves).

Uses

IVUS, as outlined above, has been the best technology, so far, to demonstrate the anatomy of the artery wall in living animals and humans. It has led to an explosion of better understanding and research on both (i) the behaviour of the atherosclerosis process, and (ii) the effects of different treatment strategies for changing the evolution of the atherosclerosis disease process. This has been important given that atherosclerosis is the single most frequent disease process for the greatest percentage of individuals living in first world countries.

Intravascular ultrasound in the coronary anatomy

While the routine use of IVUS during percutaneous coronary intervention does not improve short term outcomes, there are a number of situations in which IVUS is of particular use in the treatment of coronary artery disease of the heart. In particular in cases when the degree of stenosis of a coronary artery is unclear, IVUS can directly quantify the percentage of stenosis and give insight into the anatomy of the plaque.

One particular use of IVUS in the coronary anatomy is in the quantification of left main disease in cases where routine coronary angiography gives equivocal results. Many studies in the past have shown that significant left main disease can increase mortality, and that intervention (either coronary artery bypass graft surgery or percutaneous coronary intervention) to reduce mortality is necessary when the left main stenosis is significant.

When using IVUS to determine whether an individual's left main disease is clinically significant, in terms of the desirability of physical intervention, the two most widely used parameters are the degree of stenosis and the minimal lumen area. A cross sectional area of $\leqslant 7$ mm^2 in a symptomatic individual or $\leqslant 6$ mm^2 in an asymptomatic individual is considered to be clinically significant and warrants intervention to improve one-year mortality. However, these exact cutoffs are up for debate and different cutoff cross-sectional areas may be used in practice depending on differing interpretations of the trial data.

Validating the efficacy of new treatments

Because IVUS is widely available in coronary catheterisation labs worldwide and can accurately quantify arterial plaque, especially within the coronary arteries, it is increasingly being used to evaluate newer and evolving strategies for the treatment of coronary artery disease, including the statins, torcetrapib and other approaches.

Tomography

Tomography is imaging by sections or sectioning, through the use of wave of energy. A device used in tomography is called a tomograph, while the image produced is a tomogram. The method is used in radiology, archaeology, biology, geophysics, oceanography, materials science, astrophysics and other sciences. In most cases it is based on the mathematical procedure called tomographic reconstruction. The word was derived from the Greek word tomos which means 'a section', 'a slice' or 'a cutting'. A tomography of several sections of the body is known as a polytomography (Fig. 12.11) .

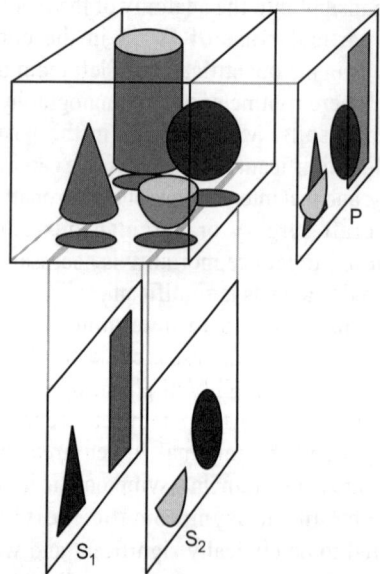

Fig. 12.11. Basic principle of tomography: superposition free tomographic cross sections S₁ and S₂ compared with the projected image P.

In conventional medical X-ray tomography, clinical staff make a sectional image through a body by moving an X-ray source and the film in opposite directions during the exposure. Consequently,

structures in the focal plane appear sharper, while structures in other planes appear blurred. By modifying the direction and extent of the movement, operators can select different focal planes which contain the structures of interest. Before the advent of more modern computer-assisted techniques, this technique, ideated in the 1930s by the radiologist Alessandro Vallebona, proved useful in reducing the problem of superimposition of structures in projectional (shadow) radiography.

Modern tomography

More modern variations of tomography involve gathering projection data from multiple directions and feeding the data into a tomographic reconstruction software algorithm processed by a computer. Different types of signal acquisition can be used in similar calculation algorithms in order to create a tomographic image. With current technology, tomograms are derived using several different physical phenomena listed in the following Table.12.1.

Table.12.1. Tomograms are derived using several different physical phenomena.

Physical phenomenon	Type of tomograph
X-rays	CT
Gamma rays	SPECT
Electron-positron annihilation	PET
Electrons	Electron tomography or 3D TEM
Ions	Atom probe

Some recent advances rely on using simultaneously integrated physical phenomena, e.g. X-rays for both CT and angiography, combined CT/MRI and combined CT/PET.

The term *volume imaging* might subsume these technologies more accurately than the term tomography. However, in the majority of cases in clinical routine, staff request output from these procedures as 2-D slice images. As more and more clinical decisions come to depend on more advanced volume visualisation techniques, the terms tomography/tomogram may go out of fashion.

Many different reconstruction algorithms exist. Most algorithms fall into one of two categories: filtered back projection (FBP) and iterative reconstruction (IR). These procedures give inexact results: they represent a compromise between accuracy and computation time required. FBP demands fewer computational resources, while IR generally produces fewer artifacts (errors in the reconstruction) at a higher computing cost.

Although MRI and ultrasound make cross sectional images they don't acquire data from different directions. In MRI spatial information is obtained by using magnetic fields. In ultrasound, spatial information is obtained simply by focusing and aiming a pulsed ultrasound beam.

Synchrotron X-ray tomographic microscopy

Recently a new technique called synchrotron X-ray tomographic microscopy (SRXTM) allows for detailed three dimensional scanning of fossils.

Virtual Image Generation from the Linear Array Image

The so called push broom images are generated by the linear array technology by which successive lines on the ground are systematically scanned. Consequently, these images have somehow a dynamic geometry in the sense that each image line has its own exterior orientation parameters leading effectively to a multi-projection image. This dynamism in geometry complicates the space resection intersection operations with rigorous mathematical models and necessitates the incorporation of the observed values for the satellite trajectory. Alternatively, the generic approach may be utilised. However, this approach has also its own shortcomings regarding the requirement of large number of the GCPs and resulted instability of the mathematical solution. In this section we propose a pre-processing stage through which a virtual single projection image is generated from the linear array image by intersecting each pixel position in the scan lines with an approximate digital elevation model (DEM) by a forward intersection approach. This is then followed by an inverse projection to the virtual

image plane and gray shade interpolation. The generated virtual image more or less satisfies the geometry of a real single projection image and hence can be treated with conventional mathematical models used in photogrammetry. The errors in the generated virtual image are partly due to the approximations of the DEM and partly due to the attitude and altitude variations of the scan lines. Assuming that the DEM error is negligible, the orientation and position variations of the scan lines may be regarded as a sort of systematic image displacement which can be handled by a rigorous self calibration or similar mathematical models. The potential of the proposed approach, as far as the impact of the relief displacement is concerned, is investigated using a simulation strategy.

Typically, two different approaches of rigorous and generic mathematical models are utilised for the geometric correction of the linear array images. The former approach to be implemented inevitably takes the form of a multi-projection model whereas with the latter method multi-projection assumption is not necessary. Thus, the main drawback of the rigorous sensor model is its complex mathematical model which requires some approximations for the exterior orientation parameters of each scan line. With the generic sensor model, although much simpler mathematical model is used, the number and distribution of GCPs are crucial. In this section an alternative approach is proposed by which a virtual image having a single projection centre is first generated using the linear array scan lines. The virtual image is then regarded as a conventional camera generated image. Space intersection is then performed on the stereo-virtual images to generate the object space coordinates. In the section that follows, the adopted procedures for the generation of the virtual image are outlined.

Virtual image generation

The geometry of the single and multi-projection imaging devices is different (Fig.12.12). The difference lies in the fact that with the single projection images the relief and tilt displacements are radial from the nadir point and iso-centre respectively. These points are unique in a single-projection image.

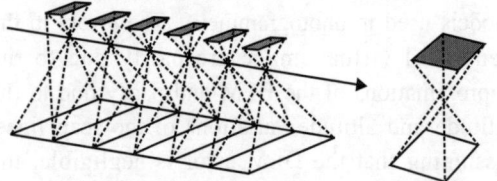

Fig.12.12. Multi and single-projection images.

With the linear array images, on the other hand, each scan line has its own nadir point and iso-centre. Therefore, there are as many nadir points and iso-centres as the number of the scan lines. Figure 12.13, visualises different geometry of these two classes of images.

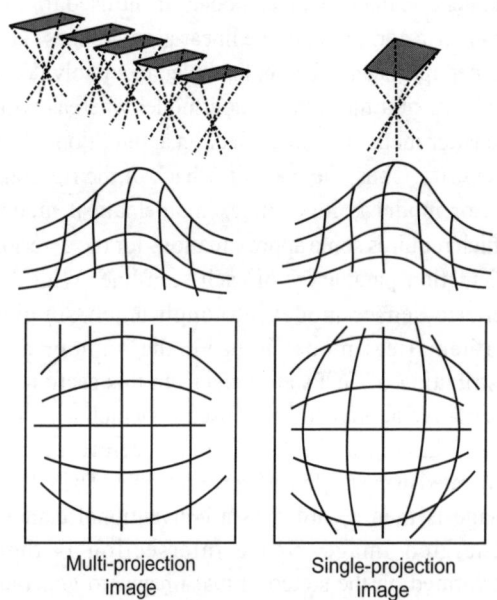

Multi-projection image   Single-projection image

Fig. 12.13. (a) Relief displacement in a multi-projection image, (b) Relief displacement in a single-projection image

With a flat terrain, in the absence of tilt displacement, the geometry of single and multi-projection images is identical, since the relief displacements of the pixels are equal. However, in a non-flat terrain as indicated in Fig. 12.13, the two classes of images have different displacement patterns. To generate a virtual single-projection image, relief variation on the ground must be taken into consideration, without which the single-projection image cannot be generated. Figure 12.14. depicts graphically the simplified relationship of the virtual single-projection image and the linear array image.

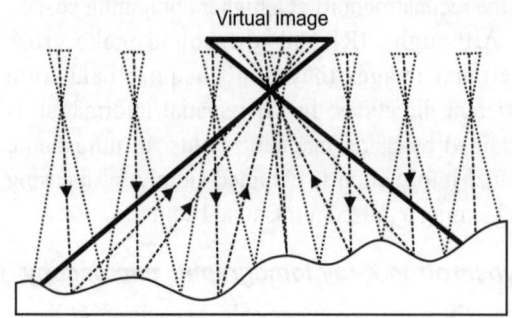

Fig. 12.14. Virtual image generated from the scan lines using a digital elevation model.

Phased Array Ultrasonics

Phased array (PA) ultrasonics is an advanced method of ultrasonic testing that has applications in medical imaging and industrial nondestructive testing, originally pioneered by Albert Macovski of Stanford University. In medicine a common application of phased array is the imaging of the heart (images of the fetus in the womb are usually made by curvilinear array, a multi-element probe that does not actually phase the signals). When applied to steel the PA image shows a slice that may reveal defects hidden inside a structure or weld.

Principle of operation

The PA probe consists of many small ultrasonic elements, each of which can be pulsed individually. By varying the timing, for instance by pulsing the elements one by one in sequence along a row, a pattern of interference is set up that results in a beam at a set angle. In other words, the beam can be steered electronically. The beam is swept like a search-light through the tissue or object being examined, and the data from multiple beams are put together to make a visual image showing a slice through the object.

Features of phased array:
1. The method most commonly used for medical ultrasonography.
2. Multiple probe elements produce a steerable, tightly focused, high-resolution beam.
3. Produces an image that shows a slice through the object.
4. Compared to conventional, single-element ultrasonic inspection systems, PA instruments and probes are more complex and expensive.
5. In industry, PA technicians require more experience and training than conventional technicians.

13

Mechanism of Electrodes

INTRODUCTION

Electrodes are used both for the measurement of bioelectric vents and to deliver current to living tissue. In the former case, the electrode current density is very low, but in the latter it is quite high. In performing these functions, an electrode may establish ohmic contact with the tissue, or the mode of communication may be capacitive. Capacitive electrodes have been used for measuring bioelectric events and for stimulation. Apart from a few specialised uses (e.g. electrosurgery and diathermy) they are fairly uncommon. The most frequently encountered electrodes establish ohmic contact with tissue via an electrolyte.

ELECTRODE–ELECTROLYTE INTERFACE

When a metallic electrode comes into contact with an electrolyte, an ion-electron exchange occurs. There is a tendency for metallic ions to enter into solution and a tendency for ions in the electrolyte to combine with the metallic electrode. Although the details of the reaction may be complex in a given situation, the net result is the existence of a charge distribution at the electrode–electrolyte interface. The spatial arrangement of the charge depends on the manner in which the electrode and electrolyte react. Several types of charge distribution have been proposed. The simplest was conceived by Helmholtz, who postulated that there exists a layer of charge of one sign tightly bound to the electrode and a layer of charge of the opposite sign in the electrolyte. The separation between the two layers of charges (often called the electrical double layer) is of course measured

in ionic dimension (Fig. 13.1a). Gouy and stern proposed different charge distributions as illustrated in Fig. 13.1b, c and d.

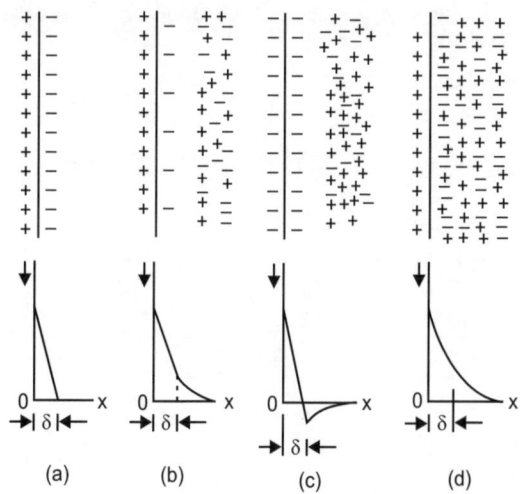

Fig. 13.1. Various configuration of charge distribution and potentials at an electrode–electrolyte interface: (a) Helmholtz, (b) Gouy, (c) Stern, (d) pure Gouy.

Parsons described electrodes in terms of the reactions at the double layer, referring to electrodes in which no net transfer of charge occurs across the metal-electrolyte interface as 'perfectly polarised.' Those in which unhindered exchange of charge is possible were called 'perfectly nonpolarisable.' Real electrodes have properties that lie between these idealised limits. MacInnes stated that the term 'electrode polarisation' is applied in two ways; first, as just stated and second, as the condition in which the electrode–electrolyte potential is altered by the passage of current.

In a conceptual sense, an electrode–electrolyte interface resembles a voltage source and a capacitor. However, it is well known that current can pass through an electrode–electrolyte interface. Therefore any electrical model for such an interface must include resistance, capacitance, and a potential. Figure 13.2 summarises this concept. Although it is easy to identify these three components, it is by no means easy to create an accurate electrical model to include them because their magnitude depends on the electrode metal, its area, the electrolyte, temperature, current density, and the frequency of current used for measurement.

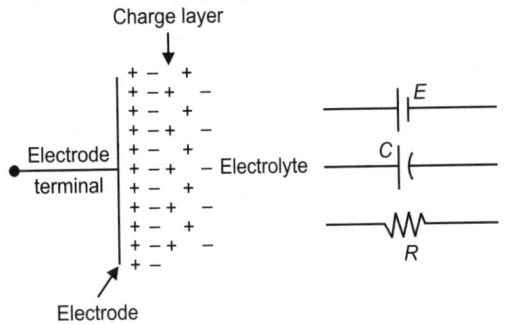

Fig. 13.2. The charge distribution at an electrode–electrolyte interface and the three circuit elements. (voltage E, capacitance C, and resistance R) that can be used to describe it in terms of an electrical model.

ELECTRODE POTENTIAL

Electrode potential, E, in electrochemistry, according to an IUPAC definition, is the electromotive force of a cell built of two electrodes:

1. On the left-hand side is the standard hydrogen electrode.
2. On the right-hand side is the electrode the potential of which is being defined.

By convention:

$$E_{Cell} := E_{Right} - E_{Left}$$

From the above, for the cell with the standard hydrogen electrode (potential of 0 by convention), one obtains:

$$E_{Cell} = E_{Right} - 0 = E_{Electrode}$$

Electrode potential is measured in volts (V).

The measurement is generally conducted using a three-electrode setup (see Fig. 13.3):

1. Working electrode.
2. Counter electrode.
3. Reference electrode (standard hydrogen electrode or an equivalent).

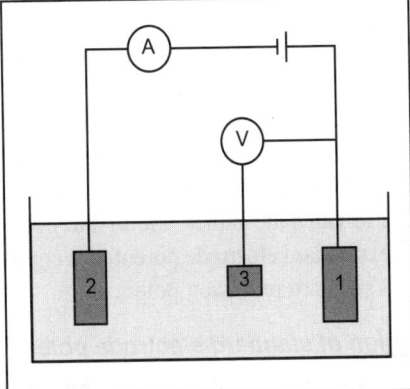

Fig. 13.3. Three-electrode setup for measurement of electrode potential.

The potential measurements are performed with the positive terminal of the electrometer connected to working electrode and the negative terminal to the reference electrode.

The measured potential of the working electrode may be either that at equilibrium on the working electrode ('reversible potential'), or a potential with a non-zero net reaction on the working electrode but zero net current ('corrosion potential', 'mixed potential'), or a potential with a non-zero net current on the working electrode.

Standard Electrode Potential

In electrochemistry, the standard electrode potential, abbreviated $E°$ or $E^{\ominus}$ (with a superscript plimsoll character, pronounced 'standard' or 'nought'), is the measure of individual potential of a reversible electrode at standard state, which is with solutes at an effective concentration of 1 mol dm^{-3}, and gases at a pressure of 1 bar. The values are most often tabulated at 25°C. The basis for an electrochemical cell such as the galvanic cell is always a redox reaction which can be broken down into two half-reactions: oxidation at anode (loss of electron) and reduction at cathode (gain of electron). Electricity is generated due to electric potential difference between two electrodes. This potential difference is created as a result of the difference between individual potentials of the two metal electrodes with respect to the electrolyte.

Although the overall potential of a cell can be measured, there is no simple way to accurately measure the electrode/electrolyte potentials in isolation. The electric potential also varies with temperature, concentration and pressure. Since the oxidation potential of a half-reaction is the negative of the reduction potential in a redox reaction, it is sufficient to calculate either one of the potentials. Therefore, standard electrode potential is commonly written as standard reduction potential.

Calculation of standard electrode potentials

The electrode potential may not be obtained empirically. The galvanic cell potential results from a *pair* of electrodes. Thus, only one empirical value is available in a pair of electrodes and it is not possible to determine the value for each electrode in the pair using the empirically obtained galvanic cell potential. A reference electrode, standard hydrogen electrode (SHE), for which the potential is defined or agreed upon by convention, needed to be established. In this case SHE is set to 0.00 V and any electrode, for which the electrode potential is not yet known, can be paired with SHE – to form a galvanic cell – and the galvanic cell potential gives the unknown electrode's potential. Using this process, any electrode with an unknown potential can be paired with either the SHE or another electrode for which the potential has already been derived and that unknown value can be established.

Since the electrode potentials are conventionally defined as reduction potentials, the sign of the potential for the metal electrode being oxidised must be reversed when calculating the overall cell potential. Note that the electrode potentials are independent of the number of electrons transferred – that is, they are set to one mole of electrons transferred — and so the two electrode potentials can be simply combined to give the overall cell potential even if different numbers of electrons are involved in the two electrode reactions. For practical measurements, the electrode in question is connected to the positive terminal of the electrometer, while SHE is connected to the negative terminal.

Standard reduction potential table

Since the values are given in their ability to be reduced, the bigger the standard reduction potentials, the easier they are to be reduced, in other words, they are simply better oxidising agents. For example, F_2 has 2.87 V and Li^+ has –3.05 V. F_2 reduces easily and is therefore a good oxidising agent. In contrast, $Li_{(s)}$ would rather undergo oxidation (hence a good reducing agent). Thus Zn^{2+} whose standard reduction potential is –0.76 V can be oxidised by any other electrode whose standard reduction potential is greater than –0.76 V (e.g. H^+(0 V), Cu^{2+}(0.16 V), F_2(2.87 V)) and can be reduced by any electrode with standard reduction potential less than –0.76 V (e.g. H_2(–2.23 V), Na^+(–2.71 V), Li^+(–3.05 V)).

In a galvanic cell, where a spontaneous redox reaction drives the cell to produce an electric potential, Gibbs free energy $\Delta G°$ must be negative, in accordance with the following equation:

$$\Delta G°_{cell} = -nFE°_{cell}$$

where n is number of moles of electrons per mole of products and F is the Faraday constant, ~96485 C/mol. As such, the following rules apply:

If $E°_{cell} > 0$, then the process is spontaneous (galvanic cell).

If $E°_{cell} < 0$, then the process is nonspontaneous (electrolytic cell).

Thus in order to have a spontaneous reaction ($\Delta G°$), $E°_{cell}$ must be positive, where:

$$E°_{cell} = E°_{cathode} - E°_{anode}$$

where $E°_{anode}$ is the standard potential at the anode (reverse the sign of the standard reduction potential value for the electrode) and $E°_{cathode}$ is the standard potential at the cathode as given in the table of standard electrode potential.

Non-standard condition

The standard electrode potentials are given at standard conditions. However, real cells may operate under non-standard conditions. Given the standard potential of the half-cell, its potential at non-standard effective concentrations can be calculated using the Nernst equation:

$$E_{\text{half-cell}} = E^\circ - \frac{RT}{nF} \ln Q$$

where Q is the reaction quotient.

The values of E° depend on temperature (except for SHE, for which the potential has been, arbitrarily, declared 0 at all temperatures) and are normally referenced to the SHE at the same temperature. For condensed phases, they are also expected to depend somewhat on pressure (see the article on equilibrium constant). For example, the standard electrode potential for Ni/NiO redox couple has been well studied because such a solid has applications in high-temperature pseudo-reference electrodes (when enclosed inside an yttrium-stabilised zirconia ceramic membrane). The half-cell reaction for this redox couple is:

$$\text{Ni} + \text{H}_2\text{O} \rightleftharpoons \text{NiO} + 2\text{H}^+ + 2e^-$$

The standard potential of Ni/NiO has been correlated for temperatures between 0 and 400°C to be approximately:

$$E^\circ(T) = -0.0003\,T + 0.1414$$

where E° is in volts, and T is in degrees Celsius.

In biochemistry, potentials are usually defined for pH 7, with the standard potential under these conditions being $E^{\circ\prime}$–also referred to as the *mid-point potential* or $E_{m,7}$ because it is the potential at which the concentrations of the oxidised and reduced forms of the redox pair are equal.

The actual redox potential for a pair at a given pH of $x\,(E_{h,\,pH = x})$ is related to the midpoint potential by:

$$E_{h,\,pH = x} = E_{m,\,pH = x} - \frac{2.3RT}{nF}\text{pH}$$

ABSOLUTE ELECTRODE POTENTIAL

Absolute electrode potential, in electrochemistry, according to an IUPAC definition, is the electrode potential of a metal measured with respect to a universal reference system (without any additional metal-solution interface).

According to a more specific definition presented by Trasatti, the absolute electrode potential is the difference in electronic energy between a point inside the metal (Fermi level) of an electrode and a point outside the electrolyte in which the electrode is submerged (an electron at rest in vacuum).

This potential is difficult to determine accurately. For this reason, standard hydrogen electrode is typically used for reference potential. The absolute potential of the SHE is 4.44 ± 0.02 V at 25°C. Therefore, for any electrode at 25°C:

$$E_{(\text{abs})}^{M} = E_{(\text{SHE})}^{M} + (4.44 \pm 0.02)V$$

where,

E is electrode potential, V.

M denotes the electrode made of metal M.

(abs) denotes the absolute potential.

(SHE) denotes the electrode potential relative to the standard hydrogen electrode.

A different definition for the absolute electrode potential (also known as absolute half-cell potential and single electrode potential) has also been discussed in the literature. In this approach, one first defines an isothermal absolute single-electrode process (or absolute half-cell process.) For example, in the case of a generic metal being oxidised to form a solution-phase ion, the process would be:

$$M_{(\text{metal})} \longrightarrow M_{(\text{solution})}^+ + e_{(\text{gas})}^-$$

For the hydrogen electrode, the absolute half-cell process would be:

$$\frac{1}{2}\text{H}_{2(\text{gas})} \rightarrow \text{H}_{(\text{solution})}^+ + e_{(\text{gas})}^-$$

Other types of absolute electrode reactions would be defined analogously.

In this approach, all three species taking part in the reaction, including the electron, must be placed in thermodynamically well-defined states. All species, including the electron, are at the same temperature, and appropriate standard states for all species, including the electron, must be fully defined. The absolute electrode potential is then defined as the Gibbs free energy for the absolute electrode process. To express this in volts one divides the Gibb's free energy by the negative of Faraday's constant.

Rockwood's approach to absolute-electrode thermodynamics is easily expendable to other thermodynamic functions. For example, the absolute half-cell entropy has been defined as the entropy of the absolute half-cell process defined above. An alternative definition of the absolute half-cell entropy has recently been published by Fang who define it as the entropy of the following reaction (using the hydrogen electrode as an example):

$$\frac{1}{2}H_{2(gas)} \rightarrow H^+_{(solution)} + e^-_{(metal)}$$

This approach differs from the approach described by Rockwood in the treatment of the electron, i.e. whether it is placed in the gas phase or in the metal.

The basis for determination of the absolute electrode potential under the Trasatti definition is given by the equation:

$$E^M(abs) = \phi^M + \Delta^M_S \psi$$

where,

E^M(abs) is the absolute potential of the electrode made of metal M, V

ϕ^M is the electron work function of metal M, V.

$\Delta^M_S \psi$ is the contact (Volta) potential difference at the metal (M)-solution (S) interface, V.

For practical purposes, the value of the absolute electrode potential of the standard hydrogen electrode is best determined with the utility of data for an ideally-polarizable mercury (Hg) electrode:

$$E^\Theta(H^+/H_2)(abs) = \phi^{Hg} + \Delta^{Hg}_S \psi^\Theta_{\sigma=0} - E^{Hg}_{\sigma=0}(SHE)$$

where:

$E^\Theta(H^+/H_2)$(abs) is the absolute standard potential of the hydrogen electrode.

$\sigma = 0$ denotes the condition of the point of zero charge at the interface.

The types of physical measurements required under the Rockwood definition are similar to those required under the Trasatti definition, but they are used in a different way, e.g. in Rockwood's approach they are used to calculate the equilibrium vapour pressure of the electron gas. The numerical value for the absolute potential of the standard hydrogen electrode one would calculate under the Rockwood definition is sometimes fortuitously close to the value one would obtain under the Trasatti definition. This near-agreement in the numerical value depends on the choice of ambient temperature and standard states, and is the result of the near-cancellation of certain terms in the expressions. For example, if a standard state of one atmosphere ideal gas is chosen for the electron gas then the cancellation of terms occurs at a temperature of 296 K, and the two definitions give an equal numerical result. At 298.15 K a near-cancellation of terms would apply and the two approaches would produce nearly the same numerical values. However, there is no fundamental significance to this near agreement because it depends on arbitrary choices, such as temperature and definitions of standard states.

Reference Electrode

A reference electrode is an electrode which has a stable and well-known electrode potential. The high stability of the electrode potential is usually reached by employing a redox system with constant (buffered or saturated) concentrations of each participants of the redox reaction.

There are many ways reference electrodes are used. The simplest is when the reference electrode is used as a half cell to build an electrochemical cell. This allows the potential of the other half cell to be determined. An accurate and practical method to measure an electrode's potential in isolation (absolute electrode potential) has yet to be developed.

Aqueous reference electrodes

Common reference electrodes and potential with respect to the standard hydrogen electrode in given below:

1. Standard hydrogen electrode (SHE) (E = 0.000 V) activity of H^+=1 (Fig. 13.4).
2. Normal hydrogen electrode (NHE) (E ≈ 0.000 V)concentration H^+ = 1.
3. Reversible hydrogen electrode (RHE) (E = 0.000 V – 0.0591 pH).
4. Saturated calomel electrode (SCE) (E = +0.242 V saturated).
5. Copper-copper(II) sulphate electrode (E = +0.314 V) (Fig. 13.5).

6. Silver chloride electrode (E = +0.197 V saturated) Fig. 13.6.

7. pH-electrode (in case of pH buffered solutions.

8. Palladium-hydrogen electrode.

9. Dynamic hydrogen electrode (DHE).

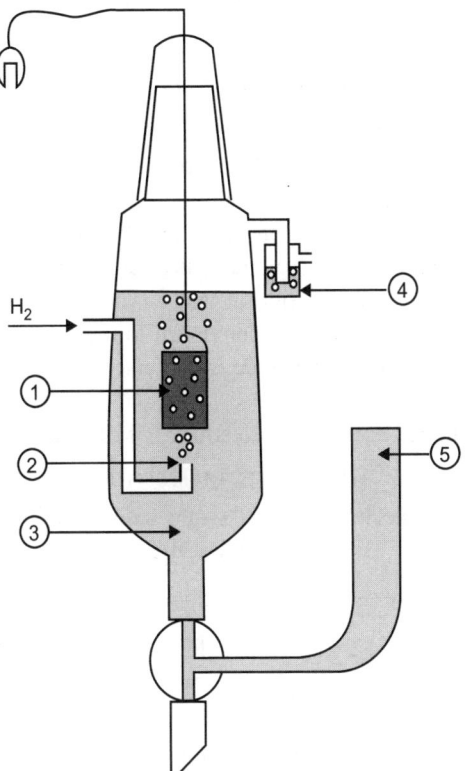

Fig. 13.4. Standard hydrogen electrode.

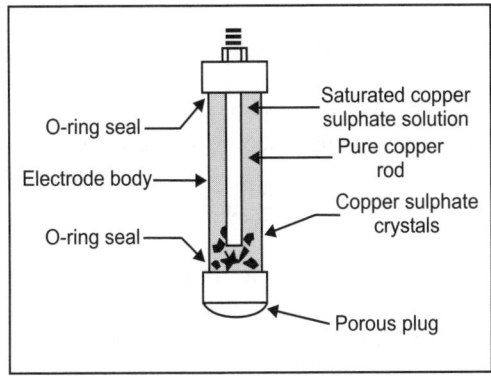

Fig. 13.5. Cu-Cu(II) reference electrode.

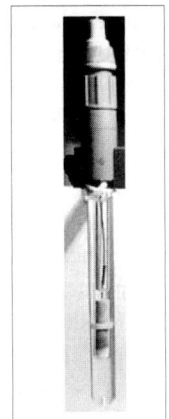

Fig. 13.6. Ag-AgCl reference electrode.

Nonaqueous reference electrodes

While it is convenient to compare between solvents to qualitatively compare systems it is not quantitatively meaningful. Much as pK_a are related between solvents, but not the same, so is the case with E°. While the SHE might seem to be a reasonable reference for nonaqueous work as it turns out the platinum is rapidly poisoned by many solvents including acetonitrile causing uncontrolled drifts in potential. Both the SCE and saturated Ag/AgCl are aqueous electrodes based around saturated aqueous solution. While for short periods it may be possible to use such aqueous electrodes as references with nonaqueous solutions the long-term results are not trustworthy. Using aqueous electrodes introduces undefined, variable, and unmeasurable junction potentials to the cell in the form of a liquid-liquid junction as well as different ionic composition between the reference compartment and the rest of the cell. The best argument against using aqueous reference electrodes with nonaqueous systems, as mentioned earlier, is that potentials measured in different solvents are not directly comparable.

A quasi-reference electrode (QRE) avoids the issues mentioned above. A QRE with Ferrocene or similar internal standard (Cobaltocene) referenced back to Ferrocene is ideal for nonaqueous work. Since the early 1960s ferrocene has been gaining acceptance as the standard reference for nonaqueous work for a number of reasons. In 1984 IUPAC recommend ferrocene (II/III) as a standard redox couple. The preparation of the QRE electrode is simple allowing a fresh reference to be prepared with each set of experiments. Since QREs are made fresh there is also no concern of improper storage or maintenance of the electrode. QREs are also more affordable than other reference electrodes.

Making a quasi-reference electrode (QRE):

1. Inserting a piece of silver wire into concentrated HCl then allow the wire to dry on a chem-wipe. This forms an insoluble layer of AgCl on the surface of the electrode and gives you a Ag/AgCl wire. Repeat dipping every few months or if the QRE starts to drift.

2. Obtain a Vycor glass frit (4 mm diameter) and glass tubing of similar diameter. Attach Vycor glass frit to the glass tubing with heat shrink Teflon tubing.

3. Rinse then fill the clean glass tube with supporting electrolyte solution and insert Ag/AgCl wire.

4. The Ferrocene (II/III) couple should lie around 400 mV versus this Ag/AgCl QRE in an acetonitrile solution. This potential will varying up to 200 mV with the specific undefined conditions. Thus adding an internal standard such as ferrocene at some point during the experiment is always necessary.

Pseudo-reference electrodes

A pseudo-reference electrode is a term that is not well defined and boarders on having multiple meanings since pseudo and quasi are often used interchangeably. There are a class of electrodes named pseudo-reference electrodes because they do not maintain a constant potential but vary predictably with conditions. If the conditions are known, the potential can be calculated and the electrode can be used as a reference. Most electrode work over a limited range of conditions, such as pH or temperature, outside of this range the electrodes behaviour becomes unpredictable. The advantage of a pseudo-reference electrode is that the resulting variation is factored into the system allowing

researchers to accurately studying systems over a wide range of conditions.

Yttria-stabilised zirconia (YSZ) membrane electrodes were developed with a variety of redox couples, e.g. Ni/NiO. Their potential depends on pH. When the pH value is known, these electrodes can be employed as a reference with notable applications at elevated temperatures.

Saturated Calomel Electrode

The Saturated calomel electrode (SCE) is a reference electrode based on the reaction between elemental mercury and mercury(I) chloride. The aqueous phase in contact with the mercury and the mercury (I) chloride (Hg_2Cl_2, 'calomel') is a saturated solution of potassium chloride in water. The electrode is normally linked *via* a porous frit to the solution in which the other electrode is immersed. This porous frit is a salt bridge.

In cell notation the electrode is written as:

$$Cl^-(4M) \mid Hg_2Cl_2(s) \mid Hg(l) \mid Pt$$

The electrode is based on the redox reaction:

$$Hg_2^{2+} + 2e^- \rightleftharpoons 2Hg(l)$$

The Nernst equation for this reaction is:

$$E = E^0_{Hg_2^{2+}/Hg} - \frac{RT}{2F} \ln \frac{1}{a_{Hg_2^{2+}}}$$

where E^0 is the standard electrode potential for the reaction and a_{Hg} is the activity for the mercury cation (the activity for a liquid is 1). This activity can be found from the solubility product of the reaction:

$$Hg_2^{2+} + 2Cl^- \rightleftharpoons Hg_2Cl_2(s), \qquad K_{sp} = a_{Hg_2^{2+}} a^2_{Cl^-}$$

By replacing the activity in the Nernst equation with the value in the solubility equation, we get:

$$E = E^0_{Hg_2^{2+}/Hg} + \frac{RT}{2F} \ln K_{sp} - \frac{RT}{2F} \ln a^2_{Cl^-}$$

The only variable in this equation is the activity (or concentration) of the chloride anion. But since the inner solution is saturated with potassium chloride, this activity is fixed by the solubility of potassium chloride. When saturated the redox potential of the calomel electrode is +0.2415 V vs. SHE, but slightly higher when the chloride solution is less than saturated.

AUXILIARY ELECTRODE

The auxiliary electrode, often also called the counter electrode, is an electrode used in a three electrode electrochemical cell for voltammetric analysis or other reactions in which an electrical current is expected to flow. The auxiliary electrode is distinct from the reference electrode, which establishes the electrical potential against which other potentials may be measured, and the working electrode, at which the cell reaction takes place.

The auxiliary electrode's potential is opposite in sign to that of the working electrode, but its current and potential are not measured. Rather, it is used to ensure that current does not run through the reference electrode (three electrode system), which would disturb the reference electrode's potential. The auxiliary electrode often has a surface area much larger than that of the working electrode to ensure that the reactions occurring on the working electrode are not surface area limited by the auxiliary electrode.

When using a three electrode cell to perform electroanalytical chemistry, the auxiliary electrode is often isolated from the working electrode using a glass frit. Such isolation prevents any by-products generated at the auxiliary electrode from contaminating the main test solution and interfering with the analytical measurement being made at the working electrode.

Auxiliary electrodes are often fabricated from electrochemically inert materials such as gold, platinum, or carbon.

Working Electrode

The working electrode, is the electrode in an electrochemical system on which the reaction of interest is occurring. The working electrode is often used in conjunction with an auxiliary electrode, and a reference electrode in a three electrode system. Depending on whether the reaction on the electrode is a reduction or an oxidation, the working electrode can be referred to as either cathodic or anodic.

Common working electrodes can consist of inert metals such as gold, silver or platinum, to inert carbon such as glassy carbon or pyrolytic carbon, and mercury drop and film electrodes (Fig. 13.7).

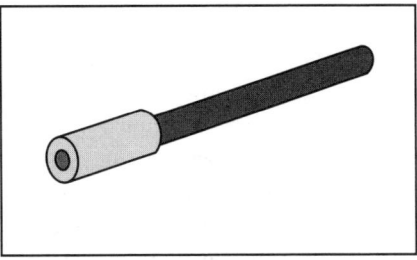

Fig. 13.7. A gold disk working electrode with a Teflon shroud insulating the disk.

Special types of working electrodes: (i) ultramicroelectrode (UME), (ii) rotating disk electrode (RDE), (iii) rotating ring-disk electrode (RRDE), (iv) hanging mercury drop electrode (HMDE), and (v) dropping mercury electrode (DME).

Reduction Potential

Reduction potential (also known as redox potential, oxidation/reduction potential or ORP) is a measure of the tendency of a chemical species to acquire electrons and thereby be reduced. Reduction potential is measured in volts (V), millivolts (mV), or E_h (1 E_h = 1 mV). Each species has its own intrinsic reduction potential; the more positive the potential, the greater the species' affinity for electrons and tendency to be reduced.

In aqueous solutions, the reduction potential is a measure of the tendency of the solution to either gain or lose electrons when it is subject to change by introduction of a new species. A solution with a higher (more positive) reduction potential than the new species will have a tendency to gain electrons from the new species (i.e. to be reduced by oxidising the new species) and a solution with a lower (more negative) reduction potential will have a tendency to lose electrons to the new species (i.e. to be oxidised by reducing the new species). Just as the transfer of hydrogen ions between chemical species determines the pH of an aqueous solution, the transfer of electrons, between chemical species determines the reduction potential of an aqueous solution. Like pH, the reduction potential represents an intensity factor. It does not characterise the capacity of the system for oxidation or reduction, in much the same way that pH does not characterise the buffering capacity.

Because the absolute potentials are difficult to accurately measure, reduction potentials are defined relative to a reference electrode. Reduction potentials of aqueous solutions are determined by measuring the potential difference between an inert sensing electrode in contact with the solution and a stable reference electrode connected to the solution by a salt bridge. The sensing electrode acts as a platform for electron transfer to or from the reference half cell. It is typically platinum, although gold and graphite can be used. The reference half cell consists of a redox standard of known potential. The standard hydrogen electrode (SHE) is the reference from which all standard redox potentials are determined and has been assigned an arbitrary half cell potential of 0.0 mV. However, it is fragile and impractical for routine laboratory use. Therefore, other more stable reference electrodes such as silver chloride and saturated calomel (SCE) are commonly used because of their more reliable performance.

Although measurement of the reduction potential in aqueous solutions is relatively straightforward, many factors limit its interpretation, such as effects of solution temperature and pH, irreversible reactions, slow electrode kinetics, non-equilibrium, presence of multiple redox couples, electrode poisoning, small exchange currents and inert redox couples. Consequently, practical measurements seldom correlate with calculated values. Nevertheless, reduction potential measurement has proven useful as an analytical tool in monitoring changes in a system rather than determining their absolute value (e.g. process control and titrations).

Standard Reduction Potential, E_0

The standard reduction potential (E_0) is measured under standard conditions: 25°C, a 1 M concentration for each ion participating in the reaction, a partial pressure of 1 atm for each gas that is part of the reaction, and metals in their pure state. The standard

reduction potential is defined relative to a standard hydrogen electrode (SHE) reference electrode, which is arbitrarily given a potential of 0.00 volts. Historically, many countries, including the United States and Canada, used standard oxidation potentials rather than reduction potentials in their calculations. These are simply the negative of standard reduction potentials, so it is not a major problem in practice. However, because these can also be referred to as 'redox potentials', the terms 'reduction potentials' and 'oxidation potentials' are preferred by the IUPAC. The two may be explicitly distinguished in symbols as E_0' and E_0.

Converting potentials between different types reference electrodes

Often a reduction potential is quoted as measured against a different reference electrode than the one desired and it becomes necessary to convert to the desired reference potential. Alternatively, it may be necessary to convert measurements to the standard reduction potential for reporting purposes. This is easily done by recognising that the observed potential represents the difference between the potential at the sensing electrode and the potential at the reference electrode, i.e.

$$E_{obs\,|\,ref} = E_h - E_{ref}$$

The voltage relationships for several different reference electrodes at 25°C can be interrelated as follows:

Reference electrode	Electrode potential with respect to SHE (mV)
Standard hydrogen electrode (SHE)	0
Saturated calomel electrode (SCE)	+241
Ag/AgCl, 1 M KCl	+236
Ag/AgCl, 4 M KCl	+200
Ag/AgCl, sat. KCl	+197

For example, if one measured 300 mV using a saturated KCl Ag/AgCl reference and wanted to refer it to the standard reduction potential (E_0) measured using an SHE reference electrode, then 197 mV should be added to the 300 mV to obtain 497 mV, since:

$$300 \text{ mV} = E_h - 197 \text{ mV}$$

it follows that

$$E_h = 300 \text{ mV} + 197 \text{ mV} = 497 \text{ mV}$$

and therefore

$$E_{obs \,|\, SHE} = E_0 = 497 \text{ mV} - 0 \text{ mV} = 497 \text{ mV}$$

Likewise, if one measured 300 mV using a saturated KCl Ag/AgCl reference and wanted to determine the corresponding measurement using an SCE reference, then given

$$300 \text{ mV} = E_h - 197 \text{ mV}$$

it follows that

$$E_h = 300 \text{ mV} + 197 \text{ mV} = 497 \text{ mV}$$

and therefore

$$E_{obs \,|\, SCE} = 497 \text{ mV} - 241 \text{ mV} = 256 \text{ mV}$$

Half cells

The relative reactivities of different half cells can be compared to predict the direction of electron flow. A higher E_0 means there is a greater tendency for reduction to occur, while a lower one means there is a greater tendency for oxidation to occur.

Any system or environment that accepts electrons from a normal hydrogen electrode is a half cell that is defined as having a positive redox potential; any system donating electrons to the hydrogen electrode is defined as having a negative redox potential. E_h is measured in millivolts (mV). A high positive E_h indicates an environment that favours oxidation reaction such as free oxygen. A low negative E_h indicates a strong reducing environment, such as free metals.

Sometimes when electrolysis is carried out in an aqueous solution, water, rather than the solute, is oxidised or reduced. For example, if an aqueous solution of NaCl is electrolysed, water may be reduced at the cathode to produce $H_{2(g)}$ and OH^- ions, instead of Na^+ being reduced to $Na_{(s)}$, as occurs in the absence of water. It is the reduction potential of each species present that will determine which species will be oxidised or reduced.

Absolute reduction potentials can be determined if we find the actual potential between electrode and electrolyte for any one reaction. Surface polarisation interferes with measurements, but various sources give an estimated potential for the standard hydrogen electrode of 4.4 V to 4.6 V (the electrolyte being positive.)

Half-cell equations can be combined if one is reversed to an oxidation in a manner that cancels out the electrons to obtain an equation without electrons in it.

Nernst equation

The E_h and pH of a solution are related. For a half cell equation (conventionally written as reduction, or with electrons on the right side):

$$aA + bB + n[e^-] + h[H^+] = cC + dD$$

The half cell standard potential E_0 is given by:

$$E_0(\text{volts}) = -\frac{\Delta G}{nF}$$

where ΔG is the Gibbs free energy change, n is the number of electrons involved, and F is Faraday's constant. The Nernst equation relates pH and E_h:

$$E_h = E_0 + \frac{0.05916}{n} \log\left(\frac{[A]^a [B]^b}{[C]^c [D]^d}\right) - \frac{0.05916h}{n} \text{pH}$$

where square brackets indicate activities and exponents are shown in the conventional manner. This equation is the equation of a straight line for E_h as a function of pH with a slope of $-0.05916\,h/n$ volt (pH has no units.) This equation predicts lower E_h at higher pH values. This is observed for reduction of O_2 to OH^- and for reduction of H^+ to H_2. If H^+ were on the opposite side of the equation from H^+, the slope of the line would be reversed (higher E_h at higher pH). An example of that would be the formation of magnetite (Fe_3O_4) from $HFeO_2^-$ (aq):

$$3 \text{ HFeO}_2^- + H^+ = Fe_3O_4 + 2 \text{ H}_2O + 2 \text{ [[e}^-\text{]]}$$

where $E_h = -1.1819 - 0.0885 \log[\text{HFeO}_2^-] + 0.0296$ pH. Note that the slope of the line is $-1/2$ the -0.05916 value above, since $h/n = -1/2$.

Many enzymatic reactions are oxidation-reduction reactions in which one compound is oxidised and another compound is reduced. The ability of an organism to carry out oxidation-reduction reactions depends on the oxidation-reduction state of the environment, or its reduction potential (E_h).

Strictly aerobic microorganisms can be active only at positive E_h values, whereas strict anaerobes can be active only at negative E_h values. Redox affects the solubility of nutrients, especially metal ions.

There are organisms that can adjust their metabolism to their environment, such as facultative anaerobes. Facultative anaerobes can be active at positive E_h values, and at negative E_h values in the presence of oxygen bearing inorganic compounds, such as nitrates and sulphates.

PLATINUM BLACK

Platinum black (Pt black) is a fine powder of platinum with good catalytic properties. The name of platinum black is due to its black colour.

Platinum black is widely used as a thin film covering solid platinum metal, forming platinum electrodes for applications in electrochemistry. The process of covering platinum electrodes with such a layer of platinum black is called 'platinisation of platinum'. The platinised platinum has a true surface area much higher than the geometrical surface area of the electrode and, therefore, exhibits catalytic action superior to that of shiny platinum.

Platinum black powder is used as a catalyst in proton exchange membrane fuel cells. In common practice, the platinum black is either sprayed or hot pressed onto the membrane or gas diffusion layer. A suspension of platinum black and carbon powder in ethanol-water solutions serves to optimise the uniformity of the coating, electrical conductivity, and in the case of application to the membrane, to prevent dehydration of the membrane during the application.

Platinum black powder can be manufactured from ammonium chloroplatinate by heating at 500°C in molten sodium nitrate for 30 minutes, followed by pouring the melt into water, boiling, washing, and reduction of the brown powder (believed to be platinum dioxide) with gaseous hydrogen to platinum black.

Process of Platinisation of Platinum Metal

Before platinisation, the platinum surface is cleaned by immersion in aqua regia (50 per cent solution, i.e.

3 volumes of 12 mol/kg of HCl, 1 volume of 16 mol/kg HNO_3, 4 volumes of water).

Platinisation is often conducted from water solution of 0.072 mol/kg of chloroplatinic acid and 0.00013 mol/kg of lead acetate, at a current density of 30 mA/cm² for up to 10 minutes. The process evolves chlorine at the anode; the interaction of the chlorine with the cathode is prevented by employing a suitable separation (e.g. a glass frit).

Smith recommends electroplating with the current density of 5 mA/cm² while reversing the polarity every 30 s for 15 minutes.

After platinisation, the electrode should be rinsed and stored in distilled water. The electrode loses its catalytic properties on prolonged exposure to air.

Platinum metal sponge

Platinum sponge is yet another form of platinum metal with a developed surface area, distinct from platinum black and platinised platinum. Platinum sponge can be obtained by strongly heating ammonium chloroplatinate. It has a gray to black colour, while its catalytic properties vary depending on the specifics of the manufacturing.

Potential of platinised platinum versus shiny platinum

In hydrogen saturated hydrochloric acid, the shiny platinum electrode is observed to assume positive potential versus that of platinum black at zero net current (+ 340 mV at room temperature). With the temperature increasing to 70 °C, the difference in potentials dropped to zero. The reason for this is not perfectly clear, although several explanations have been proposed.

SILVER CHLORIDE ELECTRODE

A silver chloride electrode is a type of reference electrode, commonly used in electrochemical measurements. For example, it is usually the internal reference electrode in pH meters. As another example, the silver chloride electrode is the most commonly used reference electrode for testing cathodic protection corrosion control systems in sea water environments.

The electrode functions as a redox electrode and the reaction is between the silver metal (Ag) and its salt — silver chloride (AgCl, also called silver(I) chloride).

The corresponding equations can be presented as follows:

$$Ag^+ + 1e^- \leftrightarrow Ag^0(s)$$

$$Ag^+ + Cl^- \leftrightarrow AgCl(s)$$

or an overall reaction can be written:

$$Ag^0(s) + Cl^- \leftrightarrow AgCl(s) + e^-$$

This reaction characterised by fast electrode kinetics, meaning that a sufficiently high current can be passed through the electrode with the 100 per cent efficiency of the redox reaction (dissolution of the metal or cathodic deposition of the silver-ions). The reaction has been proved to obey these equations in solutions with pH's of between 0 and 13.5.

The Nernst equation below shows the dependence of the potential of the silver-silver(I) chloride electrode on the activity or effective concentration of chloride-ions:

$$E = E^0 + \frac{RT}{F} \ln a_{Cl^-}$$

The standard electrode potential E^0 against standard hydrogen electrode is 0.230 V ± 10 mV. The potential is however very sensitive to traces of bromide ions which make it more negative. (The more exact standard potential given by an IUPAC is 0.22249 V, with a standard deviation of 0.13 mV at 25°C.)

Commercial reference electrodes consist of a plastic tube electrode body. The electrode is a silver wire that is coated with a thin layer of silver chloride, either physically by dipping the wire in molten silver chloride, or chemically by electroplating the wire in concentrated hydrochloric acid.

A porous plug on one end allows contact between the field environment with the silver chloride electrolyte. An insulated lead wire connects the silver rod with measuring instruments. A voltmeter negative lead is connected to the test wire. The reference electrode contains potassium chloride to stabilise the silver chloride concentration.

The potential of a silver:silver chloride reference electrode with respect to the standard hydrogen electrode depends on the electrolyte composition (Table 13.1).

Table 13.1. Reference electrode potentials.

Electrode	Potential $E^0 + E_{lj}$	Temperature coef.
	(V) at 25°C	(mV/°C) at around 25°C
SHE	0.000	0.000
Ag/AgCl/Sat. KCL	+0.197	−1.01
Ag/AgCl/3.5 mol/kg KCl	+0.205	−0.73
Ag/AgCl/1.0 mol/kg KCl	+0.235	+0.25
Ag/AgCl/0.6 mol/kg KCl	+0.25	–
Ag/AgCl (seawater)	+0.266	–

Note: E_{lj} is the potential of the liquid junction between the given electrolyte and the electrolyte with the activity of chloride of 1 mol/kg.

The electrode has many features making is suitable for use in the field:

1. Simple construction.
2. Inexpensive to manufacture.
3. Stable potential.
4. Non-toxic components.

They are usually manufactured with saturated potassium chloride electrolyte, but can be used with lower concentrations such as 1 mol/kg potassium chloride. As noted above, changing the electrolyte concentration changes the electrode potential. Silver chloride is slightly soluble in strong potassium chloride solutions, so it is sometimes recommended the potassium chloride be saturated with silver chloride to avoid stripping the silver chloride off the silver wire.

When appropriately constructed, the silver chloride electrode can be used up to 300°C. The standard potential (i.e. the potential when the chloride activity is 1 mol/kg) of the silver chloride electrode is a function of temperature as follows (Table 13.2):

Table 13.2. Temperature dependence of the standard potential of the silver/silver chloride electrode.

Temperature	Potential E^0
°C	V versus SHE at the same temperature
25	0.22233
60	0.1968
125	0.1330
150	0.1032
175	0.0708
200	0.0348
225	–0.0051
250	–0.054
275	–0.090

Bard and other give the following correlations for the standard potential of the silver chloride electrode as a function of temperature (where t is temperature in °C):

$E^0(V) = 0.23695 - 4.8564 \times 10^{-4}t - 3.4205 \times 10^{-6}t^2 - 5.869 \times 10^{-9}t^3$ for $0 < t < 95°C$.

The same authors also give the fit to the high-temperature potential, but it appears to contain a typographic error. The corrected fit, which reproduced the data in the table above is:

$E^0(V) = 0.23735 - 5.3783 \times 10^{-4}t - 2.3728 \times 10^{-6}t^2 - 2.2671 \times 10^{-9}(t + 273)$ for $25 < t < 275°C$.

An extrapolation to 300°C gives E^0 of –0.138 V.

STANDARD HYDROGEN ELECTRODE

The standard hydrogen electrode (abbreviated SHE), also called normal hydrogen electrode (NHE), is a redox electrode which forms the basis of the thermodynamic scale of oxidation-reduction potentials. Its absolute electrode potential is estimated to be 4.44 ± 0.02 V at 25°C, but to form a basis for comparison with all other electrode reactions, hydrogen's standard electrode potential (E^0) is declared to be zero at all temperatures. Potentials of any other electrodes are compared with that of the standard hydrogen electrode at the same temperature.

Hydrogen electrode is based on the redox half cell:

$$2H^+(aq) + 2e^- \longrightarrow H_2(g)$$

This redox reaction occurs at platinised platinum electrode. The electrode is dipped in an acidic solution and pure hydrogen gas is bubbled through it. The concentration of both the reduced form and oxidised form is maintained at unity. That implies that the pressure of hydrogen gas is 1 bar and the concentration of hydrogen in the solution is 1 molar. The Nernst equation should be written as:

$$E = \frac{RT}{F} \ln \frac{a_{H^+}}{(p_{H_2}/p^0)^{1/2}}$$

or

$$E = \frac{2.303RT}{F}\text{pH} - \frac{RT}{2F} \ln p_{H_2}/p^0$$

where,

1. a_{H^+} is the activity of the hydrogen ions, $a_{H^+} = f_{H^+} C_{H^+}/C^0$.
2. p_{H_2} is the partial pressure of the hydrogen gas, in pascals, Pa.
3. R is the universal gas constant.
4. T is the temperature, in kelvins.
5. F is the Faraday constant (the charge per a mole of electrons), equal to $9.6485309*10^4$ C mol^{-1}.
6. p^0 is the standard pressure 10^5 in Pa.

The choice of platinum for the hydrogen electrode is due to several factors:

1. Inertness of platinum (it does not corrode).
2. the capability of platinum to catalyse the reaction of proton reduction
3. A high intrinsic exchange current density for proton reduction on platinum.
4. Excellent reproducibility of the potential (bias of less than 10 μV when two well-made hydrogen electrodes are compared with one another.

The surface of platinum is platinised (i.e. covered with platinum black) because of:

1. Necessity to employ electrode with large true surface area. The greater the electrode true area, the faster electrode kinetics
2. Necessity to use electrode material which can adsorb hydrogen at its interface. Platinisation improves electrode kinetics.

Nevertheless, other metals can be used for building electrodes with a similar function, for example, palladium-hydrogen electrode. Table 13.3 shows comparison of exchange current density for proton reduction.

Table 13.3. Comparison of exchange current density for proton reduction reaction in 1 mol/kg H_2SO_4.

Electrode material	Exchange current density $-log_{10}(A/cm^2)$
Palladium	3.0
Platinum	3.1
Rhodium	3.6
Iridium	3.7
Nickel	5.2
Gold	5.4
Tungsten	5.9
Niobium	6.8
Titanium	8.2
Cadmium	10.8
Manganese	10.9
Lead	12.0
Mercury	12.3

Interference

Because of the high adsorption activity of the platinised platinum electrode, it's very important to protect electrode surface and solution from the presence of organic substances as well as from atmospheric oxygen. Inorganic ions that can reduce to a lower valency state at the electrode also have to be avoided (e.g. Fe^{3+}, CrO_4^{2-}). A number of organic substances are also reduced by hydrogen at a platinum surface, and these also have to be avoided.

Cations that can reduce and deposit on the platinum can be source of interference: silver, mercury, copper, lead, cadmium and thallium.

Substances that can inactivate ('poison') the catalytic sites include arsenic, sulphides and other sulphur compounds, colloidal substances, alkaloids, and material found in living systems.

The scheme of the standard hydrogen electrode:
1. Platinised platinum electrode.
2. Hydrogen blow.

3. Solution of the acid with activity of $H^+ = 1$ mol kg^{-1}.
4. Hydroseal for prevention of the oxygen interference.
5. Reservoir through which the second half-element of the galvanic cell should be attached. The connection can be direct, through a narrow tube to reduce mixing, or through a salt bridge, depending on the other electrode and solution. This creates an ionically conductive path to the working electrode of interest.

COPPER-COPPER(II) SULPHATE ELECTRODE

The copper-copper(II) sulphate electrode is a type of reference electrode, based on the redox reaction with participation of the metal (copper) and its salt-copper(II) sulphate. It is used for measuring electrochemical potential and is the most commonly used reference electrode for testing cathodic protection corrosion control systems.

The corresponding equation can be presented as follow:

$$Cu^{2+} + 2e^- \longrightarrow Cu^0 \, (metal)$$

This reaction characterised by fast electrode kinetics, meaning that a sufficiently high current can be passed through the electrode with the 100 per cent efficiency of the redox reaction (dissolution of the metal or cathodic deposition of the copper-ions).

The Nernst equation below shows the dependence of the potential of the copper-copper(II) sulphate electrode on the activity or concentration copper-ions:

$$E = 0.337 + \frac{RT}{2F} \ln a_{Cu^{2+}}$$

Commercial reference electrodes consist of a plastic tube holding the copper rod and saturated solution of copper sulphate. A porous plug on one end allows contact with the copper sulphate electrolyte. The copper rod protrudes out of the tube. A voltmeter negative lead is connected to the copper rod.

The potential of a copper copper sulphate electrode is +0.314 volt with respect to the standard hydrogen electrode.

DYNAMIC HYDROGEN ELECTRODE

A dynamic hydrogen electrode (DHE) is a reference electrode, more specific a subtype of the standard hydrogen electrodes for electrochemical processes by simulating a reversible hydrogen electrode with an approximately 20 to 40 mV more negative potential.

A separator in a glass tube connects two electrolytes and a small current is enforced between the cathode and anode.

Applications of hydrogen electrode:

1. *In situ* reference electrode for direct methanol fuel cells.
2. Proton exchange membrane fuel cells.

Reversible Hydrogen Electrode

A reversible hydrogen electrode (RHE) is a reference electrode, more specific a subtype of the standard hydrogen electrodes for electrochemical processes and differs from the standard hydrogen electrode by the fact that the measured potential does not change with the pH so that they can be directly used in the electrolyte.

The name refers to the fact that the electrode is in the actual elektrolyte solution and not separated by a salt bridge. The hydrogen ion concentration is therefore not 1, but corresponds to that of the elektrolyte solution; in this way we can achieve a stable potential with a changing pH value. The potential of the RHE correlates to the pH value:

$$E_0 = 0.000 - 0.059 \text{ pH}$$

In general, for hydrogen electrodesthe reaction is:

$$E = E_{00} + \frac{RT}{F}\left(\ln\left(\left[a\text{H}_3\text{O}^+ \right]\right) - \frac{1}{2}\ln\left(p[\text{H}_2]\right)\right)$$

Here E_{00} is the standard potential (this is by definition equal to zero), R is the universal gas constant, T the absolute temperature and F is the Faraday constant.

Surges occur in the electrolysis of water which means that the required cell voltage due to kinetic inhibition higher is than the equilibrium potential. The voltage increases with increasing current density at the electrodes. The measurement of equilibrium potentials is therefore possible without power.

The reversible hydrogen electrode is a fairly practical and reproducible electrode 'standard.' The term refers to a hydrogen electrode immersed in the electrolyte solution actually used.

The benefit of that electrode is that no salt bridge is needed:

1. No contamination of the electrolyte by Cl^- or SO_4^{2-}.
2. No diffusion potentials at the electrolyte bridge (liquid junction potential). This is important at temperature different to 25°C.
3. Long time measurements possible (no electrolyte bridge means no maintenance of the bridge).

Palladium-Hydrogen Electrode

The palladium-hydrogen electrode (abbreviation: Pd/H_2) is one of the common reference electrodes used in electrochemical study. Most of its characteristics are similar to the standard hydrogen electrode (with platinum). But palladium has one significant feature — the capability to absorb (dissolve into itself) molecular hydrogen.

Electrode operation

Two phases can coexist in palladium when hydrogen is absorbed:

1. Alpha-phase at hydrogen concentration less than 0.025 atoms per atom of palladium
2. Beta-phase at hydrogen concentration corresponding to the non-stoichiometric formula $PdH_{0.6}$.

The electrochemical behaviour of a palladium electrode in equilibrium with H_3O^+ ions in solution parallels the behaviour of palladium with molecular hydrogen:

$$\frac{1}{2}H_2 = H_{ads} = H_{abs}$$

Thus the equilibrium is controlled in one case by the partial pressure of fugacity of molecular hydrogen and in other case — by activity of H^+-ions in solution:

$$E = E^0 + \frac{RT}{F}\ln\frac{a_{H^+}}{\left(p_{H_2}\right)^{1/2}}$$

When palladium is electrochemically charged by hydrogen, the existence of two phases is manifested by a constant potential of approximately +50 mV compared to the reversible hydrogen electrode. This potential is independent of the amount of hydrogen absorbed over a wide range. This property has been utilised in the construction of a palladium/hydrogen reference electrode. The main feature of such electrode is an absence of non-stop bubbling of molecular hydrogen through the solution as it is absolutely necessary for the standard hydrogen electrode.

MICROELECTRODES

Microelectrodes are used for: (i) potential recording, (ii) current injection, and (iii) introduction into the cell of ionselective resins for measuring potential or determining the free concentration of cytosolic constituents. (i) and (ii) are the procedures underlying conventional microelectrode recording, voltage-clamping and patch-clamping. This section will be restricted to considering the fundamentals of reliable and accurate measurement of membrane potentials and the experimental manipulation of membrane potential by injection of current.

Making Microelectrodes

One definition of a microelectrode (ME) might be: 'an electrode constructed with a tip having the dimensions of the order of a micrometer (1 μm)'. Usually this means a glass micropipette of the type pioneered by Ling and Gerard, which is filled with an electrolyte solution to act as a conductor of electricity.

Glass MEs are made by heating a capillary until molten, when it is stretched; while the glass is still plastic but cooling down, the tip draws out, breaks and separates.

1. By hand: This is not recommended because of lack of reproducibility, although great artists can heat a capillary in a bunsen and pull out a fine tip.

2. Vertical puller: This usually has a nichrome filament and a 2 stage pull-the first by gravity, the second electromagnetic. This is fine for MEs up to about 30 to 40 MΩ. In our

experience these pullers are less effective for making fine-tipped microelectrodes for use on small cells.

3. Horizontal puller 1 (Livingstone type): These pullers are gear driven and have a platinum foil heating element. They are good for fine tips (ME resistance can be 30–300 MΩ) but this type of puller produces rather long wispy shanks.

4. Horizontal puller 2 (Brown-flaming, Ensor, industrial science): These pullers usually have a platinum or nichrome heating element with a range of preheat times and a 1 or 2 stage pull. The Brown-Flaming has a gas jet which cools the heater rapidly. Good reproducibility can be achieved with these pullers, but setting them up correctly is time consuming. They are generally good for fine MEs with resistances up to 300–500 MΩ and short shanks.

Filling Microelectrodes

Glass microelectrodes are usually filled with a salt solution. The composition of the solution can be determined by the individual experimenter and depends on the experimental protocol. Nowadays, the preferred method of filling is to pull electrodes from capillary that has a glass-fibre fused into the lumen. When the ME is pulled the lumen shape is preserved up to the tip. Using fibre-containing capillary, MEs can be backed-filled with small amounts of solution. The solution tracks down the channels formed either side of the fibre right down to the tip. Bubbles do form but don't occlude the lumen completely. The exception is when a bubble forms directly in front of an Ag/AgCl sintered pellet in a perspex ME holder. This is easy to remedy.

One should realise, however, that other forms of ME than this exist and that even with what might be considered to be a micropipette there are alternatives to an electrolyte solution as a conductor. Thus, micropipettes have been filled with molten Wood's metal which solidifies to give a continuous metal conductor (in our experience, simultaneously cracking the insulating glass envelope.), or have been drawn over single carbon (graphite) fibres around 7 mm in diameter to form a ME with a carbon conductor. These manufacturing techniques produce electrodes with impedances of 200 kW to 2 MW. Similar values are obtained with glass or varnish-coated tungsten MEs which have been electrolytically etched to a fine tip; it is possible to electroplate the tips with other metals for positional marking (e.g. iron, which can be visualised by the Prussian Blue reaction) or for lower noise and reduced polarisation. All these MEs which use non-electrolyte filling as the electrical conductor have high DC resistances, however, and are employed in extracellular recording and stimulation; in this recording mode they are used for registering the occurrence rather than the accurate wave form of signals (for example, neuronal discharges). An exception to the latter statement is the use of carbon fibre electrodes to measure redox potentials of oxidisable compounds in biological tissues. Metal electrodes behave electrically in moist preparations as if they are a small resistance in series with a larger resistance and parallel capacitance: they are not suitable for measuring standing DC potentials. They do, however, have low noise at the frequencies where most of the power from action potential signals is concentrated. Consequently, a good signal-to-noise ratio is obtained when they are used for extracellular recordings, better than that of electrolyte-filled micropipettes.

Electrolyte-filled (usually with NaCl) micropipettes are also used for extracellular recording of neuronal discharges since they can also faithfully reproduce the potential wave-form down to DC levels. Frequently, these MEs are used to measure potentials set up by synaptic current flow across the resistance of the extracellular space. By considering the potential gradient and its spatial derivative within a tissue, the location of sinks and sources of current can be used to pinpoint synaptic regions within the tissue and this technique is known as current density analysis.

Connection of Microelectrodes to Recording Circuit

The preparation and the electrode are both wet; electronic circuitry is dry and has metallic conductors.

Plain metal/liquid interfaces display junction potentials and can produce gas (hydrogen and oxygen) if current is passed through them. The latter is particularly annoying since the presence of gas bubbles on the electrode simulates the insertion of a capacitance in the circuit at the liquid/metal junction, thereby limiting DC recording. (Hence the reason that metal MEs are not used for intracellular recording). Connections are therefore made to the recording circuit via non-polarisable reversible electrodes. Silver/silver chloride (Ag/AgCl) electrodes exchange electrons for Cl$^-$ ions in solution. They are usually employed in the form of silver wire coated with silver chloride or a sintered pellet of metallic silver and powdered AgCl pressed around a silver connecting wire. The pellets have the advantages of large current carrying capacity and stability to light. Stability is obviously of prime importance in measuring membrane potentials as is the property of reversibility, i.e. the property whereby the passage of current in either direction through the electrode does not alter the potential difference between the metal and the solution. The Ag/AgCl reference electrode is reversible and of constant potential because AgCl is sparingly soluble and therefore the solution is saturated with respect to AgCl; the concentration of Ag$^+$ ions in solution is inversely proportional to the [Cl$^-$] (from the definition of solubility product) and as a result the potential EAg of metal relative to the solution is given by $E_{Ag} = \text{Const} - RT/F \ln[Cl^-]$ (from the Nernst expression for the electrode potential of a metal). Differences in [Cl$^-$] in the solutions composing these 'half-cells' lead to a standing potential which should not vary unless [Cl$^-$] does at either electrode. If, in the course of an experiment, [Cl$^-$] does vary (for instance, as a result of changing the bathing medium in an *in vitro* preparation) then the AgCl reference electrode should be interfaced to the preparation by means of a salt bridge which will maintain a constant [Cl$^-$], avoids damage to the AgCl electrode and toxic effects of Ag in the bath. The salt bridge comprises 1–2 per cent agar in 0.15 M NaCl, or with continuous bath perfusion, concentrated KCl may be used to minimise junction potentials. Normally the ME tip itself forms the other salt bridge, with a AgCl wire inserted in the ME barrel, but to equalise the reference electrode potentials exactly an additional salt bridge may be used at the back of the ME, with a AgCl pellet in the ME holder.

AgCl pellet electrodes can be purchased cheaply and are available as discs or pellets, some small enough to insert in the back of wide bore ME glass. There are 3 widely used procedures for chloriding Ag wires; for each the wire must be clean. (i) electrolytic coating is done by connecting 2 wires immersed in 0.1 M HCl to the poles of a 1.5 V battery and passing current for 20 minutes or so, reversing the polarity at regular intervals, resulting in a uniform but fragile grey coat, (ii) wires may be dipped in molten AgCl (requiring an intense gas/air or gas/oxygen torch and crucible) to produce a tough coating, and (iii) Ag wires kept in hypochlorite-based bleach become coated with AgCl, and can be changed frequently if necessary.

Junction Potentials

There is a potential difference set up at the interface between two salt solutions of different ionic composition or concentration by differing diffusional flux of anions and cations across the boundary: this is a liquid junction or diffusion potential. It is described, for a single solute, by equations in the form

$$V = \frac{u - v}{u + v} \frac{RT}{F} \ln \frac{c_1}{c_2}$$

where u is the mobility of the cations in solution and v is the mobility of the anions and c_1 and c_2 are the solute concentrations on opposite sides of the interface. R is the gas constant, T, the temperature and F is Faraday's Constant. Equations for the junction potential in more complex cases are given by Barry and Lynch. Junction potentials develop:

1. As a result of different anionic and cationic mobilities.
2. Different solute concentrations develop between the bath solution and reference salt bridge if these differ, and a modified form of junction potential, termed a tip potential, exists across the ME tip. They cannot be eliminated

but the correct electrode configuration ought to aim to stabilise them with respect to experimental solution changes or to reduce them by trying to equalise u and v. A reference salt bridge of 150 mM NaCl and agar is suitable if the composition of the bath is constant.

Experiments in which changes of ionic composition are imposed are often made to determine reversal potentials, and precision is important if permeability ratios are to be derived. The junction potential change at the reference boundary can be minimised by a continuously renewed 2–3 M KCl junction. K^+ and Cl^- have similar mobilities in aqueous solution. Moreover, with high concentrations of KCl, diffusion of KCl from the salt bridge predominates and potential changes due to alterations in salt concentration in the bath are small. A small continuous outflow of KCl solution, generated by 1–2 cm hydrostatic pressure through a 2–5 mm tip, prevents dilution within the bridge by the bath solution and the resulting generation of a concentration gradient and junction potential within the salt bridge and reference electrode itself. However, leakage of KCl into the solution bathing the preparation can lead to unwanted changes of ionic composition, so downstream siting and perfusion of the bath are essential. If this cannot be done, the electrode arrangement can be used to measure junction potentials at the tip of a NaCl bridge when the bath solution is changed in the absence of the preparation, and the results used to correct the membrane potentials recorded when the NaCl bridge is used as reference.

A second problem arises when kinetic measurements of membrane potential response to ionic changes are made, or when the bath solution is changed locally (i.e. not at the reference), for instance with a puffer pipette or similar device. In both cases a junction potential will exist within the bath, even if only transiently, between the recording site and the reference, and will contribute to the potential recorded. As an example, when recording the timecourse of Cl-evoked potential changes by fast perfusion in skeletal muscle fibres, Hodgkin and Horowicz used differential recording with respect to a blunt ME placed adjacent to the recording site to avoid transient Cl⁻ junction potentials along the bath.

Tip Potentials

The surface chemistry of the glass is complex: at the tip of a ME it is believed that a restriction of anionic mobility is established. As a result of this, the liquid junction potential is altered by properties of the electrode tip. This is the tip potential (TP). The TP is abolished by breakage of the tip. It can be measured by measuring the potential change when the tip is broken, or by registering the potential change when an electrode of similar manufacture and filling solution, but with its tip broken is added in parallel between the input of the measuring device and the solution bathing the ME tip TPs are (i) of negative sign, up to −70 mV with electrodes filled with 3 M KCl and tested in physiological saline, (ii) abolished when inside and outside solutions are the same, (iii) larger in higher resistance electrodes, (iv) may vary widely in magnitude between otherwise similar electrodes, (v) can often be reduced by filling MEs with acidic solutions, and (vi) can be reduced and even reversed in sign by addition of small concentrations of polyvalent ions (e.g. thorium, $Th4^+$) and high concentrations, 10–100 mM $[Ca^{2+}]$, to the bathing solution.

The TP is the main source of uncertainty in measuring membrane potential because it changes depending on the immediate ionic environment into which the tip is placed. Adrian studied some properties of TPs of KCl-filled MEs and the change in TP when the tip was in 100 mM NaCl or 100 mM KCl (to simulate cell impalement). The TP is smaller on going from extracellular to intracellular solution, the difference becoming larger the larger the initial potential. For a TP of −5 mV, the error is about 2 mV. Roughly speaking, TP is proportional to ME resistance, and inversely proportional to salt concentration of the external solution. The change in TP in going from one solution to another is proportional to the size of the TP. Thus, if possible, MEs with the smallest resistance, and therefore small

TP, should be selected. Adrian used MEs filled by the method of boiling; subsequently it has been shown that the method of ME filling and also the time after filling influences TPs. Smaller TPs are observed with the fibre-filling method (e.g. MEs made from filament glass) and with immediate usage.

Clearly, the problem of TP is complex and unpredictable and possibly for this reason is largely ignored in the majority of research reports. Generally speaking, TP is negative and the effect on impalement is to estimate a more positive value of the resting potential as the TP becomes more positive inside the cell. Measurement of the TP requires use of a KCl bridge between AgCl electrodes at both the reference and ME connections. The potential is initially zeroed with KCl connections into the bath solution and the TP recorded as the additional potential when the ME is introduced. A system with differential recording between ME and reference and KCl junctions to permit measurement of TP (or junction potentials of salt bridges introduced in place of the ME).

Previous paragraphs have been included as an introduction to the wider range of ME usage; the recording techniques to be described are not dependent on a need to know the absolute value of potential. Even in the case of extracellular field potential analysis it is the difference of potential within the preparation that is of interest and any offsets or error potentials in the recording circuitry are of no consequence provided that they are fixed. It is, however, important to realise that using electrodes in aqueous solution to measure potentials is by no means as theoretically straight forward as putting a voltmeter across the terminals of an electronic component. The theoretical basis of potential measurement in aqueous solution is discussed lucidly by Finkelstein and Mauro.

Measuring Membrane Potentials Using Microelectrodes

The electronic amplifier used to record potentials via MEs should have the following characeristics:

1. Input resistance should be at least 100–1000 times the ME resistance in order to measure the full signal at the ME tip and draw negligible current from the signal source.

2. Low leakage current. The current flowing into or out of the input terminal of the amplifier should be less than that which would cause a 1 mV drop across the ME or the cell input resistance.

3. Response time should be adequate: with a good response time there are ways of overcoming the low-pass filtering properties of a voltage recording set-up.

Capacitance compensation

The low pass filtering properties of the microelectrode and its amplifier are due to inevitable capacitances between the microelectrode and ground (Fig. 13.8). C_t, the transmural capacitance can be minimised by (i) thick pipette walls (glass pipettes can be made thicker by coating with a layer of Sylgard (Corning), and (ii) a low solution level in the bath to reduce the effective transmural area. C_s, the stray capacitance from the microelectrode and amplifier input to ground (that is, the microscope, bath, stand, etc.) can be reduced by minimising the length of the ME and connecting wire and by driving the shield of the connecting wire with a low impedance signal from the output of the ME amplifier (Fig. 13.9). C_a, the input capacitance of the amplifier should be negligible if the amplifier is chosen to have a good response time as suggested. C_{tot} is the total summed capacitance.

Once C_{tot} is minimised it can be compensated for by using a feedback circuit ofen described as 'negative' capacitance (Fig. 13.10). This positive feedback circuit provides the current lost through C_{tot}, preventing a potential drop across the electrode resistance. Good compensation clearly depends on the rapidity with which the feedback circuit can supply current. The fully compensated rise time is proportional to the geometric mean of the rise time of the recording amplifier and the rise time of the uncompensated circuit. This suggests that the best strategy is (i) to minimise stray capacitance, and (ii) use a head-stage amplifier with a fast rise time. Overcompensation of input capacitance results in damped oscillations at the leading edge of potential steps and finally in continuous oscillation.

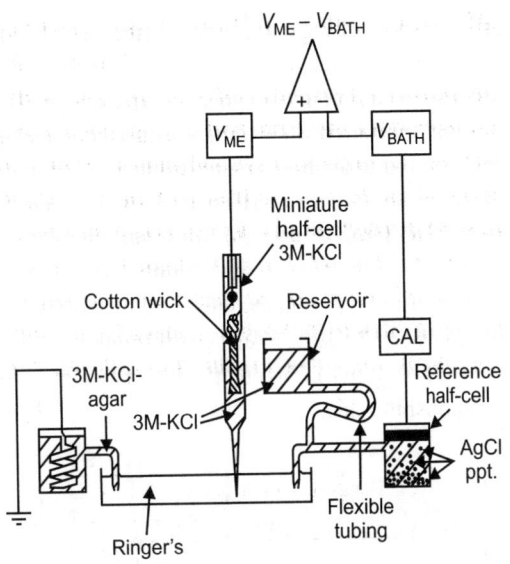

Fig. 13.8. An arrangement of electrodes permitting measurement of TP or junction potentials in a perfusion bath. The potentials of the reference half electrode and miniature KCl half cell are zeroed with respect to ground with the cotton wick in the bath. Placing the wick into the back of the ME introduces an additional potential due to the TP. During an experiment with changes in the bath composition the flowing KCl reference maintains a constant bath potential. Juction potentials with respect to normal Ringer can be measured by substituting a blunt pipette containing Ringer for ME and changing the bath solution. The calibrator CAL can be used to offset the standing membrane potential to look at small changes, e.g. synaptic potentials at high gain without high pass filtering.

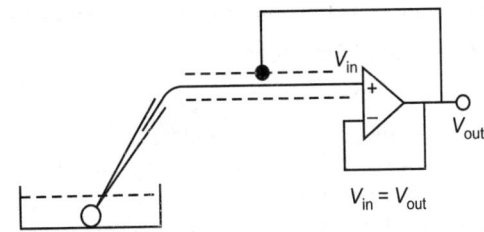

Fig. 13.9. A low-impedance driven shield to reduce C, the stray capacitance to ground.

Manipulating Cell Membrane Potentials

Experimental protocols often require the manipulation of membrane potential (for example, to test passive membrane properties such as input resistance by passing current into the cell). With two MEs in the same cell, one electrode can be dedicated to voltage recording, the other to current injection. This is the preferred method, but simultaneous current injection and voltage recording through a single ME can be achieved-one needs a way of eliminating the potential difference between ME barrel and ME tip caused by the voltage drop due to current flowing through the ME resistance (R_{ME}). These two potentials can be large (i.e. 1 nA through a 50 MΩ electrode = 50 mV). Two methods are available for accomplishing this.

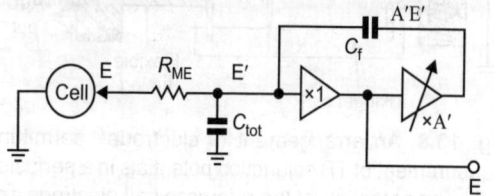

Fig. 13.10. The potential across C_f is $A'E'-E' = E'(A'-1)$ and the current across C_f is $C_f' \times de/dt'(A'-1)$. To compensate for the current loss across the capacitance to ground when E' is changing with time ($C_{tot} \times dE'/dt$) the gain of amplifier A' is adjusted so that $C_f (A'-1) = C_{tot}$. In this way current is supplied to the input of the amplifier, equal and opposite to the loss through C_{tot}. Another way of regarding this is that of adding *negative capacitance* in parallel with C_{tot}. The effectiveness of a negative capacitance circuit is such that the fully compensated rise time of a circuit is approximately twice the geometric mean of the amplifier's rise time and the uncompensated circuit's rise tim.

Bridge balance circuits

The modern analogues of the Wheatstone bridge circuitry formerly used for eliminating $E = IR_{ME}$ are still known as bridge balance circuits, though they are not strictly bridge circuits. Nowadays it is usual to subtract electronically from the voltage output a scaled proportion of the input signal driving the current injection circuit (current pump). The circuit in Fig. 13.11 does just this.

The amplifier gains can be scaled so that the ME resistance can be read off the dial of the BAL potentiometer in MΩ, for example; this is one simple way to measure ME resistance.

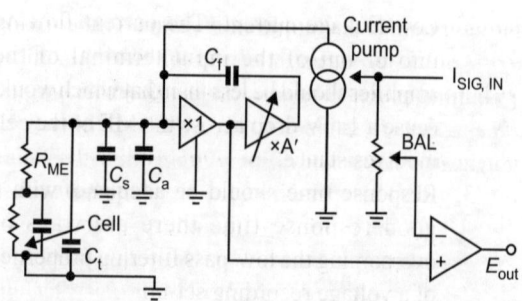

Fig. 13.11. A circuit to compensate for the potential drop across a ME due to passage of current. The current pump will pass a current proportional to the command voltage and independent of the electrode resistance. The command voltage is therefore scaled and subtracted from the ME potential. The circuit assumes that the ME has a linear current-voltage relation (i.e. obeys Ohm's law). This may not always be true, and should be checked.

Possible artefacts arise from incorrect balancing or the inability to balance the bridge with certainty. First, the method depends on R_{ME} not changing during passage of current through the ME. One should, if possible, use MEs with linear current-voltage (I-V) relationships, or restrict the current to a range of values over which the I-V relation is more or less linear. Second, one cannot compensate completely for the capacitance distributed in the transmural elements comprising the ME tip (C_t). In poor recording conditions, for example deep immersion of the ME in the bath, the frequency response of the recording system is compromised to such an extent that the charging of the cell membrane capacitance cannot be accurately judged (Fig. 13.12).

Discontinuous current injection method

This is an alternative to bridge balance and eliminates one source of artefact-that of non-linearity of the ME I-V relation. Instead of injecting continuous current, pulses are injected. Figure 13.13 shows the principle of the single-electrode switched current clamp. If the membrane time constant is large compared to the electrode time constant, charge will be stored on the membrane capacitance (time constant $C_m \times R_m$,), whereas the potential due to IR_{ME} (time constant $C_{tot} \times R_{ME}$) decays rapidly. If the voltage is sampled and held between time points $S (V_{S\&H})$ at a time when IR_{ME} is zero, only V_m, the true membrane potential is measured and the change in V_m approximates that which would be seen in the normal bridge balance case with a continuous current of one half the amplitude (Fig. 13.13b). Obviously, the approximation is better the higher the pulse frequency.

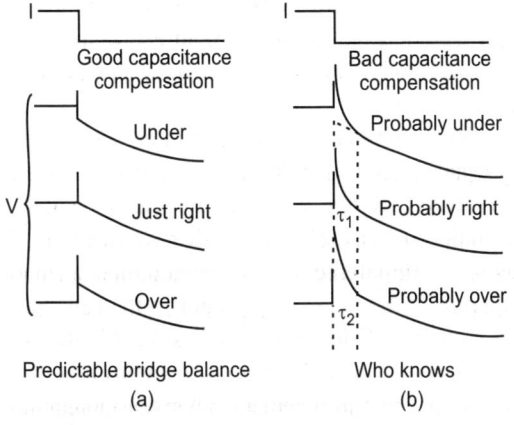

Fig. 13.12. Incorrect capacitance compensation can lead to spurious balance of the ME resistance.

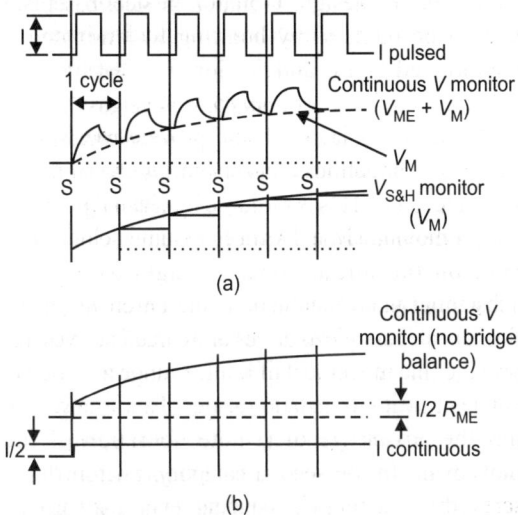

Fig. 13.13. The principle of the single-electrode switched current clamp is shown. In (a) current pulses lead to rapid charging of the ME RC network. The slower charging of the cell membrane RC network leads to a smaller signal which is sampled some time after the end of a current pulse when the charge on RCME has decayed. (b) illustrates the point that the pulsed current is equivalent to a continuous current of half the pulse amplitude which (a) causes a voltage drop across RME (b) charges the membrane capacitance.

The voltage due to current passage down the ME does not appear and furthermore, since one monitors voltage after IR_{ME} has decayed, any change in R_{ME} during current passage is of no consequence, provided that the current pump can deliver a truly constant current. Clearly, for rapid switching rates capacity neutralisation is important. In addition, the noncompensated C_t must be minimised to allow fast settling. Artefacts encountered with this method of 'balancing' electrode resistance stem largely from inadequate capacity compensation or using too high a pulse frequency. These are illustrated in Fig. 13.14.

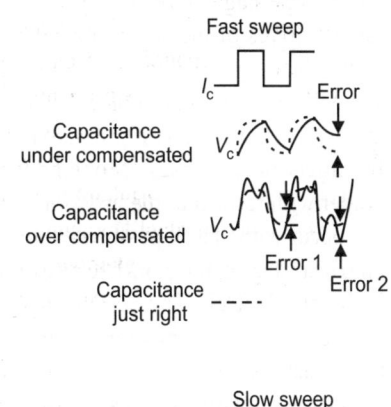

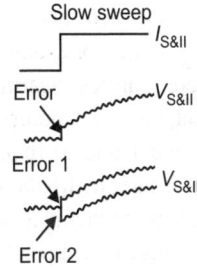

Fig. 13.14. Artefacts which can arise from inappropriate use of the switched clamp. (I_c, V_c are continuous monitor outputs; $I_{S\&H}$, $V_{S\&H}$ are sampled outputs).

If the capacity compensation is correctly adjusted and the ME is clearly settling within a half cycle time then the VS & H (sample and hold) should exhibit no step with the onset of current injection. To help settling times asymmetric duty cycles may be employed (e.g. 25 per cent current injection, 75 per cent settling time). In these cases the current I, delivered with a duty cycle of D is equivalent to a constant current of $I \times D$.

Mechanical Stability

The interaction between ME (or patch pipette) and cell needs to be stable on a submicron scale to avoid damage to the cell membrane and consequent excessive current leakage. There are two symptoms of mechanical problems, slow drift of the ME tip with respect to cell, and faster vibrations.

Drift can arise from the following causes.

1. The cell or tissue may move in the bath, a problem that can usually be simply remedied (except when recording from muscle). The bath may move with respect to the microscope stage, remedied by servicing the ratchet drives of the stage movement or by adding locking screws or some other device.

2. The ME may move in its holder, either axially or laterally, particularly if pressure is applied for injection purposes. Movement of the holder with respect to the micromanipulator can occur with plastic push-in arrangements onto headstage connectors because of 'creep' in the plastic itself. The best arrangement is to secure the ME holder to the micromanipulator directly.

Drift in the micromanipulator can occur between slider assemblies, for example loose rack and pinion drives, screw drives, bearing races or dovetails. If the manipulator is not mounted with flat surfaces then drift can occur due to rocking movements. If the manipulator uses hydraulic drives these are subject to drift because of thermally induced expansion of the fluid, so in this case temperature stability is important.

Vibration of the ME tip with respect to the cell can be minimised by the following precautions. The source of vibration is usually floorborne and is eliminated by working on a solid floor, as close as possible to solid ground or at least a supporting wall. Wooden or other unstable flooring can be avoided by sitting the baseplate assembly on brackets bolted to a supporting wall (a cheaper and more effective remedy than an airtable). Vibration reaching the baseplate supports can be filtered by compliant mounts, such as cycle tubes, pneumatic cushions (supplied by optical manufacturers) or regulated compressed air isolation tables, with a heavy table top (total mass 200–500 kg). Generally low frequencies are transmitted more effectively than high through this arrangement; roughly the product of mass and compliance determines the high frequency cut-off. There are two important points to note, that lateral vibration may be as prominent as vertical, and that isolation tables are tuned to a low frequency, 1–2 Hz, to achieve damping and may exagerate inputs in that range.

The combined transmitting microscope stage-baseplate-micromanipulator-ME holder-ME connections make a system of levers with great potential for vibration, or transmitting small movements to the ME-cell impalement. The connections from the fulcrum of the micromanipulator to the cell should be as short, stiff and light as is feasible. Lightweight, e.g. piezo-driven manipulators mounted on the stage may be the best arrangement, otherwise more remote mounting requires manipulators of massive construction to achieve stability and precision, such as the Huxley design. Vibration in steel baseplates should be damped by bonding to laminated or compressed board and flexion avoided by using sufficient thickness or honeycomb designs.

Micromanipulators should provide precision of movement, much less than 1 mm, with stability in the same range. This is achieved by either lightweight design moving short distances mounted close to the cell, on the microscope or stage, or by more substantial units mounted on the baseplate. In the former category piezo drives or hydraulic drives may provide fine movement of limited range mounted on compact optical translation stages. This arrangement has the advantage of remote operation of fine movement. In the second category, micrometer or screw drives acting via reducing levers may provide fine movement in only vertical or, in the Huxley design, all three axes. Baseplate mounting of a coarse unit with a remotely operated fine control is often used.

Microscopy

The experimental microscope is an important part of an ME or patch clamp system, often an essential mechanical component as well as a means for seeing the cell.

Generally, ME (and patch clamp) technique is improved by seeing the tip and cell clearly during impalement or seal formation, and there are a number of examples of significant advances in the application of ME measurements resulting from better optics. The iontophoretic studies of postsynaptic mechanism at the skeletal endplate and autonomic ganglia used Nomarski differential interference contrast (DIC) optics to see synaptic elements clearly. The same optical system with infrared video microscopy can be used to see and record from soma or dendritic elements in brain slices. DIC and fluorescence microscopy are used to identify cell types and developmental stages when investigating changes in electrophysiological properties. The use of indicators for intracellular ion concentrations requires good optics for fluorescence microscopy.

Some general considerations are given here. Good optical resolution requires a good microscope objective, particularly as high a numerical aperture (NA) as is practicable. 'Resolving power', the separation of 2 distinct points, is proportional to 1/NA. The practical restriction in an upright microscope is mechanical, because high NA is achieved by decreasing the distance between objective lens and specimen. An upright microscope is essential for work in thick specimens such as tissue slices or embryos and the minimum working distance for placing MEs is about 1.5 mm. The best NA currently available with this working distance is 0.75 in a 40× water immersion objective (Zeiss 0.75 W 40×), although water immersion objectives exist with NA 0.9 or 1 but shorter working distance. For single cells dispersed or in culture an inverted microscope can be used. If the chamber base is made of a thin coverslip working distance is no longer a problem (the ME or pipette comes from above) and the maximum NA obtainable with an oil immersion objective, 1.3–1.4, can be used. Illumination of the specimen should also be with as high an NA condenser as possible; the same restriction of working distance means that a condenser of NA 0.9 can be used with upright microscopy (good illumination is important in thick specimens) but only 0.5–0.6 with inverted.

Contrast methods such as phase contrast, DIC or Hoffman greatly improve the visibility of thin cells and small structures on large cells, and one or other of these is really necessary. Phase contrast is inexpensive and adequate for single cells, but for thicker specimens DIC optics are favoured. CCD TV cameras are also inexpensive and convenient.

For fluorescence microscopy the brightness of the specimen increases with the NA^2 and decreases with $1/(magnification)^2$, so high NA low magnification objectives are often used for microspectrofluorimetry.

ELECTRODES AND ELECTROLYTES

When metallic electrodes are placed on the surface of the body, contact is made via electrolytic solutions. If the electrodes are to be left in place for extended periods, evaporation of the solution takes place. To prevent such an occurrence, it is sometimes possible to locate the electrodes in body cavities and use the fluids in these regions as electrolytic conductors; sometimes the cavities can serve as containers for the electrolytes. Although not all the body cavities can be employed in unanesthetised subjects, consideration should be given to using the nose, ear, mouth, axilla, navel, rectum, vagina, and urethra. Often electrodes in these and other areas can be combined with other transducers, such as electrical thermometers or acoustic pickups. Sometimes the metallic cases of these devices can serve as active, indifferent, or ground electrodes.

Electrode jellies and pastes were developed during the early string-galvanometer days of electro-cardiography when investigators were anxious to eliminate the cumbersome immersion electrodes, which required that the subject be seated with both hands and feet in saline-filled buckets. Study was begun of the behaviour of electrodes consisting of sheets of metal wrapped in saline-soaked bandages and applied to the skin. Since the string galvanometer was activated by the electrical current that would flow as a result of the potential differences appearing on the body surface during cardiac activity (ECG), large electrodes and strong electrolytes were needed to obtain a low-resistance contact with the subject.

About 1935, when electrode pastes and jellies began to replace the saline-soaked pads, the characteristics of several of the earliest electrode jellies were investigated by Bell. Using lead electrodes (14 × 5 cm) on human subjects, they measured the DC resistance and 300 Hz impedance with the following substances under the electrodes: (i) 1 per cent saline, (ii) a paste of saline, glycerine, water, and pumice, (iii) soft green soap, and (iv) electrode jelly that contained crushed quartz. They found that when the electrodes were wrapped in gauze, soaked in 1 per cent saline, and applied to the subjects, the DC resistance was highest (3080 Ω). With the other three preparations in direct contact with the electrodes and skin, the resistances were 2010, 2040, and 1100 Ω, respectively. By analysing their results, Bell and his colleagues quickly found that the presence of an abrasive reduced the resistance considerably. They were able to show that the resistance with green soap was reduced by a factor of 3 when crushed quartz was added and the mixture rubbed into the skin. They also found that by lightly rubbing the dry skin with glass paper (fine sandpaper) and applying the electrolyte, they could obtain very low and extremely stable DC resistance and impedance values. This early observation demonstrated the need for abrasives in electrode pastes and jellies.

A modern reappraisal of traditional electrode jellies for recording the ECG was presented by Lewes, who called attention to the fact that strong electrolytes were essential in the string-galvanometer days, when the electrode–subject resistance had to be in low-kilohm range, but with the advent of electronic instruments with high input impedance the need for a low electrode resistance had disappeared. To prove his point the recorded more than 4000 ECGs with instruments of high input impedance the need for a low electrode resistance had disappeared. To prove his point he recorded more than 4000 ECGs with instruments of high input impedance (2–4 MΩ), using a remarkable variety of substances as electrode jellies. The recordings made with each substance were compared with those obtained with standard electrode jelly. The substances used were lubricating compounds (K-Y jelly, Lubrifax), culinary compounds (mayonnaise, french mustard, tomato paste), and toilet preparations (hand cream and tooth paste). All these substances are poor conductors, and all produced ECGs indistinguishable from those taken with standard electrode jelly.

From studies such as those just reported, it can be seen that two types of electrode preparation are now in use. One has low resistivity and originated in the days when it was necessary to obtain a low-resistance contact with the subject. Such preparations are still used for recording bioelectric events and must be used when electrodes are used to pass current, as in the case of stimulation or defibrillation. The other type of electrode electrolyte that is available is high in resistivity and resembles skin lotion. Such preparations are suitable for recording bioelectric events with modern equipment, which has an adequately high input impedance. Such preparations should never be used with stimulating or defibrillating electrodes.

The electrodes, and the electrolyte used with them, must not be considered to be independent of the recording equipment to which the electrodes are connected.

Although most of the commercially available electrode pastes are satisfactory for recording a variety of bioelectric events, various authors have presented their own recipes. Among these are Jenks and Graybiel, Bell, Marchant and Jones, Thompson and Patterson, Shackel, Lykken, Edelberg and Burch, Asa, and Fascenelli. Figure 13.15 shows electrodes and electrolytes interface.

Interface between Materials

In this section we extend those ideas to describe the electrical phenomena which result when dissimilar materials are placed in contact-in particular we discuss what happens when a metal electrode is placed in an ionic solution, but the ideas developed are equally applicable when solids with different properties are in contact, as in a semiconductor junction for example.

The boundary between the dissimilar materials is like a semipermeable membrane; some of the ion species present can diffuse from one material to the other. The electrical conditions at the interface are

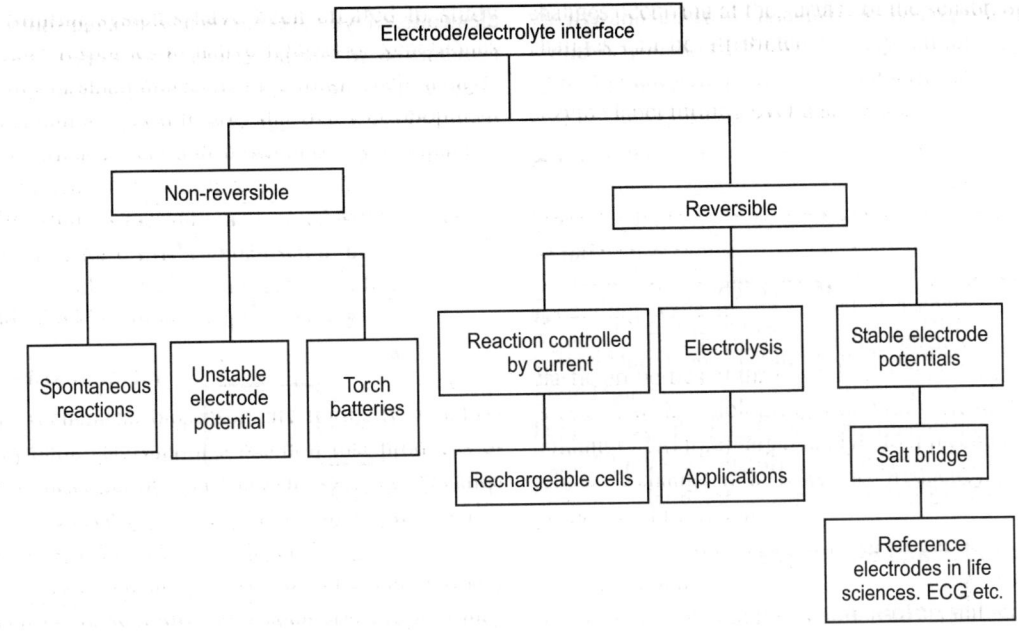

Fig. 13.15. Electrodes and electrolytes interface.

determined by the same basic conditions that we used when discussing membrane potentials, namely:

1. Bulk neutrality.
2. Zero current density if the external electric circuit is not complete.

Motion of ions through the interface is determined by these electrical conditions and by the possible chemical reactions which can occur at the interface. The chemical reactions play a role analogous to that of the permeabilities in determining the transfer of ions through semipermeable membranes.

For example, when copper is placed in a copper sulphate solution the chemical reaction which takes place at the surface of the copper is:

$$Cu \rightleftharpoons Cu^{2+} + 2e^-.$$

This chemical equation expresses the idea that a copper atom (Cu) can become a doubly charged copper ion (Cu^{2+}) by giving up 2 electrons (e^-), a change indicated by the right-pointing arrow. The left-pointing arrow indicates that the reaction can go the other way: a copper ion can pick up two electrons to become a neutral atom. In this reaction the only ion which can cross the interface is Cu^{2+}. Consequently the zero current condition corresponds to a zero flow

of ions across the interface, just as if the interface were a semipermeable membrane permeable only to Cu^{2+} ions. Hence a charge double layer builds up to give a Nernst equilibrium at the interface.

By contrast if magnesium is placed in acid the reaction is:

$$Mg + 2H^+ \rightleftharpoons H_2 + Mg^{2+};$$

a magnesium atom (Mg) in the metal combines with two hydrogen ions (H^+) in the solution, releasing a molecule of hydrogen gas (H_2) and leaving a doubly charged magnesium ion (Mg^{2+}) in solution. In this case two species of ions can cross the interface. The interface potential mediates the reaction in the sense that it ensures that the currents carried by H^+ and Mg^{2+} ions cancel out. The interface behaves like a membrane which has different permeabilities to Mg^{2+} and H^+ ions.

EMF and Potential Difference

Chemical reactions between metals and electrolytes can be exploited to produce electrical energy from chemical energy. The chemical reactions are responsible for producing charge separation at the boundaries between solid metal and a solution containing its ions. We can describe this energy conversion process in terms of an abstract quantity called EMF (symbol ξ). As noted in chapter E2 EMF can be defined as the energy per charge given to a system of charges. Once they are separated the charged particles create an electrostatic field and its associated potential difference. If you look at a static situation such as the separated charge on the $+$ and $-$ terminals of a battery, the PD between the terminals must be equal to the EMF which created it: $V = \xi$. (That equality no longer holds if you extract energy from the battery by putting it in a circuit and letting current through it.) Since the quantity that is measured in practice is the potential difference, we shall discuss the effects of EMFs in terms of potentials.

Electrodes and Electrolytes

Electrode potentials

If you put strips of two different metals into an appropriate electrolyte solution you are likely to find that a potential difference appears between the two strips. The system is a galvanic cell, commonly known as a battery. The potential difference is produced by an EMF associated with the chemical reactions between both the metals and the electrolyte. The interface between each piece of metal and the electrolyte solution forms an electrode. Electrodes are always used in pairs. It is impossible to make voltage measurements or pass current into an electrolyte without using two electrodes.

A simple example is a piece of copper (Cu) and a piece of zinc (Zn) both partly immersed in the same dilute solution of copper sulphate ($CuSO_4$). The copper becomes about 1 volt positive with respect to the zinc. The potential change occurs in two steps at the electrode-electrolyte interfaces, not in the bulk solution (Fig. 13.16). Both metals are negative relative to the electrolyte, but the potential of the zinc is more negative than that of the copper. So the copper is positive with respect to the zinc.

It is impossible to measure these absolute electrode potentials directly because you can't make contact with the electrolyte without using another electrode. If you introduce a third electrode the problem is still there because you don't know its electrode potential. However the cell potential, which is the difference between the two electrode potentials, can be measured directly.

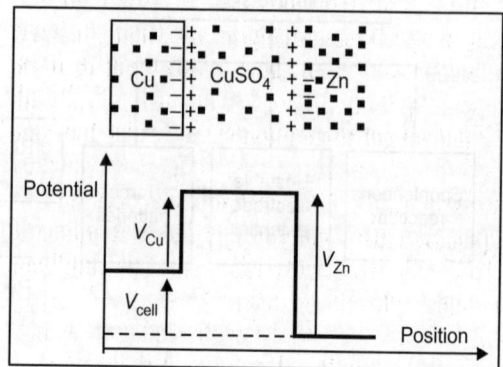

Fig. 13.16. Potential distribution in a cell on open circuit. The cell potential is the difference between the potential changes at the two interfaces. Note that the actual values of the individual potentials V_{Cu} and V_{Zn} cannot be measured; only the difference $V_{cell} = (V_{Cu} - V_{Zn})$ can be found.

Metal–electrolyte electrode

The chemistry, electrode potential, and other characteristics of an electrode depend not only on the solid electrode material, but also on the solution in which it is placed. Strictly the electrode is not just the metal, but the combination of the metal and the solution. Thus for example, when copper is placed in a copper sulphate solution we refer to a copper–copper sulphate electrode.

Nernst equilibrium potential

The chemistry of the electrode reaction is such that neither electrons in the metal nor negative ions in the solution cross the interface. The physical processes at the interface between the metal and a solution of its ion are similar to those that occur when a single ion diffuses through a semipermeable membrane. The tendency of metal ions to diffuse from the electrode to the electrolyte (i.e. from a strong 'solution' to a weaker solution) or the other way is balanced by the potential difference across the interface, creating a Nernst equilibrium. The potential of a metal electrode relative to a solution of its own ion might be modelled using the Nernst Equation:

$$V_{metal} - V_{solution} = \frac{kT}{ze} \ln\left(\frac{C_{solution}}{C_{metal}}\right)$$

where, $C_{solution}$ is the concentration of metal ions in the electrolyte and C_{metal} is the effective concentration of ions in the solid electrode. One trouble with this model is that we cannot accurately assign a theoretical value to C_{metal}, nor can it be measured. So the equation needs to be manipulated into a useable form. The first step is to introduce a standard reference value for concentrations, C_{ref}, and to split the right hand side of the equation into two terms:

$$V_{solution} = \frac{kT}{ze} \ln\left(\frac{C_{solution}}{C_{ref}}\right) + \frac{kT}{ze} \ln\left(\frac{C_{ref}}{C_{metal}}\right)$$

$$= \frac{kT}{ze} \ln\left(\frac{C_{metal}}{C_{ref}}\right) + \frac{kT}{ze} \ln\left(\frac{C_{solution}}{C_{ref}}\right)$$

Next, we hide the troublesome idea of the concentration of ions in the solid metal by labelling the first term as the standard electrode potential, $V_{electrode}$ and looking for a way of measuring it. The second term could be called a concentration potential. The equation is now:

$$V_{metal} - V_{solution} = V_{electrode} + \frac{kT}{ze} \ln\left(\frac{C_{solution}}{C_{ref}}\right)$$

$$... (13.1)$$

where we have written:

$$V_{electrode} = -\frac{kT}{ze} \ln\left(\frac{C_{metal}}{C_{ref}}\right) \text{—not the minus sign!}$$

There are some important interpretations to be made about this equation. Firstly it says that there are two things that contribute to an electrode potential: (i) a contact between a metal and a solution of its own ion, and (ii) the concentration of that ion in the solution. We can now talk about those two contributions separately, but first we need to specify a value for the reference concentration. The universally accepted value is one mole per litre: $C_{ref} = 1$ mol.L^{-1}.

Now for the problem of measuring the standard electrode potential. We have already seen that it can't be measured directly, because you need another electrode which has its own, unknown, electrode potential. The problem is solved by carefully specifying a standard reference electrode, so that all other electrode potentials can be referred to it. The chosen standard is a device called the standard hydrogen electrode. (See the right hand side of Fig. 13.17). The metal electrode consists of platinum metal coated with platinum black (colloidal platinum), which absorbs and holds gaseous hydrogen. The lower part is immersed in an exactly 1 molar solution of hydrogen ions (H$^+$) while the upper part is surrounded by hydrogen gas. Hydrogen gas is continually bubbled through the arrangement.

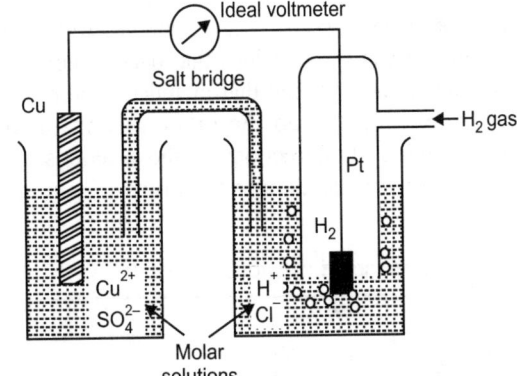

Fig. 13.17. Measurement of a standard electrode potential. The electrode to be measured is in a molar solution of its own ion. That solution is electrically connected to a standard hydrogen electrode by a salt bridge. The concentrations of the metal ions in the left hand cell and the hydrogen ions on the right must both be equal to 1.00 mol.L^{-1}.

It is often said that the electrode potential of the hydrogen electrode is defined to be zero, but that is not strictly true because the potential difference between metal electrode and electrolyte is really unknown. It is better to say that all other electrode potentials are the potential difference that you get when you make them into a galvanic cell with a hydrogen electrode.

You don't always have to use a hydrogen electrode. Once the electrode potential of one metal has been measured relative to the hydrogen electrode, you can use that electrode as a reference for other electrodes. The standard electrode potential could be either positive or negative, depending on the chemical reaction that occurs at the electrode when it is included in a cell with a hydrogen electrode. If atoms of metal X lose electrons and go into solution, the chemical reaction could be

$$X \longrightarrow X^+ + e^-$$

or

$$X \longrightarrow X^{2+} + 2e^- \quad \text{etc.}$$

On the other hand ions might come out of solution:

$$X^+ + e^- \longrightarrow X \quad \text{etc.}$$

The reaction and the sign of the standard electrode potential depend on what happens when the electrode is made into a complete cell with a hydrogen electrode. Table 13.4 shows some examples. Although this table shows the reactions that occur when the electrode is part of a cell that includes a hydrogen electrode, they can go the other way in other arrangements. The directions of the reactions are determined by the thermodynamics of energy conversion.

Table 13.4. Standard electrode potentials.

Electrode	Electrode reaction	$V_{electrode}$/volt
Sodium	$Na \longrightarrow Na^+ + e^-$	−2.72
Magnesium	$Mg \longrightarrow Mg^{2+} + 2e^-$	−1.55
Zinc	$Zn \longrightarrow Zn^{2+} + 2e^-$	−0.76
Hydrogen	$H_2 \longrightarrow 2H^+ + 2e^-$	− 0.00
Copper	$Cu^{2+} + 2e^- \longrightarrow Cu$	+0.34
Silver	$Ag^+ + e^- \longrightarrow Ag$	+0.80

Electrode processes

Equilibrium can be reached if the metal electrode is held by an insulator so that there is no external current path (Fig. 13.18). The electrolyte in the solution is partially dissociated into positive metal ions and negative ions which both move through the solution in random thermal motion. Some of the metal ions strike the metal plate and some of those collect electrons from the metal, so they remain on the surface as neutral atoms. So the plate gains positive charge and the solution loses positive charge.

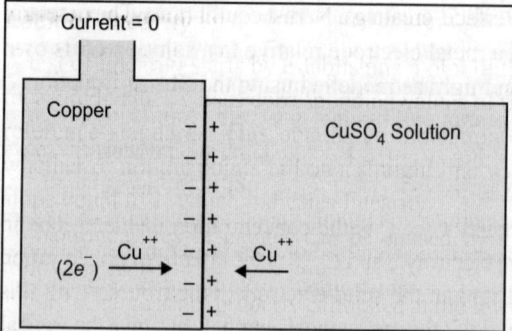

When a copper plate is placed in copper sulphate solution, copper ions are simultaneously dissolved from and deposited on the metal plate:

$$Cu \rightleftharpoons Cu^{2+} + 2e^-$$

If the plate is insulated, a charge double layer rapidly builds up on the interface, thus equalising the rates of dissolving and deposition. The copper is in Nernst equilibrium.

Fig. 13.18. Copper-copper sulphate electrode with no current.

Metal atoms can also dissolve off the plate; they become ionised and diffuse into solution so that the plate gains negative charge and the solution gains positive charge. When the metal plate is first put into the electrolyte the rate at which positive ions flow from the metal into the solution is greater than the rate at which ions are deposited on the metal from the solution–because the concentration of ions is much greater in the metal than in the solution. So the solution gains excess positive charge, leaving behind on the metal plate an excess of negative charge. A charge double layer forms at the interface, and the resulting electric field across the boundary encourages the deposition of positive ions from the solution and discourages the metal atoms of the plate from going into the solution. An equilibrium is rapidly reached in which the plate is negative with respect to the solution, and the rate of deposition of metal ions is equal to the rate at which metal atoms dissolve from the plate. In this equilibrium the ions form and recombine at the same rate, and the mass of the plate does not change.

Currents through electrodes

When current enters the metal plate from an external circuit, diffusion to and from the metal still leaves a net negative charge on the plate but the process is no longer self-limiting. Electrons flow out of the plate to the external circuit, and there is a corresponding flow of positive ions from the metal to the electrolyte. This flow of ions is no longer balanced by the deposition of ions from the solution; when charge flows into the metal plate, the metal dissolves. The rate at which the metal dissolves is controlled by the current (Fig. 13.19).

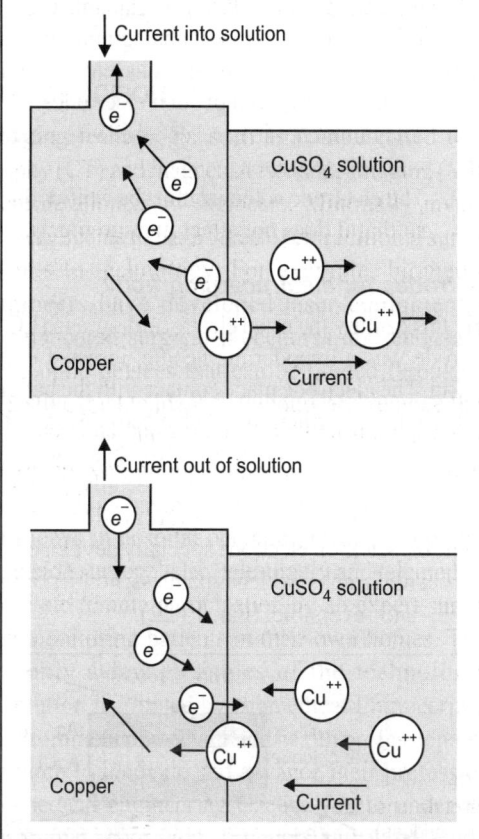

Fig. 13.19. Current in copper-copper sulphate electrode. Current is carried by Cu^{2+} ions in the solution and by electrons in the metal.

Exactly the opposite happens when there is a current out of a metal electrode to an external circuit. Electrons flow into the plate and a corresponding amount of metal is deposited, again at a rate controlled by the current. In a situation like this, where the rate and direction of the reaction are totally determined by the current, we say the electrode process is electrochemically reversible. Basically, a reversible electrode is one which can pass current without altering its chemical environment.

Non-reversible electrodes

To see what happens if the metal of the solid electrode and the metal ions in solution are different consider the example of a zinc electrode in copper sulphate solution. Zinc ions (Zn^{2+}) diffuse into the solution, and copper ions (Cu^{2+}) diffuse from the solution on to the zinc plate (Fig. 13.20).

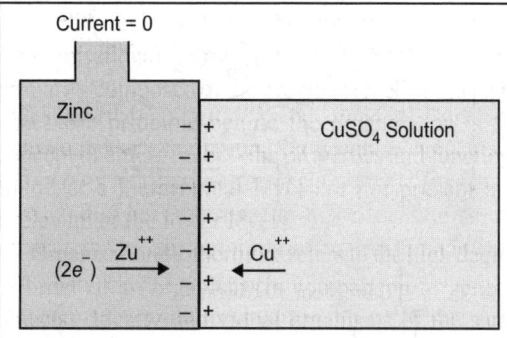

When a zinc plate is placed in $CuSO_4$ solution, zinc ions are dissolved and copper ions are simultaneously deposited on the plate.

$$Zn \rightarrow Zn^{2+} + 2e^-$$
$$Cu^{2+} + 2e^- \rightarrow Cu$$

If the plate is insulated, a charge double layer rapidly builds up, thus equalising the rates of these two reactions. There is no equilibrium, but a continuing transfer of zinc to the solution and copper to the plate.

Fig. 13.20. Zinc-copper sulphate electrode -no current.

A charge double layer builds up to give a steady state in which the copper ions are deposited at the same rate as the zinc ions dissolve. The plate gets coated with copper and the electrolyte becomes contaminated with zinc. The potential difference across the interface is such that there is no net current flow across the interface. However, unlike the case of the copper-copper sulphate electrode, there is a net flow of copper ions to the zinc plate, which is balanced by a net flow of zinc ions from the plate.

When there is current into the zinc plate from an external circuit the zinc dissolves even more rapidly (Fig. 13.21). A current into the zinc electrode corresponds to a flow of electrons from the electrode to the external circuit, and a flow of zinc ions from the zinc plate to the electrolyte. When the current is reversed the deposition of copper is speeded up, and dominates the flow of zinc ions into the electrolyte. This process is not electrochemically reversible.

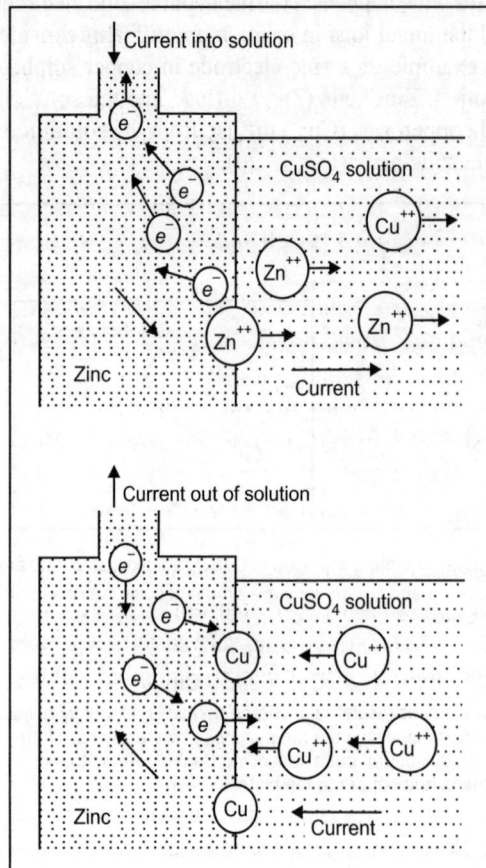

Fig. 13.21. Current through a zinc-copper sulphate electrode. External current into the zinc electrode corresponds to a flow of electrons from the electrode, and a flow of zinc ions from the zinc plate to the electrolyte. The electrode is not electrochemically reversible. Current from the solution to the metal is carried by copper ions in the solution and by electrons in the metal. Copper is deposited on the zinc plate.

Reversible electrodes

In the examples above the distinction between the reversible copper-copper sulphate electrode and the non-reversible zinc-copper sulphate electrode is clear. Copper won't contaminate the copper sulphate,

whereas zinc will. A considerable research effort has been expended in developing suitable electrodes for various purposes; electrodes for making biological measurements, electrical batteries, etc. In many of these the property of electrochemical reversibility is an important consideration.

Bioelectrodes

Bioelectrodes are specifically designed to make electrical contact with a living organism, e.g. for electrocardiographs, electroencephalographs, making electrical measurements on living cells, etc. Two vital characteristics are required of such electrodes:

1. They must not irritate, or otherwise interact with the specimen.
2. The electrode potential must be well-defined, so that it does not affect measurements.

Electrodes for electrocardiography

Early this century the usual electrocardiograph (ECG) electrode was a hypodermic needle, inserted under the skin. The electrode made contact with the patient, but it also hurt. Furthermore such electrodes satisfied neither of the above criteria. Nowadays contact is made to the patient's skin with specially designed electrodes. One very satisfactory design is a disposable stick-on electrode specially developed for electrocardiography, which is painless, non-irritating, reliable–and reversible. (Fig. 13.22).

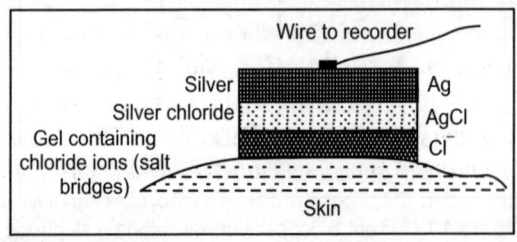

Fig. 13.22. Structure of a disposable ECG electrode (schematic). The silver chloride layer forms a reversible electrode with the chloride-containing gel. The gel makes a compatible bridge to human tissue.

The electrode consists of silver foil coated with silver chloride ($AgCl$). A proprietary gel containing chloride (Cl^-) ions provides an electrically conducting path between the silver chloride and the skin. A chloride electrolyte is desirable for this application as it is compatible with chloride ions in the body tissues and perspiration.

The actual electrode in the device-the contact between a solid and a solution-is the silversilver chloride interface. The electrode reaction is:

$$Ag + Cl^- \rightleftharpoons AgCl + e^-$$

The electrode is a reversible chloride electrode. The interfaces between the silver chloride and the proprietary contact paste, and between the contact paste and the skin, have contact potentials resulting from the diffusion of ions. In practice the potentials across these interfaces are low and, more importantly, they change very little with changes of current during the measurement process. This is particularly important in operating theatres where stray currents passed through the electrodes by cardiac defibrillators must not prevent immediate observation of the electric signals from the heart.

Calomel electrodes

Chloride is a very common ion in living organisms, so many bioelectrodes are based on it. One example is the calomel electrode. (Calomel electrodes were used to measure the potential across the membrane in the experiments on ion diffusion in video lecture E4, and in the cell potential measurements.

This electrode consists of calomel (mercurous chloride, Hg_2Cl_2) in contact with mercury. The electrode reaction is:

$$Hg_2Cl_2 + 2e^- \rightleftharpoons 2Hg + 2Cl^-.$$

This is another reversible electrode. It is linked to the organism to be investigated by a salt bridge containing a saturated solution of potassium chloride. In the electrodes used to study membrane potentials this salt bridge is contained in a bundle of fibres. In the electrodes used for measuring plant cell potentials it is contained within the very fine glass tube which is inserted into the cells. This bridge acts in the same way as the paste used to establish contact between the electrocardiograph electrode and the skin. The combination of a reversible electrode and a compatible salt bridge is often used as a reference electrode. Such reference electrodes are widely used in the life sciences.

Batteries

In the individual cells of batteries, electrode potentials are exploited to realise the conversion of chemical energy into electrical energy; each cell with its pair of electrodes is a source of EMF. The open-circuit cell potential, (which is equal to the EMF) is equal to the difference in the two electrode potentials. There are hundreds of chemically stable electrodes which can be used to make batteries.

The classic example is a relatively simple system known as the Daniell cell, one of the earliest practical batteries (Fig. 13.23). It usually consists of two half-cells, one copper-copper sulphate electrode and one zinc-zinc sulphate electrode, separated by a porous wall, usually an earthenware pot. It performs the same function as the salt bridge-keeping the different electrolytes substantially apart while still providing a conducting path for sulphate ions to diffuse through.

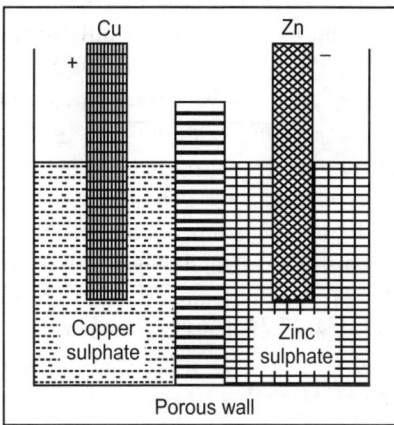

Fig. 13.23. Daniell cell.

Net electrical energy is delivered by the pair of chemical reactions: zinc going into solution and releasing electrons and copper coming out of solution by picking up electrons. We can use the table of electrode potentials (Table 13.3) to predict the cell voltage if both electrolytes are molar solutions (other concentrations will give different values):

Zinc electrode	$Zn \longrightarrow Zn^{2+} + 2e^-$;	$V_{Zn} = -0.76$ V.
Copper electrode	$Cu^{2+} + 2e^- \longrightarrow Cu$;	$V_{Cu} = +0.34$ V.
Total	$Zn + Cu^{2+} \longrightarrow Zn^{2+}$ $+ Cu$;	$V_{cell} = V_{Cu} - V_{Zn}$ $= 1.10$ V.

This calculation shows that the copper is positive with respect to the zinc. There is no way of measuring the potential in the electrolytes.

Nicad Battery

The nickel-cadmium battery (often called a Nicad battery) is a fully rechargeable cell frequently used in cordless power tools, calculators, and portable electronic instruments. The positive electrode of a fully charged nicad cell consists of nickel oxide hydroxide supported on a nickel frame, while the negative electrode is cadmium metal. Both these electrodes are reversible in the potassium hydroxide electrolyte (Fig. 13.24).

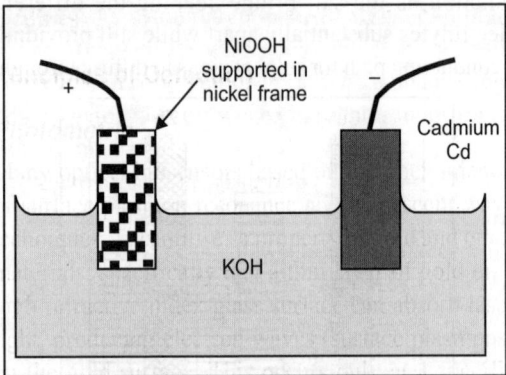

Fig. 13.24. The Nicad battery.

Negative electrode

The reaction at the negative electrode is the simpler. When no current is drawn a nernst equilibrium exists, the reaction being self-limited by the build-up of negative charge on the electrode.

$$Cd + 2OH^- \rightleftharpoons Cd\,(OH)_2^{2-}.$$

When the cell is supplying current to an external circuit, electrons flow from this electrode, and the reaction proceeds to form cadmium hydroxide-the cadmium is oxidised to cadmium hydroxide.

$$Cd + 2OH^- \xrightleftharpoons[\text{charge}]{\text{discharge}} Cd(OH)_2 + 2e^-.$$

When the cell is being charged this reaction is reversed. Electrons are supplied to the cadmium electrode, and the hydroxide is reduced back to metallic cadmium.

Positive electrode

The positive electrode is a hydrated oxide of nickel. During discharge it is reduced to divalent nickel hydroxide.

When no current is drawn a Nernst equilibrium exists, positive charge building up on the electrode:

$$NiOOH + H_2O \rightleftharpoons Ni(OH)_2^+ + OH^-.$$

When the cell is supplying current to an external circuit, electrons flow into the anode from the external circuit and the reaction proceeds to form nickel hydroxide:

$$NiOOH + H_2O + e^- \xrightleftharpoons[\text{charge}]{\text{discharge}} Ni(OH)_2 + OH^-.$$

Thus, during the discharge of this cell cadmium is oxidised to its hydroxide whereas the hydrated nickel oxide is reduced to nickel hydroxide. The potassium hydroxide electrolyte is unchanged during the cell reaction; its purpose is to provide plenty of OH^- ions which are exchanged between the electrodes, but not used up.

Both electrodes of a nicad cell are electrochemically reversible in the same electrolyte a property which simplifies the construction of practical nicad cells.

Concentration cells

We have seen that electrode potentials, as described by Eq. 13.1, can be explained as having two parts one contribution from a standard electrode potential and another arising from the concentration of the electrolyte . That model suggests that we ought to be able to get a net cell voltage by using two electrodes with the same metal and electrolyte and a salt bridge (or a porous pot) with different electrolyte concentrations in the two compartments. Such a device, which is called a concentration cell, works but the voltage is often small (Fig. 13.25).

Example: A concentration cell consists of two silver-silver nitrate electrodes with 1.0 molar silver nitrate in one compartment and 0.10 molar on the other side. When we write down the difference between the electrode potentials, the standard electrode potentials cancel out and we are left with the difference in concentration potentials, from Eq. 13.1:

$$V_{cell} = \frac{kT}{ze}\ln\left(\frac{C_1}{C_{ref}}\right) - \frac{kT}{ze}\ln\left(\frac{C_2}{C_{ref}}\right)$$

$$= \frac{kT}{ze}\ln\left(\frac{C_1}{C_2}\right)$$

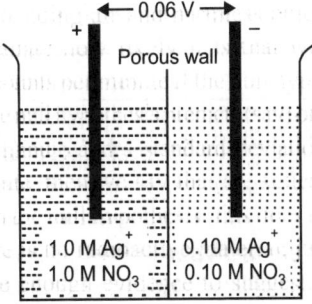

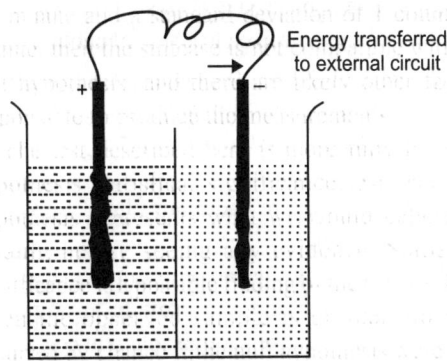

Fig. 13.25. A concentration cell.

Supposing that the temperature is 20°C or 293 K and given that $z = 1$ for the silver ion, you might remember that the factor in front of the log function is about 25 mV. Putting in the ratio of concentrations gives a potential of 25 mV × ln (10) which is equal to 58 mV or about 0.06 V–not much of a battery but you could improve it by increasing the concentration ratio.

Remember that this result is the potential difference between the electrodes when they are not connected to an external circuit— the cell just sits at a potential difference of 58 mV and there is a chemical equilibrium. When you draw energy from the cell by

completing the circuit the chemical reactions start up to supply the energy, and the potential difference between the terminals will drop. The reactions proceed in a direction that will try to equalise the concentrations of silver ions in the two compartments That can be achieved by moving electrons along the external connecting wire from the low concentration electrode to the high concentration side, so that silver ions can pick up electrons and come out of solution as silver atoms. An equal amount of silver goes into solution on the low concentration side.

Summary of principles: electrodes and cells

1. Electrode potential = standard electrode potential + concentration potential.
2. Standard electrode potential = cell potential with molar electrolytes and hydrogen reference electrode.
3. Cell potential = difference in electrode potentials.

Electrolysis

Electrolysis is the process in which electric currents from an external source supply the energy necessary to make a chemical reaction take place. It is just the opposite of what occurs in a battery, where the energy of a chemical reaction is converted into electrical energy. Although electrolysis occurs in charging and discharging a battery, the term electrolysis is usually used only when the primary interest is in the chemical products of the process.

Consider two copper electrodes in a copper sulphate solution. The reaction caused by a current is simply the transfer of copper from one electrode to the other. This very simple system — two electrodes of the same metal in an electrolyte containing that metal's ion- illustrates the principles of electrolysis, and permits us to investigate further the subtleties of electrode processes.

First, take the case where there is no current. Each electrode is in Nernst equilibrium with the electrolyte. Diffusion of ions from each plate establishes a negative charge on the plate. The resulting charge double layer limits the rate of diffusion of ions from the plate so that it is equal to the rate of diffusion of ions from the electrolyte to the plate.

If we arbitrarily take the potential of the copper sulphate electrolyte as zero, then each copper electrode will be at some negative potential relative to that, i.e. at the appropriate Nernst equilibrium value for the particular electrolyte concentration and temperature. The observable quantity—i.e. the measured cell voltage—is the difference of these two equal Nernst potentials, i.e. 0 V. When a source of EMF is connected to the cell, one plate is made positive with respect to the other, so there is a current through the cell, as Cu^{2+} ions. As a result copper is removed from the positive plate, and deposited on the negative plate.

By maintaining this potential difference across the cell we have considerably changed the potential distribution in the cell. This applied voltage, V_{cell}, is equal to the sum of three components. (Fig. 13.26).

1. There is an interface potential at the positive electrode which is less than the Nernst value. The rate at which copper dissolves is greater than the rate at which it is deposited on the electrode. So there is a net flow of copper into the electrolyte.

2. At the negative electrode the interface potential now exceeds the Nernst value, and there is a net flow of Cu^{2+} ions from the solution to the electrode, where a deposit of copper is built up.

3. There is a potential gradient across the electrolyte and an associated electric field within the electrolyte which drives the flow of Cu^{2+} ions between the electrodes.

The difference between the Nernst equilibrium potentials and the actual potential difference at the electrode when there is an electric current is called the overpotential of the electrode. These overpotentials and the resistive potential drop across the cell must be established to make the reaction proceed. However they represent wasted energy. They can be minimised by suitable cell design and a low electrolysis rate, but some potential difference is required, and hence some energy must be dissipated to make the process proceed at a finite speed.

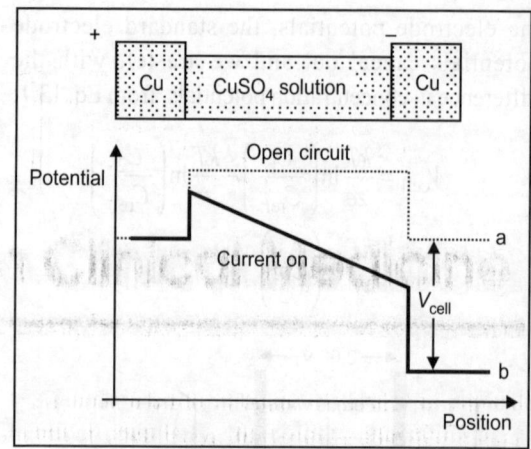

Fig. 13.26. Variation of potential through an electrolytic cell: (a) no current (light line), (b) current causes transfer of copper between electrodes (heavy line).

Applications of electrolysis

Electroplating

Electrolysis may be used to deposit a thin but tough layer of a selected metal on to a base of another metal, either for protection or decorative purposes. Examples include the following:

1. Cutlery is plated with silver to give an attractive finish.
2. Steel parts are cadmium plated to prevent corrosion.
3. Steel car fittings are chromium plated both to prevent rust and provide an attractive finish. To make a tough adherent coating the fitting is plated with nickel before the chromium plating.

In electroplating, the object to be coated is the negative electrode of an electrolytic cell, and the positive electrode and electrolyte are chosen to deposit the desired material.

Electropurification of metals

Electrolysis is also used for the purification of certain metals. Of particular importance is the electropurification of copper. The impure metal is the positive electrode of an electrolytic cell, and pure metal is deposited on the negative electrode. Impurities either dissolve in the electrolyte, or fall as sludge to the bottom of the tank. The cell potential is adjusted so that copper is deposited out in preference to other metallic ions.

BIOCATALYTIC ELECTRODES

Biocatalytic membrane electrodes, the result of modern biotechnology, represent one of the most exciting applications of immobilised enzymes and other biocatalysts, Although at first a laboratory curiosity, they now become a well-used analytical technique due to their simple construction, reliability, and adaptability for continual *in vitro* and *in vivo* analyses. Often, the same internal indicator element can be used for the determination of several different substances, if a set of the respective biocatalytic membranes are available. The analyses are easily reproducible and timesaving, since such operations as incubation, development of colouration, and centrifugation connected with other methods are not needed.

However grandiose the development of biosensors has been in the last decade, these devices enter only slowly into practical use, which may be due to the fact that technical personnel are not used to them or mistrust them, being accustomed primarily to prevailing optical methods. The number of analyses of blood glucose performed by the hitherto most widespread glucose oxidase electrode in the United States is at present estimated to about 10 per cent. The situation is to some extent similar to that of ion-selecive electrodes; these met with a broad application only after about 15 years following Simon's discovery of the valinomycin electrode for potassium ions in 1969. Biocatalytic electrodes will undoubtedly bring new developments in chemical analysis based on molecular recognition elements and in the course of time will find their place in laboratories as have the present glass pH electrode, also as detectors of chromatographic columns, and so on, and in addition, in human therapy.

In an effort to increase the stability of enzyme membranes, attention is at present turned toward enzymes of thermophile organisms. Technical development tends to automated flow-through analysers (FIAs) equipped with miniature biosensors

for simultaneous determination of several analytes. In this trend one can also estimate that semicoductors sensitive to different ions (ISFETs) and dissolved gases will compete with conventional electrochemical detectors. The first semiconductor sensors equipped with enzyme reaction layers are known and a multifunctional biosensor with a single biochip has already been constructed, making possible simultaneous analysis of glucose, urea, and potassium ions. But further technical improvement will be necessary to make these means fulfil the exacting demands of routine analytical and clinical laboratories.

Preparation of the Electrode Enzyme Layer

For a successful construction of the enzyme electrode it is necessary to choose a suitable enzyme that reacts readily with the substance to be determined, and which, by means of a suitable technology, must be immobilised onto the respective sensor capable of monitoring the enzyme reaction that is going on. In case the enzyme is not commercially available, it must be isolated in die proper purity. Rapid growth in the number of recognised enzymes and the reactions associated with them ensures that a wide variety of enzyme electrodes are now available for determining specific reactants. Depending on the nature of the enzyme, the type of internal sensor, and the species to be determined, a variety of physical and chemical immobilisation procedures have been employed. The importance of the technique of enzyme immobilisation is documented by the fact that to a considerable extent it determines the availability, lifetime, and analytical qualities of the sensor. Chemically immobilised enzymes are often less sensitive to inactivation by heat, pH shifting, and inhibitors; only the most powerful and irreversible inhibitors can actually influence their activity, which frequently persists for many successive analyses. Preparation of enzyme membranes is the subject of many patents, particularly in Japan.

Use of a free soluble enzyme

An active layer consisting of a soluble enzyme has been used especially at the initial stages of the development of enzyme electrodes, but in some cases it is also used for monoenzyme and multienzyme systems. This is the simplest method of physical immobilisation of an enzyme, and consists of capturing it on the surface of the measurement section of an electrochemical sensor by means of the dialysis membrane. This ensures free diffusion of the substrate and reaction products, whereas the macromolecular enzyme remains a component of the sensing device. Soluble enzymes face a serious challenge when attempts are made to utilise them for the analysis of complex mixtures such as waste-water, extracts, and blood. They can be affected by activators, inhibitors, temperature, pH, and so on. For good sensor function it is important that the reaction layer of the sensor contain an excess (> 10 U) of enzyme; these effects can then be minimised or eliminated.

To achieve a highly active reaction layer on the probe, either a concentrated enzyme solution or a paste prepared from the crystalline of lyophilised preparation is used. The appropriate amount is spread in a thin layer onto the center of a piece of cellophane, 20 to 25 μm thick, which in turn is put on the sensing part of the electrochemical probe, and usually fixed with a rubber O-ring and stretched without folds or air bubbles. For delimiting the regular thickness of the enzyme layer, we found it advantageous to insert in it a piece of a nylon net (25 mesh/mm^2). The enzyme solution can also be dropped into porous material (such as cigarette paper or a millipore type GS filtering membrane), which is then covered with the dialysis membrane. The electrode is kept in an appropriate buffer between uses.

Enzyme adsorption on supports

In some instances free soluble enzyme can be bound to an inert support by adsorption. Glutamate dehydrogenase and creatinine deiminase were adsorbed by standing in enzyme solution at 4°C for 24 hours with wet polyvinyl chloride membranes, with recoveries of 4.2 and 28.9 per cent, respectively, to create a creatinine specific sensor. At 4°C they retained 80 to 85 per cent of initial enzyme activity for 6 months. Bacterial glucose dehydrogenase has rapidly been adsorbed together with Meldola blue

(as electron transfer mediator) on the surface of a carbon electrode having a quick response; similarly, glucose oxidase was adsorbed within 5 min on palladium/gold-sputtered graphite, and fungal laccase can be adsorbed onto porous carbon or on soot.

Gel-entrapment technique

High-molecular-weight enzymes can be immobilised effectively by physical entrapment into the synthetic or natural gel matrix; some examples are given below.

Acrylamide polymers

Acrylamide polymers have met with wide-spread use. A mixture containing 121 mg of acrylamide, 23 mg of N,N'-methylenbisacrylamide, 0.1 mg each of potassium persulphate and riboflavin, and about 1000 units of enzyme per cubic centimeter of water was layered onto the tip or bulb of the electrode previously covered with a thin nylon net; all pores of net must be saturated. Polymerisation takes place in a nitrogen gas atmosphere by irradiating with a mercury lamp for about 30 to 60 minutes, after which time a dry, hard-layer is formed; 1 cm^3 of the solution is enough for several sensors. Irradiation by cold nonisothermal plasma in electrical discharges can be used for the polymerisation process instead of chemical initiators.

Enzyme immobilisation by gel entrapment is sometimes inadequate because of continuous protein washout from the polymer. For protection the enzyme layer may be covered with a dialysis membrane to prevent leaching of enzyme into buffer, in which the electrode is stored between uses. It is, however, possible to anchor the enzyme into hydrophillic gel covalently, for which the copolymerisation of polyacrylamide with N-acryloxysuccinimide was utilised. The conditions must, however, be optimalised empirically. Simultaneous protection from inactivation by coenzyme under oxygen exclusion and at low temperature resulted in about 50 per cent retention of glutamate dehydrogenase activity.

Gelatine layers

Gelatine layers are made as follows 5 per cent gelatine solution in 37°C distilled water is mixed together with the enzyme solution in a ratio of about 1:1 and poured onto a cellulose acetate film support. After drying for 48 hrs at 4°C the membranes are removed from the support, cut into appropriate pieces, and fixed to the tip of the electrode by means of a dialysis membrane and an O-ring.

Agar and calcium alginate gels

Agar gels (3.5 to 4 per cent) have been used, successfully to immobilise fungal laccase or whole microbial cells into a layer formed between two glass plates. Calcium alginate gels are also used occasionally to immobilise individual enzymes or cell organelles. The layer of 7 per cent sodium alginate and biocatalyst solution (3:2) is gently immersed into 0.1 M calcium chloride; after 30 minute the gel is washed with buffer to remove excess calcium salt.

Cross-linking method

Bifunctional reagents form intermolecular connections during the reaction with enzymes, giving rise to insoluble reticulum in which a considerable part of the enzyme activity is retained. In the preparation of enzyme membranes particularly, the easily accessible glutaraldehyde proved useful in reacting with the ε-amino groups of lysyl residues. The reaction was optimalised for a number of enzymes by Broun. Loss of enzyme activity is usually reduced when the enzyme is cross-linked with an inert protein rich in lysine (about 50 mg of bovine serum albumin or gelatine per cubic centimeter), which reduces direct contact of the enzyme with glutaraldehyde, thus protecting the enzyme against denaturation. Numerous modifications for the cross-linking of enzymes are now available.

Reticulation on the electrode

A buffered solution of the proper amounts of enzyme, albumin, and diluted glutaraldehyde is rapidly mixed and the measurement section of the electrode is dipped into the mixture under rotation until a coating is obtained. To keep the membrane adherent, a nylon net is usually fastened around the electrode with a rubber O-ring prior to coating. Excess of aldehyde is washed out with water or neutralised by immersing the electrode in the glycine solution. Gelatine can substitute for serum albumin as the protecting agent provided that the reticulation is carried out by dipping

the electrode or a glass plate with a dry enzyme gelatine coating into a 2.5 per cent glutaraldehyde solution. It is of interest that the concentration of oxygen in the gelatine membrane is roughly 20 times higher than it is in water for the same partial pressure. During measurement the intermembrane oxygen is consumed, which renders the oxidase substrate assay independent of the amount of oxygen in the sample solution tested.

An expensive enzyme can be spared when its solution in admixture with albumin is deposited directly on the measuring part of the electrode. After rapid mixing with the appropriate volume of glutaraldehyde, solidification takes place and homogeneous film is formed.

A new method of preparing 50 μm-thick uniform membranes directly on the surface of a glass or Pt electrode was described by Tor and Freeman. From a copolymer of acrylamide (70 per cent) and methylacrylamide (30 per cent), hydrazide was prepared whose 25 per cent solution is mixed with the enzyme (cholinesterase, urease, or penicillinase). The electrode bulb is dipped into the mixture, and as soon as the coating dries in air, a thin opaque film is cross-linked by dipping into 1 per cent glyoxal. The membrane adheres strongly to the electrode surface, but to avoid cracks, it must not be touched mechanically. The preparation lasts about 2 hrs and the stable storage period is 2 to 6 months.

Separate enzymic membrane

As pNH$_3$ or pO$_2$ electrodes form the basis of several enzyme electrodes, changing the biocatalytic layer would be advisable to obtain enzyme electrodes for different analytes. Flexible membranes obtained by coating the polyamide net with a reticulum are advantageus in that they can be dried after use, and if necessary, they can repeatedly be mounted to the electrochemical sensor. A simple and broadly applicable procedure used extensively in our studies is as follows: Portions of the mixture of buffered enzyme (pH 7, free of ammonium salt), 10 per cent bovine serum albumin (or 5 per cent gelatine), and 2 per cent glutardialdehyde are rapidly deposited on marked areas of a stretched nylon net (25 mesh/mm^2, fibre thickness 40 µm) and spread using a plastic rod on both sides. After drying in a horizontal position, the membranes are storable at 4°C for months; in some cases they can be delivered to other users by mail. The amount of membrane components has been optimised for electrodes incorporating single enzymes (pea seedling diamine oxidase, mushroom polyphenol oxidase, squash L-ascorbate oxidase, maize polyamine oxidase, pig plasma ceruloplasmin), or a mixture of other enzymes (pea diamine oxidase and bacterial L-lysine decarboxylase, almond emulsion and/glucose oxidase, or yeast invertase, kidney mutarotase, and glucose oxidase); 50 µL of the mixture containing 5 to 25 enzyme units per square centimeter is sufficient, and 50 to 100 aldehyde molecules per molecule of protein are needed for reticulation as calculated from the composition of different optimised enzyme membranes.

Some enzymes were also allowed to reticulate on pig small intestine wall 'hydrolysed with chymotrypsine or pepsine, on the matrix of a polycarbonate ultrafiltration membrane, on a silane-treated polycarbonate membrane, or inside a Millipore filter. In the last case the membrane was gold coated to improve contact with the polarographic anode, but a limited lifetime was achieved. By co-cross-linking of several enzymes with plasma albumin and glutaraldehyde on a glass plate in the presence of ferrite particles, magnetic mono- and bienzyme membranes were manufactured, which permits the membrane to be fastened on an electrode bearing a cylinder magnet without an O-ring.

Spare porous particles

This method is suitable for enzymes of low specific activity. To a solution of the enzyme (about 15 to 50 mg protein per milliliter) in a 10 mM phosphate buffer (pH 6.8), 2 per cent glutardialdehyde is admixed to a final concentration of 0.2 per cent. The mixture is rapidly frozen at –30°C and stored in a refrigerator, where it is left to melt for several hours at 4°C. Spongy yellowish reticulum is homogenised, centrifuged, and washed with buffer. A small part of a dense suspension is attached to the electrode surface by means of cellophane and an O-ring. A disadvantage of this method is the fact that it is difficult to achieve a reproducible thickness of the biocatalytic layer.

Photo-cross-linking procedure

A photo-cross-linking procedure was used to immobilise lactate oxidase and lactate dehydrogenase. A mixture 1:1:30 by weight of both enzymes and polyvinyl alcohol bearing stilbazolium groups (8 wt per cent aqueous solution, pH 7.0) was spread on a Teflon plate and dried for 12 hrs at 4°C. The thickness of the enzyme layer was adjusted by changing the amount of the mixture. The dried film was removed from the plate and irradiated with a xenon arc lamp (30 mV/cm^2) for 5 min on each side, The membrane was stored in 0.1 M phosphate buffer, pH 7.0, at 4°C.

Covalent attachment on supports

Chemical bonding of enzymes onto various matrices, although still promising, is usually tedious or necessitates skilled manipulation. An important prerequisite of the often multistep reaction sequence is to obtain a stable enzyme layer mechanically and catalytically. Four examples of the covalent attachment procedure are described.

Binding on collagen

For the construction of sensors sensitive to various saccharides, methanol, and cholesterol, Coulet and his group used a membrane of highly polymerised insoluble collagen which was activated in there steps. Carboxy groups were first acid esterified with methanol, then treated with hydrazine, and finally, treated with nitrous acid; the acylaside formed reacts with enzyme under mild conditions. Within 4 days enzyme membranes were obtained which exhibit mechanical resistance and stability in a-buffer (2 years at 4°C) as well as in the dry state. For bienzyme membranes, a method was developed to bind the two enzymes on both sides asymmetrically, which is sometimes advantageous over randomly coimmobilised enzymes (e.g. for maltose and other disaccharide measurements). Membranes that are more stable mechanically can be obtained by co-cross-linking of the mixture of collagen and polyvinyl alcohol with epichlorohydrin. On the reticulum thus formed, glucose oxidase can be bound by means of glutaraldehyde either directly or after previous introduction of aminoethyl groups into matrix.

Recent improvement in membrane technology have led to commercial products that can replace the collagen matrix. Immunoaffinity membranes Posidyne NAZ require activation by the azide procedure, and preactivated Pall Biodyne A immunoaffinity membranes (BIA membranes) are capable of binding glucose oxidase or oxalate Oxidase directly in an extremely simple and fast way. With the latter, 400 assays of glucose and 150 assays of oxalate can be performed within 50 and 120 days, respectively.

Binding on Nylon Net

For constructing sensitive superprobes on the basis of pO_2 and pNH_3 electrodes, Mascini used a fine nylon net. The mild chemical binding process covers activation of the nylon material with dimethylsulphate, following sequential reaction with lysine, glutaraldehyde, and enzyme. The preparation lasts almost 1 day and the resulting enzyme membranes show improved mechanical properties and analytical characteristics when used for the determination of sugars, ascorbic acid, cholesterol, alcohol, or urea. They can be fixed on the probe surface several times without damage. Another activation method for covalent linkage of glucose oxidase and ascorbate oxidase comprises treatment of a surface-hydrolysed nylon net with cyclohexylisocyanide, glutaraldehyde, and enzyme.

Binding on cellulose triacetate

A solution containing a mixture of cellulose triacetate, glutaraldehyde, and 1,8-diamino-4-aminomethyloctane in the ratio 5:1:4 (by weight) was spread on a glass plate and dried for 3 days. The dried film was removed from the support and first activated by 1 per cent glutaraldehyde in 0.1 M phosphate buffer at pH 7.7. Loading with enzyme(s) was carried out by immersing the activated layer in an enzyme solution (1 mg per milliliter of 0.1 M phosphate buffer, pH 7.4) for 12 hrs at 4°C. The enzyme membrane was stored in phosphate buffer at pH 7 and 4°C.

Binding on carbon electrodes

Every type of compact enzyme membrane increases the sensor response time because of the diffusion barrier. To obtain extremely thin coatings, attempts were also made to fix enzymes directly on the electrode surface in a convenient and reproducible fashion. Perhaps the most successful example is the modification of a graphite electrode by attaching specific molecules to its surface. Glucose oxidase and L-amino acid oxidase have been linked covalently with a cyanuric chloride yielding sensors with both superior response times and linear ranges as well as with good stability (20 to 30 days). However, in the flow system with an electrode containing glucose oxidase attached on the surface of the reticulated vitreous carbon using a carbodiimide method, the current varied nonlinearly with glucose concentration. A very stable membrane-free glucose sensor was obtained by covalent binding of enzyme on graphite followed by absorption of N-methylphenaziniun ion as the mediator necessary for electron transfer. Another approach—attaching glucose oxidase apoenzyme through flavine adenine dinucleotide (FAD) covalently bound to the glassy carbon electrode-failed because the reconstituted enzyme activity amounted to only about 0.2 per cent of the immobilised FAD. On the other hand, successful results were achieved when glucose oxidase was bound, probably through its carbohydrate moiety, onto a glassy carbon electrode incorporating (3-aminophenyl)boronic acid.

Configurations of Biocatalytic Electrodes

A biochemical electrode utilising biocatalysis can be designed for every substance, which, although itself electrochemically inert, is subject to enzyme reaction in which an electroactive substance (product, cosubstrate, coenzyme) participates and whose electrochemical detection can be related to the concentration of analyte:

$$\text{Analyte (+ effector)} \xrightarrow{\text{Biocatalyst}} \text{Product(s)}$$

This conversion can sometimes be achieved only by using more enzymes or by using biocatalytically active systems on a higher level of integration.

Today's state of knowledge and experience indicates that it is possible to present a hierarchy of various biological mediators for constructing biocatalytic electrodes:

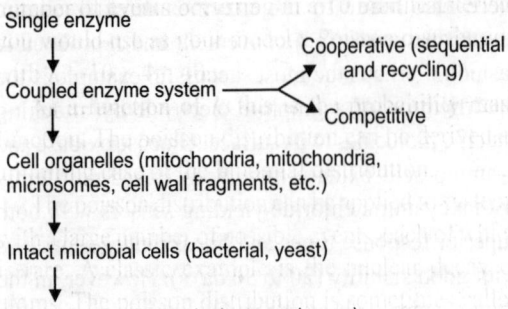

Single and multiple-enzyme electrodes

In single- and multienzyme sensors, the enzymes proved most useful were those that do not require expensive coenzyme for their action. Notable among these are various hydrolases (urease, arginase, amidases, glycosidases, esterases), lyases (e.g. amino acid decarboxylase and deaminases), dehydrogenases, and particularly, terminal oxidases with firmly bound prosthetic groups. The latter include flavoprotein enzymes containing flavine adenine dinucleotide (FAD), such as glucose oxidase, L- and D-amino acid oxidase, plant polyamine oxidase, and so on, and quinoprotein enzymes containing methoxatine (pyrroloquinoline quinone, PQQ), such as *Acinetobacter* glucose dehydrogenase, *Pseudomonas* alcohol dehydrogenase, and some bacterial, plant, and plasma amine oxidases. Using NAD⁺ dependent dehydrogenases, it proved useful in some cases to immobilise tile coenzyme behind chemically modified dialysis membrane or by covalent linkage to dextrane. The possibilities of electrochemical detection of analyte after enzymic conversion are often varied, which can be demonstrated by two single enzyme reactions catalysed with highly specific urease and glucose oxidase.

The only substrate of urease is urea, which is hydrolysed according to the equation:

$$\text{Urea} + H_2O \xrightarrow{\text{Urease}} 2NH_3 + CO_2 \qquad ...(13.2)$$

The reaction products are contained in an aqueous medium, according to pH, in equilibrium with NH_4^+ and HCO_3^- ions. From that fact it follows that for determining urea, urease can be immobilised to different types of electrochemical transducers; indeed, a number of urease sensors have been constructed: (i) on the basis of the potentiometric gas NH_3 and gas CO_2 electrodes, (ii) on ammonium ion-sensitive glass or nonactin membrane electrodes, (iii) on antimony pH electrode, and (iv) on the basis of a special conductimetric electrode.

An example of a reaction requiring oxygen as a cosubstrate is the oxidation of glucose:

$$\beta\text{-D-Glucose} + O_2 + H_2O \xrightarrow[\text{Oxidase}]{\text{Glucose}} \qquad ...(13.3)$$
$$\text{Gluconic acid} + H_2O_2$$

Here the possibilities of constructing enzyme electrodes are even more varied. Glucose can be determined amperometrically as well as potentiometrically by immobilising glucose oxidase: (i) on a Clark pO_2 sensor poised at –650 mV versus Ag–AgCl for detecting oxygen consumption, (ii) on a platinum anode poised at 600 to 650 mV versus Ag–AgCl or at 600 to 750 mV versus SCE for detecting hydrogen peroxide, (iii) on a pH electrode for detecting gluconic acid or on a potentiometric platinum or porous graphite electrode, (iv) on iodide ISE for detecting hydrogen peroxide which is consumed for oxidation of iodide added into the medium in 10^{-4} M concentration.

$$H_2O_2 + 2J^- + 2H^+ \longrightarrow J_2 + 2H_2O \qquad ...(13.4)$$

and (v) on a platinum or carbon paste anode poised at 400 mV versus SCE for detecting hydroquinone formed from *p*-benzochinone replacing oxygen:

$$\beta\text{-D-Glucose} + \text{P-benzoquinone} + H_2O \qquad ...(13.5)$$
$$\xrightarrow[\text{Oxidase}]{\text{Glucose}} \text{Gluconic acid} + \text{Hydroquinone}$$

Further oxygen-independent systems exploit the ability of mould glucose oxidase and bacterial quinoprotein glucose dehydrogenase to utilise chemical electron transfer mediators. Finally, NAD⁺ dependent glucose dehydrogenase from *Bacillus* sp.

has also been used for the construction of a glucose sensor.

Some bioorganic compounds can be determined electrochemically only if two or more enzymes cooperate during the sequence conversion of analyte A through intermediate B to the product P:

$$A \xrightarrow{E_1} B \xrightarrow{E_2} P \qquad ... (13.6)$$

This is the principle of metabolic chains. As example will serve to illustrate the determination of sucrose, which can be detected by means of the glucose oxidase if the following reactions precede the detection of glucose [see (Eq. 13.3)]:

$$Sucrose \xrightarrow{Invertase} \alpha\text{-D-Glucose} + \beta\text{-D-Fructose} \qquad ... (13.7)$$

$$\alpha\text{-D-Glucose} \xrightarrow{Invertase} \beta\text{-D-Glucose} \qquad ... (13.8)$$

For sucrose, self-contained bioelectrodes have been constructed that monitor either O_2 consumption or the production of H_2O_2. Their drawback is the fact that they are sensitive to both sucrose and glucose. To remove the interference by glucose, Scheller and Renneberg equipped an amperometric anode sensing hydrogenperoxide with a double catalytic membrane; in the first membrane, which contains only glucose oxidase and catalase glucose is consumed, so that only sucrose enters the second membrane, which contains glucose oxidase and invertase. Up to 2 mM glucose can be tolerated.

In determining creatinine, the interference due to creatine is eliminated by using the bioamperometric method; on the first anode three enzymes are immobilised: creatinine amidohydrolase, creatine amidinohydrolase, and sarcosine oxidase; on the second anode the first enzyme is omitted. The first anode is sensitive to both creatinine and creatine, the second to creatine; the difference in current signals thus relates to the creatinine. The geometry of the two internal sensors as well as the diffusion properties of their membranes should, of course, be equal.

Recently, a 'second-generation' compact biamperometric enzyme electrode has been constructed that enables the proper substrate and the interfering one to be determined simultaneously. It was applied for the determination of the essential amino acid lysine, which is degraded in the biosensor reaction layer by two enzyme-catalysed steps with the consumption of oxygen.

$$L\text{-lysine} \xrightarrow[\text{(B. cadaveris)}]{\text{L-lysine decarboxylase}} Cadaverine + CO_2 \qquad ... (13.9)$$

$$Cadaverine \xrightarrow[+ O_2]{\substack{\text{Diamine oxidase} \\ \text{(pea seedling)}}} \Delta^1\text{-piperideine} + NH_3 + H_2O_2 \qquad ... (13.10)$$

This bienzyme electrode, based on the Clark oxygen cell, has the advantage over the later-single-enzyme potentiometric pCO_2 electrode of short response and recovery times. However, the decarboxylation product cadaverine can also be present in the sample (e.g. silages, some fodders) so that overestimated values of L-lysine are obtained. We over came this difficulty by using special equipment called a differential oximeter, designed in our laboratory. The detector is a bipolar Clark oxygen electrode composed of two cathodes and one common Ag-AgCl reference electrode. The cathodes are tightly covered with a two-compartment enzyme membrane: one part consists of L-lysine decarboxylase and diamine oxidase; the other one containing heat-inactivated L-lysine decarboxylase, exhibits only diamine oxidase activity. The double Clark electrode produces two current signals, one of which relates to the sum of L-lysine and diamine, the other, to the interfering diamine only. The electronic module makes it possible to subtract both current signals so that the content of both substances, L-lysine and diamine, can be determined simultaneously using a double-line recorder. The analysis takes about 5 min, including calibration. The device can also be used for analysing the mixture of other metabolic couples, such as amygdalin +glucose. Some examples of very sensitive bienzyme electrodes in whose membrane a combination of enzymes results in the recyclisation of the substrate and thus in chemical amplification of the electrode signal are dealt with in chapter.

The viability of electrode assembling based on the competition of two enzymes catalysing different reactions for one common substrate was demonstrated by the determination of toxicologically important antipyretic drug aminopyrine. The membrane of the pO_2 electrode consists of coimmobilised catalase and horseradish peroxidase in a gelatine layer and the reaction scheme for this determination is as follows:

$$H_2O_2 \xrightarrow[\text{Aminopyrine}]{\substack{\text{Catalase} \\ \text{Peroxidase}}} \begin{array}{l} (1/2)O_2 + H_2O \\ \\ \text{Product} + H_2O \end{array} \qquad \text{... (13.11)}$$

A defined amount of hydrogen peroxide is added to the air-saturated buffer medium. It diffuses into the elecrode membrane, where it is destroyed by catalase, thus inducing an increase in the oxygen reduction current; after the addition of aminopyrine, the peroxidase competes additionally with catalase for peroxide and the oxygen current is decreased according to analyte concentration. Other peroxidase substrates are possibly also detectable in this way.

Cell organelle-based electrodes and hybrid electrodes

Subcellular organelles such as mitochondria, microsomes, or membrane fragments contain, in their structures, naturally immobilised sets of biocatalysts capable of mediating important transformations of organic substances. For example, liver microsomes containing a monooxigenase cytochrome P-450 system metabolises a wide variety of drugs and other xenobiotics by a mixed-function hydroxylase reaction (SH = substrate):

$$SH + O_2 + NADPH + H^+ \xrightarrow{\text{P-450}}$$
$$S-OH + NADP^+ + H_2O \qquad \text{... (13.12)}$$

To develop a sensor for drug measurement, aniline was chosen by Schubert as a model substance: rabbit liver microsomes were entrapped into the gelatine layer and fixed on the rotating graphite disk electrode; in the presence of NADPH, aniline is transformed to p-aminophenol, which can be oxidised electro-chemically to quinoneimine at 250 mV versus SCE. A linearity of response was obtained up to 0.5 mM

aniline concentration. Gelatine membrane–immobilised microsomes were also combined with a convential Clark-type oxygen probe and employed for the measurement of coenzyme NADPH up to 1 mM. Further configurations with microsomal P-450 have also been discussed; however, all these electrodes do not permit application to routine analysis, due to low selectivity, and further work will be necessary to improve the sensitivity and reproducibility of sensor operation.

Broken *Escherichia coli* cells and membrane vesicles were also co-immobilised with gelatine by tanning with 2 per cent glutaraldehyde and fixed onto an oxygen sensor; the electrode utilises bacterial respiratory chain and was employed for measuring NADH, NADPH, D-and L-lactate, succinate, L-malate, 3-glycerophosphate, or pyruvate in the range 1 to 50 mM. When present in a mixture it was possible to discriminate among these metabolites by changing enzyme activities using various carbon sources for bacterial growth, thermal treatment, or selective inhibitors.

Mitochondria prepared by fractional centrifugation of pig kidney homogenates were coupled with a gas NH_3 electrode to monitor l-glutamine; the sensor appeared to be more stable (10 days) than that containing isolated glutaminase (1 day). The physical integrity of mitochondria has to be preserved by osmotic adjustment of the appropriate buffer. Nevertheless, even better characteristics of the glutamine sensor were reported with immobilised bacterial cells or with thin kidney slices.

In bioprobes termed 'hybrid electrodes' the biocatalyst consists of isolated enzyme immobilised together with cell organelles, whole microbial cells, or even tissue sections within a single or sandwiched reaction layer capable of converting the analyte in more steps into electrochemically measurable species. Such devices have been constructed, e.g. for assaying coenzyme NAD$^+$, urea, and creatinine. Rate liver microsomes which are singly applied for coenzyme NADPH measurements can be coupled with the action of pure dehydrogenases to monitor glucose-6-phosphate, ATP, or isocitrate. An attempt was also made to assemble a hybrid electrode for aniline by co-immobilisation of liver microsomes with glucose oxidase on a graphite electrode; the system can replace expensive NADPH otherwise needed for aniline hydroxylation, by hydrogen peroxide formed from the enzymatic oxidation of glucose, but the fivefold lower sensitivity makes the peroxide-dependent reaction rather unattractive.

Microbial electrodes

Micro-organisms are generally excellent producers of enzymes, which were used extensively in various types of biosensors, 'as reviewed recently. A novel approach to the development of bioselective electrodes was reported in 1977 from Rechnitz's laboratory, where paste of living bacterial cells was fixed in place of isolated enzymes on the surface of the electrochemical sensor to form a 'microbial electrode' which functions in a manner similar to that of a conventional enzyme electrode. The first analytes were L-aspartic acid and L-arginine, but later Rechnitz and co-workers developed a useful membrane electrode for L-glutamine by coupling intact cells of Sarcina lutea with an ammoniasensing probe instead of unstable enzyme glutaminase. This empirical approach proved to be very fruitful, and since then many other bioselective microbial probes have been described in which living bacterial or yeast cells were used as biological transducers to permit determinations of various inorganic and bioorganic substances, amino acids, vitamins, antibiotics, and pollutants. Most bacterial electrodes have utilised strains exhibiting specific deaminase activity in conjunction with an ammonia-sensing electrode; the remaining ones are usually based on oxygen, carbon dioxide, or hydrogen sulphide probes. In most cases the paste of cells is simply supported onto the indicator sensor by means of acetylcellulose or dialysis membrane.

The use of microbial cells in potentiometric and amperometric electrodes offers several advantages over conventional enzyme electrodes, the principal ones being construction simplicity, low cost, and increased electrodes, lifetime (2 to 3 weeks) due to the natural enzyme environment inside the cell; there is also a possibility of the regeneration of the microbial,

layer by storing the electrode in appropriate nutrient medium when it is not in operation; the use of cells as biocatalysts represents the only possibility of constructing such devices for determining compounds for which the relevant enzyme has not yet been isolated or when the complex reaction sequence is not completely understood; furthermore, the application of cells would be particularly superior to those cases in which expensive cofactors are required or when a multistep conversion of the analyte is needed to produce an electrochemically measurable product, since the appropriate cell represents a package of enzymes and cofactors needed for any of its metabolic reactions. This has been demonstrated with a microbial sensor for the determination of nitrate or nitrilotriacetic acid.

In some instances the complexity of cellular metabolism can be advantageous when the multistep degradation leads to enhanced electrode sensitivity. For example, 2 mol of ammonia is formed by Pseudomonas sp. per mole of L-histidine, 1 mol in the initial histidine-ammonia-lyase reaction and the 1 mol in later steps connected with the production of L-glutamic acid. The multistep degradation of organic substances forms the basis of microbial sensors that enable the biological oxygen demand (BOD) in waste-water to be determined automatically within a few minutes.

On the other hand, the microbial electrode may be less favourable compared with the conventional enzyme electrode with respect to specificity, response time, and reproducibility. In most instances the analytical usefulness of the electrode depends on selection of the appropriate microbial strain: the respective applicable enzyme is often substrate inducible and sterile media of appropriate composition are required for cultivation. Some microbial electrodes suffer from selectivity when interfering assimilable substances are present in the sample analysed. Thus an ammonia-sensitive nitrifying bacteria/pO_2 sensor also responded to glucose and other nutrients, so that the addition of antibiotics such as chloramphenicol in the sample solution was required.

Tissue-based electrodes

It was Rechnitz's group that introduced tissue as a biocatalyst into the analysis via electrochemical device. Thin tissue slices now appear to be the system of choice for workers untrained in enzymology. They are attractive because of material availability and the often high content of analytically applicable enzyme. The slice technique also obviates the need for tedious enzyme purification followed by artificial immobilisation if the relevant enzyme is not available commercially. Other enzymes present in tissue need not be unfavorable to sensor selectivity when the electrochemical detector and working conditions as for pH and buffer composition are carefully selected or when undesirable metabolic pathways are selectively inhibited. Because of the complexity of the tissue biocatalytic layer, it is obvious that step-by-step optimisation with regard to the principal variables and response characteristics for every new type of electrode is needed.

Arnold and Rechnitz illustrated the effectiveness of this strategy by enhancing the selectivity of guanine-sensitive rabbit liver slice/pNH$_3$ electrode using borate buffer containing Mn^{2+} ions to eliminate guanosine phosphorylase and adenosine deaminase activity, respectively. In another case interferences caused by adenosine mono-, di-, and triphosphate (AMP, ADP, and ATP) were suppressed with inhibitors of alkaline phosphatase and AMP deaminase present in the intestinal mucosa cells used as the active layer of adenosine-sensitive electrode. It appears, however, that in most electrodes a very limited number of substances actually interfere. Glutamine electrode containing pig kidney slice for example, gave only light potential change with asparagine out of 13 compounds tested as potential interferants.

One type of tissue can mediate the analysis of more analytes provided that it is coupled with different electrochemical transducers. A thin liver slice was used for the determination of guanine and hydrogen peroxide, a squash tissue slice for determining L-glutamate and L-ascorbate, and banana pulp tissue for determining dopamine and oxalate,

respectively. The use of plant material in conjunction with electrochemical transducers is a relatively new prospect. Fruits, leaves, blossoms, and seeds are already employed for biosensor purposes, but the great diversity of natural material suggests that many additional bioelectrodes should be feasible. Very recent results from our laboratory have shown good applicability of walnut pericarp slices, insect hemolymph, and the latex juice from dandelion or other plants for amperometric detection of phenols.

Until recently a series of tissue-based Potentiometric and amperometric electrodes were developed as efficient devices in analysing a number of bioorganic substances. A tracing of responses of a phenol-sensing electrode after repeated addition of the catechol into stirred bulk solution is shown as an example in Fig. 13.27. In most cases the operational lifetime is surprisingly high, evidently due to the unchanged internal conditions for respective enzymes entrapped in the natural support structure. Arnold and Rechnitz made an extensive comparative study with four different types of glutamine electrodes whose active layer was composed of isolated glutaminase, cells of *Sarcina flava*, pig kidney mitochondria, and pig kidney tissue. The tissue containing probe exerted the highest useful lifetime (30 days) as well as other improved analytical characteristics.

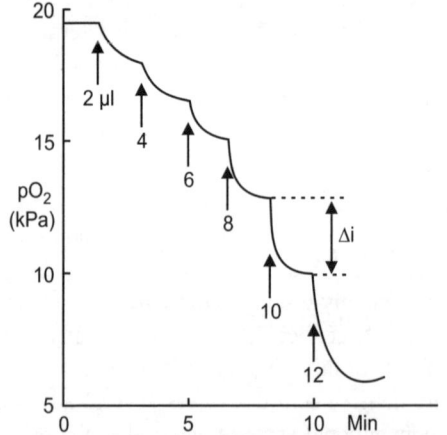

Fig. 13.27. Calibration of a phenol-sensing probe composed of a Clark oxygen electrode and mushroom tissue slice, 150 μm thick. Each step corresponds to addition of 2 to 12 μL of 20 mM catechol, into 3 mL of 0.1 M phosphate buffer at pH 7 and 30°C.

It is usually very easy to replace the slice, which partially lost its respective enzyme activity after repeated analysis. In every case a recalibration of the electrode is necessary. Phenol oxidating slices, for example, possess a short operation lifetime due to staining by chinone polymerisation products. It is, however, often possible to store spare slices for long periods in appropriate preservatives. An impressive example is the possibility of storage of the active segments of squash or cucumber peel containing ascorbate oxidases as long as 1 year in 50 per cent glycerol. This makes it possible to bridge the seasonal vegetation period sufficiently.

Enzyme immunoelectrodes

Immunochemical reactions belong to the most specific reactions of the living matter. As the interaction between the antiody and the antigen would not give any direct effect useful for electrochemical detection, one of the approaches is to couple it with any enzymic reaction supplying electroactive species (Fig. 13.28); this method represents an electrochemical counterpart of the ELISA procedure. Although hitherto-describe sensors for the determination of antigens and haptens of pharmacological importance are encouraging due to their sensitivity and selectivity, their manufacture, compared with current enzyme electrodes, is more difficult, since it is necessary to have available not only the specific antibody, but also an antigen or antibody with a chemically linked marker enzyme, which is most frequently catalase, peroxidase, or glucose oxidase.

A common assay procedure is as follows: A membrane with bound antibody (*Ab*) is placed onto an amperometric or potentiometric probe. The probe is then immersed in the buffered mixture of nonlabelled antigen (*Ag*) to be assayed and a known amount of enzyme-labeled antigen (E-*Ag*); two competitive reactions take place at the electrode membrane during the bathing period:

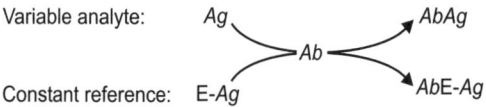

Variable analyte: Ag → AbAg
                        Ab
Constant reference: E-Ag → AbE-Ag

When adsorption equilibrium is reached, the probe is thoroughly washed to remove the unspecifically adsorbed antigens, and then it is put in solution containing substrate for determining the initial rate of reaction catalysed by the enzyme complexed on the electrode membrane. The electrode signal changes with increasing concentrations of the nonlabelled antigen.

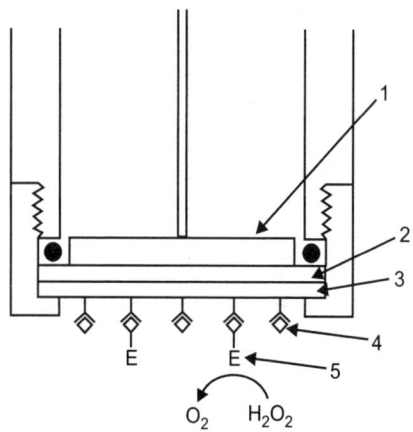

Fig. 13.28. Scheme of the enzyme immunoelectrode based on membrane-bound antibody and its mode of operation: 1. Platinum cathode. 2 Oxygen-permeable plastic membrane. 3 Antibody-coupled membrane. 4 Antigen (analyte). 5 Catalase-labelled antigen as the reference.

For determining human chorion gonadotropin (HCG), an important pregnancy marker, the entire complex of proteins of the respective antiserum was chemically bound in three steps to the membrane consisting of acetyl cellulose and bromoacetyl cellulose. The antibody-bound membrane was then firmly fixed onto the Teflon membrane of an oxygen probe. The calibration was performed by measuring oxygen production from 5 mM hydrogen peroxide after a 30-min incubation of the probe in a mixture of various amounts of nonlabelled hormone with a constant amount of catalase-labelled hormone (prepared by conjugating HCG with catalase using ghitaraldehyde). The antibody-bound membrane was replaced for each measurement owing to time-consuming regeneration. 0.02 to 100 IU HCG can be measured, one unit being 1.4×10^{-7} g. On the same principle, tumor antigen α-fetoprotein was also assayed in the range 10^{-8} to 10^{-11} g/mL.

If a low-molecularweight organic substance is to be determined it must first be linked to a protein, such as beef serum albumin, since only in the function of hapten is it capable of producing formation of the necessary specific antibody in the blood of the immunised animal. Thus very low theofylline concentrations were determined highly specifically. The drug sensor was composed of an oxygen electrode and antibody-coupled nylon net membrane. The assay procedure involved the competitive immunochemical reaction of the membrane antibody with catalase-labeled theophylline. The sensitivity of this method (5×10^{-8} to -5×10^{-7} M) is equal to that of radioimmunoassay or enzyme immunoassay.

In another case, specific antibodies against hepatitis B surface antigen were labelled with glucose oxidase and immobilised onto a gelatine membrane fixed over an oxygen probe. The response of the sensor immersed in a standard glucose solution is directly proportional to the oxygen consumption and to the hepatitis B surface antigen' over the range 0.1 to 100 μg/L.

Potentiometric detection was also used for determining hepatitis B antigen. This time the antibody was labelled with peroxidase and immobilised on gelatine membrane by the sandwich technique. The enzyme activity is followed by means of an iodide-selective electrode from the decrease in iodide concentration in the presence of hydrogen peroxide. The potential change is proportional to the enzyme activity and thus also to the concentration of antigen that need not be purified. The linearity holds for the range 0.5 to 50 μg/L, and 0.1 μg/L can still be detected reproducibly. The method is quicker than most immunochemical techniques and the results are in a good agreement with radioimmunoanalysis.

14

Ventilation and Ventilators

INTRODUCTION

This chapter presents an overview of the structure and function of mechanical ventilators. Mechanical ventilators, which are often also called respirators, are used to artificially ventilate the lungs of patients who are unable to naturally breathe from the atmosphere. The very early devices used bellows that were manually operated to inflate the lungs. Today's respirators employ an array of sophisticated components such as microprocessors, fast response servo valves and precision transducers to perform the task of ventilating the lungs. The changes in the design of ventilators have come about as the result of improvements in engineering the ventilator components and the advent of new therapy modes by clinicians. A large variety of ventilators are now available for short-term treatment of acute respiratory problems as well as long-term therapy for chronic respiratory conditions.

IRON LUNG

An iron lung is a machine that enables a person to breathe when normal muscle control has been lost or the work of breathing exceeds the person's ability. It is a form of medical ventilator. Properly, it is called a negative pressure ventilator.

Method and Use

Humans, like many other animals, breathe by negative pressure breathing: the rib cage expands and the diaphragm pulls down, expanding the chest cavity. This causes the pressure in the chest cavity to decrease, and the lungs expand to fill the space. This,

in turn, causes the pressure of the air inside the lungs to fall (it becomes negative, relative to the atmosphere), and air flows into the lungs from the atmosphere: inhalation. When the chest cavity is contracted, the reverse happens and the person exhales. If a person loses part or all of the ability to control the muscles involved, breathing becomes difficult or impossible.

The person using the iron lung is placed into the central chamber, a cylindrical steel drum. A door allowing the head and neck to remain free is then closed, forming a sealed, airtight compartment enclosing the rest of the person's body. Pumps that control airflow periodically decrease and increase the air pressure within the chamber, and particularly, on the chest. When the pressure is below that within the lungs, the lungs expand and atmospheric pressure pushes air from outside the chamber in via the person's nose and airways to keep the lungs filled; when the pressure goes above that within the lungs, the reverse occurs, and air is expelled. In this manner, the iron lung mimics the physiological action of breathing: by periodically altering intrathoracic pressure, it causes air to flow in and out of the lungs. The iron lung is a form of noninvasive therapy.

Modern Usage

Positive pressure ventilation systems are now more common than negative pressure systems. Positive pressure ventilators work by blowing air into the patient's lungs via intubation through the airway; they were used for the first time in Blegdams Hospital, Copenhagen, Denmark during a polio outbreak in

1952. It proved a success and soon superseded the iron lung throughout Europe.

The iron lung now has a marginal place in modern respiratory therapy. Most patients with paralysis of the breathing muscles use modern mechanical ventilators that push air into the airway with positive pressure.

These are generally efficacious and have the advantage of not restricting patients' movements or caregivers' ability to examine the patients as significantly as an iron lung does.

However, negative pressure ventilation is a truer approximation of normal physiological breathing and results in more normal distribution of air in the lungs. It may also be preferable in certain rare conditions, such as Ondine's curse, in which failure of the medullary respiratory centres at the base of the brain result in patients having no autonomic control of breathing.

At least one reported polio patient, Dianne Odell, had a spinal deformity that caused the use of mechanical ventilators to be contraindicated. Thus, there are patients who today still use the older machines, often in their homes, despite the occasional difficulty of finding the various replacement parts. Biphasic cuirass ventilation is a modern development of the iron lung, consisting of a wearable rigid upper-body shell (a cuirass) which functions as a negative pressure ventilator.

MEDICAL VENTILATOR

A medical ventilator may be defined as any machine designed to mechanically move breatheable air into and out of the lungs, to provide the mechanism of breathing for a patient who is physically unable to breathe, or breathing insufficiently (Fig. 14.1).

While modern ventilators are generally thought of as computerised machines, patients can be ventilated indefinitely with a bag valve mask, a simple hand-operated machine.

Ventilators are chiefly used in intensive care medicine, home care, and emergency medicine (as standalone units) and in anesthesia (as a component of an anesthesia machine).

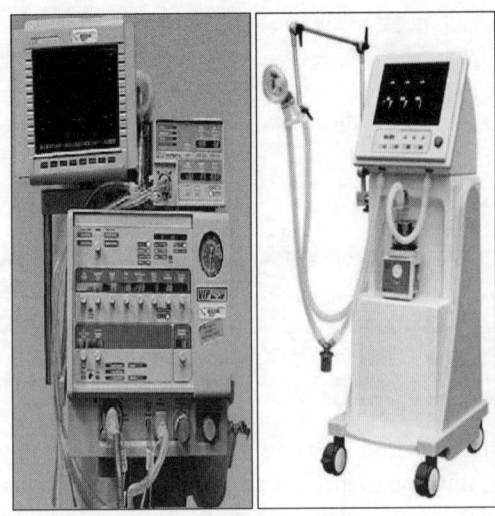

Fig. 14.1. Medical ventilator.

Function

In its simplest form, a modern positive pressure ventilator consists of a compressible air reservoir or turbine, air and oxygen supplies, a set of valves and tubes, and a disposable or reusable 'patient circuit'. The air reservoir is pneumatically compressed several times a minute to deliver room-air, or in most cases, an air/oxygen mixture to the patient. If a turbine is used, the turbine pushes air through the ventilator, with a flow valve adjusting pressure to meet patient-specific parameters. When overpressure is released, the patient will exhale passively due to the lungs' elasticity, the exhaled air being released usually through a one-way valve within the patient circuit called the patient manifold. The oxygen content of the inspired gas can be set from 21 per cent (ambient air) to 100 per cent (pure oxygen). Pressure and flow characteristics can be set mechanically or electronically.

Ventilators may also be equipped with monitoring and alarm systems for patient-related parameters (e.g. pressure, volume, and flow) and ventilator function (e.g. air leakage, power failure, mechanical failure), backup batteries, oxygen tanks, and remote control. The pneumatic system is nowadays often replaced by a computer-controlled turbopump.

Modern ventilators are electronically controlled by a small embedded system to allow exact adaptation of pressure and flow characteristics to an individual patient's needs. Fine-tuned ventilator settings also serve to make ventilation more tolerable and comfortable for the patient. In Germany, Canada, and the United States, respiratory therapists are responsible for tuning these settings while biomedical technologists are responsible for the maintenance.

The patient circuit usually consists of a set of three durable, yet lightweight plastic tubes, separated by function (e.g. inhaled air, patient pressure, exhaled air). Determined by the type of ventilation needed, the patient end of the circuit may be either noninvasive or invasive. Noninvasive methods, which are adequate for patients who require a ventilator only while sleeping and resting, mainly employ a nasal mask. Invasive methods require intubation, which for long-term ventilator dependence will normally be a tracheotomy cannula, as this is much more comfortable and practical for long-term care than is larynx or nasal intubation.

Life-critical system

Because the failure of a mechanical ventilation system may result in death, it is classed as a life-critical system, and precautions must be taken to ensure that mechanical ventilation systems are highly reliable. This includes their power-supply provision.

Mechanical ventilators are therefore carefully designed so that no single point of failure can endanger the patient. They usually have manual backup mechanisms to enable hand-driven respiration in the absence of power. Some systems are also equipped with compressed-gas tanks and backup batteries to provide ventilation in case of power failure or defective gas supplies, and methods to operate or call for help if their mechanisms or software fail.

High frequency percussive ventilation

High-frequency percussive ventilation (HFPV) began to be used in selected centres in the 1980s. It is a hybrid of conventional mechanical ventilation and high-frequency oscillatory ventilation. It has been used to salvage patients with persistent hypoxemia when on conventional mechanical ventilation or, in some cases, used as a primary modality of ventilatory support from the start.

Mechanical ventilation

In medicine, mechanical ventilation is a method to mechanically assist or replace spontaneous breathing.

This may involve a machine called a ventilator or the breathing may be assisted by a physician or other suitable person compressing a bag or set of bellows. Traditionally divided into negative-pressure ventilation, where air is essentially sucked into the lungs, or positive pressure ventilation, where air (or another gas mix) is pushed into the trachea (Fig. 14.2).

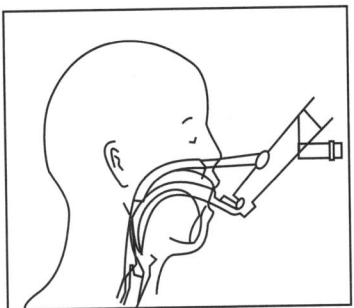

Fig. 14.2. Nasotracheal intubation.

It can be used as a short term measure, for example during an operation or critical illness (often in the setting of an intensive care unit). It may be used at home or in a nursing or rehabilitation institution if patients have chronic illnesses that require long-term ventilatory assistance.

Owing to the anatomy of the human pharynx, larynx and esophagus and the circumstances for which ventilation is required then additional measures are often required to 'secure' the airway during positive pressure ventilation to allow unimpeded passage of air into the trachea and avoid air passing into the esophagus and stomach. Commonly this is by insertion of a tube into the trachea which provides a clear route for the air. This can be either an endotracheal tube, inserted through the natural openings of mouth or nose or a tracheostomy inserted through an artificial opening in the neck. In other circumstances simple airway maneuvres, an oropharyngeal airway or laryngeal mask airway may be employed. If the patient is able to protect their own airway such as in noninvasive ventilation or negative-pressure ventilation then no airway adjunct may be needed. Mechanical ventilation is often a life-saving intervention, but carries many potential complications including pneumothorax, airway injury, alveolar damage, and ventilator-associated pneumonia.

In many healthcare systems prolonged ventilation as part of intensive care is a limited resource (in that there are only so many patients that can receive care at any given moment). It is used to support a single failing organ system (the lungs) and cannot reverse any underlying disease process (such as terminal cancer). For this reason there can be (occasionally difficult) decisions to be made about whether it is suitable to commence someone on mechanical ventilation. Equally many ethical issues surround the decision to discontinue mechanical ventilation.

Negative pressure machines

The iron lung, also known as the Drinker and Shaw tank, was developed in 1929 and was one of the first negative-pressure machines used for long-term ventilation. It was refined and used in the 20th century largely as a result of the polio epidemic that struck the world in the 1940s. The machine is effectively a large elongated tank, which encases the patient up to the neck. The neck is sealed with a rubber gasket so that the patient's face (and airway) are exposed to the room air.

While the exchange of oxygen and carbon dioxide between the bloodstream and the pulmonary airspace works by diffusion and requires no external work, air must be moved into and out of the lungs to make it available to the gas exchange process. In spontaneous breathing, a negative pressure is created in the pleural cavity by the muscles of respiration, and the resulting gradient between the atmospheric pressure and the pressure inside the thorax generates a flow of air (Fig. 14.3).

In the iron lung by means of a pump, the air is withdrawn mechanically to produce a vacuum inside the tank, thus creating negative pressure. This negative pressure leads to expansion of the chest, which causes a decrease in intrapulmonary pressure, and increases flow of ambient air into the lungs. As the vacuum is released, the pressure inside the tank

equalises to that of the ambient pressure, and the elastic coil of the chest and lungs leads to passive exhalation. However, when the vacuum is created, the abdomen also expands along with the lung, cutting off venous flow back to the heart, leading to pooling of venous blood in the lower extremities. There are large portholes for nurse or home assistant access. The patients can talk and eat normally, and can see the world through a well-placed series of mirrors. Some could remain in these iron lungs for years at a time quite successfully.

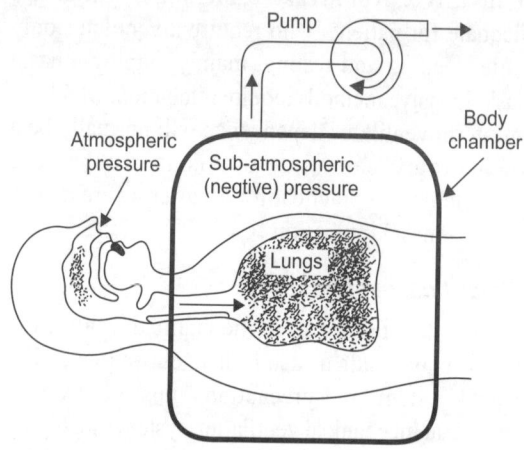

Fig. 14.3. A simplified illustration of a negative-pressure ventilator.

Today, negative pressure mechanical ventilators are still in use, notably with the Polio Wing Hospitals in England such as St. Thomas' (by Westminster in London) and the John Radcliffe in Oxford. The prominent device used is a smaller device known as the cuirass.

The cuirass is a shell-like unit, creating negative pressure only to the chest using a combination of a fitting shell and a soft bladder. Its main use is in patients with neuromuscular disorders who have some residual muscular function. However, it was prone to falling off and caused severe chafing and skin damage and was not used as a long term device. In recent years this device has resurfaced as a modern polycarbonate shell with multiple seals and a high pressure oscillation pump in order to carry out biphasic cuirass ventilation.

Positive pressure machines

The design of the modern positive-pressure ventilators were mainly based on technical developments by the military during World War II to supply oxygen to fighter pilots in high altitude. Such ventilators replaced the iron lungs as safe endotracheal tubes with high volume/low pressure cuffs were developed. The popularity of positive-pressure ventilators rose during the polio epidemic in the 1950s in Scandinavia and the United States and was the beginning of modern ventilation therapy. Positive pressure through manual supply of 50 per cent oxygen through a tracheostomy tube led to a reduced mortality rate among patients with polio and respiratory paralysis. However, because of the sheer amount of manpower required for such manual intervention, mechanical positive-pressure ventilators became increasingly popular (Fig. 14.4).

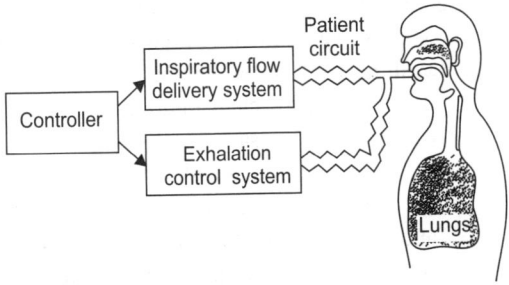

Fig. 14.4. A simplified diagram of the functional blocks of a positive-pressure ventilator.

Positive-pressure ventilators work by increasing the patient's airway pressure through an endotracheal or tracheostomy tube. The positive pressure allows air to flow into the airway until the ventilator breath is terminated. Subsequently, the airway pressure drops to zero, and the elastic recoil of the chest wall and lungs push the tidal volume—the breath—out through passive exhalation.

This is an example of a neonatal (infant) ventilator.

INDICATIONS FOR USE

Mechanical ventilation is indicated when the patient's spontaneous ventilation is inadequate to maintain life. It is also indicated as prophylaxis for imminent collapse of other physiologic functions, or ineffective gas exchange in the lungs. Because mechanical ventilation only serves to provide assistance for breathing and does not cure a disease, the patient's underlying condition should be correctable and should resolve over time. In addition, other factors must be taken into consideration because mechanical ventilation is not without its complications.

Common medical indications for use include:

1. Acute lung injury (including ARDS, trauma).
2. Apnea with respiratory arrest, including cases from intoxication.
3. Chronic obstructive pulmonary disease (COPD)
4. Acute respiratory acidosis with partial pressure of carbon dioxide (pCO_2) > 50 mmHg and pH < 7.25, which may be due to paralysis of the diaphragm due to Guillain-Barré syndrome, Myasthenia Gravis, spinal cord injury, or the effect of anaesthetic and muscle relaxant drugs.
5. Increased work of breathing as evidenced by significant tachypnea, retractions, and other physical signs of respiratory distress.
6. Hypoxemia with arterial partial pressure of oxygen (PaO_2) with supplemental fraction of inspired oxygen (FiO_2) < 55 mm Hg.
7. Hypotension including sepsis, shock, congestive heart failure.
8. Neurological diseases such as muscular dystrophy amyotrophic lateral sclerosis.

TYPES OF VENTILATORS

Ventilation can be delivered via:

1. Hand-controlled ventilation such as:
   (a) Bag valve mask.
   (b) Continuous-flow or anaesthesia (or T-piece) bag.
2. A mechanical ventilator. Types of mechanical ventilators include:
   (a) Transport ventilators: These ventilators are small, more rugged, and can be powered pneumatically or via AC or DC power sources (Fig. 14.5).
   (b) ICU ventilators: These ventilators are larger and usually run on AC power

(though virtually all contain a battery to facilitate intra-facility transport and as a back-up in the event of a power failure). This style of ventilator often provides greater control of a wide variety of ventilation parameters (such as inspiratory rise time). Many ICU ventilators also incorporate graphics to provide visual feedback of each breath (Fig. 14.6).

(i) NICU ventilators: Designed with the preterm neonate in mind, these are a specialised subset of ICU ventilators which are designed to deliver the smaller, more precise volumes and pressures required to ventilate these patients.

(c) PAP ventilators: These ventilators are specifically designed for noninvasive ventilation, this includes ventilators for use at home, in order to treat sleep apnea.

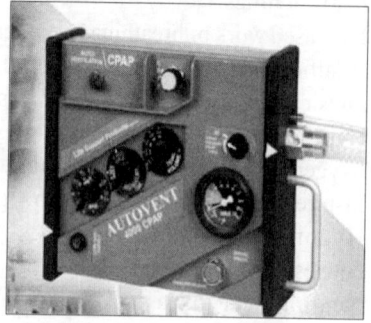

Fig. 14.5. Transport ventilators.

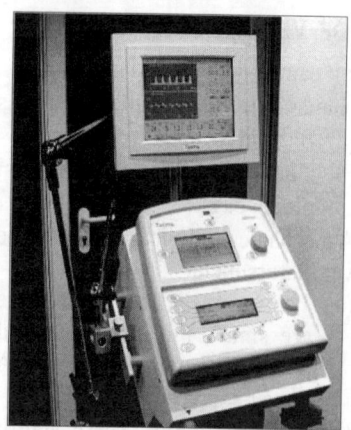

Fig. 14.6. ICU ventilators.

Modes of Ventilation

Conventional ventilation

The modes of ventilation can be thought of as classifications based on how to control the ventilator breath. Traditionally ventilators were classified based on how they determined when to stop giving a breath. The three traditional categories of ventilators are listed below. As microprocessor technology is incorporated into ventilator design, the distinction among these types has become less clear as ventilators may use combinations of all of these modes as well as flow-sensing, which controls the ventilator breath based on the flow-rate of gas versus a specific volume, pressure, or time.

Breath termination

Modes of ventilation are classified by the means that they determine the inspired breath is complete. This is sensed by either pressure or volume.

1. Volume ventilation: A predetermined tidal volume (V_t) is set for the patient and is delivered with each inspiration. The amount of pressure necessary to deliver this volume will fluctuate from breath to breath based on the resistance and compliance of the patient and ventilator circuit. If the tidal volume is set at 500 ml, the ventilator will continue to inspire gas until it reaches its goal. Upon completion of the inspired volume, the ventilator will open a valve allowing the patient to passively exhale.

2. Pressure ventilation: A predetermined peak inspiratory pressure (PIP) is determined based on the patients condition and pathophysiology. The ventilator will flow gas into the patient until this set pressure is reached. Upon reaching the preset PIP, the ventilator allows for passive exhalation. Caution and close observation must be given in this mode due to potential for either hypo-ventilation or hyperventilation because the tidal volume is variable.

Several manufactures have incorporated features from both of theses modes in an attempt to accommodate patients needs. These modes are flow-variable, volume-targeted, pressure-regulated, time-limited modes (for example, pressure regulated volume control – PRVC). This means that instead of providing an exact tidal volume each breath, a target volume is set and the ventilator will vary the inspiratory flow at each breath to achieve the target volume at the lowest possible peak pressure. The inspiratory time (T_i) limits the length of the inspiratory cycle and therefore the I:E ratio. Pressure regulated modes such as PRVC or Auto-flow (Draeger) can most easily be thought of as turning a volume mode into a pressure mode with the added benefit of maintaining more control over tidal volume than with strictly pressure-control.

Breath initiation

The other method of classifying mechanical ventilation is based on how to determine when to start giving a breath. Similar to the termination classification noted above, microprocessor control has resulted in a myriad of hybrid modes that combine features of the traditional classifications. Note that most of the timing initiation classifications below can be combined with any of the termination classifications listed above.

1. Assist control (AC): In this mode the ventilator provides a mechanical breath with either a preset tidal volume or peak pressure every time the patient initiates a breath. Traditional assist-control used only a preset tidal volume—when a preset peak pressure is used this is also sometimes termed Intermittent Positive Pressure Ventilation or IPPV. However, the initiation timing is the same—both provide a ventilator breath with every patient effort. In most ventilators a back-up minimum breath rate can be set in the event that the patient becomes apnoeic. Although a maximum rate is not usually set, an alarm can be set if the ventilator cycles too frequently. This can alert that the patient is tachypneic or that the ventilator may be autocycling (a problem that results when the ventilator interprets fluctuations in the circuit

due to the last breath termination as a new breath initiation attempt).

2. Synchronised intermittent mandatory ventilation (SIMV): In this mode the ventilator provides a preset mechanical breath (pressure or volume limited) every specified number of seconds (determined by dividing the respiratory rate into 60 seconds—thus a respiratory rate of 12 results in a 5 second cycle time). Within that cycle time the ventilator waits for the patient to initiate a breath using either a pressure or flow sensor. When the ventilator senses the first patient breathing attempt within the cycle, it delivers the preset ventilator breath. If the patient fails to initiate a breath, the ventilator delivers a mechanical breath at the end of the breath cycle. Additional spontaneous breaths after the first one within the breath cycle do not trigger another SIMV breath. However, SIMV may be combined with pressure support. SIMV is frequently employed as a method of decreasing ventilatory support (weaning) by turning down the rate, which requires the patient to take additional breaths beyond the SIMV triggered breath.

3. Controlled mechanical ventilation (CMV): In this mode the ventilator provides a mechanical breath on a preset timing. Patient respiratory efforts are ignored. This is generally uncomfortable for children and adults who are conscious and is usually only used in an unconscious patient. It may also be used in infants who often quickly adapt their breathing pattern to the ventilator timing.

4. Pressure support ventilation (PSV): When a patient attempts to breathe spontaneously through an endotracheal tube, the narrowed diameter of the airway results in higher resistance to airflow, and thus a higher work of breathing. PSV was developed as a method to decrease the work of breathing in-between ventilator mandated breaths by providing an elevated pressure triggered by spontaneous

breathing that 'supports' ventilation during inspiration. Thus, for example, SIMV might be combined with PSV so that additional breaths beyond the SIMV programmed breaths are supported. However, while the SIMV mandated breaths have a preset volume or peak pressure, the PSV breaths are designed to cut short when the inspiratory flow reaches a percentage of the peak inspiratory flow (e.g. 10–25 per cent). New generation of ventilators provides user-adjustable inspiration cycling off threshold, and some even are equipped with automatic inspiration cycling off threshold function. This helps the patient ventilator synchrony. The peak pressure set for the PSV breaths is usually a lower pressure than that set for the full ventilator mandated breath. PSV can be also be used as an independent mode.

5. Continuous positive airway pressure (CPAP): A continuous level of elevated pressure is provided through the patient circuit to maintain adequate oxygenation, decrease the work of breathing, and decrease the work of the heart (such as in left-sided heart failure — CHF). Note that no cycling of ventilator pressures occurs and the patient must initiate all breaths. In addition, no additional pressure above the CPAP pressure is provided during those breaths. CPAP may be used invasively through an endotracheal tube or tracheo-stomy or noninvasively with a face mask or nasal prongs.

6. Positive end-expiratory pressure (PEEP): It is functionally the same as CPAP, but refers to the use of an elevated pressure during the expiratory phase of the ventilatory cycle. After delivery of the set amount of breath by the ventilator, the patient then exhales passively. The volume of gas remaining in the lung after a normal expiration is termed the functional residual capacity (FRC). The FRC is primarily determined by the elastic qualities of the lung and the chest wall. In many lung diseases, the FRC is reduced due to collapse of the unstable alveoli, leading to a decreased surface area for gas exchange and intrapulmonary shunting, with wasted oxygen inspired. Adding PEEP can reduce the work of breathing (at low levels) and help preserve FRC.

Airway Pressure Release Ventilation (APRV)

APRV begins from an elevated baseline (called P_{high} or measured high pressure) and achieves tidal ventilation with a brief release of the P_{high}. This brief release allows CO_2 removal through passive exhalation secondary to elastic recoil. The exhalation time (T_{low}) is shortened to usually less than one second to prevent alveolar derecruitment and collapse — it is essentially CPAP with a brief release.

Ever increasing empirical evidence and clinical experience is showing that APRV is the primary mode of choice when ventilating a patient with ARDS or acute lung injury (ALI). Advantages to APRV ventilation include: decreased airway pressures, decreased minute ventilation, decreased dead-space ventilation, promotion of spontaneous breathing, almost 24 hours a day alveolar recruitment, decreased use of sedation, near elimination of neuromuscular blockade, optimised arterial blood gas results, mechanical restoration of FRC (functional residual capacity), a positive effect on cardiac output (due to the negative inflection from the elevated baseline with each spontaneous breath), increased organ and tissue perfusion, potential for increased urine output due to increased renal perfusion.

A patient with ARDS on average spends 8 to 11 days on a mechanical ventilator; APRV may reduce this time significantly and therefore reduce the incidence of VAP (ventilator acquired pneumonia), a risk that increases with each hour an intubated patient spends on the ventilator (VAP rate is 100 per cent at 100 days on the vent) and carries with it a near 50 per cent mortality rate. So, hospitals that are reporting a 0 per cent incidence of VAP, may be improperly coding or improperly reporting.

A controlled clinical trial testing APRV against the current ARDSNet protocol must be initiated.

High Frequency Ventilation (HFV)

High-frequency ventilation refers to ventilation that occurs at rates significantly above that found in natural breathing (as high as 240–900 'breaths' per minute).

Within the category of high-frequency ventilation, the three principal types are high-frequency jet ventilation (HFJV), high-frequency flow interruption (HFFI), and high-frequency oscillatory ventilation (HFOV) (Fig. 14.7).

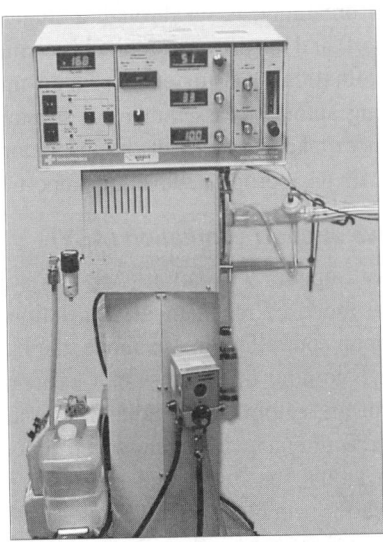

Fig. 14.7. High-frequency ventilator.

High Frequency Jet Ventilation employs a endotracheal tube adaptor in place for the normal 15 mm ET tube adaptor. A high pressure 'jet' of gas flows out of the adaptor and into the airway. This jet of gas occurs for a very brief duration, about 0.02 seconds, and at high frequency: 4–11 hertz. Tidal volumes ≤ 1 ml/kg are used during HFJV. This combination of small tidal volumes delivered for very short periods of time create the lowest possible distal airway and alveolar pressures produced by a mechanical ventilator. Exhalation is passive. Jet ventilators utilise various I:E ratios—between 1:1.1 and 1:12—to help achieve optimal exhalation.

Conventional mechanical breaths are sometimes used to aid in reinflating the lung. Optimal PEEP is used to maintain alveolar inflation and promote ventilation-to-perfusion matching. Jet ventilation has

been shown to reduce ventilator induced lung injury by as much as 20 per cent.

'HFFI' operates similarly to a conventional ventilator, providing increased circuit pressure during the inspiratory phase and dropping back to PEEP during the expiratory phase.

In 'HFOV' the pressure wave is driven by an electromagnetically controlled diaphragm similar to a loudspeaker. Because this can rapidly change the volume in the circuit, HFOV can produce a pressure that is lower than ambient pressure during the expiratory phase. This is sometimes called 'active' expiration. In both types of high-frequency ventilation the pressure wave that is generated at the ventilator is markedly attenuated by passage down the endotracheal tube and the major conducting airways.

This helps protect the alveoli from volutrauma that occurs with traditional positive pressure ventilation. Although the alveoli are kept at a relatively constant volume, similar to CPAP, other mechanisms of gas exchange allow ventilation (the removal of CO_2) to occur without tidal volume exchange. Ventilation in HFOV is a function of frequency, amplitude, and I:E ratio and is best described graphically as the area under the curve of an oscillatory cycle. Amplitude is analogous to tidal volume in conventional ventilation; larger amplitudes remove more CO_2. Seemingly paradoxical, lower frequencies remove more CO_2 in HFOV whereas in conventional ventilation the opposite is true. As frequency decreases, there is less attenuation of the pressure wave transmitted to the alveoli. This results in increased mixing of gas and thus ventilation. I-time is set as a percentage of total time (usually 33 per cent). Amplitude is a function of power and is subject to variability due to changes in compliance or resistance. Therefore, power requirements may vary significantly during treatment and from patient to patient. Patient characteristics and ventilator settings determine whether $PaCO_2$ changes may be more sensitive to amplitude or frequency manipulation. In HFOV, mean airway pressure (MAP) is delivered via a continuous flow through the patient circuit which passes through a variable restriction valve (mushroom valve) on the expiratory limb.

Increasing the flow through the circuit and/or increasing the pressure in the mushroom valve increases MAP. The MAP in HFOV functions similarly to PEEP in conventional ventilation in that it provides the pressure for alveolar recruitment.

Noninvasive ventilation (Noninvasive Positive Pressure Ventilation or NIPPV)

This refers to all modalities that assist ventilation without the use of an endotracheal tube. Noninvasive ventilation is primarily aimed at minimising patient discomfort and the complications associated with invasive ventilation. It is often used in cardiac disease, exacerbations of chronic pulmonary disease, sleep apnea, and neuromuscular diseases. Noninvasive ventilation refers only to the patient interface and not the mode of ventilation used; modes may include spontaneous or control modes and may be either pressure or volume modes.

Some commonly used modes of NIPPV include:

1. Continuous positive airway pressure (CPAP).
2. Bi-level positive airway pressure (BIPAP). Pressures alternate between inspiratory positive airway pressure (IPAP) and a lower expiratory positive airway pressure (EPAP), triggered by patient effort. On many such devices, backup rates may be set, which deliver IPAP pressures even if patients fail to initiate a breath.
3. Intermittent positive pressure ventilation (IPPV) via mouthpiece or mask.

Proportional assist ventilation (PAV)

Proportional assist ventilation (PAV) is a form of synchronised ventilator support based upon the Equation of motion in which the ventilator generates pressure in proportion to the instantaneous patient effort. Unlike other modes of partial support, there is no target flow, tidal volume or pressure. PAV's objective is to allow the patient to attain ventilation and breathing pattern his ventilatory control system desires. The main operational advantages of PAV are automatic synchrony with inspiratory efforts, exhalation and adaptability to change in ventilatory demand.

Proportional assist ventilation plus

Proportional assist ventilation plus (PAV) + (Puritan Bennett – 840 ventilator range, Proportional pressure support — PPS (Drager Evita series) and Respironics BiPAP Vision PAV, are commercially available implementations of PAV which automatically amplify the patient's own spontaneous effort to breathe by increasing airway pressure during inspiration proportionally to a set amplification factor. In PAV+, the level of amplification, thus the level of work of breathing, is set through a single setting (%support) and the pressure applied is continuously and automatically adjusted based on measures (including automatic assessment of Elastance and Resistance) taken throughout the inspiratory cycle to maintain an appropriate level of support.

Adaptive support ventilation (ASV)

Adaptive Support Ventilation (ASV) is a positive pressure mode of mechanical ventilation that is closed-loop controlled. In this mode, the frequency and tidal volume of breaths of a patient on the ventilator are automatically adjusted based on the patient's requirements. The lung mechanics data are used to adjust the depth and rate of breaths to minimise the work rate of breathing. In the ASV mode, every breath is synchronised with patient effort if such an effort exists, and otherwise, full mechanical ventilation is provided to the patient.

ASV technology was originally described as one of the embodiments of US Patent No. 4986268. In this invention, a modified version of an equation derived in physiology in 1950 to minimise the work rate of breathing in man, was used for the first time to find the optimum frequency of mechanical ventilation. The rationale was to make the patient's breathing pattern comfortable and natural within safe limits, and thereby stimulate spontaneous breathing and reduce the weaning time. A prototype of the system was built by the inventor in late 1980s. The inventor is Dr. Fleur T. Tehrani who is a university professor in the US. Shortly after the Patent was issued in 1991, Hamilton Medical, a ventilator manufacturing company, contacted the inventor and discussed marketing the technology with her. Some years later, Hamilton Medical marketed this closed-loop technique under license of this Patent as ASV.

Since the issuance of the Patent, a number of articles have been published by the inventor and her colleagues that are related to the invention, and some of them describe further advancements of the closed-loop techniques presented in the Patent.

Neurally Adjusted Ventilatory Assist (NAVA)

Neurally adjusted ventilatory assist (NAVA) is a new positive pressure mode of mechanical ventilation, where the ventilator is controlled directly by the patient's own neural control of breathing. The neural control signal of respiration originates in the respiratory centre, and are transmitted through the phrenic nerve to excite the diaphragm.

These signals are monitored by means of electrodes mounted on a nasogastric feeding tube and positioned in the esophagus at the level of the diaphragm. As respiration increases and the respiratory centre requires the diaphragm for more effort, the degree of ventilatory support needed is immediately provided.

This means that the patient's respiratory centre is in direct control of the mechanical support required on a breath-by-breath basis, and any variation in the neural respiratory demand is responded to by the appropriate corresponding change in ventilatory assistance.

CHOOSING AMONGST VENTILATOR MODES

Assist-control mode minimises patient effort by providing full mechanical support with every breath. This is often the initial mode chosen for adults because it provides the greatest degree of support. In patients with less severe respiratory failure, other modes such as SIMV may be appropriate. Assist-control mode should not be used in those patients with a potential for respiratory alkalosis, in which the patient has an increased respiratory drive. Such hyperventilation and hypocapnia (decreased systemic carbon dioxide due to hyperventilation) usually occurs in patients with end-stage liver disease, hyperventilatory sepsis, and head trauma. Respiratory alkalosis will be evident from the initial arterial blood

gas obtained, and the mode of ventilation can then be changed if so desired.

Positive end expiratory pressure may or may not be employed to prevent atelectasis in adult patients. It is almost always used for pediatric and neonatal patients due to their increased tendency for atelectasis.

High frequency oscillation is used most frequently in neonates, but is also used as an always alternative mode in adults with severe ARDS. Pressure regulated volume control is another option.

Initial Ventilator Settings

The following are general guidelines that may need to be modified for the individual patient.

Tidal volume, rate, and pressures

1. For adult patients and older children:
   (a) Tidal volume (T_v) is calculated in millilitres per kilogram. Traditionally 10 ml/kg was used but has been shown to cause barotrauma, or injury to the lung by overextension, so 6 to 8 ml/kg is now common practice in ICU. Hence a patient weighing 70 kg would get a TV of 420–480 ml. In adults a rate of 12 strokes per minute is generally used.
   (b) With acute respiratory distress syndrome (ARDS) a tidal volume of 6–8 ml/kg is used with a rate of 10–12 per minute. This reduced tidal volume allows for minimal volutrauma but may result in an elevated pCO_2 (due to the relative decreased oxygen delivered) but this elevation does not need to be corrected (termed permissive hypercapnia).
2. For infants and younger children:
   (a) Without existing lung disease — a tidal volume of 4–8 ml/kg to be delivered at a rate of 30–35 breaths per minute
   (b) With RDS—decrease tidal volume and increase respiratory rate sufficient to maintain pCO_2 between 45 and 55. Allowing higher pCO_2 (sometimes called permissive hypercapnia) may help prevent ventilator induced lung injury .

As the amount of tidal volume increases, the pressure required to administer that volume is increased. This pressure is known as the peak airway pressure. If the peak airway pressure is persistently above 45 cmH$_2$O (4.4 kPa) for adults, the risk of barotrauma is increased and efforts should be made to try to reduce the peak airway pressure. In infants and children it is unclear what level of peak pressure may cause damage. In general, keeping peak pressures below 30 cmH$_2$O (2.9 kPa) is desirable.

Monitoring for barotrauma can also involve measuring the plateau pressure, which is the pressure after the delivery of the tidal volume but before the patient is allowed to exhale. Normal breathing pattern involves inspiration, then expiration. The ventilator is programmed so that after delivery of the tidal volume (inspiration), the patient is not allowed to exhale for a half a second. Therefore, pressure must be maintained in order to prevent exhalation, and this pressure is the plateau pressure. Barotrauma is minimised when the plateau pressure is maintained < 30–35 cmH$_2$O.

Sighs

An adult patient breathing spontaneously will usually sigh about 6–8 times per hour to prevent microatelectasis, and this has led some to propose that ventilators should deliver 1½–2 times the amount of the preset tidal volume 6–8 times per hour to account for the sighs. However, such high quantity of volume delivery requires very high peak pressure that predisposes to barotrauma. Currently, accounting for sighs is not recommended if the patient is receiving 10–12 ml/kg or is on PEEP. If the tidal volume used is lower, the sigh adjustment can be used, as long as the peak and plateau pressures are acceptable. Sighs are not generally used with ventilation of infants and young children.

Initial FiO$_2$

Because the mechanical ventilator is responsible for assisting in a patient's breathing, it must then also be able to deliver an adequate amount of oxygen in each breath. The FiO$_2$ stands for fraction of inspired oxygen, which means the percent of oxygen in each breath that is inspired. (Note that normal room air has ~21 per cent oxygen content). In adult patients who can tolerate higher levels of oxygen for a period of time, the initial FiO$_2$ may be set at 100 per cent until arterial blood gases can document adequate oxygenation. An FiO$_2$ of 10 per cent for an extended period of time can be dangerous, but it can protect against hypoxemia from unexpected intubation problems. For infants, and especially in premature infants, avoiding high levels of FiO$_2$ (>60 per cent) is important.

Positive end-expiratory pressure (PEEP)

PEEP is an adjuvant to the mode of ventilation used to help maintain functional residual capacity (FRC). At the end of expiration, the PEEP exerts pressure to oppose passive emptying of the lung and to keep the airway pressure above the atmospheric pressure. The presence of PEEP opens up collapsed or unstable alveoli and increases the FRC and surface area for gas exchange, thus reducing the size of the shunt. For example, if a large shunt is found to exist based on the estimation from 100 per cent FiO$_2$, then PEEP can be considered and the FiO$_2$ can be lowered (<60 per cent) in order to maintain an adequate PaO$_2$, thus reducing the risk of oxygen toxicity.

In addition to treating a shunt, PEEP may also be useful to decrease the work of breathing. In pulmonary physiology, compliance is a measure of the 'stiffness' of the lung and chest wall. The mathematical formula for compliance (C) equals change in volume divided by change in pressure. The higher the compliance, the more easily the lungs will inflate in response to positive pressure. An under-inflated lung will have low compliance and PEEP will improve this initially by increasing the FRC, since the partially inflated lung takes less energy to inflate further. Excessive PEEP can however produce overinflation, which will again decrease compliance. Therefore, it is important to maintain an adequate, but not excessive FRC.

Indications

PEEP can cause significant haemodynamic consequences through decreasing venous return to the right heart and decreasing right ventricular function. As such, it should be judiciously used and is indicated for adults in two circumstances.

1. If a PaO$_2$ of 60 mmHg cannot be achieved with a FiO$_2$ of 60 per cent.
2. If the initial shunt estimation is greater than 25 per cent.

If used, PEEP is usually set with the minimal positive pressure to maintain an adequate PaO$_2$ with a safe FiO$_2$. As PEEP increases intrathoracic pressure, there can be a resulting decrease in venous return and decrease in cardiac output. A PEEP of less than 10 cmH$_2$O (1 kPa) is usually safe in adults if intravascular volume depletion is absent. Lower levels are used for pediatric patients. Older literature recommended routine placement of a Swan-Ganz catheter if the amount of PEEP used is greater than 10 cmH$_2$ for hemodynamic monitoring. More recent literature has failed to find outcome benefits with routine PA catheterisation when compared to simple central venous pressure monitoring.

If cardiac output measurement is required, minimally invasive techniques, such as oesophageal doppler monitoring or arterial waveform contour monitoring may be sufficient alternatives. PEEP should be withdrawn from a patient until adequate PaO$_2$ can be maintained with a FiO$_2$ < 40 per cent. When withdrawing, it is decreased through 1–2 cmH$_2$O decrements while monitoring haemoglobin-oxygen saturations. Any unacceptable haemoglobin-oxygen saturation should prompt reinstitution of the last PEEP level that maintained good saturation.

Positioning

Prone (face down) positioning has been used in patients with ARDS and severe hypoxemia. It improves FRC, drainage of secretions, and ventilation-perfusion matching (efficiency of gas exchange). It may improve oxygenation in >50 per cent of patients, but no survival benefit has been documented.

Sedation and paralysis

Most intubated patients receive intravenous sedation through a continuous infusion or scheduled dosing to help with anxiety or psychological stress. Sedation also helps the patient tolerate the constant irritation of the endotracheal tube in their mouth, pharynx and trachea. Without some form of sedation and analgesia, it is common for patients to 'fight' the ventilator. This fighting increases work of breathing and may cause further lung injury. Daily interruption of sedation is commonly helpful to the patient for reorientation and appropriate weaning. These interruptions are frequently described as 'sedation vacations' and have been shown to reduce the time patients stay on mechanical ventilation.

HUMIDIFIERS FOR USE WITH AUTOMATIC LUNG VENTILATORS

The ventilation of a patient for prolonged periods with room air or cylinder gases when the air-conditioning action of the nasal passages is bypassed by an endotracheal or tracheotomy tube is likely to result in a marked drying of bronchial and alveolar secretions. Depletion of this mucosal moisture increases the viscosity of the mucous layer, slows its movement and reduces ciliary action. The build-up of solidifying secretions can significantly affect the airway resistance. In order to avoid these complications, a humidifier is usually attached to the output of the ventilator in order to add water vapour to the inspired gas delivered to the patient (Fig. 14.8).

In the past, the commonest type of humidifier for use with ventilators has been the 'bubbler' type. In principle, this is simply a container of water thermostatically maintained at about body temperature and through which each expired tidal volume from the ventilator is bubbled to pick-up water vapour. British Standard 4494 specifies the operation of humidifiers for use with breathing machines. Over the minute volume range of 5 to 20 litres per minute, the output from the humidifier should contain not less than 53 mg of water vapour per litre (a relative humidity of not less than 75 per cent at 37°C) at the end of a one meter length of 22 mm bore corrugated rubber tubing when the input gas temperature is in the range 10 to 25°C. The gas temperature at the point of entry to the patient must not

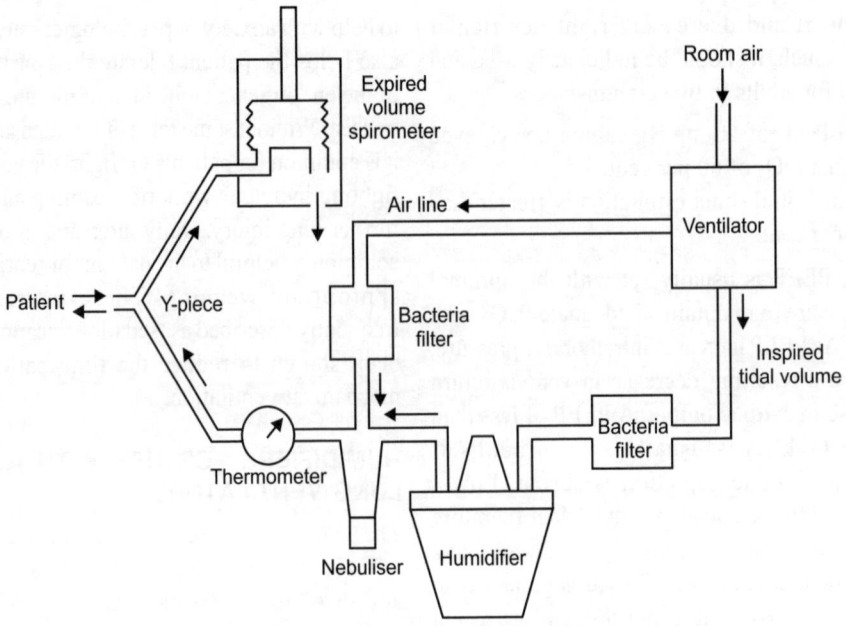

Fig. 14.8. The connection of a humidifier and a nebuliser to a ventilator.

exceed 39°C at any time and the resistance to flow of the humidifier should not exceed 30 mm of water at a steady flow of 30 litres per minute.

Considerable improvements have been made in the design of bubbler type humidifiers, for example, in the version incorporated in the Type AV3 intensive care ventilator by Philips Medical Systems Ltd. This is a two tank design which has a low and constant compressible volume with a plug-in sterilisable water bath unit. A thermostat controls the water bath temperature and as an additional safeguard, a thermistor senses the temperature of the humidified gas supplied to the patient. This can be set between 27° and 37°C. Other forms of humidifier include the 'scent-spray' type. A fine jet of water produced by a vibrator pump and a jewelled orifice is caused to impact on to a metal tube where it forms a fine mist of water vapour which is entrained by the passing tidal volume going to the patient. The humidifier uses a maximum rate of 20 ml of water per hour and it can hold 500 ml.

Assuming that the incoming gas to the humidifier is dry and the water vapour content of the humidified gas is 6 per cent by volume at 37°C, for an 8 litre minute volume the humidifier is supplying 400 ml of water vapour per minute. At 37°C, 1 ml of liquid water is equivalent to 1400 ml of vapour so this represents a consumption of 20 ml of water per minute.

This type of humidifier is compact and can be mounted adjacent to the inspiratory valve which with the expiratory valve may be mounted in a valve block close to the patient. In order to prevent the condensation of water vapour from causing the disk valves to stick, Dräger electrically heat the valve block to 40°–45°C. The Dräger Spiromat 661 ventilator is provided with a concentric delivery hose arrangement with the inner tube carrying the humidified air to the patient. This is a heat exchanger system, the warm expired air which surrounds the inner tube helps to prevent condensation of the water vapour contents of the inspired air. The fact that the lumen of the inspiratory hose of a ventilator can be smaller than that of the expiratory hose also led Bushman and Robinson to the design of a double-lumen concentric ventilator hose. In many types of ventilator, the expired gas is returned to the machine and passes through the expiratory port and valve and often a tidal and minute volume measuring device. Since this part of the ventilator is normally at room temperature, a considerable condensation of water vapour may occur when a humidifier is in use. This can cause a lightweight mica disk valve to stick and also give rise to false readings with turbine or vane type volume meters. Hence, it may be necessary to heat these devices to about 45°C to prevent the condensation of water in them or to provide drainage facilities and to employ materials which will not take up water.

A number of ventilators are fitted with ultrasonic humidifiers. Radio frequency power is supplied to a concave piezoelectric transducer made of a ceramic material. This results in the transducer vibrating at an ultrasonic frequency of the order of 1.4 MHz. The concave shape of the ceramic focuses the ultrasonic waves into a container full of sterile water. The resulting intense agitation of the water gives rise to the production of a fine mist of water particles which are claimed to have a close range of drop sizes. This helps to achieve a uniform penetration of the lungs. A powerful ultrasonic humidifier can produce copious amounts of water and care must be taken in its use with patients. One possible regime is to use a bubbler humidifier and an ultrasonic humidifier for alternate hours. Care must also be taken to ensure that any radio frequency field from an ultrasonic humidifier will not effect pacemakers and other apparatus used by the patient.

Nebulisers

Humidifiers, except those of the ultrasonic types, are basically designed to produce a maximum amount of water vapour with a minimum amount of particulate water. This is in contrast to nebulisers which are designed to generate a maximum output of particles of medication in a desired size range. There may be a considerable overlap in function between a humidifier and a nebuliser, the difference often being one of degree. Nebulisers are frequently used in conjunction with a patient-triggered assistor for the administration of drugs such as bronchodilators in the form of an aerosol. Other forms of aerosol therapy use mucolytic, proteolytic or antibiotic aerosols. A heated aerosol of hypertonic saline, with or without propylene glycol, can be employed for sputum induction of for the removal of thick bronchial plugs.

15

Anaesthesia and Anaesthesia Equipment

INTRODUCTION

Anaesthesia, has traditionally meant the condition of having sensation (including the feeling of pain) blocked or temporarily taken away. This allows patients to undergo surgery and other procedures without the distress and pain they would otherwise experience. Another definition is a 'reversible lack of awareness', whether this is a total lack of awareness (e.g. a general anaesthetic) or a lack of awareness of a part of the body such as a spinal anaesthetic or another nerve block would cause. Anaesthesia is a pharmacologically induced reversible state of amnesia, analgesia, loss of responsiveness, loss of skeletal muscle reflexes and decreased stress response.

VOLATILE ANAESTHETIC

The volatile anaesthetics are a class of general anaesthetic drugs. They share the property of being liquid at room temperature, but evaporating easily for administration by inhalation (some experts make a distinction between volatile and gas anaesthetics on this basis, but both are treated in this chapter, since they probably do not differ in mechanism of action). All of these agents share the property of being quite hydrophobic (i.e. as liquids, they are not freely miscible with in water, and as gases they dissolve in oils better than in water).

The ideal volatile anaesthetic agent offers smooth and reliable induction and maintenance of general anaesthesia with minimal effects on other organ systems. In addition it is odourless or pleasant to inhale; safe for all ages and in pregnancy; not metabolised; rapid in onset and offset; potent; and safe for exposure to operating room staff. It is also cheap to manufacture; easy to transport and store, with a long shelf life; easy to administer and monitor with existing equipment; stable to light, plastics, metals, rubber and soda lime; nonflammable and environmentally safe.

None of the agents currently in use is ideal, although many have some of the desirable characteristics. For example, sevoflurane is pleasant to inhale and is rapid in onset and offset. It is also safe for all ages. However, it is expensive (approximately 3 to 5 times more expensive than isoflurane), and approximately half as potent as isoflurane.

Anaesthetists administer these agents using an anaesthetic vaporiser attached to an anaesthetic machine. Agents stored as liquids and administered by vaporiser include:

1. Diethyl ether: Pungent smelling and extremely flammable; still used in the Third World.
2. Chloroform: Now abandoned for clinical use
3. Trichloroethylene: Now abandoned for clinical use.
4. Halothane (N01 AB01): Sweet smelling, slow onset and offset, potent, risk of hepatitis with repeated use.

DEPTH OF ANAESTHESIA

Despite the widely different anaesthetic agents that are in use, it is possible to identify signs that indicate the depth of anaesthesia. The estimation of depth rests on variety of physical signs, which include the response to stimuli.

Perhaps the best two generalising statements that can be made relative to the depth of anaesthesia are: (i) the central nervous system depression increases progressively from the highest centres (e.g. cortex) to the lowest (e.g. spinal cord), and (ii) respiration (which is also a phenomenon of the central nervous system) is progressively depressed. Thus, general anaesthesia extends from a depression of the sensitivity to painful stimuli to respiratory arrest.

The signs used to identify the depth of anaesthesia are type and rate of respiration, pupillary size and response to light, eyeball movements, corneal reflex, muscle tone, and often the patellar tendon reflex. Inspiration is achieved by contraction of the muscles of the rib cage and diaphragm; expiration results from the relaxation of these muscles and the elastic recoil of the lungs and thorax. Thus, respiration has two components, thoracic and diaphragmatic. Contraction of the dome-shaped diaphragm causes the abdomen to move outward. Therefore, the two signs of respiration are thoracic and abdominal movements. With progressively increasing depth of anaesthesia, respiratory rate decreases, followed by a delay between the thoracic and abdominal components. With deeper anaesthesia, the thoracic component becomes more depressed and ultimately disappears, leaving only the abdominal component. Finally, with very deep anaesthesia, the abdominal component disappears when the respiratory centre is paralysed.

The eyes provide several types of useful information relative to the depth of anaesthesia. The pupil is constricted by parasympathetic activity and dilated by sympathetic activity. In addition, pupillary constriction in response to light is a reflex. Since deepening anaesthesia depresses reflexes, the absence of this light reflex is often used as an indicator of depth of anaesthesia. It is important to note that profound hypoxia also causes wide dilation of the pupils; however, this state is easily differentiated from increased sympathetic activity by noting the other signs of anaesthesia. In some species, and with many anaesthetics, the eyeballs oscillate with light anaesthesia. Perhaps the most frequently used eye sign is the corneal reflex. If the cornea is tapped very lightly, the eyelid blinks; this protective reflex is fairly

resistant to anaesthesia. Another sign of general anaesthesia is progressive lowering of body temperature due to depression of the hypothalamic temperature-regulation centre. The decrease in temperature is related to the depth and duration of anaesthesia. For this reason, special care must be taken to prevent excessive heat loss from subjects who are under anaesthesia for prolonged periods. Although the signs and responses just described are all used to estimate the depth of anaesthesia, no single sign can be relied on, since different anaesthetics often have slightly different effects and may enhance or attenuate the various signs and responses. In addition, preanaesthetic medication often enhances or abolishes some of the signs. It is customary to use premedication to obtain a smooth induction and remove the side effects of some anaesthetics.

GUEDEL'S CLASSIFICATION

Since the invention of anaesthesia in 1846, assessment of its depth was a problem. To determine the depth of anaesthesia, anaesthetist must rely on a series of physical signs of the patient. In 1847, John Snow and Francis Plomley attempted to describe various stages of anaesthesia, but Arthur E. Guedel in 1937 described a detailed system which was generally accepted. This classification was designed for use of a sole inhalational anaesthetic agent, ether, with patients usually premedicated with morphine and atropine. Until that time, muscle relaxants were not used during anaesthesia and intravenous induction agents were not common.

Introduction of neuromuscular blocking agents (tubocurarine) in 1942 changed the concept of anaesthesia as it could produce temporary paralysis (a desired feature for surgery) without deep anaesthesia. Most of the signs of Guedel's classification depend upon the muscular movements (including respiratory muscles), and paralysed patients' traditional clinical signs were no longer detectable when such drugs were used. Since 1982, ether is not used in United States. Now, because of the use of intravenous induction agents with muscle relaxants and discontinuation of ether, Guedel's classification is regarded as obsolete. Depth of anaesthesia can now be measured using a BIS monitor.

Stages of Anaesthesia

Stage I: (Stage of Analgesia or the stage of Disorientation): from beginning of induction of anaesthesia to loss of consciousness.

Stage II: (Stage of Excitement or the stage of Delirium): from loss of consciousness to onset of automatic breathing. Eyelash reflex disappear but other reflexes remain intact and coughing, vomiting and struggling may occur; respiration can be irregular with breath-holding.

Stage III: (Stage of Surgical anaesthesia): from onset of automatic respiration to respiratory paralysis. It is divided into four planes:

1. Plane I — from onset of automatic respiration to cessation of eyeball movements. Eyelid reflex is lost, swallowing reflex disappears, marked eyeball movement may occur but conjunctival reflex is lost at the bottom of the plane.
2. Plane II — from cessation of eyeball movements to beginning of paralysis of intercostal muscles. Laryngeal reflex is lost although inflammation of the upper respiratory tract increases reflex irritability, corneal reflex disappears, secretion of tears increases (a useful sign of light anaesthesia), respiration is automatic and regular, movement and deep breathing as a response to skin stimulation disappears.
3. Plane III — from beginning to completion of intercostal muscle paralysis. Diaphragmatic respiration persists but there is progressive intercostal paralysis, pupils dilated and light reflex is abolished. The laryngeal reflex lost in plane II can still be initiated by painful stimuli arising from the dilatation of anus or cervix. This was the desired plane for surgery when muscle relaxants were not used.
4. Plane IV — from complete intercostal paralysis to diaphragmatic paralysis (apnoea).

Stage IV: from stoppage of respiration till death. Anaesthetic overdose cause medullary paralysis with respiratory arrest and vasomotor collapse. Pupils are widely dilated and muscles are relaxed.

In 1954, Artusio further divided the first stage in Guedel's classification into three planes.

1. 1st plane: The patient does not experience amnesia or analgesia.
2. 2nd plane: The patient is completely amnesic but experiences only partial analgesia.
3. 3rd plane: The patient has complete amnesia and analgesia.

STANDARDS FOR BASIC ANAESTHETIC MONITORING

These standards apply to all anaesthesia care although, in emergency circumstances, appropriate life support measures take precedence. These standards may be exceeded at any time based on the judgment of the responsible anaesthesiologist. They are intended to encourage quality patient care, but observing them cannot guarantee any specific patient outcome. They are subject to revision from time to time, as warranted by the evolution of technology and practice. They apply to all general anaesthetics, regional anaesthetics and monitored anaesthesia care. This set of standards addresses only the issue of basic anaesthetic monitoring, which is one component of anaesthesia care. In certain rare or unusual circumstances: (i) some of these methods of monitoring may be clinically impractical, and (ii) appropriate use of the described monitoring methods may fail to detect untoward clinical developments. Brief interruptions of continual (Note that 'continual' is defined as 'repeated regularly and frequently in steady rapid succession' whereas 'continuous' means 'prolonged without any interruption at any time.') monitoring may be unavoidable. These standards are not intended for application to the care of the obstetrical patient in labour or in the conduct of pain management.

Standard I

Qualified anaesthesia personnel shall be present in the room throughout the conduct of all general anaesthetics, regional anaesthetics and monitored anaesthesia care.

Objective

Because of the rapid changes in patient status during anaesthesia, qualified anaesthesia personnel shall be continuously present to monitor the patient and provide anaesthesia care. In the event there is a direct known hazard, e.g. radiation, to the anaesthesia personnel which might require intermittent remote observation of the patient, some provision for monitoring the patient must be made. In the event that an emergency requires the temporary absence of the person primarily responsible for the anaesthetic, the best judgment of the anaesthesiologist will be exercised in comparing the emergency with the anaesthetised patient's condition and in the selection of the person left responsible for the anaesthetic during the temporary absence.

Standard II

During all anaesthetics, the patient's oxygenation, ventilation, circulation and temperature shall be continually evaluated.

Oxygenation

Objective

To ensure adequate oxygen concentration in the inspired gas and the blood during all anaesthetics.

Methods

1. Inspired gas: During every administration of general anaesthesia using an anaesthesia machine, the concentration of oxygen in the patient breathing system shall be measured by an oxygen analyser with a low oxygen concentration limit alarm in use.

2. Blood oxygenation: During all anaesthetics, a quantitative method of assessing oxygenation such as pulse oximetry shall be employed. When the pulse oximeter is utilised, the variable pitch pulse tone and the low threshold alarm shall be audible to the anaesthesiologist or the anaesthesia care team personnel. Adequate illumination and exposure of the patient are necessary to assess colour.

Ventilation

Objective

To ensure adequate ventilation of the patient during all anaesthetics.

Methods

1. Every patient receiving general anaesthesia shall have the adequacy of ventilation continually evaluated. Qualitative clinical signs such as chest excursion, observation of the reservoir breathing bag and auscultation of breath sounds are useful. Continual monitoring for the presence of expired carbon dioxide shall be performed unless invalidated by the nature of the patient, procedure or equipment. Quantitative monitoring of the volume of expired gas is strongly encouraged.

2. When an endotracheal tube or laryngeal mask is inserted, its correct positioning must be verified by clinical assessment and by identification of carbon dioxide in the expired gas. Continual end-tidal carbon dioxide analysis, in use from the time of endotracheal tube/laryngeal mask placement, until extubation/removal or initiating transfer to a postoperative care location, shall be performed using a quantitative method such as capnography, capnometry or mass spectroscopy. When capnography or capnometry is utilised, the end tidal CO_2 alarm shall be audible to the anaesthesiologist or the anaesthesia care team personnel.

3. When ventilation is controlled by a mechanical ventilator, there shall be in continuous use a device that is capable of detecting disconnection of components of the breathing system. The device must give an audible signal when its alarm threshold is exceeded.

4. During regional anaesthesia and monitored anaesthesia care, the adequacy of ventilation shall be evaluated by continual observation of qualitative clinical signs and/or monitoring for the presence of exhaled carbon dioxide.

Circulation

Objective

To ensure the adequacy of the patient's circulatory function during all anaesthetics.

Methods

1. Every patient receiving anaesthesia shall have the electrocardiogram continuously displayed from the beginning of anaesthesia until preparing to leave the anaesthetising location.
2. Every patient receiving anaesthesia shall have arterial blood pressure and heart rate determined and evaluated at least every five minutes.
3. Every patient receiving general anaesthesia shall have, in addition to the above, circulatory function continually evaluated by at least one of the following: palpation of a pulse, auscultation of heart sounds, monitoring of a tracing of intra-arterial pressure, ultrasound peripheral pulse monitoring, or pulse plethysmography or oximetry.

Body temperature

Objective

To aid in the maintenance of appropriate body temperature during all anaesthetics.

Methods

Every patient receiving anaesthesia shall have temperature monitored when clinically significant changes in body temperature are intended, anticipated or suspected.

ANAESTHETIC MACHINE

The anaesthetic machine (or anaesthesia machine in America) is used by anaesthesiologists to support the administration of anaesthesia. The most common type of anaesthetic machine in use in the developed world is the continuous-flow anaesthetic machine, which is designed to provide an accurate and continuous supply of medical gases (such as oxygen and nitrous oxide), mixed with an accurate concentration of anaesthetic vapour (such as isoflurane), and deliver this to the patient at a safe pressure and flow. Modern machines incorporate a ventilator, suction unit, and patient-monitoring devices. Figure 15.1 shows the simple schematic of an anaesthesia machine.

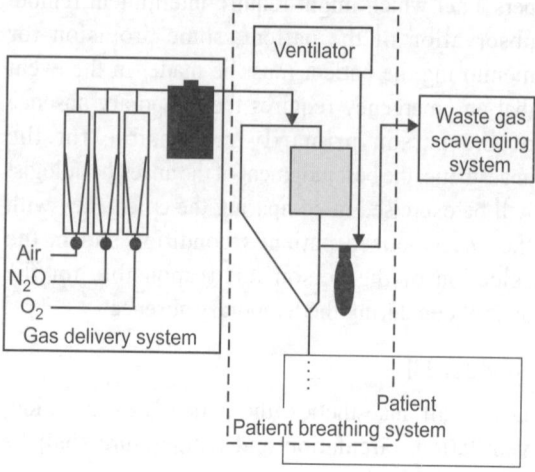

Fig. 15.1. Simple schematic of an anaesthesia machine.

The anaesthetic machine is usually mounted on antistatic wheels for convenient transportation.

Simpler anaesthetic apparatus may be used in special circumstances, such as the TriService Apparatus, a simplified anaesthesia delivery system invented for the British armed forces, which is light and portable and may be used effectively even when no medical gases are available. This device has unidirectional valves which suck in ambient air which can be enriched with oxygen from a cylinder with the help of a set of bellows. A large number of draw-over type of anaesthesia devices are still in use in India for administering an air-ether mixture to the patient, which can be enriched with oxygen. But the advent of the cautery has sounded the death knell to this contraption, due to the explosion hazard.

Components of a Typical Machine

A modern machine typically includes the following components:

1. Connections to piped hospital oxygen, medical air, and nitrous oxide. Pipeline

pressure from the hospital medical gas system (wall outlet) should be around 400 kPa (60 psi; 4 atmospheres).

2. Reserve gas cylinders of oxygen, air, and nitrous oxide attached via a specific yoke with a Bodok seal. Older machines may have cylinder yokes and flow meters for carbon dioxide and cyclopropane. Many newer machines only have oxygen reserve cylinders. The regulators for the cylinders are set at 300 kPa (45 psi; 3 atmospheres). If the cylinders are left on and the machine is plugged into the wall outlet, gas from the wall supply will be used preferentially, since it is at a higher pressure. In situations where pipeline gases are not available, machines may safely be used from cylinders alone, provided fresh cylinders are available.

3. A high-flow oxygen flush which provides pure oxygen at 30 litres/minute.

4. Pressure gauges, regulators and 'pop-off' valves, to protect the machine components and patient from high-pressure gases (referred to as 'barotrauma').

5. Flow meters (rotameters) for oxygen, air, and nitrous oxide, which are used by the anaesthesiologist to provide accurate mixtures of medical gases to the patient. Flow meters are typically pneumatic, but increasingly electromagnetic digital flow meters are being used.

6. One or more anaesthetic vaporisers to accurately add volatile anaesthetics to the fresh gas flow.

7. A ventilator.

8. Physiological monitors to monitor the patient's heart rate, ECG, noninvasive blood pressure and oxygen saturation (additional monitors are generally available to monitor end-tidal CO_2, temperature, arterial blood pressure central venous pressure, etc.). In addition, the composition of the gases delivered to the patient (and breathed out) is monitored continuously.

9. Breathing circuits, most commonly a circle attachment, or a Bain's breathing system, which are breathing hoses connected to a anaesthesia face mask.

10. A heat and moisture exchanger (HME) with or without bacteria-viral filter (HMEF).

11. Scavenging system to remove expired anaesthetic gases from the operating room. Scavenged gases are usually vented to the atmosphere.

12. Suction apparatus.

There is generally a small work bench built into the machine where airway management equipment is kept within ready reach of the anaesthetist.

Gas Blending and Vapourisation System

The basic anaesthesia machine utilises primary low pressure gas sources of 345 kPa (50 psig) available from wall or ceiling column outlets and secondary high pressure gas sources located on the machine as pictured schematically in Fig. 15.2. Tracing the path of oxygen in the machine demonstrates that oxygen comes from either the low pressure source or from the 15.2 MPa (2200 psig) high pressure yokes via cylinder pressure regulators and then branches to service several other functions. First and foremost, the second stage pressure regulator drops the O_2 pressure to approximately 110 kPa (16 psig) before it enters the needle valve and the rotameter type flowmeter. From the flowmeter O_2 mixes with gases from other flowmeters and passes through a calibrated agent vaporiser where specific inhalation anaesthetic agents are vaporised and added to the breathing gas mixture. Oxygen is also used to supply a reservoir canister that sounds a reed alarm in the event that the oxygen pressure drops below 172 kPa (25 psig). When the oxygen pressure drops to 172 kPa or lower, then the nitrous oxide pressure sensor shut-off valve closes and N_2O is prevented from entering its needle valve and flowmeter and is therefore eliminated from the breathing gas mixture. In fact, all machines built in the US have pressure sensor shut-off valves installed in the lines to every flowmeter, except oxygen, to prevent the delivery of hypoxic gas mixture in the event of an oxygen pressure failure.

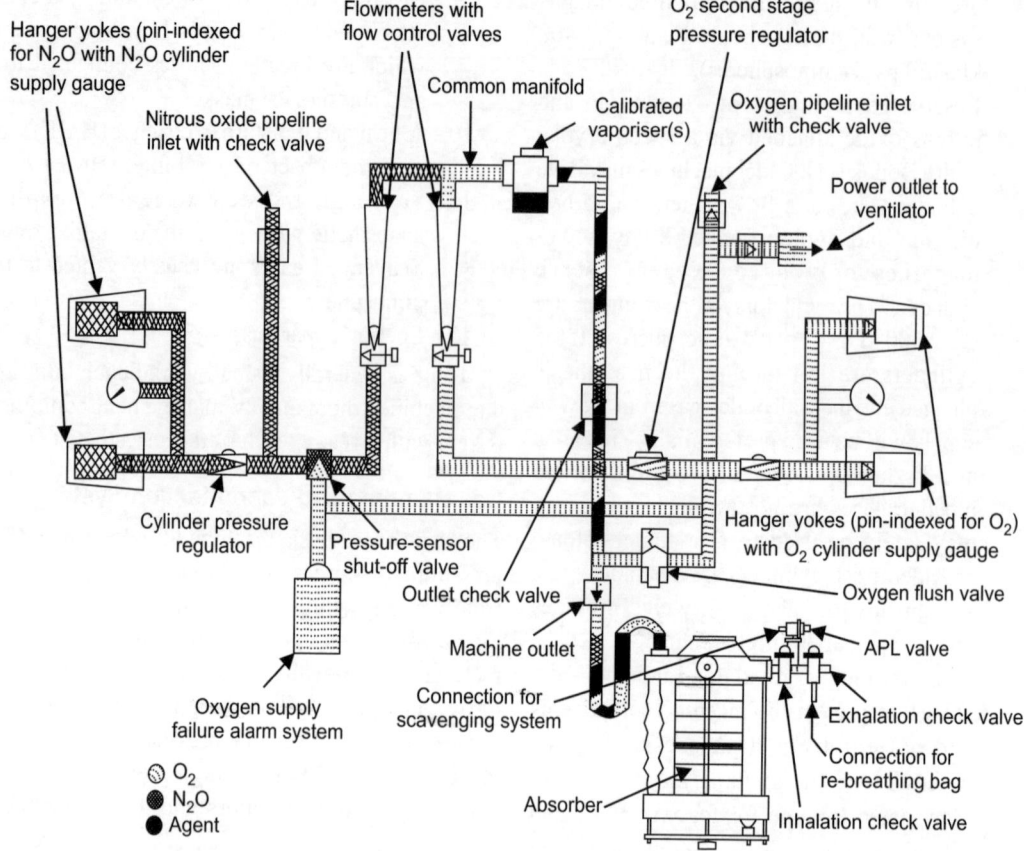

Fig. 15.2. Schematic diagram of gas piping within a simple two-gas (oxygen and nitrous oxide) anaesthesia machine.

Oxygen may also be delivered to the common gas outlet or machine outlet via a momentary normally closed flush valve that typically provides a flow of 65 to 80 litres of O_2 per minute directly into the breathing circuit. Newer machines are required to have a safety system for limiting the minimum concentration of oxygen that can be delivered to the patient to 25 per cent.

The flow paths for nitrous oxide and other gases are much simpler in the sense that after coming from the high pressure regulator or the low pressure hospital source, gas is immediately presented to the pressure sensor shut-off valve from where it travels to its specific needle valve and flowmeter to join the common gas line and enter the breathing circuit. Currently all anaesthesia machines manufactured in the US use only calibrated flow-through vaporisers, meaning that all of the gases from the various flowmeters are mixed in the manifold prior to entering the vaporiser. Any given vaporiser has a calibrated control knob that, once set to the desired concentration for a specific agent, will deliver the concentration to the patient. Some form of interlock system must be provided such that only one vaporiser may be activated at any given time.

Figure 15.3 schematically illustrates the operation of a purely mechanical vaporiser with temperature compensation.

This simple flow-over design permits a fraction of the total gas flow to pass into the vaporising chamber where it becomes saturated with vapour before being added back to the total gas flow.

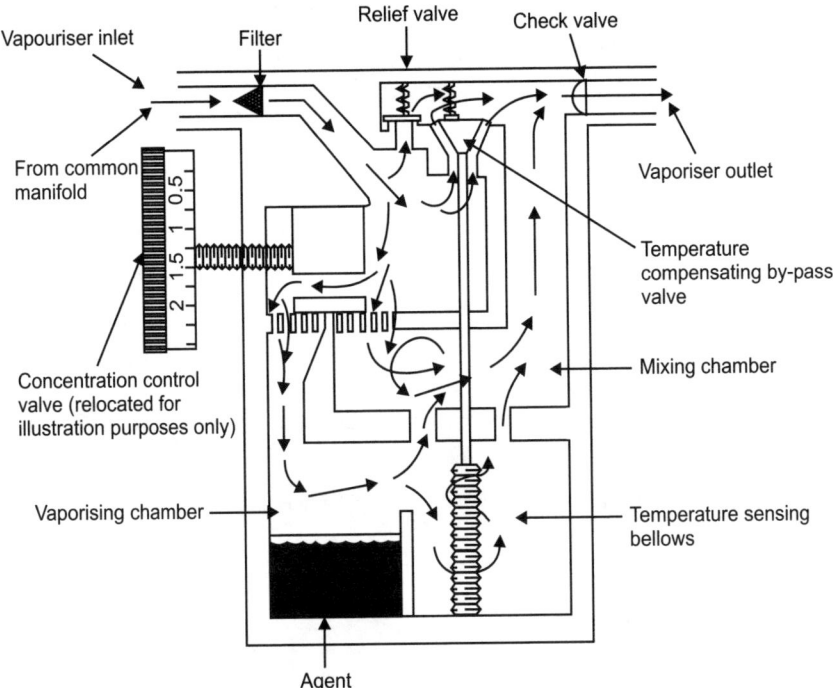

Fig. 15.3. Schematic diagram of a calibrated in-line vaporiser that uses the flow-over technique for adding anaesthetic vapour to the breathing gas mixture.

Since vaporisation is an endothermic process, anaesthetic vaporisers must have sufficient thermal mass and conductivity to permit the vaporisation process to proceed independent of the rate at which the agent is being used.

BREATHING CIRCUITS

The concept behind an effective breathing circuit is to provide an adequate volume of a controlled concentration of gas to the patient during inspiration and to carry the exhaled gases away from the patient during exhalation. There are several forms of breathing circuits which can be classified into two basic types; (i) open circuit, meaning no re-breathing of any gases and no CO_2 absorber present; and (ii) closed circuit, indicating presence of CO_2 absorber and some rebreathing of other gases. Figure 15.4 illustrates the Lack modification of a Mapleson open circuit breathing system. There are no valves and no CO_2 absorber. There is great potential for the patient to re-breath their own exhaled gases unless the fresh gas inflow is 2 to 3 times the patient's minute volume. Figure 15.5 illustrates the most popular form of breathing circuit, the circle system, with oxygen monitor, circle pressure gauge, volume monitor (spirometer) and airway pressure sensor. The circle is a closed system or semi-closed when the fresh gas inflow exceeds the patient's requirements. Excess gas evolves into the scavenging device and some of the exhaled gas is re-breathed after having the CO_2 removed. The inspiratory and expiratory valves in the circle system guarantee that gas flows to the patient from the inspiratory limb and away from the patient through the exhalation limb. In the event of a failure of either or both of these valves, the patient will re-breath exhaled gas that contains CO_2, which is a potentially dangerous situation.

There are two forms of mechanical ventilation used during anaesthesia: (i) volume ventilation, where the volume of gas delivered to the patient remains constant regardless of the pressure that is required; and (ii) pressure ventilation, where the ventilator

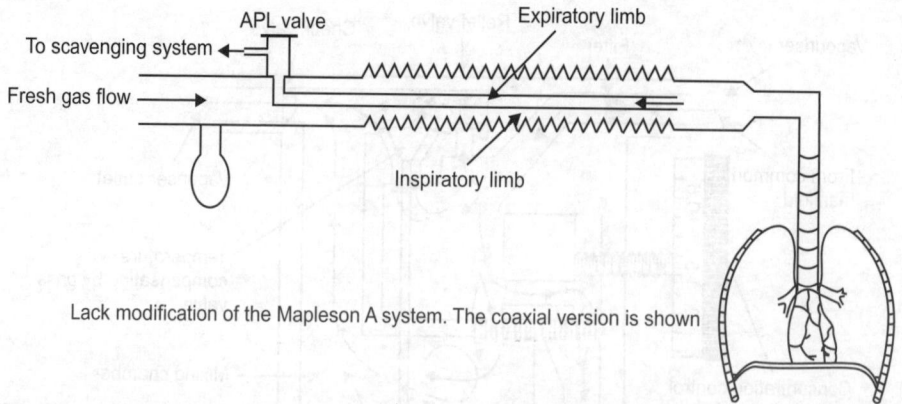

Lack modification of the Mapleson A system. The coaxial version is shown

Fig. 15.4. An example of an open circuit breathing system that does not use unidirectional flow valves or contain a carbon dioxide absorbent.

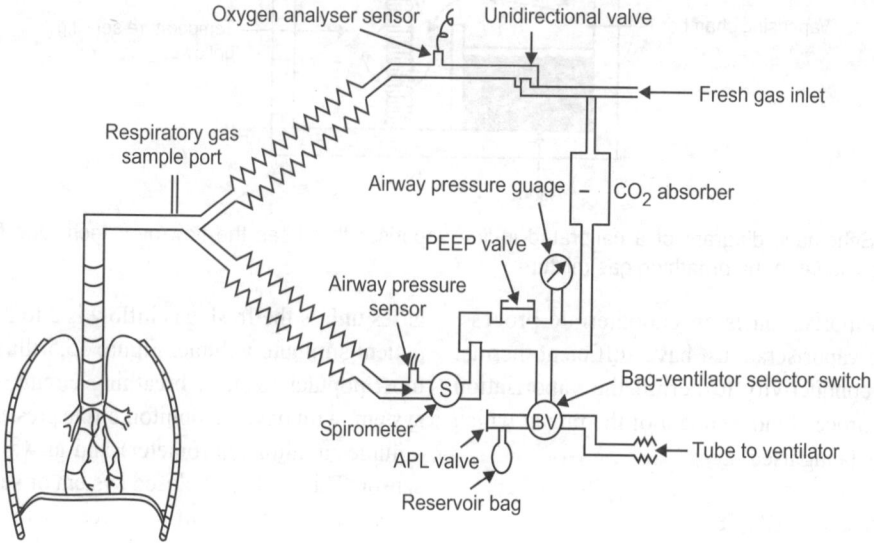

Fig. 15.5. A diagram of a closed circuit circle breathing system with unidirectional valves, inspired oxygen sensor, pressure sensor and CO_2 absorber.

provides whatever volume to the patient that is required to produce some desired pressure in the breathing circuit. Volume ventilation is the most popular since the volume delivered remains theoretically constant despite changes in lung compliance. Pressure ventilation is useful when compliance losses in the breathing circuit are high relative to the volume delivered to the lungs.

Humidification is an important adjunct to the breathing circuit because it maintains the integrity of the cilia that line the airways and promote the removal of mucus and particulate matter from the lungs. Humidification of dry breathing gases can be accomplished by simple passive heat and moisture exchangers inserted into the breathing circuit at the level of the endotracheal tube connectors or by elegant dual servo electronic humidifiers that heat a reservoir filled with water and also heat a wire in the gas delivery tube to prevent rain-out of the water before it reaches the patient. Electronic safety measures must be included in these active devices due to the potential for burning the patient and the fire hazard.

GAS SCAVENGING SYSTEMS

The purpose of scavenging exhaled and excess anaesthetic agents is to reduce or eliminate the potential hazard to employees who work in the environment where anaesthetics are administered, including operating rooms, obstetrical areas, special procedures areas, physician's offices, dentist's offices and veterinarian's surgical suites. Typically more gas is administered to the breathing circuit than is required by the patient, resulting in the necessity to remove excess gas from the circuit. The scavenging system must be capable of collecting gas from all components of the breathing circuit, including adjustable pressure level valves, ventilators and sample withdrawal type gas monitors, without altering characteristics of the circuit such as pressure or gas flow to the patient. There are two broad types of scavenging systems as illustrated in Fig. 15.6. The open interface is a simple design that requires a large physical space for the reservoir volume and the closed interface with an expandable reservoir bag and which must include relief valves for handling the cases of no scavenged flow and great excess of scavenged flow.

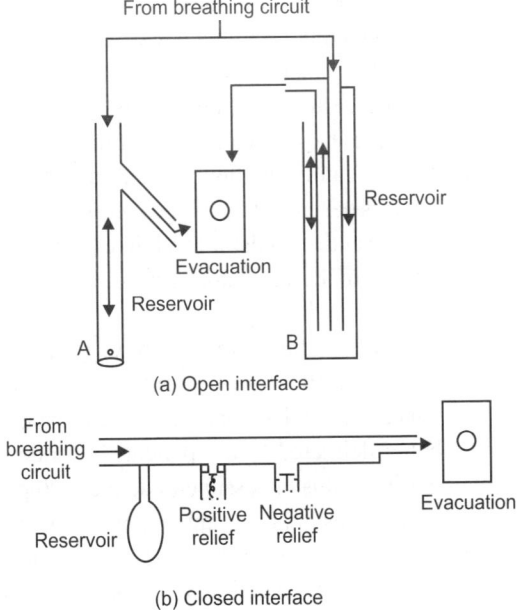

From breathing circuit

Reservoir

Evacuation

Reservoir

A   B

(a) Open interface

From breathing circuit

Positive relief   Negative relief

Reservoir

Evacuation

(b) Closed interface

Fig. 15.6. Examples of open and closed gas scavenger interfaces. The closed interface requires relief valves in the event of scavenging flow failure.

Trace gas analysis must be performed to guarantee the efficacy of the scavenging system. The National institutes of occupational safety and health (NIOSH) recommends that trace levels of nitrous oxide be maintained at or below 25 parts per million (ppm) time weighted average and that halogenated anaesthetic agents remain below 2 ppm.

Anaesthesia Gas Machine

The function of any breathing circuit is to deliver oxygen and anaesthetic gases, and eliminate carbon dioxide. Carbon dioxide may be eliminated by either washout with adequate fresh gas flow (FGF), or by soda lime absorption (Table 15.1).

The breathing system can be either:

1. Closed (fresh gas inflow exactly equal to patient uptake, complete rebreathing after carbon dioxide absorbed, and pop-off closed).
2. Semi-closed (some rebreathing occurs, FGF and pop-off settings at intermediate values).
3. Semi-open (no rebreathing, high fresh gas flow [higher than minute ventilation]).

Open systems have no valves, no tubing: for example open drop ether, or a nasal cannula. In either, the patient has access to atmospheric gases.

Non-rebreathing (Mapleson) breathing circuits

All non-rebreathing (NRB) circuits lack unidirectional valves and soda lime carbon dioxide absorption: thus, the amount of rebreathing is highly dependent on fresh gas flow (FGF) in all. Work of breathing is low in all (no unidirectional valves or soda lime granules to create resistance). Figure 15.7 shows the Mapleson D and Bain NRB circuit.

How do NRB's work? During expiration, fresh gas flow (FGF) pushes exhaled gas down the expiratory limb, where it collects in the reservoir (breathing) bag and opens the expiratory valve (pop-off or APL). The next inspiration draws on the gas in the expiratory limb. The expiratory limb will have less carbon dioxide (less rebreathing) if FGF inflow is high, tidal volume (VT) is low, and the duration of the expiratory pause is long (a long expiratory pause

Table 15.1. Function of breathing circuit.

Mode	Reservoir (breathing bag)	Rebreathing	Example
Open	No	No	Open drop
Semi-open	Yes	No	Nonrebreathing circuit, or Circle at high FGF (> VE)
Semi-closed	Yes	Yes, partial	Circle at low FGF (< VE)
Closed	Yes	Yes, complete	Circle (with pop-off valve [APL] closed)

is desirable as exhaled gas will be flushed more thoroughly). All NRB circuits are convenient, lightweight, easily scavenged. One objection is that the circuit must be reconfigured between cases, with the possibility of error.

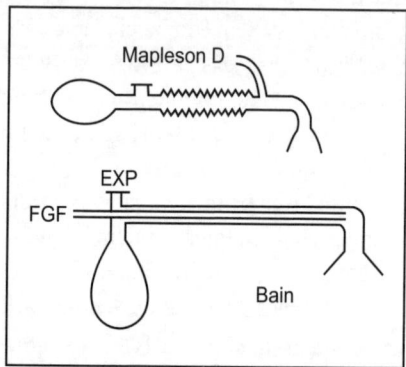

Fig. 15.7. The Mapleson D and Bain NRB circuit.

Minimum FGF In practice, most anaesthetists will provide a minimum 5 L/min for children on up to adults to prevent rebreathing (or 2–3 × minute ventilation [VE], whichever is greater).

The Bain circuit is a 'coaxial' Mapleson D- the same components, but the fresh gas flow tubing is directed within the inspiratory limb, with fresh gas entering the circuit near the mask. Fresh gas flow requirements are similar to other NRB circuits. The Bain has been shown to add more heat and humidity to inhaled gases than other Mapleson circuits.

Closed-circuit circle

System advantages and disadvantages
Circle advantages:
1. Constant inspired concentrations.
2. Conserve respiratory heat and humidity.

3. Useful for all ages (may use down to 10 kg, about one year of age, or less with a pediatric disposable circuit).
4. Useful for closed system or low-flow.
5. Low resistance (less than tracheal tube, but more than a NRB circuit).

Circle disadvantages:
1. Increased dead space.
2. Malfunctions of unidirectional valves.

Safety Features of Modern Machines

Based on experience gained from analysis of mishaps, the modern anaesthetic machine incor-porates several safety devices, including:

1. An oxygen failure alarm (also known as 'oxygen failure warning device' or OFWD). In older machines this was a pneumatic device called a Ritchie whistle. Newer machines have an electronic sensor.
2. Nitrous cutoff: the flow of medical nitrous-oxide is dependent on oxygen pressure. This is done at the regulator level. In essence, the nitrous-oxide regulator is a 'slave' of the oxygen regulator.
3. Hypoxic-mixture alarms (hypoxy guards or ratio controllers) to prevent gas mixtures which contain less than 21 per cent oxygen being delivered to the patient. In modern machines it is impossible to deliver 100 per cent nitrous oxide (or any hypoxic mixture) to the patient to breathe. Oxygen is automatically added to the fresh gas flow even if the anaesthetist should attempt to deliver 100 per cent nitrous oxide. Ratio controllers usually operate on the penumatic

principle or are chain linked. Both are located on the rotameter assembly, unless electronically controlled.

4. Ventilator alarms, which warn of disconnection or high airway pressures.
5. Interlocks between the vaporisers preventing inadvertent administration of more than one volatile agent concurrently.
6. Alarms on all the above physiological monitors.
7. The pin index safety system prevents cylinders being accidentally connected to the wrong yoke.
8. The NIST (noninterchangeable screw thread) system for pipeline gases, which prevents piped gases from the wall being accidentally connected to the wrong inlet on the machine.
9. Pipeline gas hoses have noninterchangeable Schrader valve connectors, which prevents hoses being accidentally plugged into the wrong wall socket.

The functions of the machine should be checked at the beginning of every operating list in a 'cockpit-drill'. Machines and associated equipment must be maintained and serviced regularly.

Older machines may lack some of the safety features and refinements present on newer machines. However, they were designed to be operated without mains electricity, using compressed gas power for the ventilator and suction apparatus. Modern machines often have battery backup, but may fail when this becomes depleted.

The modern anaesthetic machine still retains all the key working principles of the Boyle's machine (a British Oxygen Company trade name) in honour of the British anaesthetist H.E.G. Boyle.

PRESSURE REGULATOR

A pressure regulator is a valve that automatically cuts off the flow of a liquid or gas at a certain pressure. Regulators are used to allow high-pressure fluid supply lines or tanks to be reduced to safe and/or usable pressures for various applications.

A pressure regulator's primary function is to match the flow of gas through the regulator to the demand for gas placed upon the system. If the load flow decreases, then the regulator flow must decrease also. If the load flow increases, then the regulator flow must increase in order to keep the controlled pressure from decreasing due to a shortage of gas in the pressure system.

A regulator includes a loading element, a measuring element, and a restricting element.

Restricting element: This element is a type of valve arrangement. It can be a globe valve, butterfly valve, poppet valve, or any other type of valve that is capable of operating as a variable restriction to the flow.

Loading element: This element is what applies the needed force to the restricting element. This can be any number of things such as a weight, a spring, a piston actuator, or more commonly the diaphragm actuator in combination with a spring.

Measuring element: This element tells us when the inlet flow is equal to the outlet flow. The diaphragm is widely used because not only is it used for measuring but as well for loading purposes.

In the Fig. 15.8 single-stage regulator, a diaphragm is used with a poppet valve to regulate pressure. As pressure in the upper chamber increases, the diaphragm is pushed upward, causing the poppet to reduce flow, bringing the pressure back down. By adjusting the top screw, the downward pressure on the diaphragm can be increased, requiring more pressure in the upper chamber to maintain equilibrium. In this way, the outlet pressure of the regulator is controlled.

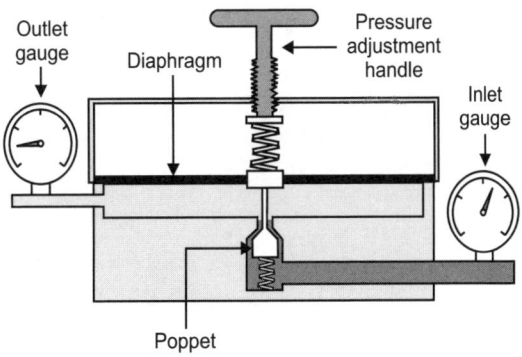

Fig. 15.8. Single-stage regulator.

Modern gas regulators can vary its operation by the use of stiffer springs, pre-amplification, velocity boosting, and lever ratio. Figure 15.9 shows two-stage regulator.

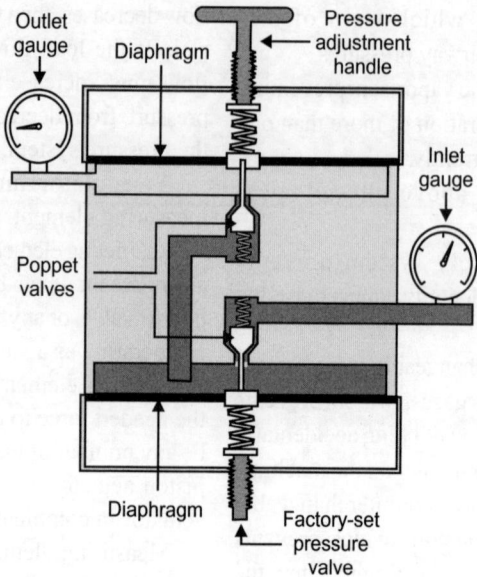

Fig. 15.9. Two-stage pressure regulator.

16

Noninvasive Measurement of Intracranial Pressure

INTRODUCTION

Raised intracranial pressure (ICP) is a life-threatening situation in which early intervention can make a substantial change in the outcome. Increased ICP may be a consequence of various etiologies, including head trauma, hydrocephalus, brain tumor, intracerebral hemorrhage, or cerebral edema. The earliest clinical symptoms of elevation in ICP are headache and decreased mental function. Other symptoms may include gaze paresis (double vision), swelling of the optic disk (papilledema), and brainstem dysfunction apparent as pupillary abnormalities and abnormal posturing. Systemic alterations may involve hypertension and tachycardia.

One of the major problems in evaluation of suspected elevation of ICP is that there is no clinical sign that provides an estimate of the degree of elevation in ICP, with the exception of extreme values of ICP in which the perfusion of the brain is compromised. Thus any noninvasive technique that can provide a reliable estimate of ICP or warning of significant elevation in ICP would be immense value in the early diagnosis and management of a potential life-threatening situation.

INTRACRANIAL PRESSURE

The normal ICP observed by placing a catheter into the lateral ventricle of the human brain and measuring the resulting pressure manometrically has an upper limit of 150 to 180 mm of cerebrospinal fluid (water) for an adult. In children the upper limit of normal may be slightly lower, from 120 to 150 mm of water. Other methods of measurement have utilised

transducers placed in the epidural or subdural space to convert the ICP directly into a voltage that is proportional to the ICP. The voltage is scaled to reflect appropriate ICP levels on a monitor.

The cranium provides a rigid container for the brain, which in the adult is nonyielding to elevations in ICP, and therefore the ICP is directly related to changes in volume of the intracranial contents. The intracranial contents consist of the brain (approximately 1500 cm³), the cerebrospinal fluid (100 to 150 cm³), and the intravascular contents (approximately 100 to 150 cm³). Therefore, changes in volume are achieved primarily by changes in cerebrospinal fluid and vascular volume. Normally, physiological changes in ICP are compensated for by displacement and increased absorption of cerebrospinal fluid and by displacement of venous blood from the brain into sinuses. As long as no permanent increase in volume occurs, the pressure-volume equilibrium will be rapidly reestablished and no long-standing increase in ICP will occur.

The pressure-volume relationship within the cranium is shown in Fig. 16.1. The relationship is described by an exponential curve. The initial horizontal portion of the curve reflects the time at which the ICP and central venous pressure are equal. As the curve rises from the horizontal with increases in intracranial volume, the residual displaceable volume is essentially exhausted, so that subsequent relatively small changes in volume will lead to large increases in ICP (P2 versus P1, Fig. 16.1). In the initial horizontal portion of the curve, it is estimated that cerebrospinal fluid is the major factor compensating for volume change by displacement into the spinal axis, accounting for 30 to 70 per cent of the volume.

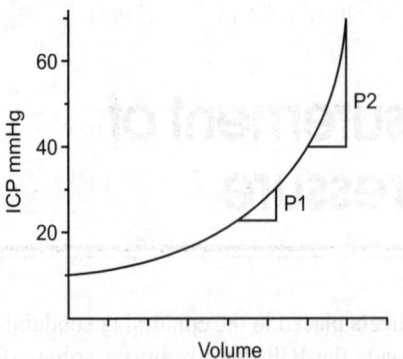

Fig. 16.1. Pressure-volume curve within the cranium. The initial horizontal portion of the curve indicates that small increases in volume can be accommodated within the cranium, without significant elevation in ICP. However, during the rising portion of the curve, similar small increases in volume will result in either small increases in ICP (P1) or large increases in ICP (P2).

When the cerebrospinal fluid buffering becomes exhausted, a change in intracranial elastance occurs and the viscoelastic properties of the subpial tissues (i.e. the brain) act as the major compensating factor. Thus interference with the circulation of cerebrospinal fluid or decreased absorption will decrease the buffering capacity of cerebrospinal fluid and the brain will be tight within the cranium. A previously well tolerated volume change may now result in a critical increase in ICP, which will cause the brain to herniate through the foramen magnum, causing death.

A series of pressure-volume curves may occur depending on the relative volumetric distribution of intracranial contents and their individual elastic properties. These elastic properties are not constant and may change with pathological processes such as cerebral edema (swelling of the brain) and brain tumors. When ICP increases to values approaching mean arterial blood pressure, there is no net perfusion of the brain. The term 'cerebral perfusion pressure' is used to differentiate the net perfusion of the brain and refers to the difference between mean arterial pressure and ICP. In experimental studies conducted in both animals and humans, measurement of cerebral perfusion pressure provides a critical value from which functional brain activity can be assessed relative to a perfusion pressure that maintains normal brain function.

TECHNIQUES FOR NONINVASIVE MEASUREMENT OF INTRACRANIAL PRESSURE

A variety of techniques have been used in attempting to measure ICP noninvasively. The first technique to be discussed utilises direct measurement of skull diameter, the second, changes in fontanelle pressure, the third technique involves measurement of changes in tension of the tympanic membrane, and the fourth technique involves changes produced in evoked potentials by ICP.

Changes in Skull Diameter

Strain gauges attached to Gardner-Wells tongs that clamp the skull laterally over the temporal bone have been used to detect variations in skull diameter as a consequence of change in ICP. Evaluations conducted in cadavers and dogs demonstrated that changes in ICP as small as 2 mm Hg could be detected. Although this technique offers some promise for evaluation of ICP, it has the limitation that the tongs penetrate the outer table of skull and is therefore not a truly noninvasive technique.

Changes in Anterior Fontanelle Pressure

In the newborn and young infants there is an opening in the cranium along the midsaggital suture in which the bone has not yet fused together. By placing a transducer in contact with the skin surface overlying the anterior fontanelle, accurate, reproducible and noninvasive measurements of ICP can be obtained. The fontanelle pressure is referenced from the bony margins adjacent to the fontanelle opening. In a study using this method of evaluation in three infants with elevated ICP who had ventricular catheters previously inserted, the fontanelle pressure was highly correlated (r = 0.962) with ICP. This technique appears to offer significant advantages over previous attempts to monitor fontanelle pressure as an index of ICP, as earlier methodology had problems with poor reproducibility, inability to correct for zero drift, and instability with patient movement or position. However, its utility is restricted to young infants and cannot be used in older children or adults.

Changes in Tympanic Membrane Tension

A third technique evaluated by Kast measures changes in ICP by detecting changes in tympanic membrane (eardrum) tension. This is accomplished by impedance audiometry techniques which measure the mechanical tension on the tympanic membrane by means of the stapedial reflex-induced displacement of the tympanic membrane. Cerebrospinal fluid and perilymph of the inner ear communicate through the cochlear aqueduct exerting pressure on the stapes footplate, which in turn is transmitted through the bony ossicles of the middle ear to the tympanic membrane. In normal subjects, following 8 s of jugular vein compression an average increase in tension of –0.128 ml at the tympanic membrane was observed. (Tympanic membrane tension was expressed as theoretical chamber size diminution in millilitres.) In cadavers, the tympanic membrane tension and cerebrospinal fluid pressure were proportional in the range of 50 to 250 mm of cerebrospinal fluid (CSF) during lumbar saline infusion.

Marchbanks also evaluated three patients with clinically diagnosed elevated ICP with the impedence audiometry technique. At least one ear from each patient displayed a reflex configuration which changed direction following a shunt operation in which the ICP was reduced to normal. This study and the previous study suggest that elevation in ICP will be transmitted as an elevation in pressure in the perilymphatic fluid in the inner ear. A primary route for the transfer of fluid pressure is through the cochlear aqueduct, which runs from the scala tympani into the subarachnoid space. If this aqueduct is fully patent, the perilymphatic hydrostatic pressure will directly reflect that of the cerebrospinal fluid.

Changes in Evoked Potentials

The evoked potential is a noninvasive measurement of the response of the brain to a sensory stimulus recorded from the scalp with standard electro-encephalogram (EEG) recording electrodes. The response is time-locked to the stimulus after a delay for conduction in the afferent pathway to the brain. The evoked potential is relatively small (0.5 to 20 µV) compared to the ongoing EEG activity (several hundred microvolts) in which it is buried, and therefore signal averaging is used to measure an evoked potential. This requires several repeated stimuli whose time-locked response is averaged to reveal the evoked potential. Signal averaging increases the signal-to-noise ratio by the square root of the number of stimuli when the noise is random in nature. A variety of sensory stimuli can be used to obtain an evoked potential. The auditory (BAEP) visual (VEP), and somatosensory (SEP) evoked potentials (Fig. 16.2) will be discussed in relation to changes in the waveform latency or amplitude with elevations in ICP. The objective of such measurements using evoked potentials is to determine if a particular pattern of change in the evoked potential correlates with a corresponding change in the ICP.

Animal studies of increased intracranial pressure

In the following studies conducted in anesthetised animals, an auditory evoked potential is produced by delivering a click or tone burst stimulus of short duration to the ear. Two types of auditory evoked potentials can be measured. The first is a short latency response occurring within the initial 10 ms and is called the brainstem auditory evoked potential (BAEP). A slightly longer latency response is called the middle latency auditory evoked potential. The somatosensory evoked potential (SEP) is produced by stimulation of a peripheral nerve with a short-duration square-wave voltage or constant-current pulse. The visual evoked potential (VEP) is produced by delivering a strobe flash or other patterned stimulus to the eyes (Fig. 16.2). Evoked potentials have been recorded in an anesthetised animal while changes in ICP were made to determine what changes in various waveform components of the evoked potential are correlated with changes in ICP.

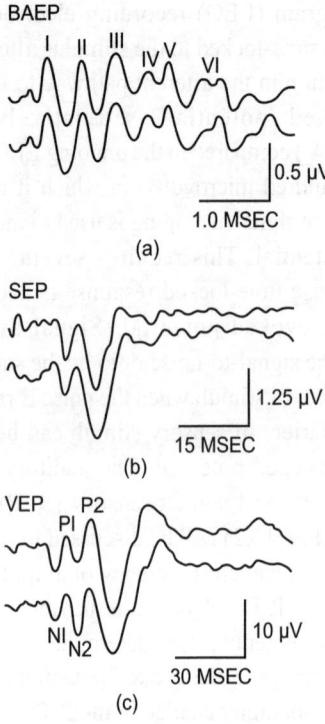

Fig. 16.2. Three different evoked potentials obtained in humans. (a) The brainstem auditory evoked potential (BAEP) obtained by delivering click stimuli to the ear and averaging 1000 responses at a vertex electrode on the scalp referenced to the ear. Six distinct positive peaks are obtained which identify signal generators in the auditory nerve (I, II), relay nuclei in the brainstem (III, IV); midbrain (V), and thalamus (VI). (b) The somatosensory evoked potential (SEP) obtained by delivering a stimulus to the posterior tibial nerve and recording from the vertex referenced to ear lobe. A total of 150 responses were averaged to produce each trace (c). The visual evoked potential (VEP) obtained by a strobe flash delivered to both eyes and recorded from the vertex referenced to ear lobe. Eight flash responses were averaged to produce a single trace. The designations N1 to N3 and P1 to P2 are used to identify peak latencies and indicate whether they are positive- or negative-going relative to the active electrode at the vertex (+) referenced to the ear lobe (–). For all three evoked potentials, two trials of each response are shown to indicate the consistency and reliability of the responses.

In an evaluation of both the SEP and the BAEP to increases in ICP produced by expansion of a balloon placed in the epidural space over the temporal area in cats, it was observed that the late components of the SEP were suppressed first, followed by the early components of the BAEP and then wave V and wave IV of the BAEP. The initial decrease in the later components of the SEP was observed at an ICP of approximately 56 mm Hg (728 mm water), at which time waves IV and V of the BAEP were also suppressed. At 78 mm Hg (1014 mm water), the SEP contained only the first positive wave, which was markedly decreased in amplitude and the BAEP showed an absence of wave V and a reduction in wave IV. These changes were observed at a time when the ipsilateral pupil became dilated, a sign that the brain was beginning to herniate. At this level of ICP there would also be a decrease in cerebral perfusion pressure if arterial pressure had not increased reflexly.

Sohmer demonstrated that when the ICP was increased to 50 mm Hg (650 mm water) in an anesthetised cat, causing an increase in mean arterial pressure which resulted in a cerebral perfusion pressure of approximately 92 mm Hg, there was a significant increase in latency of wave IV of the BAEP. When ICP was further elevated to pressures approaching the mean arterial pressure, the cerebral perfusion pressure gradually decreased and the EEG activity was absent (isoelectric) at an average cerebral perfusion pressure of 24 mm Hg. However, the BAEP at 24 mm Hg remained largely unaltered with only a slight increase in wave IV latency. When cerebral perfusion pressure was decreased further, the BAEP became isoelectric or absent when the average cerebral perfusion pressure reached 7 mm Hg. Thus the brainstem components of the BAEP became isoelectric at much greater decrements in cerebral perfusion pressure than the EEG. This finding demonstrated that the BAEP pathway in the cat is still capable of generating a response even at very low levels of cerebral perfusion pressure, which would be deleterious to maintaining normal brain function.

This observation was confirmed by Sutton who demonstrated that neither the SEP nor the BAEP showed significant changes until the ICP was markedly elevated (75 to 100 mm Hg) and cerebral perfusion pressure was compromised. The middle latency auditory cortical response to a tone burst stimulus was found to decrease in amplitude at ICP values of about 30 to 40 mm Hg (390 to 520 mm water) in the cat. These studies in the anesthetised cat would thus suggest that the BAEP is not a sensitive enough monitor of changes in ICP to be useful in clinical evaluations of suspected elevation in ICP. The middle latency auditory evoked potential may prove more useful as a noninvasive sensor to detect significant elevations in ICP since latency changes appear at lower levels of raised ICP.

In a rabbit model of hydrocephalus produced by intracisternal injection of kaolin, a significant-increase in latency of the auditory evoked response was observed at 250 mm water. Amplitude decreases and increases in interpeak latency were observed at 700 mm water, which is an approximately threefold elevation in ICP from normal.

Human studies of hydrocephalus

In the following studies, evoked potentials have been used to assess changes in waveform which are correlated with increases in ICP or clinical syndromes which typically involve significant elevation in ICP in humans. The condition of hydrocephalus may be caused by an obstruction of cerebrospinal fluid flow through the ventricles (noncommunicating hydrocephalus) or there may be a decrease in absorption of cerebrospinal fluid (communicating hydrocephalus). As described in the discussion of intracranial pressure, either of these situations will reduce the cerebrospinal fluid buffering capacity and lead to increased ICP.

Brainstem auditory evoked potentials

Abnormalities in the BAEP of humans have been observed in patients with hydrocephalus. Edwards showed increases in latency and decreases in amplitude of waves I and V—in particular, wave V/I amplitude ratio in a study of 16 hydrocephalic babies. Kraus found 80 per cent of patients with hydrocephalus to show some form of BAEP abnormality, consisting of either prolonged I-V interwave latency or reduced wave V/I amplitude ratio (33 per cent). These results have been confirmed in subsequent studies.

Thus abnormalities in BAEP have been demonstrated in hydrocephalus when the patient is symptomatic for elevation in ICP, but in none of the previous studies was an actual measurement of ICP performed to be correlated with the BAEP abnormality. It should be realised that the BAEP only examines a pathway through the brain which is localised primarily within the brainstem (waves II to IV), midbrain (wave V), and thalamus (wave VI) of the diencephalon and therefore, a priori, should not be expected to be sensitive to slight elevations in ICP since cortical structures are not evaluated primarily by the BAEP. On the other hand, the middle latency auditory evoked response may prove to be more sensitive to changes in ICP as it would be expected to reflect alterations in cortical areas. At high levels of raised ICP sufficient to cause brainstem herniation, changes in wave V latency have been found to provide warning of impending herniation.

Visual evoked potentials

The visual evoked potential (VEP) in which a flash stimulus was used has been evaluated by several investigators in studies of patients with hydrocephalus. In contrast to the BAEP, the VEP is carried in visual pathways which relay in the lateral geniculate nucleus of the diencephalon and then project by geniculocalcarine fibres to the visual cortex. The latter pathway passes around the border of the lateral ventricles on each side of the brain, and thus alterations in ventricular size or brain swelling would be expected to cause compression or alteration in function of these fibres. The effect of compression of the visual projection fibres would be apparent as increases in latency or possibly decreases in amplitude of the VEP.

In the long-term management of hydrocephalus, a shunt is frequently placed to remove excess cerebrospinal fluid by directing it into the peritoneal cavity by a catheter. There are failures in the shunt as the catheter tip becomes obstructed or the shunt valve becomes non functional which will result in elevation of ICP. If such changes are not detected at an early stage, permanent visual loss may occur or serious compromise of brain function may result.

Therefore, a technique that can provide early warning of shunt malfunction and elevation in ICP would be of considerable value.

The VEP has proven to be quite a valuable diagnostic tool in early recognition of raised ICP in hydrocephalus. Initial studies by Sklar in patients with hydrocephalus demonstrated abnormalities of VEP latency, susceptibility to fatigue and asymmetries. After shunt revision to reduce the ICP, VEP abnormalities were observed to decrease. In several patients in which there was clinical progression of the hydrocephalus, the VEP abnormalities became more pronounced. In a subsequent study of infants with hydrocephalus there was an increase in latency of the prominent positive wave P2, which normally occurs at approximately 100 ms latency following the flash (Fig.16.2c), compared to age-matched controls. Following shunt procedures in these infants, the P2 wave latency was observed to decrease in latency.

In adult patients with hydrocephalus who also demonstrated papilledema (swelling of the optic disk due to prolonged increase in ICP), it was shown that the use of a counterphase grating patterned visual stimulus to produce a VEP resulted in increased latencies only if hydrocephalic ventricular enlargement was present, whereas normal VEPs were found in patients with papilledema but without hydrocephalus. Reduction in VEP latency was observed following shunt revision and corresponded to a reduction of ventricular size in patients with hydrocephalus.

In a single case report involving a premature infant (28 weeks gestational age) who developed hydrocephalus and was managed with an Ommaya reservoir from which CSF could be removed, it was observed that VEP latency was reduced following sequential removal of CSF which also was associated with reduction of ventricular size. A shunt was inserted at 15 weeks of age and was revised at 36 weeks. Immediately following decompression of the ventricular portion of the shunt, a latency decrease of 19 ms was observed, suggesting that significant compression of the optic radiation fibres of the visual pathway had occurred before shunt revision.

In a study of 84 hydrocephalic children aged between 2 days and 15 years, an increase in the latency of the primary positive wave (P2) was observed only when increase in ventricular size was accompanied by increased head size. Following placement of a shunt in patients younger than 4 months, 4 of 12 showed some reduction in VEP latency, although 8 of 12 did not. Of these, 7 were reexamined between 6 and 12 months later and normal VEP latencies were found in 5 cases, although in 2 cases latencies remained prolonged. In children aged between 4 and 24 months who had persistent ventriculomegaly (enlarged ventricles) and had been shunted, the VEP showed an increase in P2 latency, whereas those patients with normal-sized ventricles had normal P2 latencies in this age group. In a further study by Guthkelch hydrocephalic infants up to 60 weeks of conceptional age showed significant changes in the maturation curve of the P2 VEP latency, particularly when their hydrocephalus was associated with an enlarged head or with infection. Increases in VEP latency were also found in 60 per cent of newborns with congenital hydrocephalus in a Japanese study of 27 newborns.

Human studies of the correlation of intracranial pressure with increases in latency of visual evoked potentials

Hydrocephalus and head trauma

To evaluate whether specific components of the VEP were altered in a systematic manner with increases in ICP, a study of hydrocephalic children was undertaken. Each child presented with symptoms and signs of raised ICP as a consequence of shunt malfunction. Two VEP components, N2 and N3, showed significant increases in latency. CT scans performed in these children showed no consistent pattern of abnormality in terms of correlation between increase in ventricular size and increased ICP. Thus, in contrast to previous studies, these findings indicated that ventricular size was not invariably a predictor of raised ICP, since even small slitlike ventricles were associated with significant elevation in ICP in some children.

In a second study, patients with shunted hydrocephalus who become symptomatic for raised ICP as a consequence of shunt malfunction were evaluated by flash-evoked VEPs shortly before the shunt was tapped or a ventriculostomy was performed to measure ICP manometrically directly. There was an increase in N2 latency which correlated directly (r = 0.9) with the magnitude of ICP measured (Fig. 16.3). Thus patients with hydrocephalus who were showing clinical/signs of raised ICP could be evaluated in a noninvasive manner with the flash-evoked VEP and an estimate of the actual ICP could be obtained.

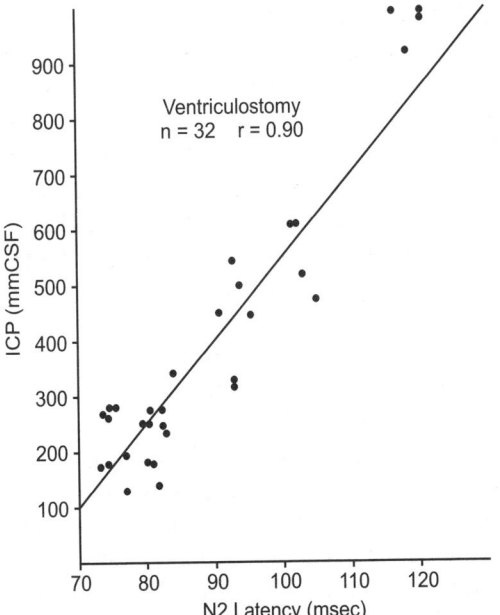

Fig. 16.3. Relationship between ICP and N2 latency of the VEP obtained with strobe flash for a group of 32 patients, in which a ventriculostomy was performed and a manometric measure of ICP was obtained. The line drawn through the points was obtained by a least-squares regression, with a correlation coefficient of r = 0.90. Each point is the average N2 latency obtained after at least four evaluations.

In patients with cerebral swelling as a consequence of severe head trauma, a study of flash-evoked VEPs performed while ICP was being measured continuously by an epidural pressure transducer defined a positive correlation (r = 0.8) of the N2

latency with ICP. A follow-up study confirmed these initial findings of an increase in N2 latency being associated with elevation in ICP. Figure 16.4 shows the correlation obtained when five patients with an epidural monitor had VEPs measured at different times when ICP varied.

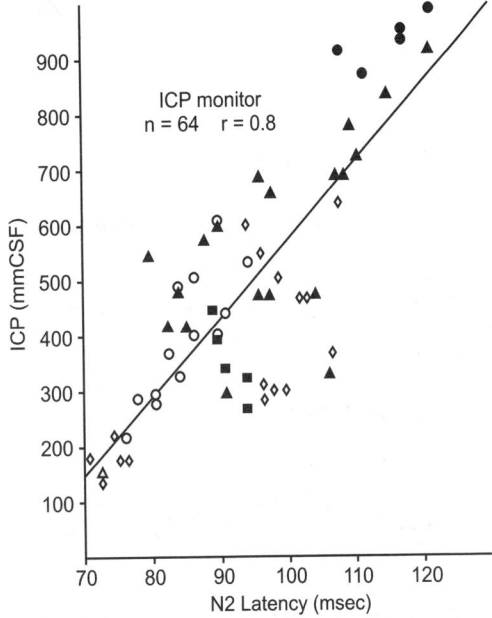

Fig. 16.4. Relationship between ICP and N2 latency of the visual evoked potential for a group of five head trauma patients (indicated by different symbols) whose ICP was being monitored by means of a fibre optic epidural pressure transducer placed through a burr hole. The range of ICP values occurred over a 5 to 10 hr. period of monitoring the visual evoked potential. The line drawn through the points is a least-squares regression fit with a correlation coefficient of r = 0.80.

The regression line drawn through the points is a least-squares fit. This regression line has the same slope as the regression line obtained with the hydrocephalus patient group (Fig. 16.3) and intersects the Y-axis in the normal range of ICP. Figure 16.5 shows the two regression lines for the two types of patients plotted on the same graph for comparison. Although the Y-intercept is different for each regression line, they both fall within the normal range of ICP. These results are not to suggest that a simple linear correlation is the best fit of the data, but simply to demonstrate that a relationship exists between the amount of N2 latency shift and the degree of elevation in ICP. Although there is more scatter of data values below 300 mm water, the more critical elevations in ICP above 300 mm water are predicted by the increase in N2 latency.

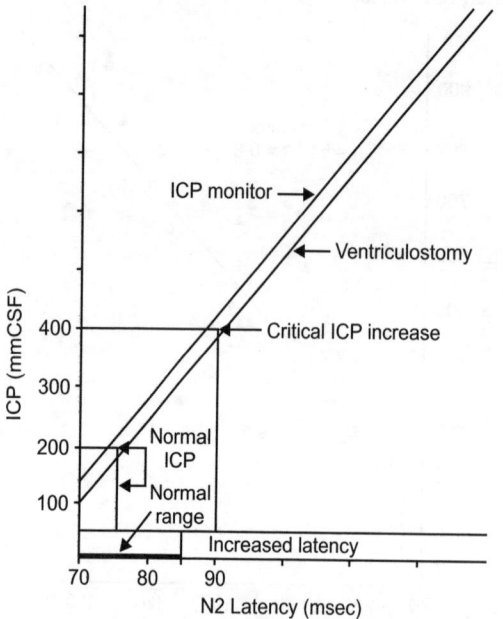

Fig. 16.5. Composite graphs showing relationship of ICP with changes in N2 latency of the visual evoked potential for both groups of patients studied in Figs 16.3 and 16.4. The regression lines have identical slopes and intersect the ordinate in the range of normal ICP for a normal N2 latency. Critical elevations in ICP were defined as N2 latencies that exceeded 90 ms, and were therefore indicative of elevations in ICP greater than 400 mm of CSF.

In evaluations of more than 1000 patients to date, no false-positive or false-negative results have been obtained using the flash-evoked VEP recorded from the vertex (Cz) referenced to ear lobe with slow stimulus rates (0.2/s) and low number of stimuli (N = 8). In each patient tested, if the N2 latency is greater than 90 ms and the P2 wave latency is greater than 110, an increase in ICP has been found.

VEPs have also been used to evaluate patients with pseudotumor cerebri, a condition presenting with symptoms of raised ICP in the absence of intracranial mass or hydrocephalus. Sorensen have

demonstrated increases in P2 latency with patternshift VEPs in these patients. A significant correlation was also observed between ICP and the P2 latency. After treatment to lower the ICP, the P2 latency decreased in patients who recovered and whose papilledema disappeared. A second study of pseudotumor cerebri patients by Pozzessere using pattern-reversal VEPs also demonstrated a latency increase when the patients were symptomatic for raised ICP with a return of the N2 latency to normal after a few days following removal of cerebrospinal fluid to lower the volume of cerebrospinal fluid present and thereby reduce the ICP.

Acute mountain sickness

One of the medical problems encountered by individuals who ascend rapidly to high altitude without sufficient acclimatisation is acute mountain sickness. The symptoms are distinguished by the onset of headache, fatigue, drowsiness, anorexia, nausea, vomiting, and sleep disturbances. The more severe form of acute mountain sickness can lead to a life-threatening condition manifested by pulmonary edema and/or cerebral edema. The early symptoms of headache, nausea, vomiting, anorexia, and sleep disturbance could be attributed to early cerebral edema (i.e. swelling of the brain).

If cerebral edema was one of the major factors responsible for acute mountain sickness, a latency shift in the N2 component of the VEP would be predicted. During the Ultima Thule Everest Expedition, Wohns reported on a 32 year-old white male who complained of severe headache, lethargy, insomnia, and lack of appetite approximately 36 hours after arriving at the base camp at 17,000 ft. A baseline study of his flash-evoked VEP showed a normal N2 latency at sea level. However, at the time the symptoms of acute mountain sickness were evident, his VEP demonstrated an N2 latency that was increased by 20 ms from his baseline value. After treatment with acetazolamide, a drug that removes water from the brain and returns it to the circulation, the symptoms lessened over the next 16 hr. and the subject returned to normal. A follow-up VEP evaluation showed that the N2 latency had also returned to baseline values. This study thus provided the first data to suggest that the neurological symptoms associated with acute mountain sickness were consistent with cerebral edema. The increase in N2 latency when the subject was symptomatic for raised ICP, followed by the return of the N2 latency to normal following treatment, suggested that the VEP was a sensitive noninvasive monitor in the diagnosis and management of cerebral edema.

DISCUSSION

Of all the various techniques that have been evaluated as noninvasive monitors of ICP, the VEP offers the most promise as a reliable technique for assessing raised ICP. The VEP has been shown to be a reliable noninvasive biosensor for ICP which has been correlated with direct measurements of ICP by ventriculostomy or with an epidural monitor. The direct correlation of N2 latency increases with ICP has also been correlated with patient's symptoms of raised ICP as well as the return of N2 latencies to normal levels following corrective measures to reduce ICP with either medication, shunt revision, or the removal of excess cerebrospinal fluid.

In this chapter four different etiologies of raised ICP, including hydrocephalus, head trauma, pseudotumor cerebri, and acute mountain sickness have all demonstrated prolonged N2 latencies when individuals showed clinical signs and symptoms of raised ICP. The mechanisms responsible for this increase in latency are not known. An increase in volume of cerebrospinal fluid would be expected to cause dilation of the ventricles, which would compress the visual projection fibres (geniculocalcarine tract), since they are located in the wall of the lateral ventricle in the posterior horn. Direct compression of nerve axons would be expected to result in alterations in the propagation of action potentials by those fibres. This could be a result of direct mechanical compression or a secondary effect due to decreased blood flow as a consequence of compression of blood vessels. These effects could account for the increase in N2 latency observed in hydrocephalus or in psuedotumor cerebri. In head trauma patients, the cerebral edema may be due to a vasogenic edema or a cytotoxic edema. In the latter case, the brain swelling is due to an increase in the intracellular fluid volume due to failure of the ATP-dependent sodium pump mechanism, causing sodium retention intracellularly and water entry into the cell in order to maintain osmotic equilibrium. With damage to neuronal cells an efflux of potassium to the extracellular fluid will occur, causing an increase in accumulation of water in the extracellular space, also further enhancing the edema process. Vasogenic edema is explained in the next paragraph, but is also an important mechanism responsible for brain swelling following head trauma.

In individuals at high altitude experiencing acute mountain sickness, the increase in N2 latency may occur as a consequence of brain edema. This occurs due to an increase in brain volume as a consequence of increased water content of the brain. Since the brain is held in a rigid container, the cranium, and encased by a relatively noncompliant membrane, the dura mater, only small increases in brain volume may occur without subsequent increase in ICP due to the pressure-volume relationship. Brain edema will also be associated with compression of visual projection fibres. At high altitudes, brain edema may be due to an increase in permeability of brain capillary endothelial cells, producing an increase in extracellular fluid volume (vasogenic edema). The edema may also be a consequence of the vasodilatory response to hypoxia at high altitude with subsequent increased cerebral blood flow. Increased cerebral blood flow during the first few days of arrival at high altitude has been demonstrated, suggesting that the vasodilatory effect of hypoxia is predominant over the vasoconstrictor effect of hypocapnia (decreased pCO_2) secondary to hyperventilation, which is commonly observed at high altitude. When strenous exercise, especially isometric exercise involved with climbing, is combined with increased cerebral blood flow and moderate hypertension at high altitude, the normal blood-brain barrier present at the endothelial cell junction may break down, leading to transcapillary and transarteriolar leakage and a nonfocal vasogenic edema ensues.

17

Chemistry and Potential Methods for *in vivo* Glucose Sensing

INTRODUCTION

The general major problems for *in vivo* sensing that should be addressed are: specificity, linearity of response, time, signal-to-noise ratio, baseline drifting, transport of glucose and its reactants and products across a protective membrane, transport of these substances and competitive reagents within the sensor, development and selection of a suitable membrane, compatibility to the body environment, effect of body on the sensor, and so on.

The study of glucose sensing has brought together the efforts of disciplines in biology; chemistry; physics; physiology; chemical, electrical, and optoelectronic engineering; and medicine. The collaborative effort to these disciplines will eventually result in an *in vivo* glucose sensor. The knowledge gained from this effort will lead to important new developments and spring-offs for other medical applications. One example would be a sensor for monitoring ageing. After all, glucose is a molecule. A basic understanding in the chemistry of glucose is essential for the development of new and reliable sensing approaches.

D-Glucose has been the most extensively studied carbohydrate because of its interesting molecular structure, its chemical and physical properties, its cardinal importance as the major source of energy for the human body, its central role in diabetes mellitus, and possibly, its role in the ageing process. Since it is one of the first substances determined in blood, many methods have been devised for its measurement. Except for the determination of pH, there are probably more methods for glucose measurement than for the determination of the levels of any other blood constituents.

Existing methods and apparatus are available for blood or urine glucose determinations in clinical laboratories and in physicians' offices for the diagnosis, monitoring, and treatment of diabetes. These methods are for short-term indications of glucose levels. They reflect only an instant in the life and activity of the diabetic patient. Recent clinical investigations suggest that monitoring long-term blood glucose levels as manifested in a glycosylated haemoglobin level would be a more reliable method for the control of diabetes.

In recent years, specialised delivery devices have been developed for programed infusion of insulin to the diabetics. These devices do not require the measurement of blood glucose level. The adequacy of such an open-loop approach for treatment of diabetes is still under evaluation. A closed-loop approach that simulates the human pancreatic actions in insulin delivery is an alternative for the control of diabetes. Such a system, when implanted into the body, would be able, accurately and continuously, to measure the glucose level, and then activate the delivery component to infuse insulin to the body as demanded by the glucose level. Thus it would be a better control system for the treatment of diabetes mellitus. For emergency or in-hospital, bedside monitoring, information concerning the glucose level for treatment with insulin is essential. Both the closed-loop approach and the bedside treatment of insulin-dependent diabetes require knowledge of blood or tissue glucose levels of the patient.

Therefore, it is imperative that a glucose sensor be made available — one that is accurate and can continuously and rapidly determine glucose levels (2.5 to 25 mmol/L or 45 to 450 mg/dL) *in vivo*.

In the following sections we present and examine some current methods for possible *in vivo* or implantable glucose sensing. It is impossible, and no attempt is made, to cover completely all possible glucose sensor developments.

ENZYMATIC REACTION

Glucose can react rapidly with substrates in the presence of a catalyst such as an enzyme. Enzymatic reactions are highly specific. Among the commonly used enzymes for glucose determination are glucose oxidase, hexokinase, and glucose dehydrogenase. Hexokinase needs a cofactor, Mg^{2+}, for catalysis, while glucose dehydrogenase needs coenzymes such as NAD^+ and NADH. Given present technology, these cofactors and coenzymes cannot be stably and permanently immobilised. Thus the use of these two enzymatic reactions for continuous, *in vivo* glucose sensing is not currently possible. Glucose oxidase, the most stable of the three, needs neither cofactors nor coenzymes. Consequently, it was the first to be considered for possible use in *in vivo* glucose sensing and since then has been studied extensively. The reaction is:

$$Glucose + O_2 \xrightarrow{\text{Glucose oxidase}} \quad \text{...(17.1)}$$
$$Glucose\ acid + H_2O_2 \quad 19\,kcal$$

Glucose concentration can be determined by measuring either the consumption of O_2 or the production of H_2O_2. The presence of a second enzyme, catalase, can enhance the rate of Eq.17.1 by catalysing the decomposition of the product, H_2O_2:

$$H_2O_2 \xrightarrow{\text{Catalase}} (1/2)O_2 + H_2O \quad 24\,kcal \quad \text{...(17.2)}$$

By combining (17.1) and (17.2), the overall reaction can be written:

$$Glucose + (1/2)O_2 \xrightarrow[\text{+ catalase}]{\text{Glucose oxidase}} \quad \text{...(17.3)}$$
$$Gluconic\ acid + H_2O \quad 43\,kcal$$

In the overall reaction, for each mole of glucose reacted, a total of 43 kcal of heat is released. This heat of reaction can be utilised for the chemical analysis of glucose and for potentially *in vivo* calorimetric glucose sensing.

POTENTIAL METHODS FOR *IN VIVO* GLUCOSE SENSING

Clinical studies have strongly suggested that a desirable method for the treatment of diabetes would be the proper delivery of exogenous insulin as demanded by fluctuations in the body's metabolism. The fluctuation of body glucose level would need to be monitored continuously by an *in vivo* glucose sensor. The instantaneous information from the glucose sensor would provide feedback to the insulin delivery system. Based on the chemical and physical properties of D-glucose described in the preceding section in general, several approaches for *in vivo* glucose sensing have been proposed: enzyme-based electrochemical, enzyme-based field-effect transistor (ENFET), enzyme-based thermoelectric, electrochemical, and optical. In this chapter we examine the feasibility of these approaches.

Enzyme-based Electrochemical Approach

Glucose sensing utilising the glucose oxidase-based electrochemical approach was first proposed by Clark and Lyons about 25 years ago. This method involves the glucose oxidase-catalysed reaction in which 1 mol of oxygen is consumed per mol of glucose oxidised, and 1 mol each of gluconic acid and hydrogen peroxide is produced (Eq. 17.1). The consumption of oxygen, the decrease in pH due to the ionisation of the gluconic acid, and the generation of hydrogen peroxide are the three possible chemical measurements that can be made to determine glucose concentration. The usual electrochemical methods for measuring the changes in oxygen, pH, or hydrogen peroxide are amperometry and potentiometry.

Amperometric electrodes

In amperometry, a potential, with respect to a stable reference electrode, is applied to the detection electrode, which is also called the working electrode.

The applied potential between these two electrodes causes an electrochemical oxidation or reduction of the measured substance at the working electrode. In this original method, employing a two electrode system, the flow of current between the working and reference electrodes may cause the reference electrode to be unstable. Therefore, modern amperometry uses a three electrode system in which the applied potential between the working and the reference electrodes causes a current to flow to a third electrode, the counter electrode. No amperometric current is allowed to flow to the reference electrode; thus the stability of the reference electrode can be assured. In both systems, if the reaction is under diffusion control, the measured amperometric currents are directly proportional to the concentration of the detected electroactive species. Clark and Lyons were first to suggest the measurement of the consumption of oxygen (Eq. 17.1) by means of a Clark amperometric oxygen electrode (often called a polarographic oxygen electrode). The sensor consists of a thin layer of glucose oxidase immobilised on the surface of the oxygen-gas electrode. The oxygen-gas sensor suffers from the fact that the measurement varies not only with the glucose concentration, but also with the oxygen level of the solution. To over come this problem, a system with two oxygen electrodes was used: one with immobilised glucose oxidase on its surface and sensing both glucose and oxygen, the other a sensing oxygen only. The concentration of glucose is then a function of the difference in the oxygen reduction currents of these two electrodes. Additionally, in biological fluids, the partial pressure of oxygen is around 85 torr, significantly lower than atmospheric oxygen. Oxygen limitation has been a problem. It can be overcome either by placing over the glucose electrode a hydrophobic membrane that is more permeable to oxygen than to glucose, by using a two-dimensional enzyme electrode, or by incorporating an 'oxygen-permeable drum in the sensor. Clark further demonstrated that the H_2O_2 produced can be amperometrically measured with a Pt electrode. This method forms the basis of the commercially available, *in vitro* glucose analyser. The technique has also been adopted for *in vitro* sensing in the Biostator glucose controller.

Various amperometric enzyme glucose sensors for *in vivo* applications have been studied. They are, however, modified designs and miniaturised versions of those originally proposed by Clark. Studies using these sensors to continuously monitor animal blood extracorporeally and also implanted in animals have been reported. Recently, Clark and his co-workers have demonstrated that a sensor with glucose oxidase immobilised with glutaraldehyde directly on a Pt surface and protected by a membrane to prevent destruction by macrophages or interference from catalase and proteolytic enzymes remains active for at least 6 months when implanted in the peritoneum of rats. Some enzyme Pt membrane units even retain usable activity for a year. These glucose sensors remain active in the peritoneal cavity for 24 to 27 days after implantation. These results are very encouraging for the development of an implantable amperometric enzyme glucose sensor. For any implanted sensor to last years (versus months), the stability of the glucose oxidase, the O_2 electrode, and the H_2O_2 electrode remains a problem.

A method of configurational cyclic voltammetry (CCV) has been developed. In this method interference by ascorbate and dissolved hydrogen oxidation currents can be suppressed, while the currents for oxidation of H_2O_2 and reduction of dissolved O_2 can be retained. Although glucose oxidase is highly specific for β-D-glucose, the enzyme sensor as a whole is not specific. Molecules such as urea and amino acids that are smaller than a glucose molecule can diffuse across the membranes intended to prevent the passage of macromolecules to the enzyme-Pt surface. These small molecules can be electrochemically oxidised at the Pt surface of the H_2O_2 electrode, causing interference signals. Furthermore, reduction products from the counter electrode may diffuse to the working electrode and be oxidised there, introducing an additional output current. The long-term stability of the reference electrode has not been determined. Compatibility of the biologically active enzyme sensor with the biological fluid, and vice versa, are additional problems.

Potentiometric enzyme electrodes

In potentiometric enzyme electrode measurement, the potential developed by the catalytic action of an enzyme on a substrate at the enzyme attached electrode is measured against a stable reference electrode. Under the condition of zero current flow, a potential difference between the enzyme-attached electrode and the reference electrode stabilises to an equilibrium value. This results in a nerstian or logarithmic relationship between the potential output and the concentration of the analyte. This potentiometric method has been used to measure glucose. Glucose oxidase and catalase are immobilised on a Pt surface. Although a nerstian response of the electrode with increasing glucose concentration has been observed, it is not reproducible. Hysteresis results when glucose concentration changes are reversed. The source of the potentiometric response is unclear. It may be involved with the oxidation or reduction of the Pt surface functional groups on the Pt surface by H_2O_2.

In principle, the pH change resulting' from the production of gluconic acid (Eq. 17.1) can be measured by potentiometry. Any appreciable change in pH should occur within or near the immobilised glucose oxidase matrix, because, in the bulk, the large volume of body fluid should be capable of buffering the pH to approximately 7.4. The measurement of a small change in local pH arising from the ionisation of the weak gluconic acid is a very difficult problem; moreover, the activity and stability of enzyme are functions of pH. Therefore, the design of the enzyme-incorporated pH electrode is crucial. If the electrode is arranged so that the pH change is confined to a very small volume around the enzyme matrix, the catalytic activity of the immobilised glucose oxidase may change with pH, producing erratic results. The stability of the enzyme for long-term *in vivo* application becomes questionable. In general, the passive nature of potentiometry , the large response time, and the constant drifting of the electrode potential preclude its usefulness for *in vivo* sensing.

Enzyme-based Field-effect Transistor Approach

Recent advances in solid-state electronics have made it possible to utilise field-effect transistors for chemical sensing. The physical principle of charge redistribution is applied for the detection of chemical changes. In its construction, the surface of the insulated gate of the field-effect transistor is coated with a chemically sensitive layer. The conductance of the channel under the insulated gate, between the source and drain electrodes, is controlled by the electrochemical potential developed at the interface between the insulated gate and the testing solution. The action on the analyte of a thin layer of enzyme immobilised on the gate surface causes chemical changes or the development of an electrochemical potential. Such a transistor is called enzyme-based field-effect transistor (ENFET). Glucose dehydrogenase has been incorporated into an ENFET with flow injection for the determination of pH changes as a method for glucose analysis. As mentioned before, the dehydrogenase requires coenzyme for catalytic activity. Therefore, it is inconceivable at the present time that the proposed glucose dehydrogenase ENFET could be used for an implantable glucose sensor.

Since glucose oxidase is very stable and does not require coenzymes, it probably would be a more suitable enzyme for the ENFET. A thin layer of cation-exchange membrane would need to be deposited on the surface of the insulated gate under the immobilised glucose oxidase layer so that the H^+ ions produced by the ionisation of the gluconic acid can be transported across the membrane to the surface of the gate. The electrochemical potential developed resulting from changes in pH can be determined potentiometrically. ENFET sensors usually produce a fast and stable response with low noise and they can easily be miniaturised. They are, however, potentiometric devices and have the inherent disadvantages of potentiometry: baseline drifting and interference from other substances present in body fluid. Also, the activity and lifetime of these sensors are limited by the stability and longevity of the enzymes.

Enzyme-based Thermoelectric Approach

A method to analyse biological substance that uses an immobilised enzyme and a thermistor to measure local temperature or heat changes arising from an enzymatic reaction has been suggested. A recent review summarises progress in this field. Since a thermistor requires the passage through it of an excitation electricity that can raise the temperature of the thermistor itself, there must' be stringent control over the ambient temperature in the order of millidegrees, if it is to be used for chemical measure-ment. Therefore, application of this method has been limited to *in vitro* chemical analysis. A thermocouple requires no excitation electricity; however, it has low sensitivity. Recently, a thin-film thermopile approach to glucose and urea sensing has been reported. Antimony and bismuth are evaporated in thin film in an alternating switchback pattern to form a series array of thermocouple junctions (e.g. 50 junctions) on a thin plastic support (Fig. 17.1). The thermoelectric sensitivity of a multiple-junction thermopile increases with the number of thermocouple junctions. It is a self-generative, differential temperature probe and does not need excitation electricity. Its thermal, common-mode rejection ratio is excellent and eliminates the need for stringent control of ambient temperature.

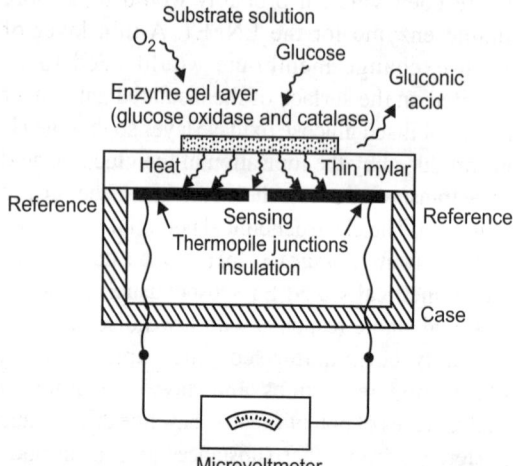

Substrate solution
O₂
Glucose
Gluconic acid
Enzyme gel layer (glucose oxidase and catalase)
Heat
Thin mylar
Reference
Sensing
Reference
Thermopile junctions insulation
Case
Microvoltmeter

Fig. 17.1. Schematic diagram of thin-film thermopile-based enzyme probe.

The enzyme-based thermoelectric glucose sensor is constructed with glucose oxidase and catalase immobilised over one set of the sensing thermoelectric junctions, whereas no enzyme is present over the reference set of junctions. A total of 43 kcal of heat is produced per mol of glucose reacted (Eq. 17.3). This heat increases the temperture of the thermoelectric junctions with the immobilised enzyme relative to the reference junctions. This temperature difference, on the order of millidegrees, generates a potential difference, or thermoelectric electromotive force (EMF), between the enzyme set and the reference set of junctions. This change in EMF is utilised for the determination of glucose concentration. In the absence of glucose, the output of the thermoelectric sensor corresponds to the electrical zero of the measuring system. Thus it is likely that only a one-point calibration is necessary if the sensor operates in the linear response region. This makes it very attractive for use as an implantable glucose sensor. The disadvantages of the thermoelectric sensor are associated with the stability and longevity of the immobilised glucose oxidase and catalase and the problem of oxygen limitation. The latter problem may be solved by combining the sensor with an oxygen-permeable drum to provide, as described in the section on the enzyme-based amperometric glucose sensor, a sufficient supply of oxygen.

Electrochemical Approach

The use of direct electrochemical reactions, without the presence of an enzyme catalyst, for glucose sensing began few years ago. Since then, almost all of the work done along this line has been limited to the concept of glucose oxidation. Oxidative currents, such as anodic peaks and anodically directed peaks of cathodic scan (also oxidative) in the cyclic voltammetry of glucose, have been the sole signals explored by electrochemists studying glucose sensors. Perhaps because this electrochemical approach was developed some 10 years after the first, and popular, glucose-oxidase-based electrochemical glucose oxidation sensing method, glucose was considered only to be oxidisable. The perspectives that glucose is an aldehyde and not only can be oxidised to an acid, but can also be reduced to an alcohol, and that this reduction and the redox couple could be utilised for sensing purpose, had to wait for another 10 years.

Self-generative electrochemical glucose oxidation

In the early work the fuel cell principle was applied to the self-generative electrochemical oxidation of glucose. The output of the fuel cell is proportional to the concentration of glucose. A number of these fuel cell sensors were implanted and evaluated. Some signs of success were seen. The method, however, proved to be impractical. The initial, high rate of glucose reaction, catalysed by the freshly prepared fuel cell anode, is strongly retarded by the gradual deterioration of the electrode. The product, gluconic acid, poisons the catalyst. Diffusion of glucose into the fuel cell catalytic layer is limited by the thickness of the layer, resulting in an intolerably long response time. Nevertheless, this initial work has inspired the development of other nonenzymatic electrochemical approaches to *in vivo* glucose sensing.

Amperometry

Amperometric and voltammetric techniques have been explored in the direct electrochemical approach. In general, the three-electrode system described previously has been used. Most of the studies employ platinised platinum for the working and counter electrodes. Some studies, however, use carbon for the counter electrode. The reference electrode is usually a Ag/AgCl electrode. The physiologic buffer solution provides sufficient chloride ions for the stability of the Ag/AgCl electrode. In amperometry, a constant potential is applied between the working and reference electrode. The observed glucose signal is the measured current flow between the working and counter electrodes or between the working electrode and a highly stable reference electrode. An inherent disadvantage of amperometry is that the catalytic activity of the working electrode gradually decreases under the applied constant potential. Lately, voltammetry, in particular cyclic voltammetry, has become the major technique adopted for sensor studies. Its major advantage is that the catalytic activity of the electrode can be restored by means of cyclic electrochemical pulsings, thus prolonging the life of the sensor.

Voltammetry

The difference between voltammetry and amperometry is that a programmed, time dependent potential waveform, instead of the constant potential of amperometry, is imposed on the working electrode. Different currents flowing between the working and counter electrodes are generated by different potentials applied to the working electrode. The operation is similar to spectroscopy, in which different spectra intensities are observed at different excitation frequencies. The programmed potential waveform is used to operate a potential sweep, from a preset lower bound potential to a preset upper bound potential. The anodic scan begins at a negative or a less positive potential (versus the reference electrode) and sweeps to a more positive one. Once the upper bound potential is reached by the anodic scan, a different scan, in the direction of decreasing potential is swept to the preset lower potential. This reversed sweep is called cathodic scan. Both anodic oxidation currents and anodically directed cathodic scan currents (also oxidative) can be observed in a complete voltammetric cycle. Commonly, these two types of currents or signals have been studied extensively for use in glucose sensing. Suitable switching, stepping, and pulsing arrangements maybe added for enhancement of electrode specificity, signal, and stability. The electrochemical approach has been considered to be nonselective. With the use of a suitable potential waveform, however, the interference of amino acids on glucose signals can be suppressed. By applying a technique of differential pulse voltammetry, interference by a low-molecular-weight substance such as urea can be reduced in the linear response range of the glucose signal.

Compensated-net-charge cyclic voltammetry

Further improvements in the cyclic voltammetric approach have led to the development of a compensated net charge (CNC) method that involves integration of the current of a cyclic voltammogram over one complete potential cycle. The method substantially improves both the sensitivity and selectivity for glucose determination in the presence of normal physiologic fluid. Interferences due to amino acids, urea, creatinine, and uric acid are significantly diminished. CNC has been applied to the study of a system with a catheter-type, high-surface-area, Pt working electrode. The system was implanted in a dog, and it functioned well for about 4 hr. Later, it did not respond to a second insulin injection and a subsequent glucose bolus. Fibrous deposits directly above the working electrode were observed.

Low-potential cyclic voltammetry

An alternative approach for the enhancement of both the selectivity and sensitivity of the working electrode is to operate the voltammetry within a narrow potential range where the glucose signals are most pronounced and where the electrode is less susceptible to interferences. Since the amino acids and carbohydrates, including glucose, urea, and so on, are all oxidisable in the high and positive potential (versus ag/AgCl) range, a desirable range for glucose sensing would be in the low and negative potential region. A systematic search for glucose oxidation and reduction signals in the low potential region with the complete cyclic voltammogram –1.00 to + 1.00 V has been done. The study has revealed two new distinct and welldefined redox current peaks of adsorbed species. At 37°C, a reduction peak occurs at –0.80 V in the cathodic scan and an oxidation peak at –0.72 V in the anodic scan (Fig. 17.2). The separation of these reduction and oxidation peaks at 37°C is 0.08 V, indicating that they are a reversible redox couple. The peak potentials of these two signals do not shift with changes in glucose concentration. A study based on the Randles-Sevcik relation has shown that the redox reaction involves a simple, direct electron-transfer process under diffusion control. The redox reaction is not complicated by any secondary chemical (nonelectrochemical) reactions. Since the reversible redox process occurs in the low potential hydrogen region, it is likely that the redox peaks are the redox of adsorbed hydrogen species generated by the interaction of the Pt surface with glucose molecules, rather than direct reduction or oxidation of glucose. This mechanism has been confirmed through the study of the cyclic voltammetry of dissolved H_2 gas in Krebs-Ringer phosphate buffer solution (KRPB). The mechanism of the glucose reversible redox reaction is given by:

$$H \cdot Pt + G-C \underset{[R]}{\overset{[O]}{\rightleftharpoons}} H^+ + Pt + G-C\overset{O}{\underset{O^-}{}}$$

Gluconate ion

A second reduction peak is present in the cathodic scan if a shorter potential range is scanned. This peak, at –0.65 V, is also glucose concentration dependent. No well-defined reversible counter (oxidative) of this peak is seen. This reduction peak could be generated by the reduction of glucose to sorbitol through the following mechanism:

(Pt electrode) Sorbitol

In actual glucose sensing, the potential range of the cycle is confined to a narrow region, –0.9 to 0.0 V or –0.9 to –0.4 V. The response time, that is, the time of a cycle, can be reduced to less than 1 min. This would be a suitable response time for monitoring the level of glucose in blood. As shown in Fig. 17.2, an inflection point occurs between the reduction peak at –0.80 V and the anodically directed peak of the cathodic scan. This inflection point is unique because its position is unchanged and it is independent of glucose concentration. It can be used as the zero of the voltammogram and for calibration of the sensor *in vivo*. Another inflection point, located near the beginning of the anodic scan, to the left of the –0.72 V anodic peak, can also be utilised for calibration of the sensor *in vivo*. The study of glucose in KRPB using this method has demonstrated that the reciprocal current outputs (both the reduction at

–0.80 V and the oxidation at –0.72 V) are linear with respect to reciprocal glucose concentration, ranging from 50 to 400 mg/dL. The linearity of the reciprocal plot indicates that the redox reaction follows Langmuir-Hinshelwood kinetics. When the method is used' to measure glucose in the dialysate of reconstituted human serum, the redox peaks are uninhibited by substances present in the dialysate. When compared with the KRPB study, the voltammogram of glucose in the dialysate appears altered, but from 100 to 200 mg/dL glucose levels, a linear response still prevails.

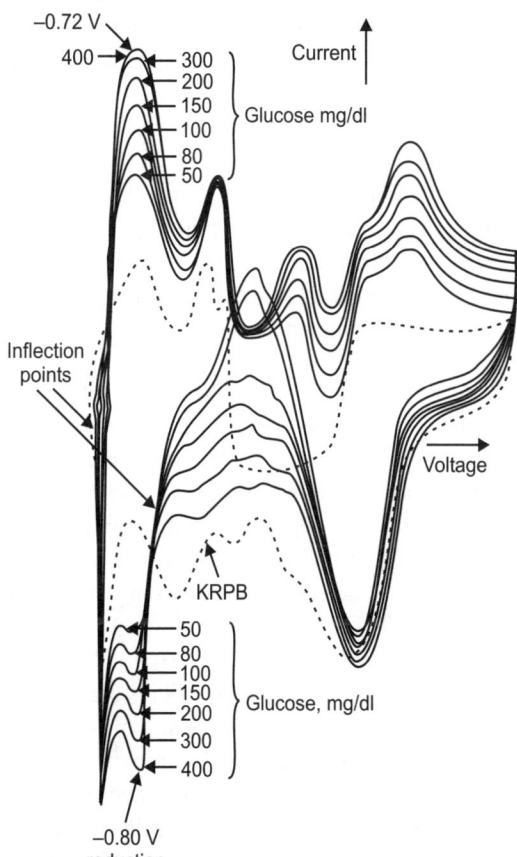

Fig. 17.2. Cyclic voltammogram of glucose in Krebs-Ringer phosphate buffer at a smooth-Pt electrode.

This sensing method needs further improvements before it can be studied *in vivo*. These include the use of a differential pulse technique to enhance selectivity and to rejuvenate the activity of the electrode, and the development of a glucose

permeable membrane to cover the electrode, preventing the passage of macromolecules that could poison the electrode and/or small molecules that could interfere with the glucose signal. Other hurdles to be overcome include the transport of glucose and its redox products across the membrane, the possible release of toxic products in the body fluid, and the potential for thrombosis caused by the production of surface charges or current leakage exterior of the sensor.

Optical Approach

Within the last decade, several innovative optical sensing methods, including methods utilising fibre optics, have been suggested and developed for *in vivo* glucose determination. The potential advantages of the optical approach over all aforementioned electrochemically related methods and the thermoelectric approach are electrically self-contained (i.e. complete absence of any electrical connections to the body), long-term stability and reliability, small size, and/or flexibility. As optoelectronic technology approaches its maturity in the next decade, the potential for its application to noninvasive and/or implantable glucose measurements becomes realisable. Several selected methods are presented briefly here. These methods are developed based on glucose's optical rotatory activity, ability to cause pH changes in the presence of an enzyme, affinity toward a lectin, and infrared absorption property.

Optical rotation methods

The measurement of glucose optical rotatory activity of a plane-polarised light of D-glucose has been used for the determination of glucose concentration in physiologic fluids such as aqueous humor and blood.

Aqueous humor glucose measurement

The concentration of glucose in the aqueous humor of the eye has been known to vary with blood glucose concentration in normal and diabetic humans. Experimental study has further demonstrated that a good relationship exists between optical rotation observed in the aqueous humor and the blood glucose concentration in the range of hypoglycemic and moderately hyperglycemic conditions (47 to 715 mg/dL), despite the presence in the aqueous humor of fructose, galactose, lactate, and sorbate. These results have led to the development of a noninvasive occular glucose sensor. In this method, continuous quantitative *in vivo* measurement of glucose in the aqueous humor can be accomplished by measuring the optical rotation of a planepolarised light directed laterally through the anterior chamber of the eye. This technique is capable of measuring extremely small rotations with an accuracy of 0.4 s of arc. It has been used to measure optical rotation of low glucose concentrations and has demonstrated linearity. A totally self-contained sensor, including the optoelectronic and telemetry components, can be incorporated into a scleral contact lens. The lens can be comfortably worn by a diabetic patient. One possible substance that may interfere is col-lagen in the cornea. Although the cornea is approximately 0.50 mm thick, it is composed of approximately 15 per cent collagen, which in the undenatured state has high birefringence and specific rotation. A major problem is the measurement of small rotation in the aqueous humor in the face of large corneal birefringence. It may be assumed that the composition of the cornea remains constant and that the constant contribution to the optical rotation can be compensated for by appropriate adjustment of the optoelectronic system. However, there are unidentified chemicals, other than glucose and protein, that contribute to the optical rotatory activity of the aqueous humor. Their fluctuation in concentration and in optical rotation may be a problem of the ocular sensor. In addition, a time constant exists for glucose transporting between the blood and the aqueous humor. This delay could cause a time lag in following absolute glucose level in the blood, although this is still a controversial question.

Blood glucose measurement

An alternative to the ocular sensor method is the direct measurement of optical rotation of glucose in the blood. The measurement can be accomplished by directly sensing the optical rotation of blood glucose as it interferes with a collimated mono-chromatic polarised laser light (ca, 780 nm) from a semiconductor diode laser. The design is a dual-diode-laser external cavity configuration. Two diode lasers are mounted facing each other across a short (ca. 1 cm long) V-groove on a silicon nitride substrate. The V-groove, covered with an ultrafiltration membrane, serves as a reservoir for glucose solution. The output is monitored as a current from a photodiode forming an optoelectronic pair with one of the diode lasers. This signal is then processed with comparator and logic circuitry. *In vitro* experiments have shown that the output from the optoelectronic pair is due to optical activity of the glucose solution, and is insensitive to the light scattered from glucose molecules. This detector would be sensitive to amino acids and other blood constituents. Interferable optical rotation contributed by these substances may be significant if the ultrafiltration membrane is not selective toward glucose. Another major problem is the efficiency of glucose transport across the ultrafiltration membrane.

Methods involving fibre optic pH measurements

Fibre optic pH sensors have been developed over the past 10 years. These small probes offer an attractive possibility for physiologic pH measurements, *in vitro* deposable, and long-term implantation purposes. The possibility of utilising fibre optic pH sensor for *in vivo* glucose determination was suggested in the early 1980. This pH sensor (Fig. 17.3) uses two single-strand optical fibres P and D (ca. 0.075 mm in diameter). The distal ends of the fibres are adjacent and parallel and fit inside a cellulose dialysis hollow fibre (0.25 mm in diameter). The proximal end of one fibre (P) is attached to a light source. The other fibre (D) is used for detection. The cellulose hollow fibre is filled with an indicator dye, phenol red, adjacent to the sealed cut ends of the optic fibre. The indicator is trapped inside the membrane by bonding it to polyacrylamide gel microspheres. Hydrogen ions diffusing 'across the cellulose fibre membrane cause the dye to change colour. The absorbance or colour change is quantitatively measured by the intensity of green light (550 nm) transmitted through the fibre optic system. Red transmission is also measured, in order to compensate for optical effects other than that of pH. It is not clear that this pH sensor truly measures absorbance rather than reflectance, since strict adherence to Beer's law was not verified. For glucose measurement, an enzyme, such as glucose oxidase, is either immobilised on the inner surface or on microspheres and filled inside the cellulose hollow fibre. The enzyme provides the needed specificity for glucose reaction and for the generation of hydrogen ions that are needed for the pH determination.

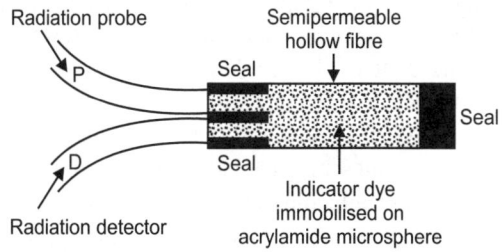

Fig. 17.3. Schematic diagram of a fibre optic pH sensor.

Recently, a fibre optic pH sensor based on energy transfer has been developed. The sensor contains a fluorosphore, eosin, and an absorber, phenol red, coimmobilised on the distal end of an optical fibre. When the eosin is excited by a laser (488 nm), where the phenol red does not absorb, it emits light in a spectral region that overlaps significantly with the adsorption spectrum of the basic form of phenol red. Nonradiative energy transfer occurs from eosin to phenol red. The amount of energy transfer increases as the pH increases, resulting in a diminishing fluorescence intensity. The changes in the absorption of phenol red as a function of pH are detected as changes in the fluorescent signal. The sensor combines the advantages of both fluorescence-based and absorptionbased sensors. It has higher sensitivity, rapid response, and greater latitude in geometric design for *in vivo* pH measurement. When incorporated with immobilised glucose oxidase, this sensor can be used for *in vivo* glucose determination. The life of these pH fibre optic glucose sensors depends on the activity and longevity of the immobilised dye, fluorosphore, eosin, and enzyme.

Fluorescence-based affinity fibre optic sensing method

A fluorescence-based affinity fibre optic sensor for monitoring various metabolites has been developed. One special application of the sensor is the *in vivo* glucose determination. The principle of the affinity sensor approach is similar to immunochemical analysis. It is based on the competitive binding between an analyte and a labelled indicator for receptor sites. In the case of the glucose sensor, the analyte is glucose; the indicator is fluorescein isothiocyanate (FITC)–dextran. Concanavalin A (con-A), a lectin, with binding sites for carbohydrates, is chosen as the receptor. The reversible bindings of the competitive reactions can be represented as follows:

$$\underset{\text{(free)}}{\text{Glucose}} + \underset{\text{(immobilised)}}{\text{Con-A}} \rightleftharpoons \underset{\text{(immobilised)}}{\text{Glucose:con-A}} \quad \text{... (17.4)}$$

$$\underset{\text{(free)}}{\text{FITC-dextran}} + \underset{\text{(immobilised)}}{\text{Con-A}} \rightleftharpoons$$
$$\underset{\text{(immobilised)}}{\text{FITC-dextran:con-A}} \quad \text{... (17.5)}$$

In a closed system for both con-A and FITC-dextran, any change in glucose concentration will cause a change in free FITC-dextran concentration. Measurement of the fluorescence of the free FITC-dextran provides a means for indirect determination of glucose. In the sensor design, the receptor con-A is immobilised on the interior wall of a hollow fibre tubing (300 μ OD × 200 μID). The tubing is then filled with FITC-dextran and sealed to an optical fibre with a design similar to that shown in Fig. 17.3. The con-A and the high-molecular-weight dextran (70,000 daltons) are confined within the hollow fibre. Only low-molecular-weight substances can pass across the pores of the hollow fibre tubing. Glucose diffuses from the exterior to the interior detector region of the tubing, and competes with the FITC-dextran for binding sites on the immobilised con-A. The displaced FITC-dextran disperses throughout the core of the hollow fibre and can then be detected by the optical fibre. The amount of fluorescence detected by the optical fibre is directly related to the amount of free FITC-dextran released from the receptor sites of the con-A bound on the hollow fibre tubing wall. The calibration response of the sensor follows the pattern for a competitive assay. A sigmoidal response curve is 'obtained for glucose concentration in the 0 to 1200 mg/dL range. A somewhat linear range of response at low glucose concentrations provides the possibility of blood glucose determination. The response time of the sensor is about 5 to 10 min. *In vivo* study-in on, line measurement of blood glucose with this sensor in a slow-bled system demonstrated fairly close correspondence between the sensor output and the actual chemical analysis. A time lag of response about 5 min is attributed to sensor response dynamics, such as the diffusin of glucose across the hollow fibre membrane (3 to 5 min) and diffusion of FITC-dextran within the tubing (5 to 10 min). The major problems with this approach are long-term stability of the con-A and the FITC-dextran and slow response. The selectivity of con-A toward other carbohydrates in the blood may not be a problem in view of that glucose contributes the most significant concentration among low-molecular-weight carbohydrates in the blood.

Infrared attenuated total reflectance spectro-scopy

A unique property of infrared attenuated total reflectance (ATR) spectroscopy is that its spectra of an analyte is independent of the sample thickness. Thus the application of multiple infrared ATR spectroscopy becomes an attractive noninvasive method for blood glucose determination through the skin. A CO_2 laser light source has been suggested for measurement of blood glucose concentration with appropriate resolution in the physiologic range. The feasibility of measuring glucose in water with the CO_2 laser system has demonstrated a resolution of 15 mg/dL. *In vitro* study of glucose in whole blood at 9.676 μm gives a resolution of 17 mg/dL. However, baseline drift of the single infrared wavelength measurement is seen. This baseline drift is attributed to the different infraredabsorbing substances other than glucose present in the blood. In fact, all blood-constituting molecules having $C = O$ stretching vibration will contribute to the infrared absorption at 9.676 μm. Since this interference is a major problem, a multiple-wavelength approach is necessary.

18

Biotelemetry

INTRODUCTION

Some of the first uses of biotelemetry systems date to the early space race, where physiological signals obtained from animals or human passengers were transmitted back to earth for analysis (the name of the medical device manufacturer Spacelabs Healthcare is a reflection of their start in 1958 developing biotelemetry systems for the early U.S. space program).

In many situations, it becomes necessary to monitor physiological events from a 'distance'. To quote a few applications:

1. Radio frequency transmissions for monitoring the health of astronauts in space.
2. Patient monitoring, where freedom of movement is desired, such as in obtaining an exercise ECG. In this instance, the requirement of trailing wires is both cumbersome and dangerous.
3. Patent monitoring in an ambulance and in other locations away from the hospital.
4. Collection of medical data from a home or office.
5. Researeh on unrestrained and unanesthetised animals in their natural habitat.
6. Use of telephone links for the transmission of ECGS or other medical data.
7. Special internal techniques, such as measuring pH or pressure in the gastrointestinal tract.
8. Isolation of an electrically susceptible patient from power-line operated ECG equipment, to protect him from accidental shock.

These applications have indicated the need from systems that can adapt the methods of measuring physiological variables to a method of transmission of resulting data. Biotelemetry (or Medical Telemetry) involves the application of telemetry in the medical field to remotely monitor various vital signs of ambulatory patients.

The means of transmitting the data from the point of generation to the point of reception can take many forms. Perhaps the simplest application of the principle of biotelemetry is the stethoscope, whereby heartbeat sounds are amplified acoustically and transmitted through a hollow-tube system to be picked up by the ear of the physician for interpretation.

PHYSIOLOGICAL PARAMETERS ADAPTABLE TO BIOTELEMETRY

Just as with hardware systems, measurements can be applied to two categories:

1. Bioelectrical parameters, such as ECG and EMG.
2. Physiological variables that require transducers, such as blood pressure, gastrointestinal pressure, blood flow and temperatures.

With the first category, a signal is obtained directly in electrical form. The second category requires some type of excitation, because the physiological parameters are eventually measured as a variation of resistance, inductance or capacitance. The differential signals obtained from these variations can be calibrated to represent pressure flow, temperature and so on, since some physical relationships do exist.

One example is ECG telemetry, the transmission of ECGS from an ambulance or site of emergency to a hospital. A cardiologist at the hospital can immediately interpret the ECG, instruct the trained rescue team in their emergency resuscitation procedures and arrange for any special treatment that may be necessary upon the patient's arrival at the hospital. In this application, the telemetry to the hospital is supplemented by two-way voice communications.

Telemetry of EEG signals also been used in studies of mentally disturbed children. The child wears a specially designed 'spaceman's helmet' with built-in electrodes, so that the EEG can be monitored without traumatic difficulties during play. In one clinic, the children are left to play with other children in a normal nursery school environment. They are monitored continuously while data are recorded.

The third type of bioelectric signal that can be telemetered is the EMG. This parameter is particularly useful for studies of muscle damage, partial paralysis problems and also in human performance studies.

One important application of telemetry is in the field of blood pressure and heart-rate research in unanesthetised animals. The transducers are surgically implanted with leads brought out through the animal's skin. A male plug is attached post-operatively and later connected to the female socket contained in the transmitter unit.

Blood flow has also been studied extensively by telemetry. Both the Doppler-type and electromagnetic-type transducers can be employed. The use of thermistors to measure temperature is also easily adaptable to telemetry. In addition to the continuous monitoring of skin temperature or systemic body temperature, the thermistor system has been found to be of use in obstetrics and gynecology. Long term studies of natural birth control by monitoring vaginal temperature, have incorporated telemetry units.

One more application is the use of the 'radio pill' to monitor stomach pressure or pH. In this application, a pill that contains a sensor plus a miniature transmitter is swallowed and the data are picked up by a remote receiver and recorded. It is interesting to note that biotelemetry studies have been performed on dogs, cats, rabbits, monkeys, deer, turtles, snakes, horses, seals and giraffes, as well as on humans.

The most common usage for biotelemetry is in dedicated cardiac care telemetry units or step-down units in hospitals. Although virtually any physiological signal could be transmitted, application is typically limited to EKG and SpO_2.

COMPONENTS OF A BIOTELEMETRY SYSTEM

A typical biotelemetry system comprises of the following essential blocks (Fig. 18.1):
1. Sensors appropriate for the particular signals to be monitored.
2. Battery-powered, patient worn transmitters.
3. A radio antenna and receiver.
4. A display unit capable of concurrently presenting information from multiple patients.
5. Animal tracking.
6. Read out device.

The transducer converts the biological variable into an electrical signal. The signal conditioner amplifies and modifies this signal for effective transmission. The transmission link connects the signal input blocks to the read-out device by wire or wireless means.

Principles of Design of a Biotelemetry System

Principles of design of a biotelemetry system are given below:
1. The telemetry system should be selected to transmit the bioelectric signals with the maximum fidelity and simplicity.
2. There should not be any constraint on the living system due to the installation of these systems and no reaction or interference from living system is desirable.
3. The size and weight of the telemetry system should be compact. For long term use units, the size and weight recommended is of the order of 1 per cent of that of the living system. For a short duration, it is about 5 per cent

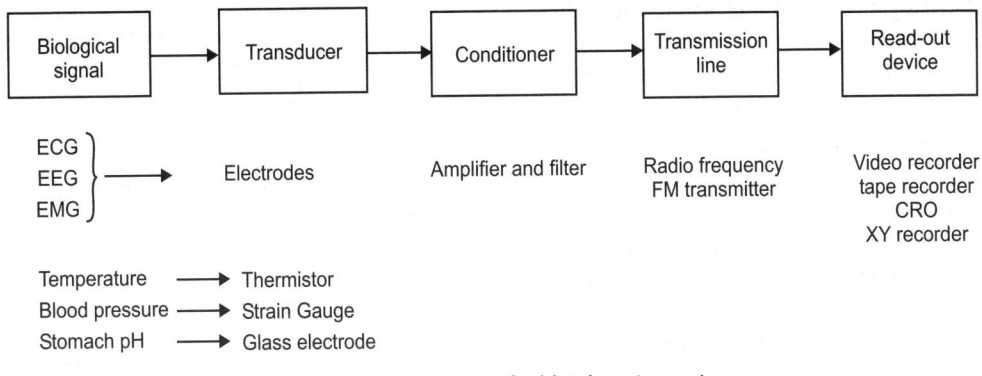

Fig. 18.1. Block diagram of a biotelemetry system.

4. Stability and reliability are essential.
5. The power consumption should be very small to extend the source lifetime in the case of implanted units.
6. For wire transmission, the shielding of the cable is a must to reduce noise levels. At the transmitter side, the amplifiers should be differential amplifiers to reject common mode interference.
7. Miniaturisation of the radio telemetering system helps to reduce noise.

Biotelemetry—Single Channel Radio Telemetry Systems

There are many types of commercial biotelemetry systems available today. To illustrate the basic principles involved in telemetry, a simple system is described. The stages of a typical biotelemetry system can be broken down into functional blocks, as shown in Fig. 18.2 for the transmitter and in Fig. 18.3 for the receiver. Physiological signals are obtained from the subject by means of appropriate transducers. The signal is then passed through a stage of amplification and processing circuits, that include the generation of a subcarrier and a modulation stage for transmission.

The receiver consists of a tuner (Fig. 18.3) to select the transmitting frequency, a demodulator to separate the signal from the carrier wave' and a means of displaying or recording the signal. The signal can also be stored in the modulated state by the use of a tape recorder, as shown in the block diagram.

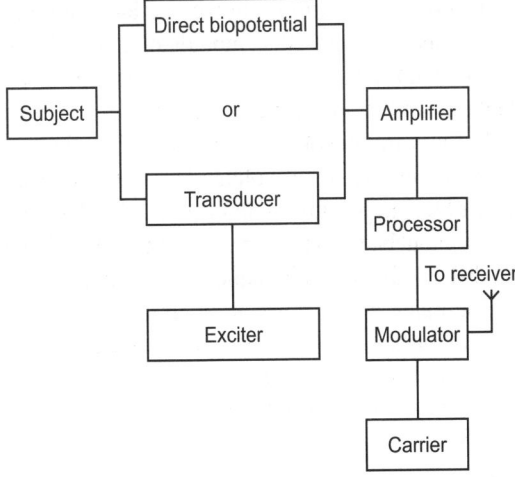

Fig. 18.2. Block diagram of a biotelemetry transmitter.

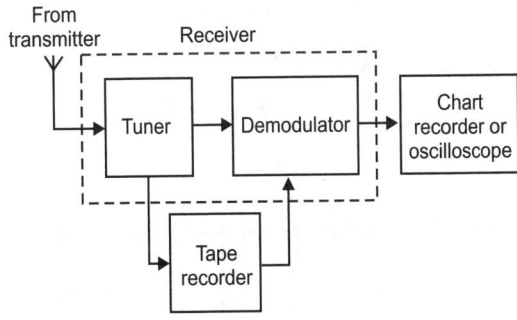

Fig. 18.3. Receiver—storage display units.

Many different types of radio-telemetry systems are being used. Their basic construction, however, is always the same. Transducers provide the signal to be transmitted and a radio-frequency (rf) carrier is modulated by the signal and fed to the radiating antenna. For short-range transmission, the antenna is often omitted, radiation being emitted by the oscillator coil as in the simple radio transmitter shown in Fig. 18.4a. The antimony/silver chloride (Sb/AgCl) electrodes that are in contact with the gastric acid represent a galvanic element that provides pH-dependent voltage modulation of the transistor. The magnesium/antimony (Mg/Sb) electrodes together with the physiologic sodium chloride (NaCl) solution form a battery providing the operating power. The capsule is swallowed and then transmits a frequency according to the sensed pH.

In most applications, however, batteries are required as well as a distinct modulator. Figure 18.4b shows an ultrahigh-frequency (UHF) tunnel-diode (TD) transmitter. Frequency modulation is achieved by the two variable capacitance diodes (CD) that are controlled by the signal voltage U_s. The frequency range of this transmitter is about 100–250 MHz, the mass without battery is less than 0.5 gram, the volume is a disk of about 5 mm diameter and 2 mm height and the range of transmission is up to about 20 m. Longer ranges are achieved by additional rf amplifiers and/or antennas, increasing the emitted power. A two-stage circuit for accomplishing this is shown in Fig. 18.5.

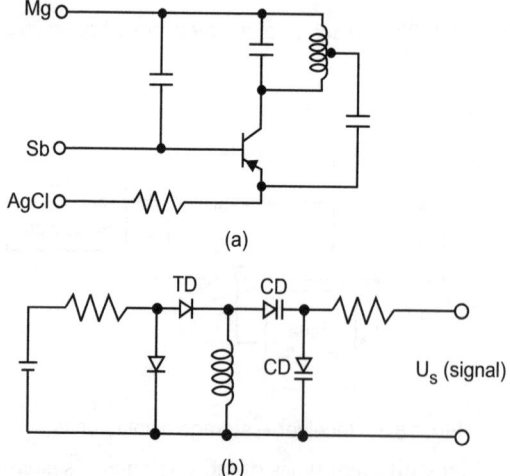

(a)

(b)

Fig. 18.4. Circuits of simple radio transmitters. (a) Single-stage electrode powered pH-transmitted, and (b) tunnel-diode battery-operated modulation stage.

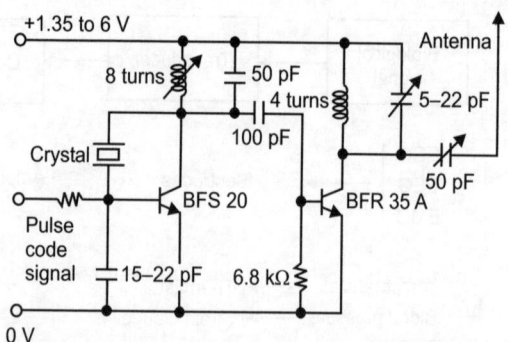

Fig. 18.5. Circuit diagram of a two-stage transmitter for pulse code telemetry. Frequency range is 100–150 MHz.

The need for short-range telemetry with an operating range of only a few feet might seem questionable. However, wireless transmission is required from totally implanted devices to eliminate any transcutaneous wires with their healing and infection problems. Transmission from the implanted system to the body surface is all that is required to solve this problem.

The range of radiotelemetry systems is affected mainly by power, frequency bandwidth and antenna gain. Environmental conditions, such as shielding by steel-concrete buildings, also influence transmission characteristics. Steel-concrete is penetrated easily only by carrier frequencies above 100 MHz.

Two principles of electromagnetic energy transmission are possible: inductions and rf radiation. Inductive coupling is effective only over very short range of several feet, whereas rf waves enable far-reaching transmission links. Inductive transmission is based on the electromagnetic coupling of two transmission coils, where the information is transferred from the primary coil to the secondary coil induction flow. Long-range transmission is based on the emission of radio waves from the transmitter antenna and the sensing of the high-frequency electromagnetic field by the receiving antenna. As induction and radio-wave systems base on dissimilar principles of transmission, optimum carrier frequencies differ greatly.

Either amplitude modulation or frequency modulation can be used in the system mentioned above. Because of reduced interference, FM transmission is often used for telemetry. In biotelemetry systems, the physiological signal is sometimes used to modulate a low-frequency carrier, called a subcarrier, often in the audio frequency range. The RF carrier or the transmitter is then modulated by the sub carrier. If several physiological signals are to be transmitted simultaneously, each signal is placed on a subcarrier of a different frequency and all the subcarriers are combined to simultaneously modulate the RF carrier. This process of transmitting many channels of data on a single RF carrier is called 'frequency multiplexing', and is much more efficient and less expensive than employing a separate transmitter for each channel. At the receiver, a multiplexed RF carrier is first demodulated to recover each of the separate subcarriers, which must then be demodulated to retrieve the original physiological signals. Either FM or AM can be used for impressing data on the subcarriers and this mayor may not be the same modulation method that is used to place the subcarriers on the RF carrier. In describing this type of system, a designation is given, in which the method of modulating the subcarriers is followed by the method of modulating the RF carrier. For example, a system in which the subcarriers are frequency-modulated and the RF carrier is amplitude-modulated is designated as FM/AM. An FM/FM designation means that both the subcarriers and the RF carrier are frequency-modulated. Both FM/AM and FM/FM systems have been used in biotelemetry, the latter more extensively.

As in AM and FM systems, the multiplexing of several channels of physiological data can be accomplished in a pulse modulation system. However, instead of frequency multiplexing, time multiplexing is used. In the time-multiplexing scheme, each of the physiological signals is sampled briefly and used to control either the amplitude, width or position of one pulse, depending on the type of pulse modulation used. The pulses representing the various channels of data are transmitted sequentially. Thus, in a typical six-channel system, every sixth data pulse represents a given channel. In order to identify the data pulses, an identifiable reference pulse is included in each set. If the sampling rate is several times higher than the highest frequency component of each data signal, no loss of information results from the sampling process.

TRANSMISSION OF BLOOD PRESSURE BY TELEMETRY

A system for monitoring blood pressure is used to illustrate the WPM method of transmission. The transducer used in this case is the flush diaphragm-type of strain-gauge transducer. Electrically, it can be represented by the bridge circuit of Fig. 18.6. Resistors R_1 and R_3 decrease, whereas R_2 and R_4 increase in value as blood pressure increases. Resistor R_b is simply for balancing or zeroing. The transducer is connected in the transmitter circuit as shown in Fig. 18.7.

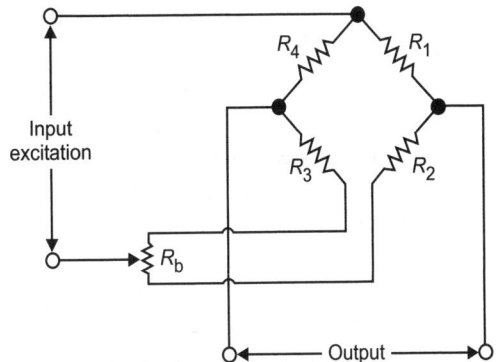

Fig. 18.6. A transducer circuit.

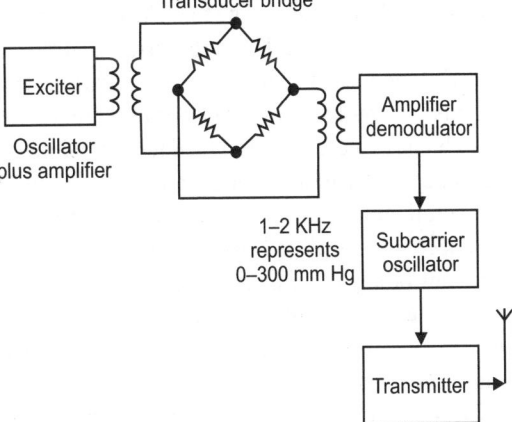

Fig. 18.7. One type of exciter-transmitter unit for blood pressure telemetry.

Either DC or AC can be used as excitation for strain-gauge bridges. When DC is used, the amplifier following the bridge must be a DC amplifier, with its associated problems of stability and drift. When AC is used, the bridge acts as a modulator and filters are required in order to recover the signal.

The exciter unit consisting of a Colpitts oscillator plus an RC coupled amplifier stage, excites the bridge with a constant voltage at a frequency of approximately 5 KHz, and is coupled to the bridge inductively. The bridge is initially balanced both resistively and capacitively so that any changes in the resistance of the arms of the bridge, due to changes in pressure on the transducer, will result in changes of the output voltage. The output voltage of the bridge is inductively coupled to a class A amplifier, the output of which is RC coupled to a class C (power) amplifier. The resulting output wave is rectified to obtain a signal representative of the pressure variation. The rectified wave is put through a resistance–capacitance filter, and the resulting voltage controls the frequency of a UJT oscillator. This is the PM subcarrier oscillator that is used to modulate the main carrier.

The system can be arranged so that there is a fairly linear relationship between the subcarrier oscillator frequency and the physiological parameter to be measured. For example, in the system for blood pressure illustrated in Fig. 18.8, a frequency range of 1 to 2 KHz represents the range of 0 to 300 mm Hg (0 to 40 KPa) pressure. The transducer action can be traced very easily. The subcarrier is used to frequency-modulate the main transmitter carrier. The carrier is transmitted at lower power on a frequency band which is specifically designed for biotelemetry. The same exciter-transmitter circuit could be used with small modifications, if the blood pressure transducer were replaced by another type or by a thermistor or any other electrical resistance device. Also the exciter–bridge combination could be replaced by a direct biopotential signal input, such as an ECG signal.

The signal transmitted at low power on the PM transmitter is picked up by the receiver, which must be tuned to the correct frequency. The audio subcarrier is removed from the RF carrier, and then demodulated to reproduce a signal that can be transformed back to the amplitude and frequency of the original data waveform. The signal can then be displayed or recorded on a chart. If it is desirable to store the data on tape for later use, the original data waveform or the modulated subcarrier signal is put on the tape. In the latter case, when playback is desired, the subcarrier signal is passed through the FM subcarrier demodulator.

MULTIPLEXING

Many applications require the transmission of various signals at the same time. For this purpose multichannel telemetry systems provide simultaneous data transfer by either frequency-division or time-division multiplexing procedures. Frequency multiplexing uses sub-carriers with various frequencies that are frequency-modulated by the measuring signal. Figure 18.8 shows a two-channel frequency-division multiplex radiotelemetry system. The sub-carriers are linearly mixed and the resulting signal modulates the main carrier. The sub-carrier frequencies must be chosen such that no overlapping of the signal-modulated spectra occurs. The receiver first demodulates the carrier signal and then separates the modulated sub-carriers by appropriate band-pass filters. Subsequent sub-carrier demodulation yields the single signals.

In a time-division multiplexing system, as shown in Fig. 18.9, the single channel are sampled periodically. If the sampling theorem is satisfied (i.e. the sampling frequency is at least twice the highest signal frequency), no information is lost. The sampling values of the different channels are then arranged side by side by a commutator that opens the transfer channel successively for the various signal channels, which results in a pulse train representing each of the channels for a certain time interval. In the receiver, another commutator demultiplexes the signal samples, which are first fed to a sample-and-hold circuit and then reconstructed by low-pass filters. To identify the single channels in the receiver, an additional channel, the frame reference signal, is transmitted to indicate the beginning of a new cycle.

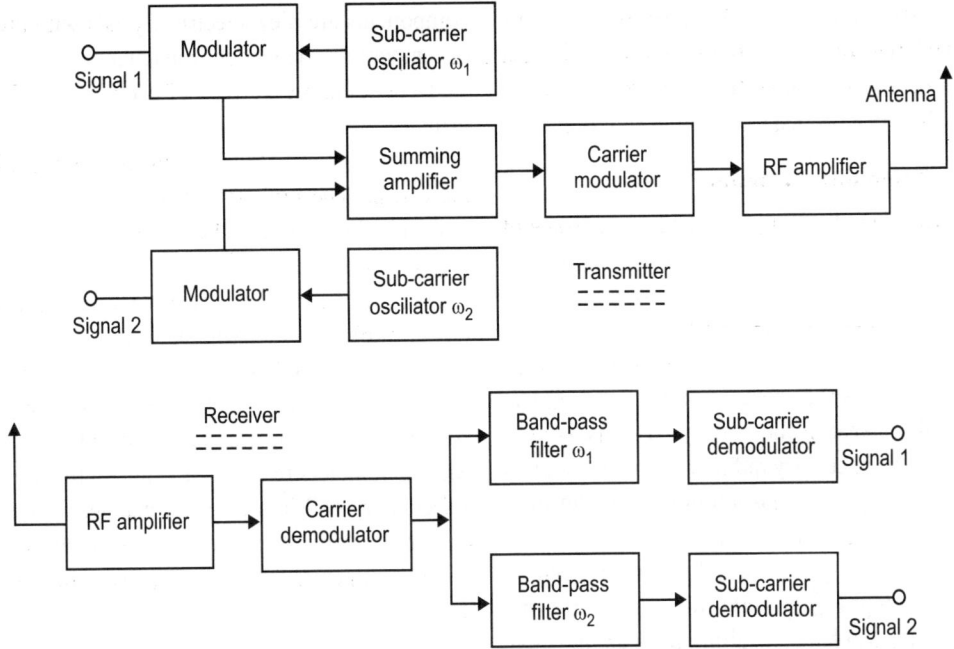

Fig. 18.8. Block diagram of two-channel frequency-division multiplex radiotelemetry system.

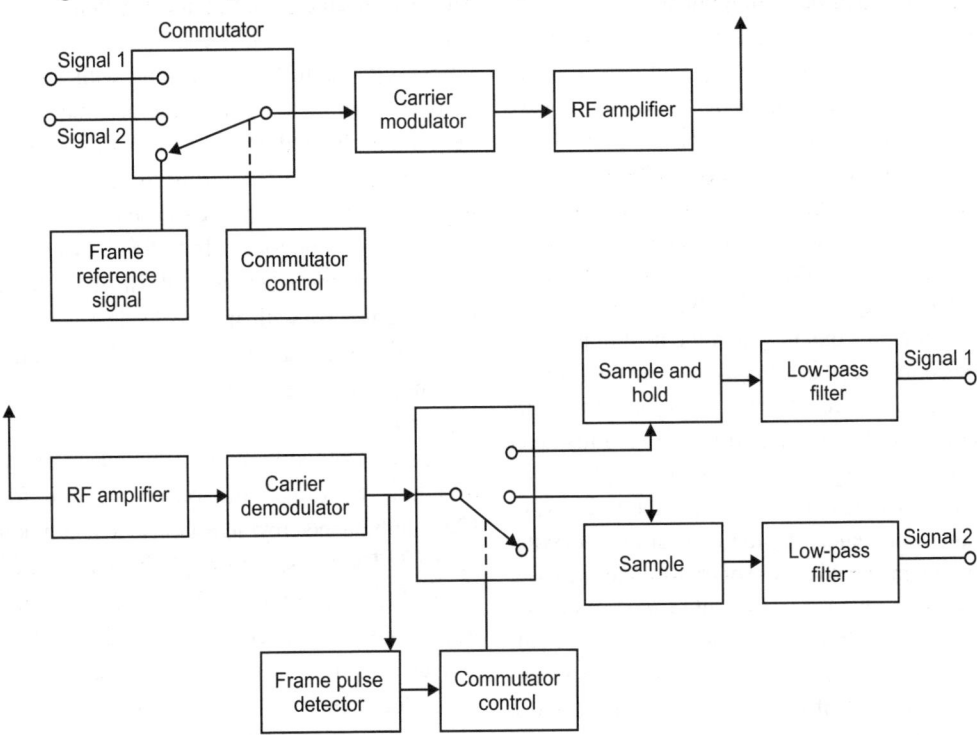

Fig. 18.9. Block diagram of two-channel time-division multiplex radiotelemetry system.

The reference signal is marked by some characteristics property, for example, a longer duration or a special amplitude. The bandwidth of the signals is determined by the sampling rate.

Passive Telemetry Systems

For control of medical implants and surveillance of patients, continuous data flow of physiological signals and functional parameters is required. Simple inductive telemetry systems are best suited for this application. However, power consumption by telemetry shortens the operating time of the implant substantially, because the battery capacity is very limited and the necessary radio-wave power is often higher than the power consumption by the intrinsic implant electronics. In this situation one can use a passive telemetry system, which does not need its own power supply, thus avoiding both lifetime reduction and problems, resulting from an inductive energy transmission into the implant (i.e. reduced reliability and additional components).

The function of passive telemetry systems is based on the coupling of two components, either by induction or by electromagnetic or ultrasonic wave fields, so that the extracorporeal component, the information receiver, changes a characteristics parameter (e.g. its impedance) according to variations of the second, implanted component's conditions. In this situation, the data transmitter operates as a modulated energy receiver. The two components can be two induction coils in which the load impedance of the secondary coil is reflected back to the primary coil, two piezoelectric crystals in which the impedance of an ultrasound-emitting transducer changes according to the load of the implanted receiver or two antennas, in which the radio-wave emission is influenced by the load of the receiving antenna. No matter what type of transmitters are used, load modulation of the implanted device can be achieved with neglible power consumption if a field-effect transistor is used as a modulation component (Fig. 18.10). This of course presumes an electric signal to be transmitted. In the case of non-electric biological signals other possible variable-load components are piezoelectric crystals with pressure or temperature-dependent capacitance.

Depending on the type of oscillator used in the primary circuit, variations of the load impedance provide either amplitude or frequency modulation of the carrier. The highest efficiency of the telemetry system is obtained when the secondary circuit is tuned to resonance.

The application of passive telemetry in an implantable pacemaker system uses inductive coupling of coils. The implanted coil alternatively serves as a secondary coil for the passive telemetry system, transmitting the intracardiac ECG as well as pacer parameters to an extracorporeal receiver or as a secondary coil in a conventional active telemetry system, by which the extracorporeal control system or programmer transmits commands to the implanted device.

Portable Telemetry Units

The rise of emergency medical technicians in the rescue services of local communities gives us an immensely useful tool in dealing with trauma and coronary victims outside of the hospital. Although very highly trained, the EMT is not a physician, so some means is often required to communicate physiological data to the local hospital where they are interpreted by a physician. In addition, two-way voice communications must be established for the EMT team to converse with and receive instructions from the physician at the hospital. Specialised communications equipment is often used to meet these requirements.

Figure 18.11 shows a portable telemetry system that has the range and power needed for the EMT/ambulance crew to establish a data link to the hospital. The transmitter might be a special unit or most often, it is a modified version of the standard walkie-talkie that is commonly used by police, fire and rescue units. The modulating signal, however, is an analog signal such as the ECG, the output of a blood pressure transducer or other physiological source.

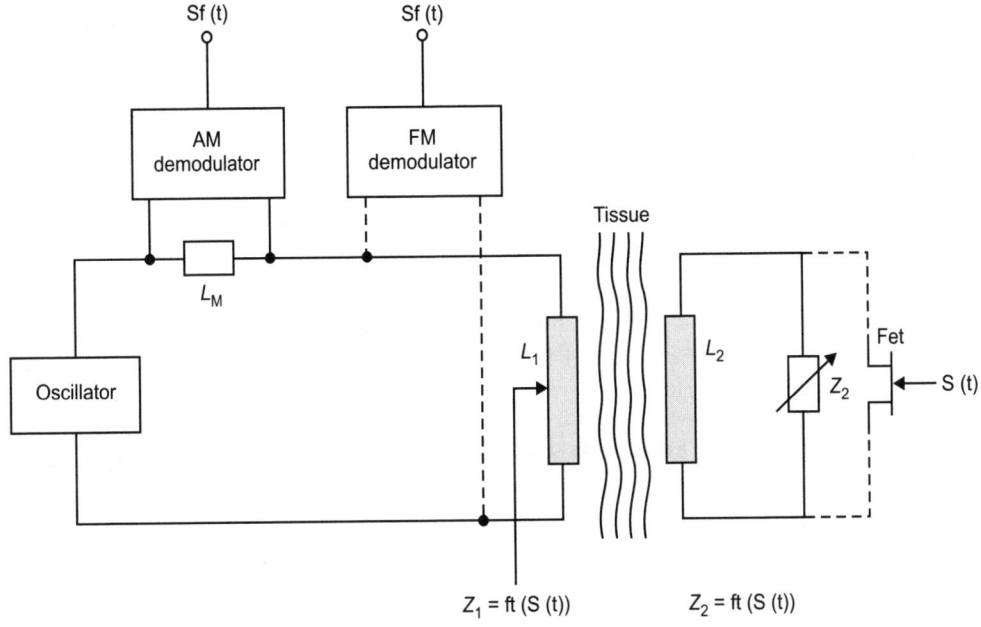

Fig. 18.10. Block diagram of passive telemetry system.

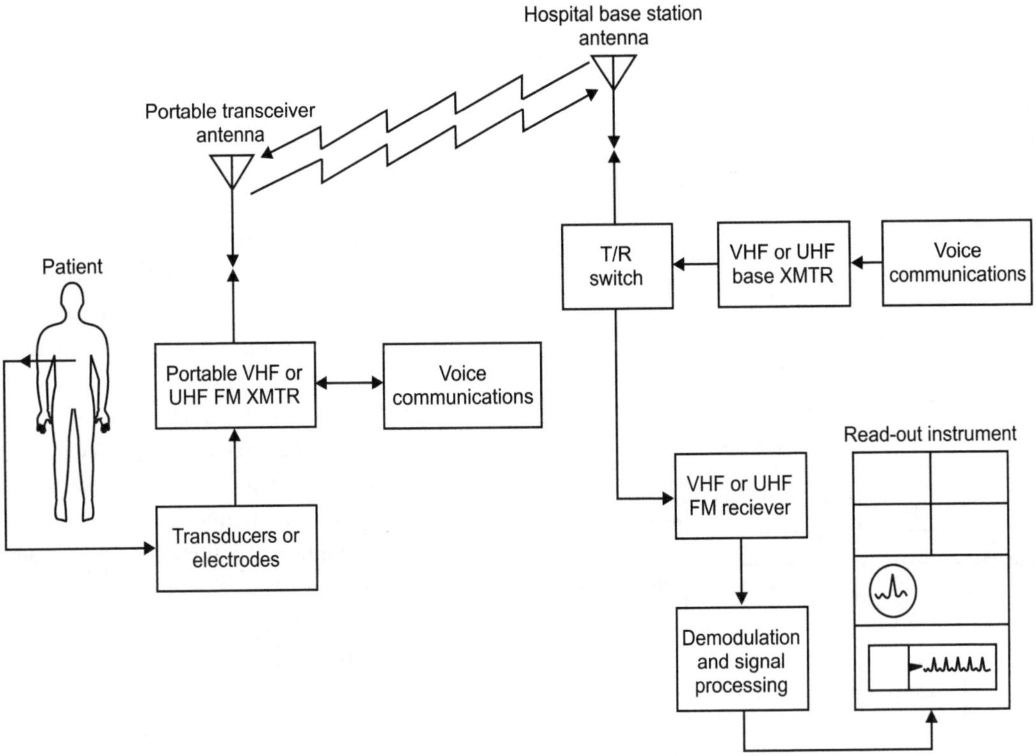

Fig. 18.11. Portable telemetry system.

The signal is transmitted over the airwaves to a base station transceiver (transmitter and receiver in the same cabinet) at the hospital. From there, the demodulation and display is similar to that of other telemetry systems. Because the size of handheld transceivers used for telemetry and voice communications is necessarily small, the available power output is low. As a result, the range is short for these units. Where the required range is greater, however, a repeater system can be used. At critical locations around the city receiver sites can pick up the small signal from the handheld units.

TRANSMISSION OF ELECTROCARDIOGRAM BY TELEMETRY

Figure 18.12 shows the block diagram of a single channel telemetry system suitable for the transmission of ECG. There are two main parts: the telemetry transmitter which consists of an ECG amplifier, subcarrier oscillator and a UHF transmitter (along with dry cell batteries), and a telemetry receiver, consisting of a high frequency unit and a demodulator, to which an electrocardiograph can be connected to record a cardioscope to display and a magnetic tape recorder to store the ECG. A heart-rate meter with an alarm facility can be provided to continuously monitor the beat-to-beat heart rate of the subject.

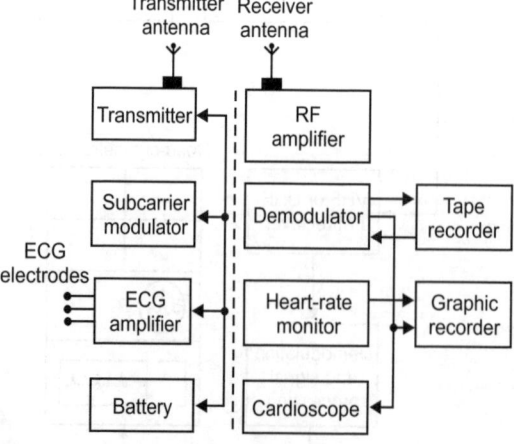

Fig. 18.12. Block diagram of a single channel telemetry system for the transmission of ECG.

It is suggested that for distortion-free transmission of ECG, the following requirements must be met:

1. The testee should be able to carry on with his normal activities, whilst carrying the instruments, without the slightest discomfort. He should be able to forget their presence after some minutes of application.
2. Motion artefacts and muscle potential interference should be kept to a minimum.
3. The battery life should be long enough so that a complete experimental procedure may be carried out.

While monitoring paced patients for ECG through telemetry, it is necessary to reduce pacemaker pulses. The amplitude of the pacemaker pulses can be as large as 80 mV compared to 1–2 mV, typical of the ECG. The ECG amplifier in the transmitter is slow and limited, so that the relatively narrow pacemaker pulses are substantially reduced in amplitude.

TELEPHONE LINKS

Although it cannot be considered to be radio telemetry, the use of the telephone system to transmit biological data is becoming quite common. One application involves the transmission of ECGS from heart patients and (particularly) pacemaker recipients. In this case, the patient has a transmitter unit that can be coupled to an ordinary telephone. The transmitted signal is received by telephone in the doctor's office or in the hospital. Tests can be scheduled at regular intervals for diagnosing the status and potential problems indicated by the ECGS.

Figure 18.13 shows a typical telephone telemetry system for transmitting and receiving medical signals. For frequency modulation, a reactance modulator has been used with a centre frequency of 1500 Hz. This frequency is modulated ±200 Hz for a 1 V peak-to-peak signal. This deviation is linear within a 1 per cent range. The demodulator consists of an audio amplifier, a carrier rejection filter, and a low pass integrator output circuit to recover the input signal. Both at the transmitting as well as receiving ends, coupling or isolation transformers are used to match the standard telephone line impedance.

Telephone lines can have noise interference. This noise will produce significant artefacts in the AM and FM modulation schemes described above.

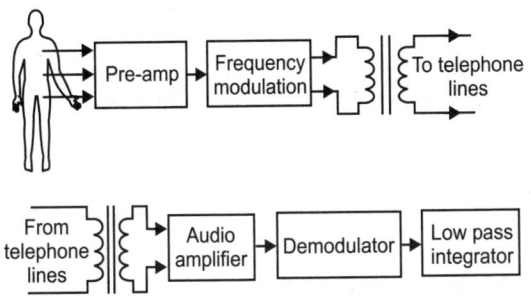

Fig. 18.13. Arrangement for the transmission of analog signals over telephone lines.

Therefore, the current practice is to use a computational facility for on-line error correction. The scheme is given in Fig. 18.14. A set of transducers and electrodes access biological data such as for temperature, breathing, heart sounds and ECG. The data is generally in analog form and in the data acquisition system (DAQ), by means of a high resolution.(12-bit) analog-to-digital converter, the data is converted to digital form. A microprocessor based system can perform some artefact rejection tasks such as nullifying drift and blocking artefactual signals which are well beyond the known range for the biomedical signal being monitored. Also, the microprocessor can time multiplex data from the different transducers, so that the information from each of the transducers is transmitted through one communication channel in the time-shared mode.

The data, now in digital form, becomes the input for a modem (acronym for Modulator-Demodulator). Modems interface the data into telephone lines according to standard protocols as, for example, TCP/IP protocol. Data transmission at 56 kbps and higher is possible. Serial, binary, asynchronous data formats are commonly used with trellis-coded modulation.

Also, an error correction facility is provided. For example, a parity check is obtained by adding to every character (formed by 7 bits) one more bit (0 or 1). At the receiving end, the parity bits are again counted and, if there is a mismatch from the input parity count,

an error is indicated and that particular small packet of data is dropped. Additional error checks are commonly incorporated to ensure that the data received is error-free.

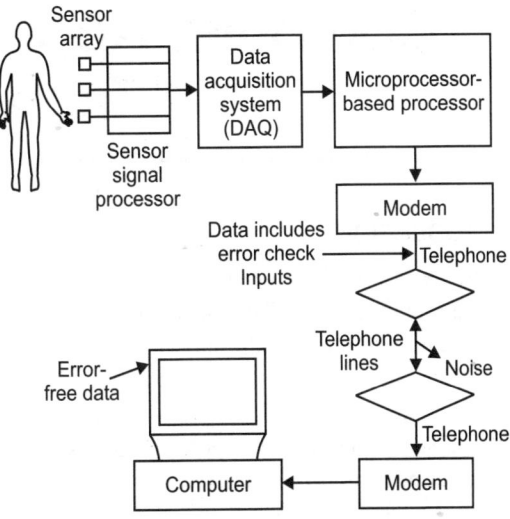

Fig. 18.14. Scheme of medical data communication through telephone line with error correction.

From the transmitting telephone, the data goes to the receiving telephone. A modem at the doctor's end, which is the receiving end, converts this data into a form which can be put through the serial part of the computer. The data is decoded by means of an algorithm and displayed in the computer monitor in numerical form as, for example, in the case of temperature and graphical form for signals like the ECG.

CURRENT TRENDS

Because of crowding of the radio spectrum due to the recent introduction of HDTV in the United States and many other countries, the FCC as well as similar agencies elsewhere have recently begun to allocate dedicated frequency bands for exclusive biotelemetry usage, for example, the Wireless medical telemetry service (WMTS). The FCC has designated the American society for healthcare engineering of the American hospital association (ASHE/AHA) as the frequency coordinator for the Wireless medical telemetry service (WMTS).

19

Computer Applications in Medical Technology

INTRODUCTION

Medicine is one field where the whole range of computer power can be and, indeed in many cases, is being used to improve the standards of diagnosis and treatment of the disease without decreasing the need for the skills of highly-trained clinical and nursing staff. The range of applications is so great that it is possible to use only a few examples to illustrate what can be done.

The computer can perform several 'on-line' and 'off line' functions which facilitate the efficient handling of voluminous data and minimises paperwork. A typical hospital information system covers the following applications areas: reservations, admissions, discharges, transfers, outpatient registration, medical records index, master index (MPI) Soundex code, personnel registration, employee databank, patient billing and accounting, surgery and other procedure scheduling, pharmacy–patient medication, diet planning and cost–benefit analysis.

CLINICAL TESTS

ECG, EEG, and EMG have been subjected to automated analysis by computer. The analog signal from the ECG is converted by ADC into a digital signal. The signal can be represented as a (Fourier) series of sine and cosine waves, each of which has frequency and amplitude term. The pattern-recognition algorithm of the computer can give an interpretation of the tracing, which is comparable to the of the expert cardiologist whose decision criteria have been incorporated into the program.

LABORATORY TEST

A laboratory system is an interactive data management system. Computerisation increases the throughput of laboratory tests, reduces transcription errors, ensures quality control, rapid performance and dissemination of test results.

The gas chromatograph mass spectrometer (GCMS) is the most powerful analytical instrument used in the clinical laboratory. High sensitivity built-in computers allow on-line recording of test results, which help in clinical decision making.

Chromosome analysis and cytological diagnosis can be achieved by the technique of syntax-directed pattern recognition.

COMPUTER-ASSISTED MEDICAL IMAGING

Nuclear medicine was the first clinical discipline to use computers in medical imaging; wherein the computer is used to supplement human performance, to store large amounts of data, quantify them and carry out memory and quantification functions that connot be accomplished by the human brain alone.

New concepts and developments in computer science and applied mathematics have made possible computer-assisted X-ray Tomography (CT), which has made a phenomenal impact on the practice of medicine. The computed CT consists of two sequential processes.

COMPUTER ASSISTED SURGERY

Computer assisted surgery (CAS) represents a surgical concept and set of methods, that use computer technology for presurgical planning, and for guiding or performing surgical interventions. CAS is also known as computer aided surgery, computer assisted intervention, image guided surgery and surgical navigation, but these terms that are more or less synonyms with CAS. CAS has been a lead in factor for the development of robotic surgery.

General Principles

Creating a virtual image of the patient

The most important component for CAS is the development of an accurate model of the patient. This can be conducted through a number of Medical imaging technologies including CT, MRI, X-rays, Ultrasound plus many more. For the generation of this model, the anatomical region to be operated has to be scanned and uploaded into the computer system. It is possible to employ a number of scanning methods, with the datasets combined through data fusion techniques. The final objective is the creation of a 3D dataset that reproduces the exact geometrical situation of the normal and pathological tissues and structures of that region. Of the available scanning methods, the CT is preferred, because MRI data sets are known to have volumetric deformations that may lead to inaccuracies. An example data set can include the collection of data compiled with 180 CT slices, that are 1 mm apart, each having 512 by 512 pixels. The contrasts of the 3D dataset (with its tens of millions of pixels) provide the detail of soft vs hard tissue structures, and thus allow a computer to differentiate, and visually separate for a human, the different tissues and structures. The image data taken from a patient will often include intentional landmark features, in order to be able to later realign the virtual dataset against the actual patient during surgery.

Image analysis and processing

Image analysis involves the manipulation of the patients 3D model to extract relevant information from the data. Using the differing contrast levels of the different tissues within the imagery, as examples, a model can be changed to show just hard structures such as bone, or view the flow of arteries and veins through the brain.

Diagnostic, preoperative planning, surgical simulation

Using specialised software, such as OsiriX, the gathered dataset can be rendered as a virtual 3D model of the patient, this model can be easily manipulated by a surgeon to provide views from any angle and at any depth within the volume. Thus the surgeon can better assess the case and establish a more accurate diagnostic. Furthermore, the surgical intervention will be planned and simulated virtually, before actual surgery takes place. Using dedicated software, the surgical robot will be programmed to carry out the pre-planned actions during the actual surgical intervention.

Surgical navigation

In computer assisted surgery, the actual intervention is defined as surgical navigation. This consists of the correlated actions of the surgeon and the surgical robot (that has been programmed to carry out certain actions during the preoperative planning procedure). A surgical robot is a mechanical device (generally looking like a robotic arm) that is computer controlled. Robotic surgery can be divided into three types, depending on the degree of surgeon interaction during the procedure: supervisory-controlled, telesurgical, and shared-control. In a supervisory-controlled system, the procedure is executed solely by the robot, which will perform the pre-programmed actions. A telesurgical system, also known as remote surgery, requires the surgeon to manipulate the robotic arms during the procedure rather than allowing the robotic arms to work from a predetermined programme. With shared-control systems, the surgeon carries out the procedure with the use of a robot that offers steady-hand manipulations of the instrument. In most robots, the working mode can chosen for each separate intervention, depending on the surgical complexity and the particularities of the case.

Applications

Computer assisted surgery is the beginning of a revolution in surgery. It already makes a great difference in high precision surgical domains, but it is also used in standard surgical procedures.

Computer assisted neurosurgery

Telemanipulators have been used for the first time in neurosurgery, in the 1980's. This allowed a greater development in brain microsurgery (compensating surgeon's physiological tremor by 10-fold), increased accuracy and precision of the intervention. It also opened a new gate to minimally invasive brain surgery, furthermore reducing the risk of post-surgical morbidity by accidentally damaging adjacent centers.

Computer assisted oral and maxillofacial surgery

Bone segment navigation is the modern surgical approach in orthognathic surgery (correction of the anomalies of the jaws and skull), in temporo-mandibular joint (TMJ) surgery, or in the reconstruction of the mid-face and orbit.

Computer assisted ENT surgery

Robotic surgery fits most of the surgeon's needs in areas with limited surgical access and requiring high-precision actions, such as middle-ear surgery.

Computer assisted orthopedic surgery

The application of robotic surgery is widespread in orthopedics, especially in routine interventions, like total hip replacement. It is also useful in pre-planning and guiding the correct anatomical position of displaced bone fragments in fractures, allowing a good fixation by osteosynthesis.

Computer assisted visceral surgery

With the advent of computer assisted surgery, great progresses have been made in general surgery towards minimal invasive approaches. Laparoscopy in abdominal and gynecologic surgery is one of the beneficiaries, allowing surgical robots to perform routine operations, like colecystectomies, or even hysterectomies. In cardiac surgery, shared control systems can perform mitral valve replacement or ventricular pacing by small thoracotomies. In urology, surgical robots contributed in laparoscopic approaches for pyeloplasty or nephrectomy or prostatic interventions.

Computer assisted radiosurgery

Radiosurgery is also incorporating advanced robotic systems. CyberKnife is such a system that has a lightweight linear accelerator mounted on the robotic arm. It is guided towards tumor processes, using the skeletal structures as a reference system (Stereotactic Radiosurgery System). During the procedure, real time X-ray is used to accurately position the device before delivering radiation beam.

Advantages of Computer Assisted Surgery

CAS starts with the premise of a much better visualisation of the operative field, thus allowing a more accurate preoperative diagnostic and a well defined surgical planning, by using surgical planning in a preoperative virtual environment. This way, the surgeon can easily assess most of the surgical difficulties and risks and have a clear idea about how to optimise the surgical approach and decrease surgical morbidity. During the operation, the computer guidance improves the geometrical accuracy of the surgical gestures and also reduce the redundancy of the surgeon's acts. This significantly improves ergonomy in the operating theatre, decreases the risk of surgical errors and reduces the operating time.

Most Notable Computer Assisted Surgery Systems

From 1989 to 2007, more than 200 CAS systems have been developed by different universities and research institutes, almost remaining experimental devices. Currently, commercially available systems approved for a clinical use are mainly VectorVision, StealthStation, DigiPointeur. All but DigiPointeur use an optical IR tracking system while DigiPointeur is an electromagnetically tracking system. The first surgical robot was called Aesop received the U.S. Food and Drug Administration (FDA) approval in 1993. It had multiple improvements and variants, such as Zeus or Hermes. The daVinci Surgical System was developed by Intuitive Surgical, derived from the Stanford Research Institute, USA. In 1997 it had received the FDA approval to assist the surgeon, and was the first Remote manipulator to have the FDA approval to perform stand-alone surgery, in 2000. It is a telesurgical system, mostly used for laparoscopic abdominal surgery. After harsh disputes and trials, the two producers merged, still under the brand name of Intuitive Surgical. Orthodoc and Robodoc are robots developed for assistance in orthopedic surgery, developed by Integrated Surgical Systems. The same company has produced Neuromate, to be used in conjunction with Orthodoc/Robodoc in neurosurgery. CyberKnife is a robot that incorporates a linear accelerator, and is used since 2001 in radiosurgery.

Ethical Issues

New and developing technologies in the medical/surgical field, and furthermore experimental devices might rise new and unforeseen risks for the patient and/or the surgical team. Ethical committees of the medical institutions have to analyse the ethical issues involved for each and every new developed device or technology. Furthermore, the high costs of the initial development of such technologies, that can be covered mostly by major hospitals, might rise questions about providing equal access to medical care for the patients.

PATIENT MONITORING IN ICU AND AUTO-MATED THERAPY

In the case of a critically ill patient, all the important physiological parameters (temperature, pulse rate, respiration rate, blood pressure, central venous pressure, heart function, lung function, urine output and blood chemistry) are transduced into electrical signals and converted through AC and DC into digital signals which are stored and analysed by the computer. Alarm signals are generated according to predetermined parameters.

The ultimate use of computers in patient care is in a closed control system, where the computer not only monitors the patient's state but is also equipped with effectors to correct any deviations from normal values.

BIOLOGICAL COMPUTERS TODAY

Biological computers today's are given below:
1. A computer made of neurons taken from leeches has been created by US scientists.

At the moment, the device can perform simple sums-the team calls the novel calculator the 'leech-ulator'.
2. But their aim is to devise a new generation of fast and flexible computers that can work out for themselves how to solve a problem, rather than having to be told exactly what to do.
3. Professor Bill Ditto, at the Georgia Institute of Technology, is leading the project and says he is amased that today's computers are still so dumb.
4. 'Ordinary computers need absolutely correct information every time to come to the right answer,' he says. 'We hope a biological computer will come to the correct answer based on partial information, by filling in the gaps itself (Fig. 19.1).'

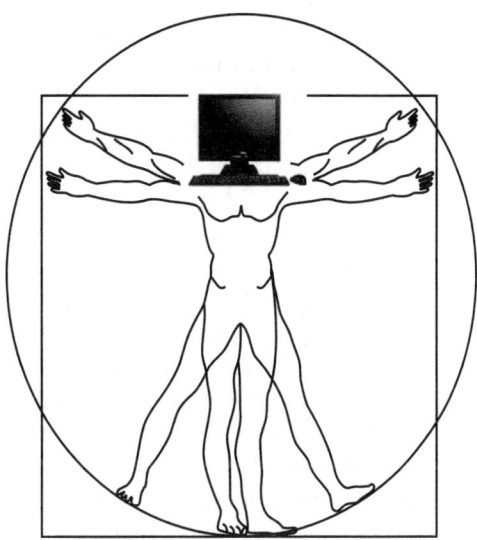

Fig. 19.1. Biological computer.

Medical Applications

Some of the medical applications are given below:
1. Scientists developed tiny implantable biocomputers
2. Molecular devices' remarkably precise scans of cellular activity could revolutionise medicine
3. Researchers at Harvard and Princeton universities have taken a crucial step toward

building biological computers, tiny implantable devices that can monitor the activities and characteristics of human cells. The information provided by these 'molecular doctors,' constructed entirely of DNA, RNA, and proteins, could eventually revolutionise medicine by directing therapies only to diseased cells or tissues.

Biological Computer Diagnoses Cancer and Produces Drug in a Test Tube

Biological computer diagnoses cancer and produces drug in a test tube are given below:

1. Weizmann Institute scientist's vision: Microscopic computers will function inside living tissues, performing diagnosis and administering treatment.

2. The world's smallest computer (around a trillion in a drop of water) might one day go on record again as the tiniest medical kit. Made entirely of biological molecules, this computer was successfully programmed to identify (in a test tube) changes in the balance of molecules in the body that indicate the presence of certain cancers, to diagnose the type of cancer, and to react by producing a drug molecule to fight the cancer cells.

3. As in previous biological computers produced in Shapiro's lab, input, output and 'software' are all composed of DNA, the material of genes, while DNA-manipulating enzymes are used as 'hardware.' The newest version's input apparatus is designed to assess concentrations of specific RNA molecules, which may be overproduced or under produced, depending on the type of cancer. Using pre-programmed medical knowledge, the computer then makes its diagnosis based on the detected RNA levels. In response to a cancer diagnosis, the output unit of the computer can initiate the controlled release of a single-stranded DNA molecule that is known to interfere with the cancer cell's activities, causing it to self-destruct.

4. In one series of test-tube experiments, the team programmed the computer to identify RNA molecules that indicate the presence of prostate cancer and, following a correct diagnosis, to release the short DNA strands designed to kill cancer cells. Similarly, they were able to identify, in the test tube, the signs of one form of lung cancer. One day in the future, they hope to create a 'doctor in a cell', which will be able to operate inside a living body, spot disease and apply the necessary treatment before external symptoms even appear.

Risk-benefit Analysis: Animated Corpse

Risk-benefit analysis: animated corpse are given below:

1. The idea of animating a corpse as in Mary's Shelly's tale. Assuming it can even be done. Benefits: Understanding the mechanics of the human physiology in a new way.

2. Risks: The general consensus might consider the idea or practice inhuman. Who would volunteer his/her body? How long would these subjects be kept 'alive.' The practice would enrage certain pro-life or pro-dead groups.

3. DQ would be LOW.

Risk-benefit Analysis: Biological Computer for Medical or Scientific Advancement

Risk-benefit analysis: Bilogical computer for medical or scientific advancement are given below:

1. Tiny 'doctors' monitoring diseases within patients and administering the correct medicines in correct doses.

2. Tiny computers: cheap to 'manufacture.' Able to run BILLIONS upon BILLIONS of calculations.

3. Risks: Technology is it's infancy. Will take some time to mature. Potential to save lives and offer a better quality of life is high.

4. DQ would be HIGH.

BIOLOGICAL BASED NANO COMPUTER REVOLUTION

As we reach the technically feasible limits of the current electronic technology of the desktop computer, a new breed of biologically based bacterial nano computers of the future may have the capacity to impact and alter desktop computing forever, through miniaturisation that could bring huge increases of computing capacity, power, storage and speed. The impact of nano technology production could not only alter how we manufacture computer components, but might spread to other forms of manufacturing as well.

In this section we will examine the current developments of bio-computing, followed by the key scientific principles and applications of molecular technology that makes this potential revolution in computing power possible. Finally we will look at how this cutting edge technology might be adopted in the future, and who would be most likely to make use of bio-computers.

Present Day Computer

Today's state-of-the-art personal computers are based on the refined technology surrounding the development of the silicon computer chip. This power was attained by leaps in miniaturisation, squeezing more and more circuits onto a single chip. Now a single printed circuit on the surface of a chip is down to 0.1 micron, about 1,000 times thinner than a human hair.

Today the computing capability of the computer chip has been embraced by consumers and industry alike in the clock speed of the PC Chip, measured in the frequency of hertz. A single hertz (Hz) is one completed cycle per second. Each cycle represents a single instruction, which may be as simple as the addition of two numbers, or one of millions of instructions created by a computer's software. 60 Hz would represent 60 cycles or instructions per second. Following this model, a megahertz is a million cycles or computations per second, and a gigahertz represents one billion cycles or computations per second. Today the state-of-the-art Pentium 4 based PC chip touts speeds up to 2000 mhz.

Bio-Chip Computer of Tomorrow

Enter the field of molecular computing, and the ability to pack billions more circuits onto a microchip than ever thought possible. Science news writer Tim McDonald asserts that 'molecules are only a few nanometers in size, and it is possible to make chips containing billions, or even trillions, of switches and components.' From this statement it would seem logical to assume that this new molecular technology has the possibility to increase the capacity of a single chip by factors measured in the millions. And if this possibility of such huge increases of a computer microchip exists, then what many would call a super computer becomes achievable.

The term supercomputer is widely used but even more widely misunderstood. In order to define what a supercomputer is, first we must leave behind the old style of measuring computing speed and power. We will speak no more of the CPU's chip speed. It is irrelevant to the new computing models we are going to explore.

Let's start fresh with a look at the most refined and efficient model of a biological supercomputer that exists today: the human brain. The human brain and our accompanying sensory biology, such as eyesight, represent a level of power and sophistication that makes even our best PCs look downright pokey. With all this fuss over desktop multimedia, here is a fact worth remembering—you are your most powerful computing asset.

Fortunately there is a body of knowledge based on the 30 year quest for robotic vision, and these statistics are revealing. Embracing a measurement in the MIPS (million instructions per second), it is thought that PC computing equivalent of human sight requires 100 million MIPS. Experimental computers achieved a few million MIPS in 1998. These were made up of thousands of PC chips and cost in the tens of millions of dollars. If we are ever to enter the realm of the super-computer, we will need to look beyond our current model of an electronically based silicon chip computer. Enter bio-chip based computing, which many scientists in a variety of disciplines believe holds the key to a new era of computers, capable of tremendous processing power and speed.

The race to engineer a new breed of machines and computers at the molecular level is well under way. The list of organisations that are actively engaged in nanotechnology research and development, as well as practical applications is impressive, including industry giants Genex, US Naval Research Labs, IBM, NEC, Hitachi, and Toshiba to name a few.

It is worth noting that even with this impressive collection of corporate R & D muscle, most scientific predictions of what types of nano-technical machines are possible are ambiguous. It is clear that computing devices are only one of many different products that are feasible. Some examples of applications for microscopic machines range from microscopic bacterial syringes — born from current bio-technology — that kill cancer cells, to pocket DNA testers, to airplane wings made of 'smart skin' material that allows the micro-surface to act as finely tuned flaps allowing for safer and more efficient flight. Other areas include data storage, inertial navigation, weapons, and a dizzying array of nano pumps, and valves.

In principal these devices will share many familiar engineering concepts used today. 'Just as ordinary tools can build ordinary machines from parts, so too can molecular tools bond molecules together to make tiny gears, motors, levers, and casings, and assemble them together to make complex machines.'

Based on the underlying principal of digital computing based on the binary code of 0's and 1's, we start to see how a single molecule capable of being in a state of 0 or 1, or On or Off, makes the possibility of molecular computing achievable, at least in theory. And since it has been proven that molecular switches can exist in several states at once, both on and off, the potential computing power grows exponentially. Combine this increased computing power with emerging miniaturised data storage technology that raises the bar of fast access to media up to terabyte capacity, and we have the makings of what we would now consider a supercomputer in a device the size of a current day PDA or smaller.

Biology and Electronics Merge

The ability to engineer and build a bio-computer lies first and foremost in the ability to merge the biological parts with the electronics into hybrid systems. Electronic computers of today simply act as routers for electrons over the 0.01 micron sized circuits of today's silicon chip. A biological PC chip, however, may allow for the same sized circuit to handle the equivalent of one thousand circuits through the development of Microelectromechanical systems, or MEMS. MEMS is the practice of combining miniaturised mechanical and electronic components.

It is widely accepted that any successful bio-chip based computer can only be built by combining the bio-chip with the latest electronic technologies, including those for display, sound, input, and connectivity. Through a wide variety of techniques currently being researched and developed, successful MEMS technology will be key to building hybrid systems containing technology based in both organically grown molecules and traditionally manufactured electronics.

Self-Assembling Materials

Manufacturing on the molecular level on a scale that would be useful is made possible by the ability for some molecules to 'self-assemble.' This ability to reproduce organically is noteworthy in many ways. Inspired by nature, this model is nothing new. But the ability to design nanotechnology based on organic molecules that build themselves once started is very new. Already successfully proving this concept are new liposomes that contain drugs for treatments of an array of diseases. There are many other areas where self-assembly has been proven to work. Some big wins include the successful design and growth of crystals starting off with a self assembling monolayer (SAM), as well as a very relevant piece to the bio-computing puzzle, Buckytubes, which are tiny self assembling graphite tubes that act as the smallest electrical wire ever known.

Universal Key

What propels the entire field of biological nanotechnology is the ability to manipulate organic matter. For the most part, any one person or group cannot own the fundamental principals that would allow for such extraordinary developments. 'The toolbox of biochemistry, the parts list—the 'kernel,' to stretch the software analogy — is shared by all organisms on the planet.'

This non-ownership factor has enormous importance. Once any biological technology is developed, anyone can take it and tweak, much like open source code for software. This model has been shown to foster innovation in the software industry, which leads us to believe it can be only good for the developing nano-machines based in biological technology.

There is the possibility of a 'democratisation' regarding the ability to design and manufacture as the technology matures. Award-winning science writer Robert Carlson believes that 'these critical technologies will first move from academic labs to large biotechnology companies to small business, and eventually to the home garage and kitchen.' Fantastic as that may seem, it is now a fact that, for instance, that many lab tests that in the past required a doctoral degree and tremendous scientific resources now come in colour coded kits any undergraduate can use successfully.

All This and Cheaper Too?

Considering a computer chip manufacturing plant costs upward of one billion dollars, the potential of biological computer chip manufacturing to be more efficient from an economic view is an important factor. The combination of cheaper and faster always gets attention, and bio-computing will be no different in that respect. But there is another aspect of this technology that could effect us in ways so profound it becomes hard to imagine.

We all know that the current model of industrialisation is a wasteful one. Aside from the obvious solutions of recycling, alternative power, and other 'green' sciences, biological manufacturing has a huge advantage, mainly that 'renewable, biological manufacturing will take place anywhere someone wants to set up a vat or plant a seed.' Once the scientific design of any given bio-pc component is

refined, it is simply grown. The drain on our planet resources and the wasteful pollution resulting from current manufacturing methods are eliminated in the process.

What Could We do with a Bio-Chip Computer?

In order to see just what the future implications of this new and exciting technology might realistically bring, let's speculate, for example, what capabilities a supercomputer the size of a watch might have. We offer this scenario; a handheld or wearable computer device capable of generating a photo-realistic 3D virtual computing environment, visually experienced by wearing glasses that project images onto the surface of the each lens. Input is provided by speaking into a tiny microphone coupled with advanced speech recognition, and sound output by a miniature earpiece.

Connectivity would be achieved by high speed wireless network access to the Internet, and your colleagues, allowing for real-time interaction and sharing of data. Then consider the exciting prospect of recording every moment and interaction each and every day of our lives, thus allowing each of us to create a virtual life history stored in digital media. Add a virtual staff of intelligent software agents able to perform research, engineering—anything a room full of highly educated and expensive employees would normally do—and we start to see the potential of this new technology.

Bio-Chip Revolution Will It Come?

As great as a bio-chip super computer sounds, and to many, including myself, the prospects of such huge advances in computing power and environments are truly revolutionary, in our opinion precious few of us will ever get to use one in our lifetime. Yes, it is possible, even probable, given the advances discussed in this section, that in the next twenty years some form of hybrid bio-chip super computer will be developed. Unfortunately there are many reasons why most of us will never even see, much less use, such an incredible device.

The silicon chip based computer provides more than enough computing power than most of the population will ever need. Unless some 'killer' application comes along that requires a quantum leap in computational power, and is widely adopted, our Pentium 4 or 5 or 10 chip will suffice quite well. Until there is a fundamental shift in the very nature of computing, most of the population running Windows 200 X on their desktop will be oblivious to the possibilities a bio-chip computer could offer.

The precious few of us who actually need the upwards of 100 million MIPS computing punch are fooling around in such focused areas as robotics and artificial intelligence — highly specialised fields that only a select few actually work in. The military might be an early adopter, but we'd never know about it unless we wore a star or two on our collar.

Glossary

Accretion	:	Growth or enlargement.
Accuracy	:	The degree to which the average value of repeated measurements approximate the true value being measured.
Active electrode	:	Electrode used for achieving desired surgical effect.
Alpha radiation	:	Particulate radiation consisting of a helium nucleus emitted from a decaying nucleus.
Ambient temperature	:	The average temperature of air surrounding the device or equipment.
Amnion	:	Thin membranous structure around fetus.
Amniotic	:	Pertaining to the amnion.
Amperometry	:	Measurements based on current flow produced in an electrochemical cell by an applied voltage.
Analog	:	A parameter which varies in a continuous, rather than incremental or discrete-step manner.
Analog meter	:	A scale and pointer meter capable of indicating a continuous range of values.
Angstrom	:	Unit of length, 1 angstrom = 10^{-10} meters.
Aorta	:	Great artery carrying blood from the left ventricle of the heart to the rest of the body.
Atrioventricular	:	Located between the upper and lower chamber of the heart.
Atrium	:	Upper chamber of the heart.
Attenuator	:	A device that reduces the amplitude or power level of a signal without introducing appreciable distortion.
Auricle	:	Chamber of the heart that receives blood from the veins.
Auto-polarity	:	The ability to measure DC values of either polarity without the need to interchange test lead connections.
Auto-zero	:	An automatic correction for offsets and drifts at zero input.
Aveolus	:	Air sac or cell in the lungs.
Average responding	:	An AC measurement obtained using a DC instrument with a rectifying input circuit calibrated in terms of the corresponding rms value. Accurate only for pure sine wave inputs.
Axon	:	Long, thin portion of a nerve cell that carries the impulse away from the main section of the cell.
Balance	:	The change in the position of an analog pointer from zero when the axis of the moving element moves from the vertical position to the horizontal positionThe balance is expressed as a percentage of the scale length.

Bandwidth	:	The frequency span where a constant amplitude input will produce a meter reading within a specified limit (usually 3 db). In controllers, the region around the set-point where control occurs.
Baud	:	Digital transmission speed in bits per second.
Beer-Lambert law	:	Principle stating that the optical absorbance of a substance is proportional to both the concentration of the substance and the path length of the sample.
Beta radiation	:	Particulate radiation consisting of an electron or positron emitted from a decaying nucleus.
Bias current	:	Current that flows out of an amplifier 's input terminals which will produce a voltage drop across the source impedance. In a perfect amplifier this error term would be zero.
Bioelectric	:	Electrical activity pertaining to a living cell.
Biophysical	:	Branch of science that applies the concepts of physical science to biology.
Brachial	:	Relating or pertaining to the arm.
Bradycardia	:	Slow heart rate.
Bronchus	:	Tube leading from trachea to either left or right lung.
Burden	:	The input impedance of a measuring circuit (expressed in ohms) or the load on the secondary of a transformer (expressed in volt-amps or watts). In potential or current transformers, burden is the maximum load the transformer can support while operating within its accuracy rating.
Calibrate	:	To determine the indication or output of a device with respect to a standard.
Capillaries	:	Smallest blood vessels in the body
Cardiac	:	Pertaining to the heart.
Cardiology	:	Study of the heart and its diseases.
Cardiovascular	:	Relating to the circulatory system.
Catheter	:	Small tube that is inserted into the body to permit injection of medications, to allow the vessel or passage open or to permit withdrawal of fluids.
Cell	:	Smallest object capable of life.
Celsius	:	Temperature scale where $0°C$ = freezing and $100°C$ = boiling point of water at sea level. Formerly known as Centigrade.
Cephalic	:	Pertaining to the head or skull.
Cerebellum	:	Large dorsal brain structure.
Cerebrum	:	Anterior portion of the brain.
Coagulation	:	Solidification of proteins accompanied by tissue whitening.
Cold junction compensation	:	A correction applied to thermocouple measurements to compensate for the temperature of the TC wire connections, so the temperature reading is only the result of the measuring TC junction.
Colligative properties	:	Physical properties that depend on the number of molecules present rather than on their individual properties.
Common mode rejection ratio (CMRR)	:	The ratio between the amplitude of a common mode signal and the amplitude of a differential signal that would produce the same output amplitude or as the ratio of the differential gain over the common-mode gain. CMRR = G_D/G_{CM}. Expressed in decibels, the common mode rejection is 20 log $_{10}$ CMRR. The common mode rejection is a function of frequency and source-impedance unbalance.

Common-mode rejection : *(CMR)*		The ability of a circuit or meter to reject a signal that appears at both input terminals with respect to ground.
Common-mode voltage : *(CMV)*		An AC or DC voltage which appears between the signal lines and circuit ground or earth.
Conformity error	:	The difference between the actual response and the ideal response to a particular stimulus.
Connector thermocouple :		A special polarised disconnect device whose current-carrying parts are of thermocouple alloy material.
Continuous positive *airway pressure* *(CPAP)*	:	A spontaneous ventilation mode in which the ventilator maintains a constant positive pressure, near or below PEEP level, in the patient's airway while the patient breathes at will.
Control mode	:	Type of control used in a feedback control system. One mode is proportional control. Two mode is proportional plus integral (reset) or derivative (rate)Three mode is proportional, integral and derivative (PID).
Controller	:	A device capable of receiving a signal from a process and regulating an input to that process in order to maintain a selected operating condition.
Conversion rate	:	The number of analog-to-digital conversions performed per second by a digital instrument.
Cornea	:	Transparent covering of the center portion of the eye.
Cortex	:	Outer layer of tissue on an organ.
Cortical	:	Pertaining to the cortex.
Count	:	One event or one increment of the least significant digit.
CPU	:	Central Processing Unit in digital computing systems. Often referred to as microcontroller or microprocessor.
Cranium	:	Portion of the skull containing the brain.
Crest factor	:	The ratio of the maximum (crest) value of a periodic function (AC voltage or current) to its RMS value.
Curare	:	Drug that produces muscular relaxation.
Cytochromes	:	Heme-containing proteins found in the membranes of mitochondria and required for oxidative phosphorylation, with characteristic optical absorbance spectra.
Cytoplasm	:	The matter inside a cell, except for the nucleus.
Damping	:	The manner in which the pointer of an analog instrument settles at its steady indication after the applied electrical energy is changed. Usually expressed as percent overshoot.
Deadband	:	The region through which an input can be varied without initiating a response.
Defibrillator	:	An electrical device used to deliver a shock to stop fibrillation of the heart.
Dendrite	:	Portion of the nerve cell that conducts impulses toward the cell.
Depolarised	:	State of being partially or totally non-polar.
Desiccation	:	Drying of tissue due to the evaporation of intracellular fluids.
Deutsche industry *norm (DIN)*	:	A set of German technical standards. Commonly used to specify panel meter sizes.
Diastole	:	Expansion of the chambers of the heart so that they may fill with blood.
Dicrotic	:	Double humped waveform.

Dielectric strength	:	The voltage that can be sustained without breakdown.
Differential input	:	An input circuit where signal high and signal low are electrically floating with respect to signal common or signal ground.
Digit	:	A measure of the display span of a meterBy convention, a full digit can assume any value from 0 through 9, a 1/2 digit will display a 0 or 1 and overrange at 2, a 3/4 digit will display up to 3 and over-range at 4. A meter with a display span of ±3999 counts is a 33/4 digit meter.
Dispersive electrode	:	Return electrode at which no electrosurgical effect is intended.
Drift	:	An unwanted change in the reading or set-point value over time, when inputs are held constant.
Dual-slope conversion	:	An analog to digital conversion technique which can provide high noise rejection.
Dysfunctional haemoglobins	:	Those haemoglobin species that cannot reversibly bind oxygen (carboxy-haemoglobin, methemoglobin and sulfhaemoglobin).
ECG	:	Electrocardiograph.
Ectopic	:	Located in other than normal position.
EEG	:	Electroencephalogram.
Electro motive force (emf)	:	An electrical potential difference which produces or tends to produce an electric current.
Electrocardiogram	:	Tracing of the electrical signals produced by the heart.
Electrode	:	Conductor used to make electrical contact between a wire and a conductive surface, such as human skin.
Electrodermograph	:	Recorder for measuring galvanic skin resistance.
Electroencephalogram	:	Recording of electrical signals produced by the brain.
Electroencephalograph	:	Machine for making electroencephalograms.
Electrogastrogram	:	Recording of simultaneous electrical and physical activity of the stomach.
Electrolyte	:	A solution in which electrical current is due to ionic mobility.
Electromyogram	:	Recording of electrical activity of skeletal muscles.
Electromyograph	:	Machine for making electromyograms.
Element	:	A circuit in a watt, VAR or PF meter that accepts one voltage and one current input.
Embolus	:	Abnormal solid or gaseous particle in the blood stream.
Embryo	:	Undeveloped stage of fetus.
EMG	:	Electromyograph; electromyogram.
EMI	:	Electromagnetic interference.
Expanded scale	:	An arrangement that expands a specific portion of an overall range to occupy a larger portion of the full-scale length than it normally would.
Explosion scale	:	An enclosure capable of withstanding an explosion of a specified gas or vapour which may occur within it and of preventing the ignition of a specified gas or vapour surrounding the enclosures by sparks, flashes, heat or explosion of the gas vapour within.
Extracellular	:	Outside of the cells.
Extracorporeal	:	Outside of the body.
Fail-safe	:	Assuming a safe operating mode in the event of a failure.

Fluorescence	:	Emission of light by an atom or molecule following absorption of a photon by greater energy. Emission normally occurs within 10^{-8} of absorption.
Fulguration	:	Random discharge of sparks between active electrode and tissue surface in order to achieve coagulation and/or desiccation.
Full scale value	:	The arithmetic sum of the two end-scale values (may not apply to some specialised meters, such as power factor). When zero is not on the scale, the full-scale value is the higher end-scale value.
Functional saturation	:	The ratio of oxygenated haemoglobin to total non-dysfunctional haemoglobins (oxyhaemoglobin plus deoxyhaemoglobin).
Gamma radiation	:	Electromagnetic radiation emitted from an atom undergoing nuclear decay.
Ground	:	Reference point for an electrical system. Often used to indicate an earth connection or negative side of a DC supply.
Grounded junction	:	A thermocouple construction where the junction is attached (grounded) to the sheath as contrasted to an ungrounded or exposed junction type.
Hemisphere	:	Half of a spherical object.
Homogeneous	:	Of the same sort.
Hydrodynamic focusing	:	A process in which a fluid stream is first surrounded by a second fluid and then narrowed to a thin stream by a narrowing of the channel.
Hypoxia	:	Inadequate oxygen supply to tissues necessary to maintain metabolic activity.
Hysteresis	:	The difference in an output or activation point due to rising vs. falling input signals.
Infarct	:	Area of necrotic tissue due to loss of blood perfusion.
Inhomogeneity	:	Not homogenous.
Input resistance (input impedance)	:	DC (or AC) resistance measured across the input terminals with signal leads disconnected.
Insulation resistance	:	The resistance measured between two insulated points on a device when a specified DC voltage is applied.
Intracellular	:	Inside of the cell.
Ion	:	Atom or molecule that carries an electrical charge, either positive or negative.
Iris	:	Coloured portion of the eye behind the cornea.
Isoelectric	:	Having the same electric charge, so cannot produce an electrical current.
Isothermal	:	A process or area that is a constant temperature.
Isotopes	:	Atoms with the same number of protons but differing numbers of neutrons.
Isotropic	:	Having the same properties in all directions.
Kelvin (K)	:	The basic temperature unit of the thermodynamic scale. 0°C= 273 K
Knife-edge pointer	:	Analog meter pointer with end flattened and turned edgewise so that the thinnest dimension or edge is seen by the observer Often used with mirror-backed scale for increased reading accuracy by elimination of parallax.
Latching (in meter relays)	:	A condition that requires the manual reset of a tripped relay. The tripped relay cannot be reset (re-energised) until the indicating pointer or display is in a non-alarm position.
Latency	:	Apparent inactivity.
Lead compensation	:	Technique for minimising or eliminating errors due to signal leads.

Least-significant digit (LSD)	:	The right most active digit of a digital display
Line rejection	:	Insensitivity to a power line frequency interference signal. Usually expressed in ₿.
Linearity error	:	A measure of the departure from a straight-line response in the relationship between two quantities, where the change in one quantity is directly proportional to a change in the other quantity Usually expressed as a maximum percent.
Lobe	:	Rounded portion of an organ.
Lumen	:	The hollow portion of a tubular organ.
Mandatory mode	:	A mode of mechanically ventilating the lungs where the ventilator controls all breath delivery parameters such as tidal volume, respiration rate, flow waveform, etc.
Manometer	:	Device used to determine gas pressures.
Measuring junction	:	That junction of a thermocouple subjected to the temperature to be measured.
Membrane	:	A thin layer of tissue.
Metabolism	:	The total of all processes required for an organism to live.
Micron	:	Unit of length, 10^{-6} meters.
Mirror scale	:	An analog meter scale with a mirror arc that enables alignment of the eyes line of sight perpendicular to the scale when taking a reading. Eliminates parallax, considerably improves reading accuracy.
Mitochondria	:	Small granules or rods.
Mitral stenosis	:	Narrowing of the oriface between left atria and ventricle.
Multivariate analysis	:	Empirical models developed to relate multiple spectral intensities from many calibration samples to known analyte concentrations, resulting in an optimal set of calibration parameters.
Myocardium	:	A muscle layer of the heart.
Myograph	:	Instrument for measurement of muscular contraction.
Necrosis	:	Death of tissue or cells.
Nephelometry	:	Measurement of the amount of light scattered by particles suspended in a fluid.
Neuron	:	Nerve cell.
Non-linearity	:	In an ideal system, the input-out relationship is linear (i.e. straight line). Any departure from straight line is expressed as non-linearity Two methods are used for measurement. The 'best straight line' approach compromises the end points and situates the line to give the most optimistic answer
Nucleus	:	Central structure (as in cells and atoms).
Occipital	:	Relating or pertaining to the rear portion of the head.
Offset current	:	The difference between two bias currents drawn by the inputs of a differential amplifier.
Offset	:	The non-zero output of a device for zero input.
Ohms per volt	:	Indication of the total terminal resistance of an analog voltmeter A 1000-ohms-per-volt meter has a resistance of 1,50,000 ohms on its 150-volt (full-scale) range, and 3,00,000 ohms on its 300-volt range. Its basic movement is a 1 mA meter.

ON-OFF control	:	Non-proportional control in which the controlled process input is either fully 'ON' or fully 'OFF' depending on whether the temperature is above or below the control point dead-band.
Operational amplifier (op-amp)	:	A very high gain DC-coupled differential amplifier with single-ended output, high voltage gain, high input impedance and low output impedance. Due to its high open-loop gain, the characteristics of an op-amp circuit only depend on its feedback network. Therefore the integrated circuit op-amp is an extremely convenient tool for the realisation of linear amplifier circuits.
OPTO-isolator	:	An isolation device that provides an electrical barrier between related circuits.
Organ	:	Group of specialised cells that perform a specific task or function.
Overload	:	The excess load beyond full-scale value that an instrument can withstand without damage or failure. Expressed as a per cent of a full-scale value.
Over-range	:	A reading that exceeds full scale.
Overshoot	:	The amount by which a meter or process exceeds the final value during a transition. Usually expressed as per cent of amplitude for a step change.
Oximetry	:	The determination of blood or tissue oxygen content, generally by optical means.
Parietal	:	Pertaining to the upper rear portion of the head.
Parts per million (PPM)	:	A convenient format to express very small numbers, such as temperature coefficients, 100 ppm is 0.01 per cent.
Patient circuit	:	A set of tubes connecting the patient airway to the outlet of a respirator.
Permeable	:	Ability to pass through pores.
Peroneal	:	Pertaining to the outer side of the lower leg.
Phase angle	:	The difference in electrical degrees by which current leads voltage in an inductive circuit or lags voltage in a capacitive circuitAlso the phase displacement between primary and secondary currents in a current transformer.
Piezoelectric	:	Electrical activity due to flexure of a crystal.
Plasma	:	The liquid portion of blood.
Plethysmography	:	Recording of volume changes due to blood flow.
Pneumatic	:	Pertaining to or operated by gases, especially air.
Pneumograph	:	Measuring instrument for recording volume changes in the thorax due to respiration.
Pneumotachygraph	:	Instrument to measure respiration rate.
Polyphase wattmeter	:	A wattmeter with 2 or 3 single-phase wattmeters mounted in the same package.
Positive end expiratory pressure (PEEP)	:	A therapist-selected pressure level for the patient airway at the end of expiration in either mandatory or spontaneous breathing.
Posterior	:	Pertaining to the rear.
Potential EMF	:	The relative voltage at a point in a circuit or in space with respect to some reference point.
Potentiometry	:	Measurement of the potential produced by electrochemical cells under equilibrium conditions with no current flow.
Power factor	:	The ratio of consumed power to apparent (volt-ampere) power in anAC circuit.
Precision	:	A measure of test reproducibility.

Pressure controlled ventilation	:	A mandatory mode of ventilation where during the inspiration phase of each breath, a constant pressure is applied to the patient's airway independent of the patient's airway resistance and/or compliance respiratory mechanics.
Pressure support	:	A spontaneous breath delivery mode during which the ventilator applies a positive pressure greater than PEEP to the patient's airway during inspiration.
Process meter	:	A panel meter with sizeable zero and span adjustment capabilities, which can be scaled for read-out in engineering units for signals such as 4–20 mA, 10–50 mA and 1–5 V.
Protoplasm	:	Substance of water, inorganic and proteinaceous material making up the parts of the cell.
PSI absolute (PSIA)	:	A pressure reading using vacuum as the reference.
PSI gauge (PSIG)	:	A pressure reading using ambient air pressure as the reference.
Psychogalvanic	:	Electrical activity produced by mental stress.
Pulmonary	:	Pertaining to the lungs.
Pulse oximetry	:	The determination of functional oxygen saturation of pulsatile arterial blood by ratiometric measurement of tissue optical absorbance changes.
Pupil	:	Variable-size aperture in the center of the eye.
Radical	:	Group of atoms that can be replaced by a single atom.
Radioisotope	:	Artificially produced radioactive element.
Range	:	The span of values over which a meter will function without entering overload condition, e.g. 0–150 VAC, 0–10 A.
Ratiometric measurement	:	A resistance measurement technique where the unknown resistance is placed in series with a known resistance.The voltage across each is measured to determine the unknown resistance.
Reactance	:	The opposition presented by capacitance and/or inductance to the passage of alternating current of a given frequency.
Rectifier-type meter	:	A DC meter equipped with a solid-state rectifier at its input to convert AC energy to DC energy. The instrument provides measurements of the average value of an AC voltage or current, and its scale is usually calibrated in terms of the RMS equivalent. Such calibration is accurate for pure sine-wave signals, but the accuracy decreases for distorted signals.
Repeatability	:	The ability of an instrument to register the same reading in successive measurements of the same input.
Resistance temperature detector (RTD)	:	A metallic sensor where resistance increases in a predictable manner with increasing temperature.
Resolution	:	The degree to which nearly equal values of a quantity can be discriminated. In digital meters, the value represented by a one-digit change in the least-significant digit.
Retina	:	Light-sensitive membrane in the eye.
Rheobase	:	Smallest electrical current that will produce stimulation.
Root mean square (RMS)	:	The square root of the mean of the square of the signal over one full cycle.
Sagittal	:	Pertaining to or parallel to the midline of the body.
Scalp	:	Skin of the head covered by hair.

Scintillation	:	The conversion of the kinetic energy of a charged particle or photon to a flash of light.
Secondary junction	:	An unwanted connection between a pair of thermocouple wires tending to produce a signal representative of the secondary junction temperature rather than the measuring junction temperature.
Self-heating	:	Internal heating of a transducer as a result of power dissipation.
Semi-permeable	:	Permeable to certain substances.
Sensitivity	:	A measure of how small an amount of concentration of an analyte can be detected.
Sensitivity	:	The minimum change in input to which a device can respond.
Serum	:	The liquid portion of blood remaining after clotting has occurred.
Settling time	:	The time required for the output to settle within a specified band of the final value when a step input change is applied.
Shield	:	A protective conductive covering that provides a least resistance path to ground for external interference.
SHUNT	:	A calibrated low resistance connected in parallel with the input terminals of an ammeter in order to enable measurement of higher currents. It can be internal or external. Typical external shunts are either 50 mV or 100 mV full scale.
Signal conditioner	:	A circuit or module which offsets, attenuates, amplifies, linearises and/or filters the signal for transmission or processing by an A/D converter. The typical output span of a signal conditioner is ±2 VDC or 4–20 mA.
Sinoatrial node	:	Collection of heart cells that functions as the natural pacemaker.
Sinus	:	Irregular cavity.
Snubber	:	A resistance/capacitor or diode/resistor network used to dissipate switching transients. Often used across high current relay contacts.
Span adjustment	:	The ability to adjust the gain of a process or meter so the display span corresponds to a specified signal span.
Specificity	:	A measure of how well a test detects the intended analyte without being 'fooled' by other substance in the sample.
Sphygmomanometer	:	Blood pressure measurement apparatus.
Spirometer	:	Measuring instrument for determining respiratory air volume.
Spontaneous mode	:	A ventilation mode in which the patient initiates and breathes from the ventilator supplied gas at will.
Spray	:	Another term for fulguration. Sometimes this waveform has a higher crest factor than that used for fulguration.
Stereotaxic	:	Precision positioning.
Synapse	:	Junction where impulse transmits from one nerve cell to another.
Synchronous motor	:	An AC motor whose speed is exactly proportional to the frequency of the applied alternating voltage.
Systemic	:	Affecting the entire body.
Systole	:	Period during which the heart contracts.
Tachycardia	:	Excessively fast heart rate.
Taut band	:	Method of suspending moving coil or moving iron vane in magnetic field. Eliminates pivot and jewel friction problems.

Temperature coefficient: (TEMPCO)		The change in a parameter produced by a change in temperature. Normally expressed in per cent/°C or ppm/°C.
Thermal gradient	:	A continuously changing temperature as a function of distance.
Thermistor	:	A semiconductor material which exhibits a known electrical resistance vs. temperature.
Thermistor	:	Electrical component that exhibits resistance changes due to temperature changes.
Thermocouple break protection	:	A means to indicate when thermocouple has failed in an open circuit condition.
Thermocouple loop resistance	:	The total resistance of the thermocouple and its extension wire.
Thermocouple	:	Device that creates a voltage proportional to temperature.
Thermocouple	:	The junction of two dissimilar metals with a voltage output proportional to temperature.
Thermopile	:	A number of thermocouples connected in series, arranged so that alternate junctions are the referenced temperature and at the measured temperature to increase the output for a give temperature diference between the measuring and reference junctions.
Thermowell	:	The housing into which an RTD or thermocouple is inserted.Allows easy removal and/or replacement.
Thoracic	:	Pertaining to the thorax.
Thorax	:	Section of the body between abdomen and neck.
Thrombus	:	Clot of blood remaining at its site of origin.
Tibia	:	Large, innermost bone of the leg.
Time constant	:	The time required for a sensor to respond to 63 per cent of its total change resulting from a step input. Five time constants are required to attain 99 per cent of the total change.
Tissue	:	Collection of similar cells that perform a specific function or take a similar form.
Torso	:	Trunk of the body.
Trachea	:	Main tube passing air from outside world to the lungs.
Transducer	:	Device that converts ener gy from one form to another for purposes of measurement or control. In this context, the ener gy converted to is usually electrical.
Tri-state output	:	A logic output which has 0, 1 and high impedance output states. For parallel connected outputs, the high-impedance state is used when the output is not active.
True RMS (TRMS)	:	The true root-mean-square value of anAC or AC-plus-DC signal. Often used to determine power of a signal.
Turbidimetry	:	Measurement of the attenuation of a light beam due to light lost to scattering by particles suspended in a fluid.
Two-wire transmitter	:	A signal conditioner in which the signal output and power input share two wires, thus minimising wiring.
Ulnar	:	Pertaining to the larger bone of the human forearm.
Utero	:	Latin dative for uterus.
Uterus	:	Organ in the female for protection and nourishment of the embryo.

Vasoconstrictors	:	Agents that narrow the blood vessels.
Vasomotor	:	Agent affecting the size of a blood vessel.
Ventricle	:	Lower chambers of the heart.
Venule	:	Small vein connected to the capillaries.
Viable	:	Able to live.
VOLT	:	The unit of electromotive force. One volt applied to a resistance of one ohm produces a current of one ampere.
Volt-amperes reactive (VAR)	:	The unit of reactive power, as contrasted to real power (watts).
Volume controlled ventilation	:	A mandatory mode of ventilation where the volume of each breath is set by the therapist and the ventilator delivers that volume to the patient independent of the patient's airway resistance and/or compliance respiratory mechanics.
WATT (W)	:	Unit of real (effective) electrical power. $W = VA \times PF$ in a sinusoidal circuit.
Zero adjustment	:	The ability to adjust a signal conditioner or meter so that zero output or zero display corresponds to a specific input signal, such as 0 V or 4 mA.

References

Anderson, K., *Bioinstrumentation and Its Principles*, Harper & Row, New York.

Arceivala, J., *Basic Concepts of Bioinstrumentation*, Marcel Dekker Inc., New York.

Berenson, C., *Application of Computer in Biomedical Engineering*, Harper & Row, New York.

Bracewell, R., *The Fourier Transform and Its Application*, Mcgraw-Hill, New York.

Christensen, D.A., *Ultrasound Bioinstrumentation*, Wiley, New York.

Cobbold, R.C., *Transducers for Biomedical Measurement*, Wiley, New York.

Cook, A.M., *Electrodes and Measurement of Bioelectric Events*, Prentice Hall, New York.

Donald. L. Wise, *Bioinstrumentation and Biosensors,* Marcel Dekker, Inc., New York.

Edward, C., *Electrical Technology*, Longman Group Ltd., London.

Faulk, B.F., *Clinical Laboratory Instruments*, Prentice Hall, New York.

Ferris, C.D., *Introduction to Bioelectrodes*, Plenum, New York.

Foster, M.A., *Magnetic Resonance in Medicine and Biology*, Pergamon, New York.

Fry, F.J., *Ultrasound: Its Application in Biology and Medicine*, Elsevier, New York.

Geddes, L.A., *Principles of Applied Biomedical Instrumentation*, Wiley, New York.

Hine, G.S., *Principles of Bioinstrumentation and Measurement*, Academic Press, New York.

Jacob Kline, *Handbook of Biomedical Engineering*, Academic Press, Inc., London.

James, A.N., *Biomedical Electronics*, Academic Press, Inc., London.

Janta, J., *Medical Physiology*, Plenum, New York.

Jolles, Z.E., *Electronic Instruments and Measurements*, Harper & Row, New York.

Joseph Carr, *Biomedical Equipment use, Maintenance and Management,* Prentice Hall, New York.

Joseph, S., *Biomedical Engineering,* Academic Press, Inc., London.

Kimmich, H.P., *Biomedical Instrumentation and Measurement*, Wiley, New York.

Lion, K.S., *Elements of Electronics and Electrical Instrumentation*, Mcgraw-Hill, New York.

Miller, H.A., *Biomedical Electrode Technology*, Academic Publishers, New York.

Murray, R.W., *Introduction to Medical Electronics*, American Chemical Society, Washington D.C.

Payne, J.P., *Medicine and Clinical Engineering*, Prentice Hall, New York.

Plonsey, R., *Bioelectric Phenomena*, Mcgraw-Hill, New York.

Rogers, D.F., *Ventilators and Humidifiers*, Wiley, New York.

Smith, H.S.*, Bioinstrumentation*, Chilton Book Company, Radnor, Pennsylvania.

Taylor, K. and Borrel, M., *Transducers and Their Importance*, McGraw-Hill, New York.

Webser, J.G., *Biomedical Instrumentation*, Wiley, New York.

Wells, P.N.T., *Ultrasonics in Clinical Diagnosis*, Harper & Row, New York.

Index